GW00650390

SK

HOMEOPATHIC APPROACH

to

DERMATOLOGY

DR. FAROKH J. MASTER

M.D. (Hom.)

Associate Editors
Dr. Priya Jani, B.H.M.S.
Dr. Pinky Bilimoria, B.H.M.S.
Dr. Farhad Adajania, B.H.M.S.
Dr. Jeenal Shah, B.H.M.S.
Dr. Jayesh Dhingreja, B.H.M.S.

SECOND REVISED EDITION

B. Jain Publishers (P) Ltd.
USA—EUROPE—INDIA

SKIN - HOMEOPATHIC APPROACH TO DERMATOLOGY

First Edition: 1993
Second Revised Edition: 2006
5th Impression: 2016

© 2006 by Dr. J. Master, M.D.

Published by Kuldeep Jain for

B. JAIN PUBLISHERS (P) LTD.
1921/10, Chuna Mandi, Paharganj, New Delhi 110 055 (INDIA)
Tel.: +91-11-4567 1000   Fax: +91-11-4567 1010
Email: info@bjain.com   Website: **www.bjain.com**

Printed in India by
B.B Press, Noida

ISBN: 978-81-319-0716-0

Preface to the Second Edition

The birth of this book was in the year 1993 (first edition). Subsequently, with support and encouragement from my colleagues in India and abroad, there was a reprint of my book in the year 1994. It has since then been acclaimed all over the world as a standard therapeutic book of dermatology.

I stress the fact, especially to younger generation, that recognition and treatment of skin disease is an important part of everybody's practice, since diseases of the skin covers 25% of the practice.

I also recommend to read more standard and reference books on dermatology like for example: Andrews' Diseases of Skin – Clinical dermatology.

This second edition has been completely re-written in light of the present day knowledge. Many chapters where homeopathic therapeutics was incomplete or not mentioned in the earlier editions have been completed or included. Many new conditions like Tuberculosis of skin, Hansen's disease, Disorders of pigmentation, Ichthyosis, Chicken pox, etc. have been included in the present edition. New cases have also been added. The peculiar symtoms of the homeopathic remedies has been described elaborately.

I sincerely acknowledge my thanks to all my extremely loving colleagues Dr. Vanmala Shroff, Dr. Jayesh Dhingreja and Dr. Trupti Pradhan who have so kindly and willingly worked for me. Their contribution has enhanced the prestige of this book.

I also thank Miss Sunita Shah for using digital camera and incorporating the photographs in Synthesis and Radar, helping me to search precise information from reference books and for her extra forbearance during my busy practice.

Finally my sincere thanks to Dr. Nandkishor Sonawane and Dr. Saudamini Suryawanshi who helped me in preparing therapeutics for this book.

Finally I thank Almighty for giving me good health, my wife Dilnavaz and my daughters Rukhshin and Mahaziver who have supported me all throughout.

Farokh J. Master, M.D. (Hom.)

24th May, 2006

"It is not only unbridled passion which damage the health of man. Living on ill-gotten money also causes ill health to some extent. Living on earnings got by unjust means causes many unknown diseases to take root in us."

It is said,

"As is the Food, So is the Mind

As is the Mind, So are the Thoughts

As is the Thought, So is the Conduct

As is the Conduct, So is the Health."

Bhagavan Sri Sathya Sai Baba

Contents

Chapter-9

Chapter-10

Chapter-11

Chapter-12

Chapter-13

Chapter-14

Chapter-34

Chapter-35

Chapter-36

Chapter-37

Chapter-1

Anatomy, Physiology, Embryology, Bacteriology and Pathology

The skin forms a protective covering over the body, a barrier or shield between the body's internal and external environments. It protects the body from physical harm of light (UV rays), heat and cold and microbial injuries.

It, with all its specialized derivatives, makes up what is called the integument (Latin *a covering*), which covers the entire surface of the body.

The human skin shows wide regional variations in structures; like the scalp, face, earlobes, back, palms and soles, etc. The thickness varies; the number of sebaceous glands, collagen fibres and vasculature differs in different parts of the integument.

ANATOMY

Gross anatomy divides the skin into hairy and non-hairy regions. Histologically, skin can be divided into 3 layers the superficial epithelial layer called the *'Epidermis'*, the underlying largely fibrous connective tissue layer called the *'Dermis or Corium'*, beneath which lies another (fatty) connective tissue layer called the *'Hypodermis or subcutaneous layer'*.

A network of linear furrows and ridges of variable sizes mark the free surface of the epidermis. On the fingers, these have a constant pattern differing in each individual; thus forming the concept of identifying a person by checking out his fingerprints (Dermatoglyphics).

STRUCTURE OF EPIDERMIS

The Epidermis, formed of non-vascular stratified epithelium, is usually of a thickness of 0.7 to 0.12 mm, except that in certain areas (like the soles of the feet and the palms), it can end up being very thick, ranging from almost 0.8 to 1.4 mm. It consists largely of **keratinocytes** (keratinizing or malpighian system) and **melanocytes** (pigmentary system) with a relatively small population of other dendritic cells, the most important of them being the **Langerhans' cells** and the **Merkel cell** or (Haaschieben) or touch cells.

Keratinocytes synthesize keratin, the most superficial part of the skin and the protein that forms the hair and the nails. *Melanocytes* form melanin and transfer it through dendritic processes to the keratinocytes to form a nuclear cap that protects it from the harmful effects of UV light. *Langerhans cells* are important antigen-processing cells. *Merkel cells* are found in the basal layer of the palms and soles, the oral and genital mucosa, the nail bed, fingertips, lips and the follicular infundibula. These Merkel cells act as slow adapting touch receptors.

The epidermis can be divided into four distinct layers stratum basale or stratum germinativum, stratum spinosum, stratum granulosum and stratum corneum.

Stratum Germinativum

This forms the deepest or the basal layer of the epidermis, composed of columnar cells. *The whole of the epidermis germinates from this stratum hence the name, 'stratum germinativum'. Any trauma to this layer would result in scarring.* More and more cells are formed and pushed off to the superficial layers. Some of the cells of the stratum germinativum contain granules of the pigment called melanin; melanoblasts or melanocytes are also found in this layer. Melanocytes of dark skin synthesize melanosomes (that form the pigmented granules) larger than those produced in light skin. Also chronic sun exposure tends to stimulate the melanocytes to produce larger melanosomes, thereby making the skin darker. Freckles result from localized increase in production of pigment by a normal number of melanocytes. Nevi are benign proliferations of melanocytes. Vitiligo results from destruction of melanocytes. In albinism, the number of melanocytes is normal, but they are unable to synthesize fully pigmented melanosomes because of defects in the enzymatic formation of melanin.

Stratum Malphigii or the Prickle Cell Layer

It is superficial to the basal cell layer and is composed of several layers of polyhedral cells connected to each other by intercellular bridges. All keratinocytes adhere together by dermosomes. Half size dermosomes occur under the surface of basal cells, which play an *important role in anchoring the epidermis to dermis*. During epidermal diseases desmosomal damage with breakdown of the cellular interconnections plays an important role.

Stratum Granulosum

It is composed of flat, fusiform cells, which are one to three layers thick. These cells contain irregular granules of keratohyaline and lysosomal enzymes and cystine rich proteins. Above the top of the prickle cell layer, near the granular cells layer, lamellar granules (keratinosomes), also known as *Odland bodies* are found, which form an *effective waterproof barrier*. The Langerhans cells are normally found scattered among keratinocytes of the stratum spinosum. These cells are also stained by gold chloride method. Functionally, Langerhans cells are of the monocyte-macrophage lineage and originate in the bone marrow. They play a role in induction of graft rejection and primary contact sensitization.

Stratum Lucidum

In palmo-plantar skin there is an additional zone, a pale wavy layer called the stratum lucidum, between the granulosum and corneum. These cells are still nucleated, and may be referred to as 'transitional' cells. This layer contains refractile drops of eleidin which is a precursor of keratin.

Stratum Corneum

It is the most superficial layer, exposed to the atmosphere, consisting of many layers of non-nucleated, flattened, cornified cells. This layer tends to become thick with constant or intermittent application of mechanical pressure. Thus it is thickest on the palms and soles but thinnest on the outer aspect of the lips, on the glans penis and the eyes. There are no organelles, no nuclei, but tonofibrils are seen embedded in a dense structureless matrix.

The Epidermal-Dermal Junction

The basement membrane zone forms the junction of epidermis and dermis. It is composed of four components – the plasma membranes of the basal cells with the specialized attachment plates; an electron-lucent zone called the lamina lucida; the basal lamina; and the fibrous components associated with the basal lamina, including anchoring fibrils, dermal microfibrils and collagen fibers.

The basement membrane zone is considered to be a porous semi-permeable filter, which permits exchange of cells and fluid between the epidermis and dermis. It further serves as a structural support for the epidermis and holds the epidermis and dermis together.

The Dermis

Dermis, fibrous and profusely supplied with blood vessels, gives support to the blood vessels and lymphatics. It has in addition free nerve endings and specialized neural structures for perception of specific sensations. It also contains mast cells that secrete histamine and other vocative amines and lymphocytes that play

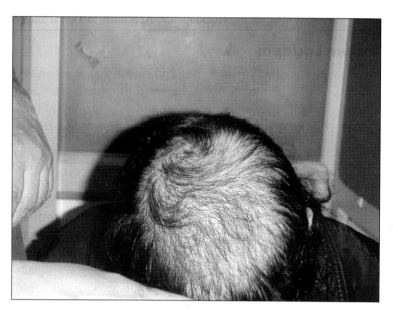

Alopecia capitis

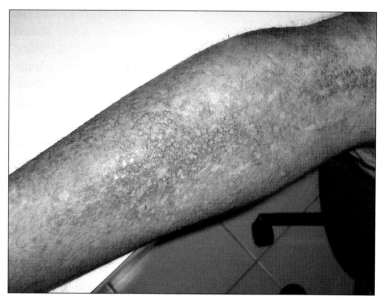

Amyloidosis of skin-1

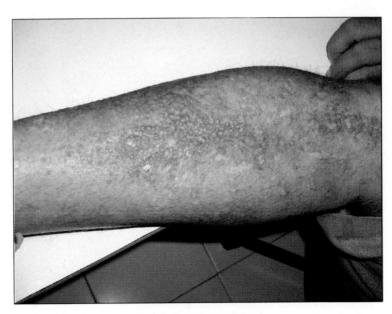

Amyloidosis of skin-2

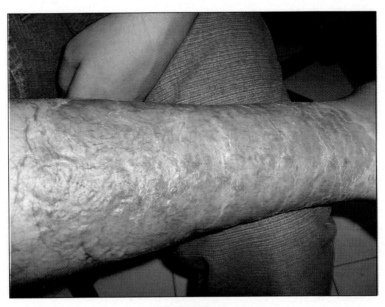

Cellulitis-1

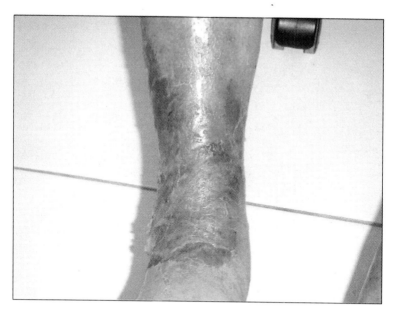

Cellulitis-2

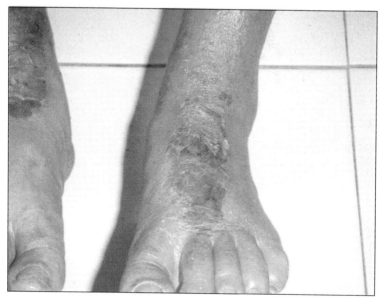

Cellulitis-3

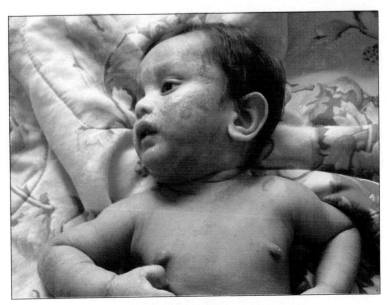

Dermatitis, atopic - baby

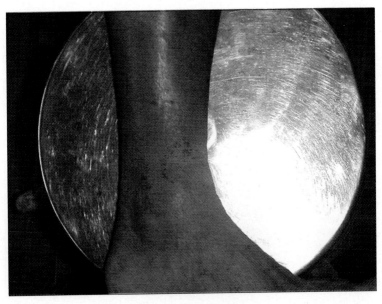

Dermatitis, statis

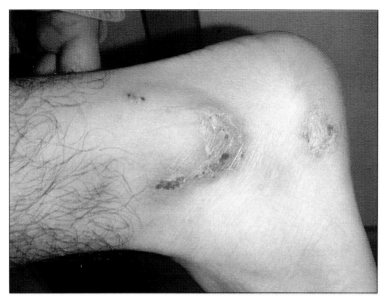

Eczema

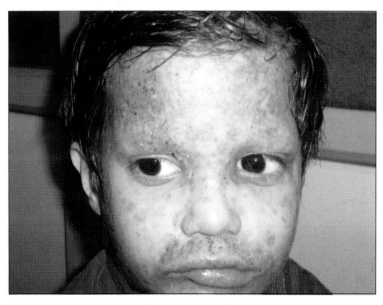

Eczema, atopic

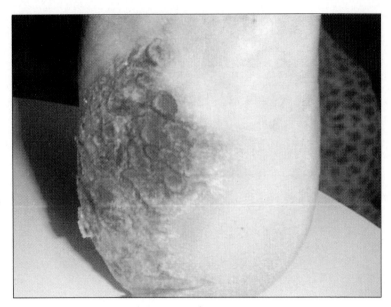

Eczema, fungal with lichenification-1

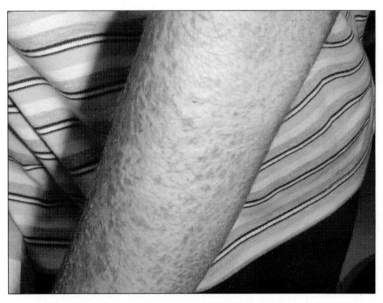

Eczema, ichthyotic

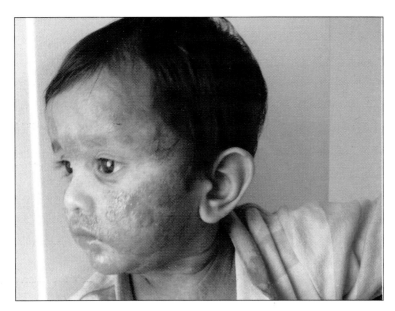

Eczema, infantile

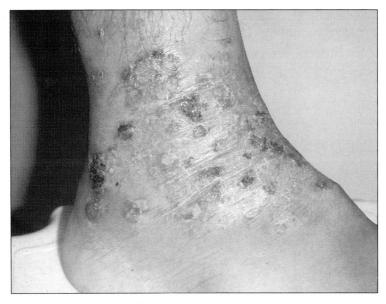

Eczema, infected-1

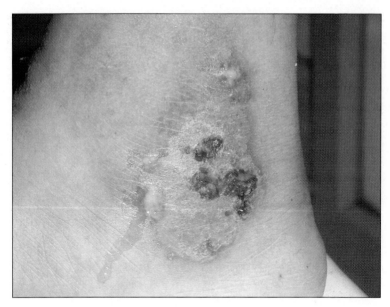

Eczema, infected-2

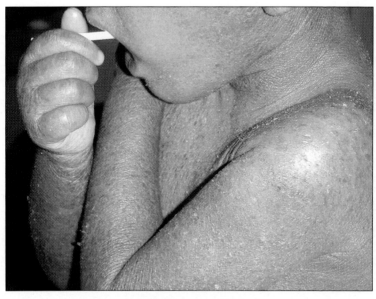

Eczema, xerotic-1

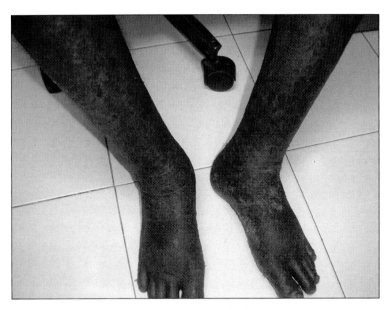

Eczema, xerotic-2

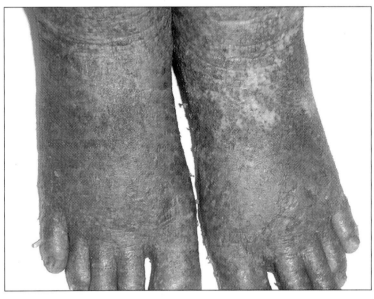

Eczema, xerotic-3

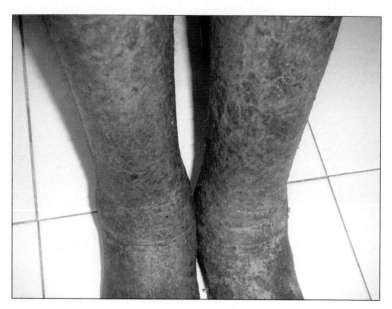

Eczema, xerotic-4

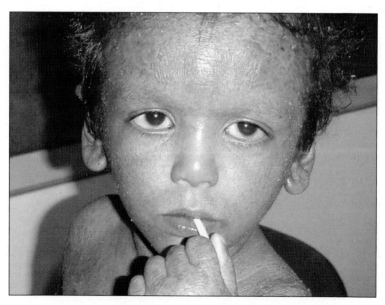

Eczema, xerotic - child-1

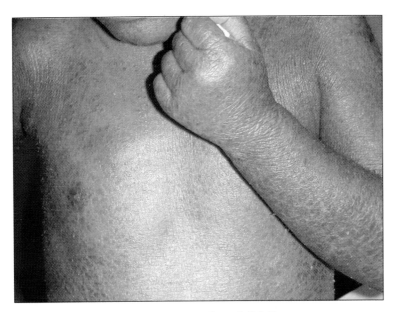

Eczema, xerotic - child-2

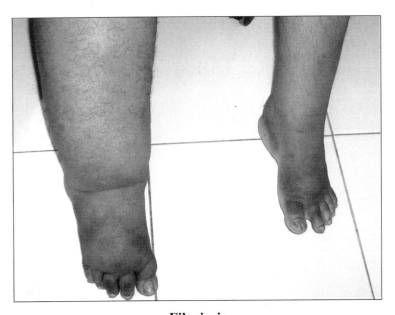

Filariasis

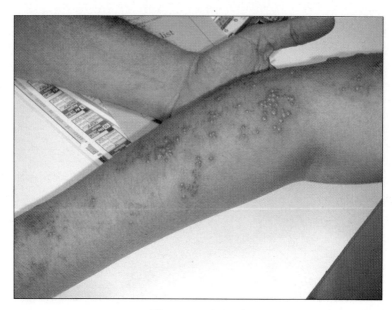

Herpes zoster-1

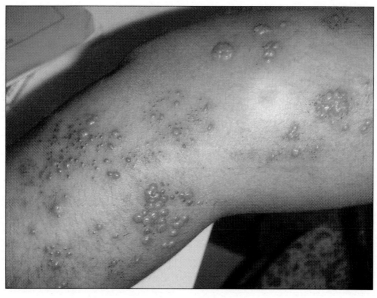

Herpes zoster-2

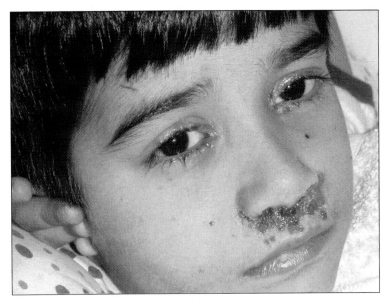

Impetigo contagiosum

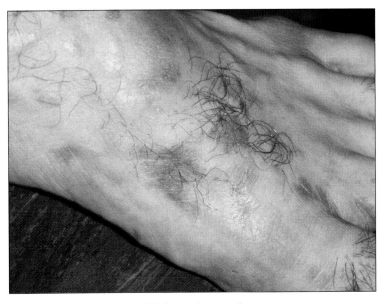

Lichen planus-1

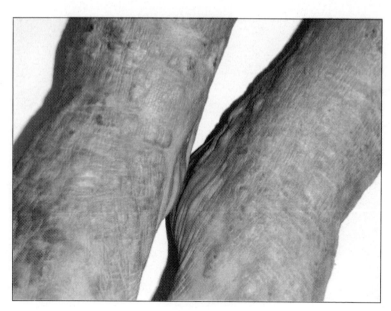

Lichen planus-2

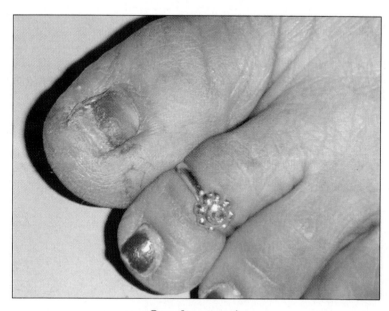

Onychomycosis

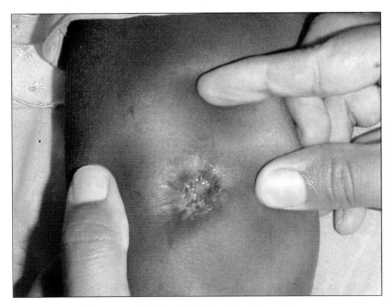

Osteomyelitis with discharging sinus

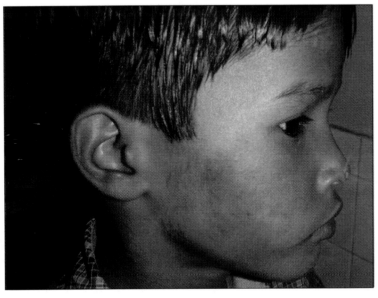

Pigmentation

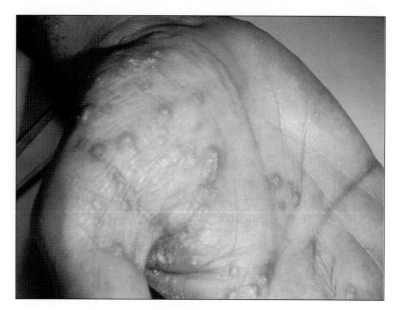

Pompholyx

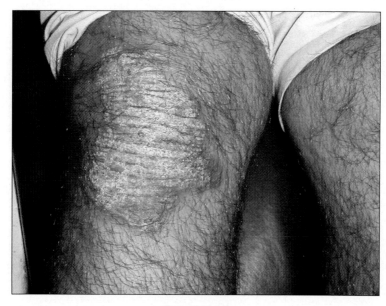

Psoriasis-1

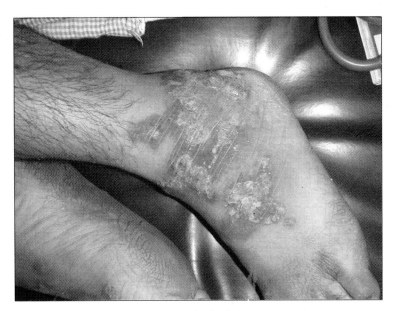

Psoriasis-3

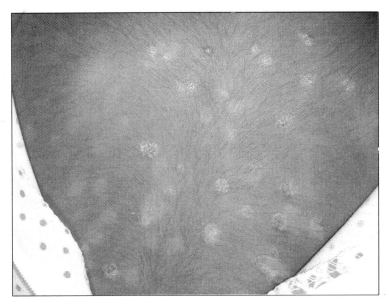

Psoriasis, guttate

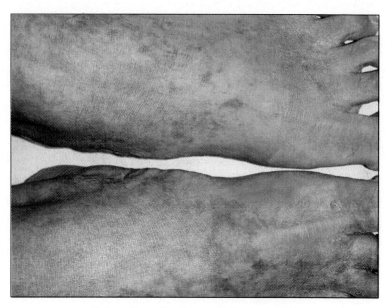

Schamberg's disease (dermatosis)

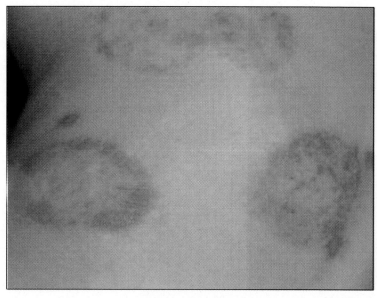

Tinea corporis

18

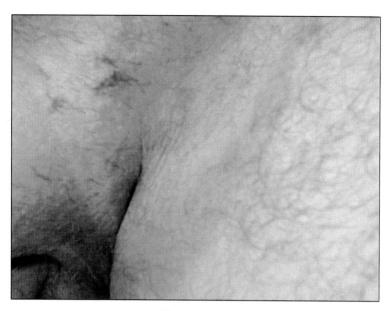

Tinea cruris

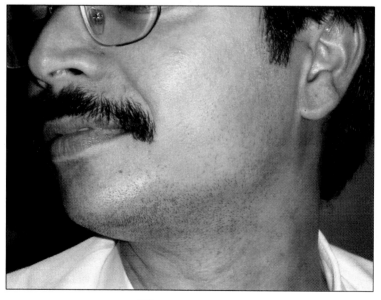

Tinea versicolor

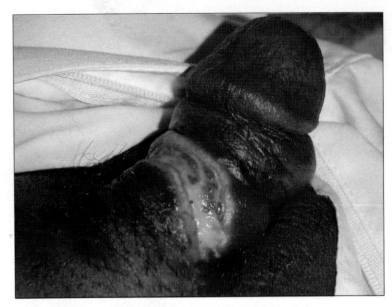

Ulcer, cancerous on penis-1

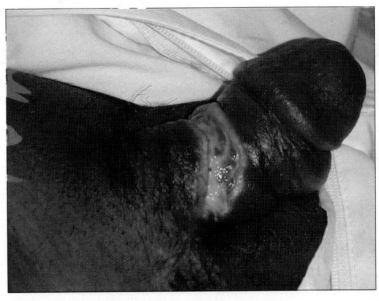

Ulcer, cancerous on penis-2

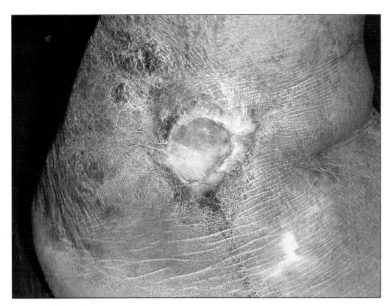

Ulcer, chronic, trophic (non healing)

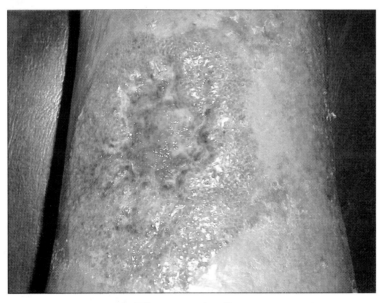

Ulcer, non-healing

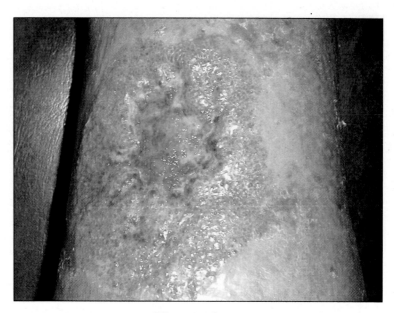

Ulcer, vericose

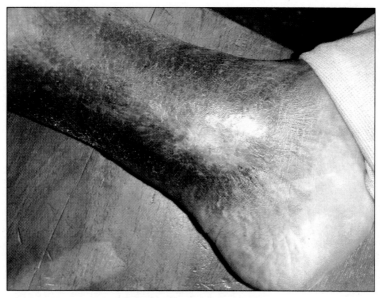

Ulcer, vericose, healed

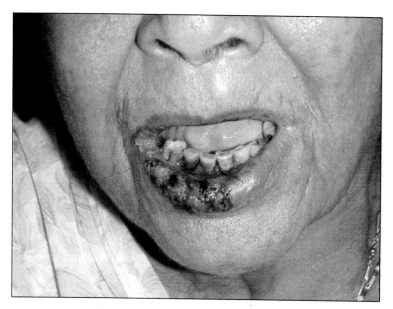

Ulcerative gingivitis and stomatitis

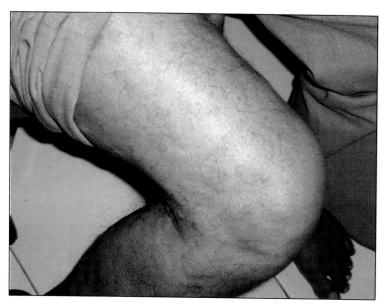

Urticaria-1

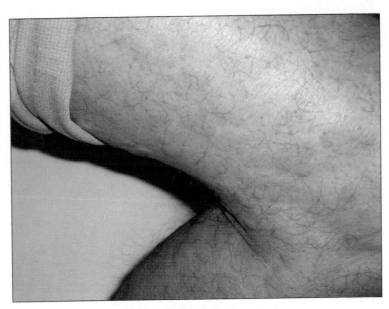

Urticaria-2

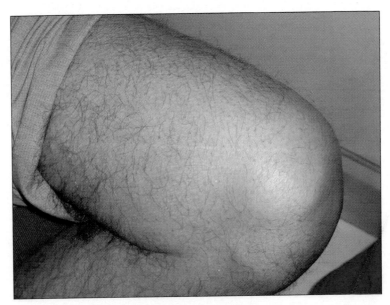

Urticaria, cured

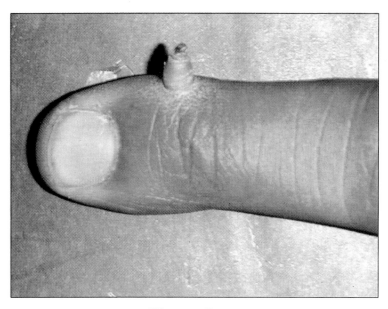

Wart on finger

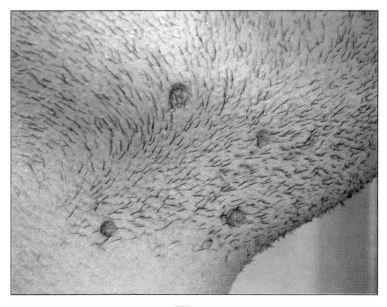

Warts

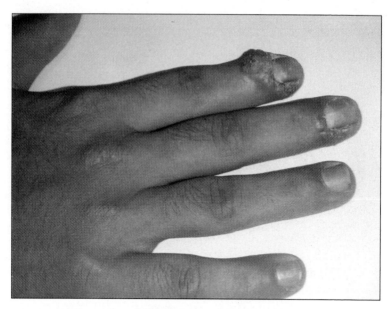

Warts around nails

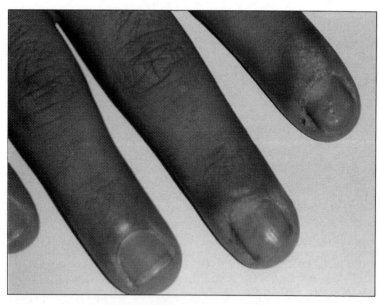

Warts around nails after medicine-1

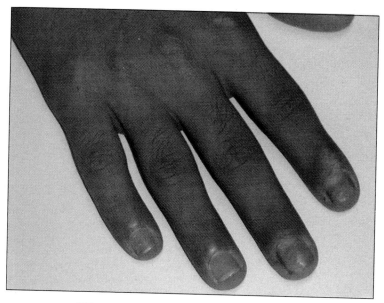

Warts around nails after medicine-2

an important immunologic role, e.g. in contact sensitivity and chronic granulomatous infections.

Dermis is mainly divided into two sections – *papillary* and *reticular* dermis. It contains connective tissue fibres, cells and all dermal appendages. Connective tissue is formed by three main components (1) collagen fibres, (2) elastic fibres, (3) ground substance.

The principle component of the dermis is *collagen,* which are fibrous proteins constituting almost 70% of the dry weight of skin. It is rich in amino acids - hydroxyproline, hydroxylysine and glycine. The collagen fibers are loosely arranged in the upper portion of the dermis (papillary) and tightly arranged in a bundle or spindle-like pattern within the lower portion of the dermis (reticular). Collagen fibers are continuously being degraded by proteolytic enzymes called collagenases, and replaced by newly synthesized fibers. The collagen is the major stress-resistant material of the skin.

The next component of the dermis, the *elastic fibers,* differ both structurally and chemically from the collagen. It consists of protein filaments and elastin, an amorphous protein. The amino acids desmosine and isedesmosine are unique to elastic fibers. Elastic fibers in the papillary dermis are fine, whereas those in the reticular dermis are coarse. The elastic fibers are of hardly any help to resist deformation and tearing of the skin, but are of importance in maintaining elasticity.

The ground substance of the dermis is composed of mucopolysaccharide acid, neutral mucopolysaccharides and electrolytes.

Connective tissue disease is a term generally used to refer to a clinically heterogeneous group of autoimmune diseases, out of which only scleroderma involves a detectable abnormality in the metabolism of collagen. Hypertrophic scar and keloid formation also reflect abnormalities in the rates of collagen synthesis and degradation. Defects in elastic tissue are seen in Marfan syndrome and pseudo-xanthoma elasticum.

Besides the structures mentioned above, in the dermis are also seen hair follicles, various type of sebaceous and sweat glands, plain muscle fibres, sensory end organs like Paccinian and Meissner's corpuscles and adipose tissue, few round cells, an occasional fibrocyte and a few pigments - carrying histocytes called melanophores.

BLOOD SUPPLY AND DRAINAGE WITHIN THE SKIN

There is a rich capillary bed in the papillary dermis and much less in the reticular dermis. Myelinated and non-myelinated sensory fibres and non-myelinated autonomic fibres supplying blood vessels and appendages richly innervate skin. In addition to superficial and deep plexuses of rich vascular supply, arterio-venous anastomosis is present in the skin. These specialized segments are known as Sucquet-Hoyer canal. Ovoid shaped smooth cells, known as glomus cells surround them, which are under the control of sympathetic nervous system. Thermoregulation is an important function of the skin vasculature.

NERVES

The dermis is rich in nerve supply. Touch and pressure are mediated by Meissner's corpuscles in the dermal papillae, especially on the palms and soles, and by the Vater-Pacini corpuscles located in the reticular portion of weight-bearing surfaces. Temperature, pain and the itchy sensations are transmitted by unmyelinated nerve fibers having their nerve endings in the papillary dermis and around hair follicles, and then pass via the dorsal root ganglia to the central nervous system.

SEBACEOUS GLANDS

The sebaceous glands, scattered all over the skin along with the hair follicles, are composed of pale-staining cells with abundant lipid in their cytoplasm, at the periphery of which are germinative cells that resemble the basal cells of the epidermis. It is from these germinative cells that the lipid-filled pale cells proliferate and are expelled into the infundibular portion of the hair follicle.

These glands are absent from the hairless portions of the body like palms, soles and sides of the feet. These glands, however, occur independently of hair follicles at certain places like the eyelids (meibomian glands), buccal mucosa, borders of the lips, the prepuce, external auditory meatus, female areolas, and around the anus. The sebaceous glands are found in greatest abundance on the face, scalp and interscapular regions. In the hairy portion of the skin the ducts of these glands open into the hair follicles, while in the non-hairy portion they open directly on the surface of the skin. The oily secretion of glands is thrown out into the hair follicles and upon the surface of the epidermis. Further, the sebaceous glands are more active at and after puberty, during menstruation and pregnancy.

SWEAT GLANDS

The sweat glands are of two types:

Eccrine Glands

The eccrine sweat unit, consisting of ordinary, small-sized sweat glands, distributed all over the skin except on the nail bed, margins of lip and glans penis, is composed of the following parts:

- The intraepidermal component opens directly onto the skin surface and is called the *spiral duct*. The duct consists of a single layer of inner or luminal cells and two or three outer rows of cells.

- The secretory acinar portion of the unit, also called as the *coil gland*, is found near the junction of the dermis and subcutaneous fat. The secretory cells are of two types glycogen-rich large pale cells (which initiate the formation of sweat) and smaller darker-staining cells (this layer actively reabsorbs sodium from the sweat to make it hypotonic by the time it reaches the skin surface). Eccrine sweat glands are most abundant on the palms, soles, forehead and axillae. Heat and emotional stress (nervous tension) tends to increase the sweating mechanism.

Apocrine Glands

They occur in the axillae, areolae, umbilicus, external auditory canal, eyelids and around the ano-genital region. These glands have their opening not at the surface epidermis, but at the upper portion of the hair follicle. The straight excretory portion of the duct opening into the hair follicle is composed of a double layer of cuboidal epithelial cells. The large coiled secretory gland is located at the junction of the dermis and subcutaneous fat and is lined by a single layer of cells, around which a layer of myoepithelial cells is surrounded. The apocrine secretion is rich in protein, carbohydrate, ammonia, lipid and iron and is odoriferous with a secondary sexual significance (pheromone). The glands start to function only after puberty.

HAIR FOLLICLE

Hair is composed of a *root* (the part embedded in the skin) and a *shaft* (the part projecting from the surface). The root of the hair at its lower end forms a bulbous enlargement, which is called the root bulb. The hair is contained in the skin in a series of invaginations called hair follicles. The hair follicle is dilated at its inner end and is known here as the hair-pit, where the hair bulb fits. The hair shaft is a dead cornified structure that extends from the follicle to above the surface of the skin. It has three components - an outer cuticle, a cortex and an inner medulla.

The hair follicle and its hair can be divided anatomically into three segments.

Infundibulum

This is the uppermost portion of the follicle, which extends from its surface opening to the entrance of the sebaceous duct.

Isthmus

This segment is the one between the sebaceous duct and the insertion of the arrector pili muscle.

Matrix

This is the most inferior portion, extending from the insertion of the muscle to the base of the follicle.

The lower bulb of the hair follicle is the site of growth. About half way up the follicle it becomes the keratinized structure devoid of living cells. The junction of these two zones (Adamson's fringe) is the level up to which keratinophilic fungi (ringworm) infect the hair, thus no permanent hair loss results in such cases.

Hair is found on almost every part of the body surface except on the palms and the soles, the dorsal surface of the terminal phalanges, the inner surface of the labia, the inner surface of the prepuce and the glans penis.

The rate of hair growth depends on mitotic activity of the cells of the bulb matrix. Hair growth and development is under endocrine control, depending on a fine balance of estrogen, androgen and gonadotrophin. Each hair follicle undergoes intermittent stages of activity and inactivity.

The basic hair colour depends on the distribution of melanosomes within the hair bulb cells. Graying of hair is a result of a decreased number of melanocytes, which produce fewer melanosomes.

Arrector pili muscles are the small bundles of plain muscle fibres, which extend from the connective tissue sheath of the hair follicles to the epidermodermal junction. When these contract under the effect of cold or emotions, they cause puckering of the skin with a hair-raising effect, which is called goose flesh. The contraction of these muscle fibres is also thought to squeeze out sebum from the duct of the sebaceous gland.

NAILS

These are semi-transparent, plate-like structures, covering the dorsal surfaces of the distal phalanges of the fingers and toes. The visible portion of the nail is called the 'nail plate', which is formed by the matrix keratinization. The proximal edge of the nail is known as the 'root' of the nail. The more opaque and rather whitish semi-lunar portion of the nail plate near its root is known as the 'lunula'. The surface of the skin on which the nail rests is known as the 'nail bed'. Skin folds called as lateral and posterior nail folds surround the lateral and the proximal borders of the nail.

A thin cuticle called the 'eponychium', which makes the exterior groove waterproof, joins the nail palate and proximal nail fold. It tends to get disrupted by extensive manicuring or washing, resulting in disease.

Fingernails grow an average of 0.1 mm per day; whereas the toenails grow at a much slower rate. Abnormalities of the nail may prove of important clinical value for cutaneous and systemic disorders.

PHYSIOLOGY

The skin is the largest immunologically active organ in the body, and its relative accessibility for basic science research has recently allowed much progress in our understanding of its multiple functions.

SKIN AS A BARRIER

- The skin tends to provide a protective barrier between the body and the environment, preventing injury and also arresting the penetration of microorganisms, harmful substances and chemicals into the body. Both minor injury to the skin as well as certain skin diseases can provide portals of entry to microorganisms, particularly streptococci or staphylococci.
- It also prevents absorbing strong radiation from the sun, by synthesizing the melanin pigment.
- Another most important function played is in preventing excessive loss of fluids and electrolytes from the surface. The skin acts as a two-way barrier to prevent the inward or outward passage of water and electrolytes. The horny layer becomes hard and brittle when the water content falls below a certain

limit, thus preventing further fluid loss. Thus in cases of severe and widespread injury to the cornified layer, death may result from dehydration or toxicity.

• The barrier is affected by many other factors, such as age, environmental conditions and physical trauma.

Temperature Regulation

By maintaining a constant body temperature, the metabolic processes will not be directly dependent on changes in the environmental temperature. Nevertheless, when exposed to extremes of temperature, heat may need to be lost or retained. Thus the skin tends to provide a sensory input to the thermo-regulatory center (hypothalamus), through the warm and cold-sensitive thermoreceptors distributed all over the skin, which allows heat loss (by radiation, conduction and by increased perspiration that cools the body) or conservation (by either inhibition of sweating or stimulation of shivering). The rich blood supply of the dermis with its system of arteriovenous shunts plays an important part in the above stated mechanism. When it is cold and we want to conserve heat, there is constriction of the arterioles; and there is flushing of the skin with perspiration when the environmental temperature rises and when one is exercising, thus ensuring greater amount of heat loss.

Mechanical Functions

Though the epidermis and its underlying fat layer plays a role in the protective function of the skin, it is the dermis that is responsible for the mechanical properties of the skin related to hard blows with blunt objects. Skin is known to have a property of elasticity for a few seconds at a time, where it can be *stretched* reversibly by 10-50%; beyond this it becomes difficult to extend. In cases of tissue-expanding techniques in skin surgery, the skin is made taut for a long time under continued stress and it gradually stretches, which is irreversible. This occurs due to the collagen fibrils. The striae seen in adolescence, pregnancy and in situations of excessive systemic corticosteroids are thought to involve a breakdown of the fibril overlap, so that there is no viscous force to limit further stretching.

On almost similar lines, another property of skin is that it can be *compressed*. If a small object is pressed into the skin, a depression is formed, with the skin becoming moulded round the object exerting the force, which remains after the object is removed. This compression is primarily due to a flow of ground substance through the dermis between the collagen fibres.

By virtue of its protein, lipid and water contents, the stratum corneum is a relatively strong, elastic tissue.

IMMUNOLOGICAL FUNCTIONS

The skin plays a vital part in immunological host defense, especially via the action of keratinocytes and Langerhans cells present in the epidermis and also by the action of T cells found in the epidermis and the dermis, usually grouped around postcapillary venules and the appendages. Antigens can be either exogenous (from external environment) or endogenous (newly formed in the cell itself).

Immunological dysfunction probably plays an important role in a wide range of skin diseases, especially the immunobullous disorders, allergic contact dermatitis, atopic dermatitis, psoriasis and cutaneous T-cell lymphoma (mycosis fungoides).

SENSORY ORGAN

Nerve endings in the skin, exist either freely or as encapsulated Meissner's or Pacinian corpuscles, which tend to direct sensations of touch, pain, warmth, cold and itch; this can then provide information regarding environmental changes to which the body can then adjust accordingly. The afferent units consist of the mechanoreceptors (which mediates touch), thermoreceptors and pain receptors (which respond only to high-threshold stimulation of either mechanical, thermal or chemical nature).

SECRETION AND EXCRETION

The eccrine glands secrete a thin, transparent watery fluid known as sweat, whereas the apocrine glands secrete a thicker, rather milky and odoriferous solution. Via sweat, besides water, we tend to excrete out the following – sodium chloride, sodium phosphate, sodium bicarbonate, keratin, a small amount of urea and certain drugs administered to the individual (for example mercury, arsenic, iodine, etc.). Sweating occurs especially in relation to thermal changes in the environment, when exercising or with different emotional conditions of fear, anger, anxiety or mental stress (where it is called as cold or mental sweating, which is under direct cerebral control).

Sebum, which is mainly composed of fatty acids and cholesterol, is secreted by the sebaceous glands. This sebum acts as a lubricant on the skin, excessive production of which leads to seborrhea and acne formation.

One other main action of the sweat and the sebum is its destructive action on the streptococci and other organisms through certain fatty acids and enzymes.

STORAGE

• Fat in the subcutaneous adipose tissue acts like a reserve store of the body's energy. It also prevents heat loss and acts as a good shock absorber.

• Almost one litre of blood is stored in the rich sub-papillary plexuses of the dermis, which can be directed to the muscles or other organs in cases of an emergency need.

• Ergosterol, the provitamin for vitamin-D, is also stored in the skin.

• There is storage of a lot of extra cellular fluid from the blood capillaries into the interstitial spaces in the dermal and hypodermal areas, whenever the hydrostatic pressure increases (This in excess leads to edema.). Also, in cases of dehydration, the water from these spaces can be drawn back into the blood, to increase its volume.

- Glucose and chloride can be stored in the skin temporarily, in cases of a sudden rise in their blood levels.

- Also, there occurs percutaneous absorption of topically applied substances which can be assessed by physiological or pharmacological means, or analyzed by chemical or histological techniques.

ABSORPTION

The skin can to some extent absorb substances dissolved in fatty solvents like vitamins and hormones, the permeability of which increases greatly when the skin is inflamed.

GASEOUS EXCHANGES THROUGH THE SKIN

Gaseous exchange through the skin in humans occurs to a very minimal extent than that in certain animals.

EMBRYOLOGY

The whole of the skin – epidermis and dermis is a unified integument organ system, but it develops from two different primitive embryonic layers- epidermis from the ectoderm and dermis from the mesoderm.

Though the epidermis and the dermis of the skin forms a unified integumentary organ, they both develop from two different primitive embryonic layers – the epidermis from the surface area of the early gastrula, i.e. the ectoderm; and the dermis and other differential structures of the epidermis (like the hair follicles) from the mesoderm. The neural crest helps in the formation of the pigment cells.

EPIDERMIS

When the foetus is *three weeks* old, the epidermis consists of only a single layer of undifferentiated or cuboidal, glycogen-filled cells.

By *4-6 weeks*, the single layer becomes differentiated into a double layer – one is the periderm or epitrichium (which is like a protective layer for the fetus before keratinization of the epidermis takes place, and is shed off in utero as the true epidermis keratinizes beneath it) and the stratum germinativum (basal layer).

By *8-11 weeks*, an intermediary layer starts to form between the periderm and the basal layer, and there is a characteristic increased glycogen secretion in all the three layers. Also a few microvillous projections start to form at the surface of the periderm, with flat polygonal cells. These microvilli of the periderm could help in the uptake of carbohydrate from the amniotic fluid. Desmosomal proteins are seen in the basal keratinocytes by the end of this stage.

By *12-16 weeks*, more layers are formed with increased glycogen both within and in-between the cells, along with numerous microvilli, and formation of the mitochondria, Golgi complexes and a few tonofilaments. Bubble-like blebs start to form from the center of the periderm cells, the surface of which then becomes dimpled and enfolded.

By *16-26 weeks*, the basal cells multiply rapidly and keep pushing the older cells towards the periderm thus causing an increase in the intermediate layer, and by 20 weeks, the prickle cells (superficial to the basal cells) form a definite stratum Malpighii. By 21 weeks, keratohyaline granules appear in the uppermost layer and form the stratum granulosum, followed by the formation of the stratum corneum due to the cornification of the most superficial cells.

The blebs of the periderm get cast off into the amniotic fluid and the early intermediate layer of cells become part of the stratum germinativum. By 20-24 weeks, the periderm layer starts to slowly separate from the embryo and is cast off as vernix caseosa along with the shed lanugo, sebum and other material.

HAIR FOLLICLES AND APOCRINE GLANDS

The beginnings of hair growth can be seen by about 9 weeks in the regions of the eyebrow, upper lip and chin. By 12 weeks hair appears over the entire body surface.

The *pregerm stage* is when there is a crowding of nuclei in the basal layer of the epidermis, which is the first sign of the formation of a hair follicle. After this comes the *hair-germ stage* where the basal cells increase in height with an elongated nucleus and this structure starts to extend downwards into the dermis. Along with this there is a multiplication of the mesenchymal cells and fibroblasts, which form the rudiment of the hair papilla beneath the hair germ; called the *hair peg*. The hair-germ continues to develop and grows obliquely downwards, becoming bulbous and gradually enveloping the mesodermal papilla. Then two *epithelial bulges* appear on the posterior wall of the follicle – the lower one is where the arrector muscle become attached and the upper one is the rudiment of the sebaceous gland. Also, a third bud appears above the sebaceous gland in many follicles, which is the rudiment of the apocrine gland.

As the bulbous hair peg extends downwards and differentiates, the first cells of the inner root sheath begin to form above the region of the matrix, which continues to grow deeper. The inner cells of the follicle grow upward into the epidermis to form the hair canal.

Hair follicles usually occur in groups of three and there is no large-scale destruction of follicles during postnatal development, only a decrease in actual density since the body surface increases; there are also no new follicles developing in an adult skin.

The hair of a foetus is fine, soft and silky – termed as lanugo, which is cast off before birth as a component of the vernix caseosa. New hair keeps developing from the hair follicles, which is shed and replaced periodically throughout life.

SEBACEOUS GLANDS

The upper epithelial bud goes on to forming a solid hemispherical protuberance on the posterior surface of the hair peg, consisting of a good amount of glycogen that is gradually lost. The cells gradually become larger and foamy accumulating lipid droplets, becoming lobulated. By 13-15 weeks, the sebaceous glands are large and functional; and after birth the size rapidly reduces and then they enlarge again after puberty to become functional.

ECCRINE GLANDS

Most of the eccrine sweat glands develop independently as solid down-growths from the epidermis. At 12 weeks, the rudiments of eccrine sweat glands are identifiable as regularly spaced undulations of the stratum germinativum. By 14-15 weeks, the tips of the eccrine sweat-gland rudiments have penetrated deeply into the dermis, and have begun to form the coils. By 3-4 months of intrauterine life, they start to appear first on the palms and soles, and come up over the rest of the body only after the fifth month. By the sixth month of fetal life, they become simple cords, which later coil and acquire lamina.

NAILS

By about 3 months (about 12 weeks) the nails start to develop as an epidermal specialization on the dorsum of the tips of the digits. By 16-18 weeks, keratinizing cells from both the dorsal and ventral matrices can be distinguished.

Under the influence of sex hormones at puberty, coarser and darker hairs appear on the pubis and axilla of both the sexes and on the face and certain regions of the trunk in the male.

MELANOCYTES

The melanocytes originate from the neural crest, the sources of which can be identified in early human embryos, but lose themselves gradually in the mesenchyme and cannot be identified before 4-6 months of gestation.

LANGERHANS CELLS

Langerhans cells are of the monocyte-macrophage lineage and originate in the bone marrow, entering the epidermis by about 12 weeks of gestation.

MERKEL CELLS

The Merkel cells appear in the basal layer of the palms and soles, lips, the oral and genital mucosa, the nail bed, fingertips, and the follicular infundibula by about 16 weeks of gestation.

DERMIS

It is formed by the mesenchymal cells, which give rise to the whole range of blood and connective tissue cells, including the fibroblasts and mast cells of the dermis and the fat cells of the subcutaneous layer. The embryonic dermis in the initial stages is very cellular, and by 6-14 weeks it consists of closely packed, spindle shaped mesenchymal cells. Three types of cells are seen in the dermis at this stage — the stellate cells, the phagocytic macrophages and the granule-secretory cells (either melanoblasts or mast cells).

Fine reticulum fibres are demonstrable by 12 weeks, which later increase in number and thickness and form the collagen fiber bundles by about 24 weeks.

Touch pads are evident on the hands and feet by the sixth week and reach maximum maturation by 15-16 weeks, after which they flatten and become indistinct.

Then the papillary and reticular layers become distinct, and by 20 weeks, connective tissue sheaths are formed around the hair follicles.

Also by 21-22 weeks of gestational period, the elastic fibers start forming and the fibroblasts are plentiful and active. The other cells that can be identified during this period are the perineurial cells, pericytes, melanoblasts, Merkel cells and mast cells.

The subcutaneous fat is apparent by the end of 12 weeks of gestation, but it becomes abundant only during the later months of fetal life.

DERMO-EPIDERMAL JUNCTION

A continuous lamina densa of the basement membrane becomes evident in the eight week of gestation, and hemidesmosomes appear in the third month.

PATHOLOGY

Hypertrophic, atrophic, inflammatory or dystrophic changes may take place in the epidermis, dermis or subcutaneous tissue or their component parts or layers.

EPIDERMIS

Hyperkeratosis

Hypertrophy of stratum corneum.

- Localized forms - corns, warts, and keratoses.
- Diffuse form - ichthyosis, keratoderma, and Pityriasis rubra pilaris.

Parakeratosis

Incompletely cornified but abnormally increased horny layer. It signifies edema of prickle cell layer, usually due to an inflammatory process, e.g. psoriasis, eczema, seborrheic dermatitis.

Dyskeratosis

Imperfect and premature keratinization taking on various shapes. It may be benign as is seen in Darier's disease (*corps ronds* and *grains* of Darier) and chronic benign pemphigus of Hailey and Hailey or it may be malignant as in epitheliomas (Bowen's disease, Paget's disease and squamous cell carcinoma).

Acanthosis

Hyperplasia of prickle cell layer. It is usually a benign process and is seen typically in chronic eczema, psoriasis, lichen planus and warts. In tuberculosis cutis verrucosus and pyoderma vegetans, acanthosis and hyperkeratosis are secondary to the disease process in the corium. Special type of acanthosis is seen in condyloma accuminatum and molluscum contagiosum; the latter exhibits molluscum bodies.

If there is atypical proliferation of prickle cells with hyperchromatic nuclei and mitotic figures (anaplasia) accompanied by loss of intercellular fibrils, malignancy must be suspected.

Spongiosis

Spongy epidermis is caused by intercellular edema (mainly prickle cell layer). With the increase of edema, collections of fluid result in intra-epidermal vesicles or bullae e.g. eczema, viral affections.

Acantholysis

Typically seen in pemphigus. Due to lysis of intercellular fibrils of basal and prickle cell layer, degenerated epidermal cells become detached, shrunken and rounded with swollen, compact, hyperchromatic nuclei (Tzarck cells). Acantholytic bulla is seen in pemphigus.

Atrophy

It is thinning of the epidermis and straightened epidermodermal junction with loss of rete ridges, e.g. senile atrophy, scleroderma, acrodermatitis atrophicans, lichen sclerosus et atrophicus, leprosy, etc. Basal cell degeneration is seen in discoid lupus erythematosus.

CORIUM

Infiltration

Polymorph nuclear cell infiltration is seen in acute inflammations; while in chronic inflammations, lymphocytes predominate. Infiltration is mainly around the blood vessels (perivascular), pilo-sebaceous apparatus and sweat glands. Epithelioid cells are seen in infective granulomata mainly tuberculosis, leprosy, Sarcoid, etc. A granuloma, histologically speaking, implies circumscribed dermal infiltration, which is usually persistent and slowly progressive. Granulomas are composed of histocytes, epithelioid cells, giant cells (Langhan's, foreign body) and plasma cells.

It is important to establish the different cells of the infiltration process, their location, number and distribution. Since these are differently affected in different disease processes, correct histological reading helps in confirmation of diagnosis.

Bullae

Dermal bullae are seen typically in dermatitis herpetiformis, erythema multiforme and epidermolysis bulla. In miliaria profunda, sweat is imprisoned in the upper part of the corium.

Collagen Tissue

It is increased in fibrosis. Increase accompanied by hyalinization and edema is seen in scleroderma. Elastic tissue is affected in elastosis, cutis laxa and pseudo-xanthoma elasticum.

Neoplasm

In the corium, it may arise from any of its constituents, viz. fibroma from fibrous tissue, leiomyoma from smooth muscle of arrector pili, neuromas from nerve fibres, lipomas from fatty tissue, etc. Then there are different types of naevi, malignant melanomas, sarcomas and reticulosis particularly mycosis fungoids, etc., tumors related to hair follicles are seen in tricho-epitheliomas, and syringomas from sweat glands.

Cysts

Sweat, sebaceous, etc.

Degeneration

Degenerative changes may affect the corium - collagen or elastic tissue or both. In stained sections, these tissues become basophilic, degenerated lumps or granules. Collagen tissue is less resistant and hence shows degenerative changes earlier than elastic tissue.

Necrobiosis

Means partial destruction of tissues – nuclei are disintegrated but the cellular structure is preserved. It is typically seen in Necrobiosis lipoidica diabeticorum.

Blood Vessels

The blood vessels of the corium are typically affected in syphilis (panarteritis with perivascular cuffing of plasma cells), Schamberg's disease, nodular vasculitis, angioma, angiokeratoma, etc.

Subcutaneous Tissue

It is affected in panniculitis, erythema nodosum, erythema induratum and Milroy's disease.

BACTERIOLOGY

Several organisms are seen as normal flora of the skin surface. The integument harbors several resident organisms like Staphylococcus albus and Coryne bacterium acnes on its surface and crevices. Pityrosporon ovale, a saprophytic fungus, is frequently found on the scalp and face. Bacteria like Streptococcus pyogenes and Staphylococcus aureus, may occasionally be found on the skin as transient flora, though they can often be demonstrated in the nose, mouth and throat. These pathogenic bacteria are also frequently found in the body particularly in the perineum. Occasionally, Candida albicans and intestinal bacteria may be seen on the skin particularly near the anus.

The various defense mechanisms of the skin protect it from any harm by these organisms under normal circumstances.

Besides this adequate daily washing and exposure to sunrays inhibits the growth of bacteria.

Under unfavorable circumstances, these defense mechanisms fail to preserve its integrity leading to various infections. Resident bacterial flora like Staphylococcus albus, which is normally non-pathogenic, may become pathogenic in persons with a defective defense mechanism.

The normal resistance of the skin is reduced in debilitating diseases like diabetes; xerodermic skin lacks the defense mechanism and is, therefore, more prone to pyoderma.

In the body folds, particularly in obese patients, where sweating is increased, pH is high, maceration is more, local temperature is raised, hence infection is frequent.

Seborrheic individuals are supposed to have altered sebaceous secretions; hence they are also prone to infections.

LABORATORY AND OTHER AIDS IN DERMATOLOGICAL PRATICE

The skin is available for close examination and clinical study; reliance on clinical acumen could never be unduly emphasized in dermatological practice. In a certain number of cases there is a definite need and indication for laboratory and other aids, either to confirm the diagnosis or to clear up doubts in case the diagnosis is not certain. But the need also arises to establish the etiology of a disease entity, and so, to establish the ultimate prognosis. *Firstly,* the homeopath must be sure of this fundamental principle before ordering any laboratory investigation. *Secondly,* only the absolutely essential laboratory investigations should be ordered. *Thirdly,* the clinician must make sure of the reliability of the laboratory reports before he bases any opinion on them.

The following are some important investigations:

Bacteriological Studies

- Smear
- Culture
- Sensitivity tests
- Vaccine

Allergy Tests

- Patch tests
- Intradermal or Scratch test
- Basophil degranulation test

Mycological Studies

- Fresh preparation
- Staining
- Culture

Biological Tests

- Tuberculin
- Lepromin
- Kveim test
- Frei test

Wood's lamp Examination

Radiological

Serological Tests for Syphilis

- Wassermann reaction
- VDRL test

Hematological Tests

- Blood routine
- ESR
- Cryoglobulin test
- Chemistry cholesterol, protein, vitamins, sugar, urea, copper, zinc, sodium, and cortisol.

Histological Examination

- Biopsy and cytological studies
- LE cell phenomenon
- Tzanck test
- Smear for cancer cell etc.
- Histochemistry
- Immunofluorescence

Miscellaneous

- Stool
- Urine routine
- Porphyrin
- 17- ketosteroid

■

Chapter-2

Cutaneous Symptoms, Signs and Diagnosis

The various diseases that affect the human skin may present similar symptoms and signs. Such identical features create problems in making a diagnosis; however in most instances the appearance of many skin lesions may be so typical and so distinctive that a glance at the patients' skin will reveal the diagnosis. Sometimes a complete history and laboratory examination including a biopsy is essential to arrive at a diagnosis.

The same disease may show variation under different conditions and in different individuals. The appearance of the lesion may be modified by previous treatment or obscured by extraneous influences. Subjective symptoms may be the only evidence of a disease, as in pruritis. In most instances, however, relying on the objective physical characteristics and location or distribution of one or more lesions that can be seen or felt makes the diagnosis.

CUTANEOUS SYMPTOMS

The common symptoms of skin diseases are itching, pain and disturbed sensations in the nature of crawling, sensation of heat, sensation of cold (tingling), anesthesia or hyperesthesia. These subjective symptoms, as much as the apparent rash are responsible for bringing the patient to the doctor for consultation.

PRURITIS (ITCHING)

Itching is defined as an unpleasant cutaneous sensation, which provokes the desire to scratch or rub the skin.

It occurs when there is a weak stimulation of the cutaneous nerves. Its intensity varies according to the disease and individual sensitivity. It may be a mere, prickling, tingling or formication, or its severity may be so intense as to be intolerable. It may be continuous or spasmodic, localized or generalized, accompanied or unaccompanied by a rash. The objective evidence of itching is a scratch mark in the form of linear excoriation.

Common causes

Scabies, pediculosis, ringworm, eczema, lichen planus, xerosis (senile pruritis), urticaria, dermatitis herpetiformis, neurodermatitis, insect bite, food allergy.

Other causes

Malignant lymphoma, diabetes mellitus, biliary obstructive disease, iron deficiency anemia, internal cancer, severe renal insufficiency, endocrinal imbalances resulting from thyroid dysfunction, menstruation and menopause.

Pruritis of the ano-genital area, especially in diabetic women, may be associated with candidia albicans infection. Uremic pruritis is generalized and occurs in severe cases in which the skin has a yellowish brown discolouration.

Intractable pruritis may be the most frequent complaint in patients receiving hemodialysis.

Factors that enhance itching

Psychic trauma, stress, absence of distractions, anxiety and fear are common exciting factors.

It is apt to be most severe at the time of undressing for bed. The ear canals, eyelids, nostrils and peri-anal area are very susceptible to pruritis.

PAIN

It may be localized to the skin as in boils and abscesses or it may radiate along a nerve as in leprotic neuritis and herpes zoster. It may be deep boring and burning as in herpes zoster, shooting as in tabes dorsalis, throbbing as in furuncles, carbuncles and cellulitis.

CRAWLING SENSATION (FORMICATION)

It is a variety of itching eg. Acarophobia.

Sensation of Heat

In dermatological practice, 'heat in the blood' or 'sense of heat (SOH)' is not uncommon. It is seen as the first sign or symptom of drug eruption, in urticaria and allergy. Lay persons even call venereal diseases as 'heat – garam' (syphilis in Arabic means heat). Ayurveda, Hippocrates and Galen have laid stress on constitution, temperament and elementary qualities like heat, cold, dryness and moisture.

It is experienced as warm sensation to feeling of burning hot, warm to hot hands and feet, uncomfortable to burning sensation in the sun, and keeping feet and hands outside the covering while sleeping. SOH is a more useful guide than leukocyte count or allergy tests in urticaria and endogenous eczema. Patients with SOH are more prone to skin diseases. May be change in eating and living habits (sattvic vegetarian diet, no spices, chillies, tea, alcohol, etc.) help to reduce SOH and hence the predisposition to allergic dermatoses.

Stinging Sensation

It is characteristic of stings of insect bites.

Hyperesthesia

Increased sensitivity, eg. Post herpetic neuralgia.

Anesthesia

Loss of sensation which may be present in patches and if dissociated (i.e. only to cold or touch or pain) is considered pathognomic of leprosy. Dissociation also occurs in syringomylia, in which the fingers may have a loss of pain and temperature sensation but preservation of tactile sensations.

The patient may notice the anesthesia himself, but usually, it is found on physical examination. The sensations tested, pertaining to skin diseases are pain sensation (pinprick), touch and temperature (hot and cold).

CUTANEOUS SIGNS

According to the nature of the pathologic process, the lesions assume more or less distinct characteristics. They may be uniform or diverse in size, shape and color and may be in different stages of evolution or of involution.

Clinically lesions are of two types – PRIMARY and SECONDARY. In case taking, primary or the original lesions are most important. The differential diagnosis centers mostly around them. The clinician must look for the primary lesion in the most recently developed eruption or at the periphery of the rash. With the passage of time, primary lesions either involute or transform or get modified into secondary lesions.

PRIMARY LESIONS

They are of the following forms macules (or patches), papules (or plaques), nodules, tumors, wheals, vesicles, bullae and pustules.

Macules

Macules are variously sized, circumscribed changes in skin colour, without elevation or depression. They may be circular, oval or irregular and maybe distinct in outline or fade into surrounding area. They are of two types: (I) Erythematous (II) Pigmentary.

A macule must be palpated for induration or infiltration, which is typical of granulomatous diseases and reticuloses. Further erythematous macules should be differentiated from purpuric macules. In the former, erythema disappears under pressure, while in the latter the redness is brighter, and does not fade under pressure.

Pigmentary merciless are differentiated into hyperpigmented or depigmented types.

Common causes of macular eruptions are:

Erythematous macules

Dermatitis, exanthemata, drug eruption, macular syphilide, erythema multiforme, tinea circianata, psoriasis, pityriasis rosea, leprosy are the commonly known causes.

Pigmentary macules

Hyperpigmented macules

Chloasma, fixed drug eruption, melanoderma, freckles, naevi, lentigines, Addison's disease.

Hypopigmentation

Leprosy, tinea versicolor, pityriasis alba.

Depigmentation

Leucoderma, vitiligo.

Papules

These are circumscribed solid elevations with no visible fluid, varying in size from a pinhead to a pea. They may be acuminate, rounded, conical, flat-topped or umbilicated and may appear white (as in milium), red (as in eczema), yellowish (as in xanthema), reddish brown (as in lupus vulgaris), or black (as in melanoma).

Plaque

A plaque is a broad papule (or confluence of papules) one or more centimeter in diameter. It is generally flat, and may be centrally depressed or even clear.

Some papules are discrete and irregularly distributed, as in papular urticaria, while others are grouped, as in lichen nitidus. Some persist as papules, whereas those of the inflammatory type may progress to vesicles and even to pustules, or may form ulcers before regression takes place. An attempt should be made to distinguish epidermic papule from dermic and mixed papules. An epidermic papule is usually superficial, dry, solid, flesh coloured; a dermic papule is usually deeper, elastic and reddish.

Common causes of papular eruptions:

Warts, Epidermal and dermal naevi, Lichen Spinulosum, Lichen scrofulosorum, Lichen planus, Drugs eruption, Eczema and eczematoides, Syphilis, Acne vulgaris, Rosacea, Chicken pox, Small pox, Prickly heat, Psoriasis and Tumour.

Papules in Lines

Warts, Psoriasis, insect bites and Lichen planus.

Nodule

Morphologically being similar to papule, they are more than 1cm in diameter (as big as a hazel nut or smaller).

Examples of nodules:

Naevi, Tuberculosis cutis, Neurofibromatosis, Sarcoid, Skin cancer, Erythema nodosum, Dermal Leishmaniasis, Xanthomatosis, Leprosy, Mycosis fungoides and Syphilis.

Tumour

They are generally soft or firm and freely movable or fixed masses of various size and shapes but is bigger than a hazel nut that is greater than 2 cm in diameter. They may be elevated or deep seated, and in some instances pedunculated. They have a tendency to be rounded and the consistency depends on the constituents of the lesion. Tumors may remain stationary indefinitely or increase in size or break down.

Examples of tumours:

Epithelioma, Naevi, Lymphosarcoma, Lipoma, Mycosis fungoides, Neurofibromas, Gumma, Secondary carcinomatosis, Keloid, Sarcoid and Xanthoma.

Vesicle (blister)

Vesicles are circumscribed epidermal elevations 1 to 10 mm in size and usually contain clear fluid. They may be pale or yellowish from serous fluid or reddish from serum mixed with blood and occasionally have deep reddish areola.

The apex may be rounded, acuminate or umbilicated as in eczema vaccination. Vesicles may be discrete, irregularly scattered, grouped as in herpes zoster or linear as in poison ivy dermatitis. They may arise directly or from a macule or papule and generally lose their identity in a short time, breaking spontaneously or developing into bullae through coalescense or enlargement or developing into pustules when the contents are of sero purulent character, the lesions are known as vesicopustules. Vesicles consist of either a single cavity (unilocular) or of several compartments (multilocular) containing fluid. On the palms, vesicles are situated rather deeply; hence their contents are discharged with difficulty. On the mucus membranes their roofs get rubbed off very easily producing erosions.

Common causes of vesicles:

Eczema, Cheiropompholyx, Dermatitis herptiformis, Herpes simplex, Herpes zoster, Impetigo, Scabies, Miliaria crystalline, Miliaria rubra, Small pox, Chicken pox, Tinea, Drug eruptions and insect bites.

Bullae

They are rounded or irregularly shaped blisters containing serous or seropurulent fluid. The only difference from a vesicle is that they are larger in size, generally larger than 1 cm. When located superficially in the epidermis, their walls are flaccid and thin and subject to rupture spontaneously or from slight injury. On rupture the remnants of the thin walls may persist and may dry to form a thin crust along with the exudate or leave a raw, moist base with the seropurulent exudate. Sub-epidermal bullae are tense and may result into ulceration and scarring.

Putting lateral pressure on the unblistered skin in a bullous eruption and having the epithelium shear off is a diagnostic maneuver referred to as Nikolsky's sign. Asboe-Hansen's sign refers to the extension of a blister to the adjacent unblistered skin when pressure is put on top of the blister.

Both these signs demonstrate the principle that in some diseases, the extent of microscopic vesiculation is more than is evident by simple inspection. These findings are useful in evaluating the severity of pemphigus vulgaris and severe bullous drug reactions. The cellular content of the bullae may be useful in confirming the diagnosis of pemphigus, herpes zoster and herpes simplex.

Common causes of bullae:

Impetigo contagiosa, Insect bite, Erythema multiforme, Epidermolysis bullosa, Pemphigus, Hydroa aestivale, Dermatitis herpetiformis and Drug eruptions.

Hemorrhagic bullae are common in pemphigus, herpes zoster, and toxic epidermal necrolysis and infrequently, lichen sclerosus et atropicus. The cellular contents of bullae may be diagnostic in pemphigus, herpes zoster and herpes simplex.

Pustule

Small elevations of the skin containing purulent material (usually necrotic inflammatory cells). They are similar to vesicles in shape and usually have an inflammatory areola. They are usually whitish or yellowish, but may be reddish if they contain blood with the pus. They may originate as pustules or may develop from papules or vesicles, passing through transitory early stages during which they are known as papulopustules or vesicopustules.

The following characters should be studied:

- The size, shape, number.
- Is the pustule discrete or confluent, epidermal or follicular, superficial or deep?
- An example of a superficial epidermal pustule is *impetigo* and of a deep epidermal pustule is *ecthyma*.
- When a pustule is in the upper part of a hair follicle, it is called *folliculitis*:
- When it is in the deeper part of a hair follicle, and involves the roof of the hair, which comes out as the core, it is called as *furunculosis (boil)*.
- When a conglomeration of boils forms a deep, dermic abscess with multiple holes on the skin through which pus is discharged, it is called as *carbuncle*.
- Pustules terminate by rupture or dessicate to form irregular yellow crusts.

Common examples of pustules:

Impetigo, Bactendes, Sycosis barbae, Furunculosis, Carbuncle, Scabies, Drug eruptions (iodides and bromides), Anthrax, Tuberculosis, Acne vulgaris, Small pox and Chicken pox.

Weals

Evanescent edematous flat elevations of various sizes caused by local dilatations of blood vessels and increased permeability resulting in localized edema. They are usually oval or of bizarre contours, whitish or pinkish and surrounded by pink areola. They may be discrete or may coalesce to form solid plaques. Itching is almost always present. Dermographism may be evident. The temporary, evanescent nature of a weal and its duration (from a

few hours to a maximum of 24 hours or so) is characteristic; it
helps to distinguish a weal from a persistent granulomatous lesions.
Weals disappear without leaving any trace of stains, scars or
atrophy.

Occasionally a weal may be surrounded by a vesicle e.g.
papular urticaria of childhood, or accompanied by bullae formation
e.g. urticaria bullosa.

Common causes of Weals:

Urticaria, Trauma, Insect bites, Urticaria pigmentosa and Drug
rashes.

SECONDARY LESIONS

Some of the important secondary lesions are scales, crusts,
erosions, ulcers, fissures and scars.

Scales (Exfoliations, Squames, Squamae)

Scales are dry or greasy laminated masses of keratitis due to
increased or abnormal formation of stratum corneum (hyper or
pan keratitis). It results from erythema or inflammation of skin or
increased dryness. These scales vary in size, some being fine,
delicate and branny, as in tinea versicolor, others being coarser, as
in eczema and ichthyosis, while still others are stratified as in
psoriasis. Large sheets of desquamated epidermis are seen in
exfoliative dermatitis, toxic epidermal necrolysis, staphylococcal
scalded skin syndrome, and scarlet fever. In psoriasis there are
silvery layer-upon-layer scales and in seborrheic dermatitis there
are greasy scales. In pityriasis rosea, the scaling is cigaratte paper
like centripetal and in pityriasis versicolor scaling is furfuraceous
or powdery. In lupus erythematous, there are adhesive scales with
nutmeg like under surface.

Common causes of scaling:

Dermatitis and eczema, Seborrheic dermatitis, Psoriasis,
Pityriasis versicolor, Exfoliative dermatitis, Tinea corporis,
Pityriasis rubra pilaris, Drug eruptions, Tinea Capitis, Ichthyosis,

Syphilis, Lichen Planus, Lupus erythematosus, Pityriasis rosea, Exanthemata following scarlet fever, Malnutrition and Pellagra.

Excoriations

Punctate or linear abrasions produced by mechanical means usually involving only the epidermis and rarely reaching the papillary layer of the dermis. Excoriations are caused by scratching with the fingernails in an effort to relieve itching in a variety of diseases (Eczema, neuro-dermatitis, scabies), by other mechanical trauma and even from constant friction. Although of various sizes and shapes, excoriations are generally smaller, linear abrasions, bright red or dark colour resulting from dried blood.

An excoriation may be superficial or deep. A crust - simple, blood or impetiginous, covers it. The longer and deeper the excoriations are, the more severe was the pruritus that provoked them.

Crust or Scab

Dried serum, pus, blood etc. usually mixed with epithelial and bacterial debris is known as a crust or a scab. They may be dry golden yellow, soft, friable and superficial as in impetigo contagiosa; yellowish as in favus; thick hard and tough as in third degreee burns, or lamellated, elevated, brown, black or green masses as in late syphilis. The latter have been described as oyster-shell (ostraceous) crusts and are known as rupia.

Common causes of crusts and scabs:

Impetigo contagiosa, Ecthyma, Ulcers, Sycosis, Seborrheic dermatitis, Eczema and dermatitis, Exanthemata-chicken pox and small pox, Herpes zoster, Kaposi's varicella form eruption, Drugs-iodides, bromides and heavy metals, Syphilis and Scratch marks.

Fissures (Cracks, Clefts)

A linear cleft through the epidermis, or rarely into dermis, caused by disease or injury. It has length but ulike an ulcer, no breadth. A fissure is usually accompanied by pain, which interferes with the use of the affected part. Because of the loss in integrity, there is risk of secondary infection. They occur most commonly where the skin is thickened and inelastic from inflammation and dryness, especially in regions subjected to frequent movement. Such areas are the tips and flexural creases of the thumbs, fingers and palms; the edges of heels; clefts between the fingers and toes, at the angles of the mouth; and about the nares, auricles and anus. When the skin is dry and sensitive, exposure to cold and wind or the action of soap and water may produce a stinging, burning sensation and fissures- chapping.

Common causes of fissures:

Chronic eczema of palms and soles, Menopausal keratoderma, Syphilitic fissures, Fissure in ano, Intertrigo and Angular stomatitis.

Erosion

Loss of all or portions of the epidermis alone, as in impetigo or herpes zoster or simplex after vesicle rupture, produces erosion.

It may or may not become crusted but it heals without a scar.

Ulcer

It is a circumscribed lesion starting from a break in the skin, reaching upto the level of dermis. It has definite length, also breadth as opposed to a fissure. A clinician should study its size, contour, depth, edge, covering crust, contents, odour and the surrounding areas of skin.

Common causes of ulcers:

Traumatic, Actinomycosis, Pyogenic, Neoplastic ulcers, Tuberculosis, Varicose ulcers, Syphilis, Trophic ulcers, Dermal Leshmaniasis, Peripheral vascular disorder, Leprosy, Metabolic disorder, Tropical ulcer, Syringomyelia and tabes, Veldt sore and Frostbite.

Causes of ulcer in mouth:

Stomatitis, Tuberculosis, Dental irritation, Syphilis, Pemphigus and Epithelioma.

Scars (Cicatrices)

New formations of connective tissue that replace loss of substance in the dermis or deeper parts as a result of injury or disease, as a part of the normal reparative and healing process. Superficial epidermal lesions heal without scarring; these are important points to be remembered in surgery and in the treatment of cutaneous lesions. In people with dark skin - Indians and Negroes - scars have a tendency to be keloidal. So, due precautions should be taken in surgery and in treatment of the burns. Scars with certain characteristics are typical of particular diseases of the skin, so that they have a diagnostic value. Those of lupus erythematosus are shiny, thin, telangiectatic and minutely pitted, corresponding to glandural orifies; those from lupus vulgaris, tough and fibrous, occasionally cord like or with scaling at the edges; those that follow burns are a mixture of thin, depressed atrophic and hypertrophic raised or fibrous lesions with keloidal tendency; those of scrofuloderma are linear and cord like; those that follow the involution of syphilis are thin, crinkled and papery. The physician should study the size, shape, colour, texture, depression or elevation of the scar – whether it is attached or free, whether there is any accompanying deformity and loss of sensations, hair, sebaceous or sweat secretions.

Common causes of scars:

Traumatic, Ecthyma, Acne necrotica and conglobata, Exanthemata - smallpox and chickenpox, Herpes zoster, Granulomata - tuberculosis, Syphilis, Leprosy, Leishmaniasis, Yaws and fungi, Varicose ulcers and Neoplasms.

Chapter-3

Certain Dermatological Terms (Special Lesions)

ALOPECIA

It implies loss of hair resulting in a bald patch. Defluvium capillorum means fall or thinning of hair without areas of complete baldness. It must be remembered that hair occurs in three stages- growing, stationary and falling. The last stage comprises a very small percentage for causes of baldness.

ATROPHY

Wasting away of skin, which appears thin with loss of elasticity, wrinkling with diminished or complete loss of hair, sweat and sebum. All destructive disease processes of the corium with intact epidermis (i.e. without ulceration) leave behind atrophy. An atrophic patch may or may not be accompanied by scaling, pigmentation and telangiectasia.

BURROW

It is a straight or tortuous, slightly elevated, flesh colour or slightly darker line found on the wrist or hand or genitals – scabies. It represents the part or tunnel of the Acarus scabies in the stratum corneum of the skin. At the deeper end of the burrow an acarus can be demonstrated.

CYST

Circumscribed collection of fluid or semi-solid substances in the skin surrounded by well-defined walls. Its size, shape, consistency, translucency, depth and whether or not it is adherent to the skin and underlined structure should be studied.

Common examples of cysts:

Sebaceous Cyst, Implantation Cyst, Dermoid Cyst, Pilonidal Cyst, Milca, Mucous Cyst, Benign Cystic Epithelium, Hydrocystoma.

COMEDONE (BLACK HEADS)

Plug at the pilo-sebaceous opening. It consists of dried sebum and epithelial debris. To begin with it is white. With the passage of time, the Sulphur of sebum is converted into sulphide and the color becomes black. Comedones are usually found on the face, shoulder, sternal region and back in acne vulgaris and acneiform eruptions due to iodides and bromides. Tar, chlorine and oils by contact, produce comedones on exposed parts like the face, arms and legs.

CIRCINATA

Circular lesions shaped like a coin or disc. If there is central clearing and spreading at the periphery the lesions are called annular.

Common examples of circinata:

Tinea circinata, Psoriasis, Impetigo, Infective eczema, Discoid dermatitis, Erythema multiforme, Lupus erythematosus, Granuloma annulare, Syphilides, Seborrhea corporis, Leprosy, Drug-eruptions, Lichen planus annularis and Pityriasis rosea.

Further special configurations may occur in different skin diseases viz half circle (arciform), multiple circles joined together (polycyclic) or circular with central dots (iris). The latter is typically seen in erythema multiforme.

ERYTHEMA

Redness of the skin due to dilatation of blood vessels. It is a common early sign of most cutaneous diseases, but may be difficult to make out in dark people.

ERYTHRODERMA

Generalized redness and infiltration of the integument as is evident in pityriasis rubra pilaris, generalized dermatitis due to drugs and reticuloses. When accompanied by scaling and exfoliation of the skin, the term exfoliation dermatitis is employed. In reality both terms mean more or less the same thing.

ERYTHEMATO-SQUAMOUS

Combination of erythema and scaling for example, psoriasis, tinea, syphilis, lichen planus, pityriasis rosea and exfoliative dermatitis.

ELEPHANTIASIS

Clinical term signifying elephant like swelling due to extreme lymphedema and fibrous hypertrophy of a part of the body. The common causes are Filariasis, Streptococcal lymphangitis and congential lymphedema. The parts commonly affected are the feet, legs and the gentalia.

GRANULOMA

Chronic swelling usually in the form of a well-defined deep seated dermic nodule. Clinically it is marked by chronic induration and scarring; histologically histiocyte infiltration in the corium is its special feature. They are very common in tropics.

There are several causes of granuloma:

Infective: Tuberculosis, Syphilis, Granuloma inguinale and lymphogranuloma inguinale, Leprosy, Yaws, Leishmaniasis, Septic, deep fugi like actinomycosis etc., Sarcoid.

Drugs: Bromides and iodides.

Neoplastic: Epitheliomas, Secondary metastasis, Reticuloses like mycosis, Fungoides, Hodgkin's disease, etc.

KERATOSIS

Circumscribed hyperplasis of the stratum corneum (horny layer) of skin of senile keratosis, arsenical keratosis and seborrheic keratosis. Keratoses have predispostion to malignancy. Follicular keratosis are seen in lichen spinulosus, keratosis follicularis, Vit. A, C, or fatty acid deficiencies, pityriasis rubra pilaris, Darie's disease, lichen planopilaris, lichen scrofulororum, etc.

KERATODERMA

It signifies diffuse plaques of hyperplasia of the stratum corneum especially of hands and feet for example tylosis, congential, arsenical, menopausal, chronic eczema, syphilis, psoriasis, avitaminosis, pityriasis rubra pilaris, etc.

KOEBNER PHENOMENON

Linear lesions produced by scratching a primary lesion which results in new lesions developing along the line of the scratch, for example lichen planus, warts and psoriasis.

LICHENOID

Violaceous or purplish, solid, firm papules resembling lichen planus but not due to it. This term is loosely used till a proper diagnosis is established. Similarly terms like pemphigoid, leucodermoid and psoriasiform have been coined to describe cutaneous lesions morphologically.

TELANGIECTASIA

It represents groups of the fine dilated capillaries. Common causes are rosacea, spider naevus, alcoholism, and liver disorder, X - ray burns.

VEGETATION

They are cauliflower like growths in moist areas like the ano-genital region, groins and axillae. If the stratum corneum is absent, vegetations look eroded-erosive vegetations. If the stratum corneum is hypertrophic, the vegetations are termed verrucous vegetations. The common causes are Condylomata lata, Pemphigus vegetans, and Pyoderma vegetans.

ZOSTERIFORM

Grouped lesions along the course of a nerve usually unilaterally. Common example is herpes zoster. But zoster form grouping may also be seen in naevi and vitiligo. Further zoster form grouping should be distinguished from linear retiform, herptiform and corynibiform grouping.

Chapter-4

Clinical Approach to Skin Disorders

IMPORTANCE OF MAKING THE RIGHT DIAGNOSIS

The point of making a diagnosis is to improve our predictive ability about the course of a disease in a particular patient and its likely response to treatment.

Three important steps in dermatological diagnosis are:

Morphological Diagnosis

Based on morphological study, localization and distribution.

Clinical Diagnosis

Establishment of the disease entity based on history and signs.

Etiological Diagnosis

Establishment of cause or causes in the individual patient.

The ultimate aim of the treating homeopath should be to establish the etiological diagnosis. Having established the diagnosis, information regarding activity, severity and acuity of the disease process (prognostic criteria) should be elicited and collected before treatment is prescribed.

PRECIS OF CASE TAKING IN DERMATOLOGY

The visibility of skin lesions sometimes tempts the untrained or inexperienced to offer a diagnosis as soon as the patient sits down, or even, with a flourish of showmanship, as the patient enters the door. It is true that some skin lesions can be diagnosed on sight with a high degree of confidence, but even in such cases a detailed history is indispensable for effectively planned management. Even when the morphological diagnosis is rapidly established, a well-planned history is essential to allow the evaluation of etiological factors, and in the many cases in which no satisfactory visual diagnosis is possible a full history may be of great value than a battery of ill-considered laboratory investigations.

History

The full history consists first of a pertinent 'screening' history which includes questions of special significance in disorders of the skin, as well as a succinct enquiry concerning major systematic symptoms, and second, of a series of questions orientated by the patient's presenting complaint in the light of the physician's experience. It is by asking the right questions that the good physician obtains the answers that assist his or her diagnosis.

Since the nature of the presenting complaint orientes the clinical history, the accuracy of the preliminary assessment is of some importance if time-consuming false trails are to be avoided. On the other hand, the full history of the skin lesions can be taken more constructively after the general medical and dermatological history.

General History

Race

The patient's race should be recorded, as it may provide information on some aspects of his or her genetic constitution, and hence on his or her predisposition to certain diseases or patterns of reaction.

Family History

Patients who suffer from any disease are more likely to have been told of relatives who have also been afflicted than if they themselves are not. A negative family history is of greater significance if the patient and his or her parents each have many siblings, than in a small family.

Geographical Factors

The patient's present and past places of residence should always be recorded. The length of time spent in each area may be important. A long visit increases the risk of significant exposure to environmental agents, but even 5min. in transit at an air terminal have allowed the inhalation of the dust-borne spores of coccidioidomycosis, or the bite of a sandfly carrying leishmaniasis.

Occupation

The occupational history should be recorded. As part of the general history, an outline of present and past employment suffices. Past occupations may be of great significance in present illnesses, especially in relation to exposure to carcinogens or metals.

Leisure Activities

Sports, hobbies and other leisure activities may involve excessive exposure to light or trauma, or to irritant or sensitizing chemicals.

Social Factors

The physician must be familiar with the living conditions, economic status and standard of nutrition of the patient, both as a guide to diagnosis and to ensure that treatment advised is realistic and practical.

Ethnic Traditions

Knowledge of the dietary habits, social conditions and religious beliefs of members of ethnic minorities, including

attitudes to disease and its treatment, may have a role in successful
disease management.

Personal History

Hobbies, special habits, etc.

Past Illnesses

Several widespread skin conditions such as urticaria,
vasculitis, guttate psoriasis and erythema multiforme can be
triggered off by viral or bacterial infections in the weeks preceding
the onset of the rash. The routine enquiry concerning past illnesses
must include details of the treatment received. Any medication
recently received should be noted, including regular or intermittent
self-medication or that received from relatives or friends.

General Health

Any specific disorder and its relation to the skin ailment.

Special History

History of presenting complaint.

Onset of Skin Lesions

The time of onset of the lesions should be determined as
accurately as possible. The date of exacerbation's or recurrences
should also be recorded.

Duration of the Complaints

The duration of the individual skin lesions is important, but
patients may give misleading answers. Basal cell carcinoma, for
example, is often noticed only when it ulcerates and the patient
will therefore report the duration of the ulcer rather than the
duration of the cancer. The periodicity is sometimes helpful, for
example when exposure to the allergen in contact dermatitis is
only intermittent. The history of the evolution may also give
diagnostic help, for example the herald spot of pityriasis rosea,
the pain for 24h before blistering in 'shingles', or the history of

severe itch and erythema for days or weeks preceding blister formation in bullous phemphigoid.

Site of Onset

The site or sites at which skin changes were first noticed is of obvious importance in diagnosis. The patient may fail to mention apparently insignificant or embarrassing lesions, and will draw attention to later and more conspicuous lesions

Primary Lesions

The patient should be asked to describe the original lesions and any subsequent changes in their appearance or character.

Manner of Spread / Extension

The course of the lesions, their rate of enlargement and the pattern of their extension or dissemination to other regions of the body should be noted.

Provoking Factors

It is often worth asking the patient whether any particular factors (e.g. heat, cold, sunlight, etc.) either exacerbate or alleviate the condition.

Eruption-active or Quiescent

Subjective symptoms

If any, also whether the symptoms preceded or followed the eruption. The presence or absence of itching, its character and its periodicity are of diagnostic importance.

Topical therapy

Self-treatment of skin lesions is almost universal, and the condition presented to the dermatologist may be concealed or replaced by the effects of inappropriate applications. The patient should be asked to describe precisely what measures have been employed.

History of any illness preceding or accompanying the skin disorder

Exploration of environmental factors

The nature of the lesions and their distribution may suggest the possible role of drugs, light or ectoparasite or of environmental, irritant or sensitizing chemicals. The most detailed interrogation may be necessary in order to establish a probable association between such factors and the skin lesions.

Psychological factors

The dermatologist will have to assess the patient's emotional state and domestic and business conflicts. The possible role of psychological factors should be thoroughly explored. They are of the greatest importance in initiating, aggravating or perpetuating a wide variety of dermatoses.

Examination

Most patients referred to the dermatologist present objective changes in the appearance or consistency of the skin. The detailed and critical analysis of these physical signs, in terms of the range of pathological processes that can produce them, will often permit an accurate morphological diagnosis. The ability to elicit cutaneous physical signs and to interpret them correctly should be acquired by every dermatologist at an early stage of training. The morphological diagnosis is merely the first step towards the final diagnosis and assessment, and not the ultimate objective. The patient should always be examined in a good light, preferably daylight. Ideally, the entire skin should be examined in every patient, and this must be insisted on wherever the diagnosis is in doubt.

Local

Inspection

*   Clinical nature of the lesions - Primary, Secondary or Special form.

- Shape and pattern of the lesions
- Distribution of the lesions - regional, general or local; grouped or polymorphous.
- Colour of the lesion
- Particular examination of scalp, mouth, nails, genitalia and feet.

Palpation

- The effect of rubbing Whereas scratching shows evident and identifiable changes, the response to rubbing is more subtle. Lesions, perhaps only one of several, become thickened and hyperkeratotic (lichenification). Hair in the area are broken and dystrophic, and the patient's nails often show a polished appearance.
- The Koebner or Isomorphic phenomenon, diascopy, etc.

General physical examination

- Patient is ill, toxic, conscious, cyanotic, febrile, anemic, debilitated or not. Mental make-up, bearing, clothes, mannerisms.

Laboratory Aids

■

Chapter-5

Localization of the Common Dermatoses

Acne vulgaris
* Face.
* Shoulders.
* Upper back.
* Chest.

Atopic dermatitis
* Eyes.
* Face.
* Neck.
* Front of elbow.
* Back of knees.

Chilblains
* Fingers.
* Toes.

Contact dermatitis
* Site of suspected contact.

Dermatitis herpetiformis
* Scapular region.

- Lower back.
- Chest.
- Forearms.

Dermal leishmaniasis
- Exposed parts.
- Face.
- Hands.
- Elbows.

Erythema multiforme
- Hands.
- Forearm.
- Face.
- Mouth.

Erythema nodosum
- Front of the legs.

Herpes simplex
- Lips.
- Genitals.

Herpes zoster
- Unilateral lesions on trunk.
- Face.
- Neck.
- Extremities.

Intertrigo
- Flexures of groins.
- Axillae.
- Inframammary region.

Lupus erythematosus (chronic)
* Butterfly distribution on face.

Lichen Planus
* Legs.
* Wrist.
* Forearms.
* Genitals.
* Mouth.

Neurodermatitis
* Back of the neck.
* Forearms.
* Legs.
* Ankles.
* Anogenital region.

Pediculosis
* Scalp.
* Trunk.
* Pubic region (according to the variety).

Pityriasis versicolor
* Chest.
* Back.
* Upper parts of arms.

Psoriasis
* Scalp.
* Elbows.
* Knees.
* Back.
* Legs.
* Nails.

Rosacea

- Central part of the face.

Scabies

- Hands (interdigital spaces, palms).
- Front of the wrists.
- Elbow.
- Penis.
- Buttocks.
- Abdomen.

Seborrheic dermatitis

- Scalp.
- Retro-auricular region.
- Eyebrows.
- Elbows.
- Sternal region.
- Inter-scapular region.
- Flexures.

Sycosis barbae

- Beard region.

Tinea cruris

- Scrotum.

Tinea pedis

- Interdigital spaces of the feet, soles.

Varicose ulcers

- Ankles (inner surface).

Rosacea erythematosis.
Lateral part of the face

Rosacea.
Seborrheic dermatitis.

Chapter-6

Regional Differential Diagnosis of Common Dermatoses

Scalp

- Diseases of hair.
- Infective eczema.
- Pediculosis.
- Pityriasis capitis.
- Psoriasis.
- Seborrheic dermatitis.
- Tinea capitis.

Face

- Acne vulgaris.
- Atopic dermatitis.
- Cholasma.
- Contact dermatitis and eczema.
- Dermal leishmaniasis.
- Herpes simplex and zoster.
- Impetigo.

- Lupus erythematosis.
- Lupus vulgaris.
- Rosacea.
- Seborrheic dermatitis.
- Sycosis.
- Vitiligo.

Nose

- Chloasma.
- Dermal leishmaniasis.
- Lupus erythematosis.
- Lupus vulgaris.
- Rhinoscleroma.
- Rosacea.

Ear

- Infective eczema.
- Leprosy.
- Seborrheic dermatitis.

Neck

- Atopic eczema.
- Contact dermatitis.
- Lichen simplex chronicus.
- Skin tags.
- Warts.

Back

- Contact dermatitis.
- Neurodermatitis.
- Sycosis nuchae.

Front

- Actinomycosis.

- Contact dermatitis.
- Pityriasis versicolor.
- Pyoderma .
- Scrofuloderma.

Lips

- Angular stomatitis.
- Cheilitis.
- Cheilitis glandularis.
- Contact dermatitis.
- Deficiency diseases.
- Lichen planus.
- Lupus erythromatosus.
- Syphilis.

Mouth

- Deficiency diseases.
- Epithelioma.
- Lichen planus.
- Pemphigus.
- Stomatitis.
- Syphilis.
- Tuberculosis.

Chest

- Acne.
- Dermatitis.
- Herpes zoster.
- Pediculosis.
- Pityriasis rosacea.
- Pityriasis versicolor.
- Seborrheic dermatitis.

Back

- Acne vulgaris (upper part).
- Dermatitis herpetiformis (scaplular region).
- Herpes zoster.
- Pemphigus.
- Pityriasis rosacea (along the ribs).
- Pityriasis versicolor.
- Psoriasis.
- Seborrheic dermatitis (interscapular region).

Armpits

- Contact dermatitis.
- Flexural psoriasis.
- Fox-Fordyce's disease.
- Hiradenitis suppurativa.
- Infective eczema.
- Seborrheic dermatitis.
- Tinea.
- Trichomycosis axillaries.

Abdomen

- Herpes zoster.
- Lichen planus.
- Pediculosis pubis.
- Pemphigus.
- Pityriasis rosacea.
- Pityriasis versicolor.
- Tinea.

Groins

- Chancroidal pulp.
- Flexural psoriasis.
- Infective eczema.

- Lymphogranuloma inguinale.
- Moniliasis.
- Scrofuloderma.
- Tinea cruris.

Anal region

- Condylomata acuminatum.
- Condylomata lata.
- Contact eczema.
- Fissure in ano.
- Neurodermatitis.
- Pruritus ani.

Genitals

- Chancre.
- Chancroid.
- Contact dermatitis.
- Epithelioma.
- Granuloma inguinale.
- Herpes progenitalis.
- Leukoplakia.
- Lichen planus.
- Lichen sclerosis et atrophicus.
- Neurodermatitis.
- Pediculosis.
- Phagedaena.
- Scabies.
- Secondary syphilis.

Arms

- Herpes zoster.
- Tinea versicolor.

Forearms

- Dermatitis herpetiformis.
- Discoid dermatitis.
- Erythema multiforme.
- Lichen planus.
- Psoriasis.
- Tinea circinata.

Elbows

- Atopic dermatitis (front).
- Dermal leishmaniasis.
- Lupus vulgaris.
- Psoriasis (back).

Hands

- Chilblains.
- Contact eczema.
- Drug allergy.
- Dyshidrosis (palms).
- Infective dermatitis.
- Keratoderma.
- Leprosy.
- Nummular eczema.
- Psoriasis.
- Pustular bacteroids.
- Raynaud's disease.
- Syphilis.
- Tinea.
- Trade eruptions.
- Tuberculosis.
- Verrucosis.
- Warts.

Thighs

* Contact dermatitis.
* Folliculitis.
* Tinea.

Knees

* Atopic dermatitis (back).
* Lupus vulgaris.
* Psoriasis (front).

Legs

* Bazin's disease.
* Discoid dermatitis.
* Erythema nodosum.
* Folliculitis.
* Henoch Schonlein purpura.
* Lichen planus.
* Neurodermatitis.
* Psoriasis.

Feet

* Actinomycosis Madurae.
* Bacteroids.
* Buerger's disease.
* Chilblains.
* Contact dermatitis.
* Discoid dermatitis.
* Dyshidrosis.
* Keratoderma.
* Leprosy.
* Neurodermatitis.
* Post traumatic infective eczema.
* Raynaud's disease.

- Tinea.
- Tuberculosis cutis verrucosus.
- Varicose ulcers.
- Warts

SYSTEMIC DISEASES PRODUCING CUTANEOUS DISORDER

Cutaneous lesions are occasionally produced by systemic disorders so they may help in the diagnosis of the latter. On the other hand a cutaneous disease may affect the internal organs. Hence it should never be forgotten that skin is an organ of the whole body and should be considered as such, in the practice of dermatology.

Important e.g. are:

Nutritional
- Pellagra, avitaminosis.

Metabolic
- Diabetes: Pruritus, moniliasis, furunculosis, carbuncle, xanthomatosis, necrobiosis lipoidica, trophic ulcers, gangrene.
- Amyloidosis cutis
- Cirrhosis: Spider naevi, sallow complexion, paper money skin, pruritus.
- Porphyrinuria: Pigmentation, haydro aestivale.
- Xanthomatosis.
- Bronze diabetes or Henochromatosis.

Endocrine
- Thyrotoxicosis: Pigmentation
- Myxedema: Alopecia, Myxedematous skin.
- Cushing's diseases: Flame shaped stria.
- Pituitary cachexia (Simmonds): Alopecia.

- Addisions disease: Pigmentation.
- Menstrual disorders: Pigmentation, chloasma, alopecia, hirsuitism.

Focal Sepsis

(In teeth, ears, sinuses, tonsils, lung, gall bladder, kidneys, prostate, etc.)
- Pyemic abscesses.
- Lupus erythematous.
- Bacteriodes.
- Rosacea.
- Discoid eczema.
- Acne vulgaris.
- Urticaria.
- Erythema multiforme.
- Dermatitis herpetiformis.
- Dyshidrosis.

Vascular disorder

- Raynaud's disease.
- PAN.
- Arteriosclerosis.
- Buerger's disease.

Carcinomatosis

- Secondaries in skin.
- Pigmentation.
- Pruritus.
- Acanthosis nigricans.

Naevi

- Hemangioma of skin: Associated with angioma of brain.
- Adenoma sebaceum: Associated with tuberous sclerosus.
- Neurofibromatosis: Associated with lesions in bones, nerves and eyes.

Collagen diseases

- Lupus erythematosus.
- Scleroderma.
- Dermatomyositis.

Fever and rashes

Chapter-7

Natural History of Disease

A good clinician and intelligent patient are of enormous help in studying natural history of disease, thereby assisting in making a correct diagnosis, because different diseases follow different and varied course depending of course, on climate, patient's resistance and virulence of disease process, etc.

A few important examples are listed below:

- Exanthemata like small pox, chicken pox, herpes zoster have limited course of 12-15 days unless secondarily infected. Pyodermas are of short duration, unless they become chronic as in folliculitis. Anthrax, tropical ulcer and pyoderma gangrenosum develop rapidly.

- In comparison fungus affections in tropical countries are common in summer and more so in warm, humid season of monsoon. In the cold weather, they become dormant to recur again in the hot weather unless properly treated. History extends over years. Scabies is more frequently seen in winter and insect bites in the summer and monsoon on exposed parts.

- Warts spread slowly by auto-inoculation except in the beard region (spread fast by shaving) and moist areas (condylomata acuminatum).

- History of dermal leishmaniasis is usually in weeks in endemic areas. Syphilitic chancre develops a few weeks after exposure while herpes progenitalis and gonorrhea within 1-3 days and chancroid in 3-5 days, granuloma venereum in 2-6 days and lymphogranuloma in 1-2 weeks. History of epithelioma on glans penis extends to months and warts only a few weeks. Syphilitic gumma has history of months, while history of tuberculosis and leprosy extends over years.

- Psoriasis has usually winter aggravation; but some cases do show summer flare-ups when prickly heat becomes psoriasiform. Seborrheic dermatitis tends to increase in autumn and spring and the history is chronic. Lichen planus has sudden or insidious onset depending upon the cause. Drug eruptions are usually acute in onset and short lived unless caused by heavy metals like arsenic or produce erythroderma-like picture.

- Amongst the neoplasms, history of basal cell epithelioma is in years, squamous cell epitheliomas in months, while malignant melanomas develop in weeks to months.

Chapter-8

Clinical Immunology and Allergy

The concept of immunity has undergone revolutionary changes and has widened the scope immeasurably.

The WHO report defines immunity as follows "The immune response comprises all the phenomenon that result from the specific interaction of cells of the immune system with antigen."

Allergic change in some form occurs in all individuals. This may be beneficial, as in the antibody response to vaccines and infective organisms, or harmful, as in anaphylactic sensitivity, delayed hypersensitivity, contact dermatitis or cytotoxic reaction.

An antigen is a substance that stimulates the formation of humoral antibody, or alters the reactivity of lymphocytes and other cells (the cell-mediated response). Two types of cells - T-lymphocytes (Thymus dependent) and B-lymphocytes (Bursa equivalent of Fabricius) mediate this.

Antigens that commonly sensitize persons to anaphylactic or to delayed-type hypersensitivity's are known as allergens.

Antigenic stimulation results in the formation of anti-bodies known as immunoglobulins, or a response by cells (e.g. lymphocytes), which, when 'primed' with antigen specificity, are referred to as immunologically competent cells, and their reaction with antigen is conveniently termed a cell-mediated response.

There are three patterns of immune responsiveness:

- Immune awareness: Immune awareness is the state of 'informed acceptance' or tolerance, in which lymphoid cells have been primed to recognize common antigens, but few specific clones and only traces of antibody are formed.

- Formation of antibody and possibly patch-test sensitivity without clinical allergy Antibody formation may occur without the individual becoming noticeably allergic. Many individuals have anti-bodies to the common substances of their environment, and show no reaction when exposed to them, for example to grass pollen, cows' milk or egg white.

- Antibody formation and cell-mediated immune responses manifested as allergy on normal exposure to the allergens, or even on exposure to very small amounts well tolerated by the general population. The term allergy designates a specific altered reactivity of the tissues to substances, compared with the response to the first exposure to the same substances, or the reactivity of other individuals of the same species not previously exposed to the substances. Allergy may develop without reexposure to the antigen if the antigen persists in the blood or tissues long enough to react with the antibody formed against it, as occurs in serum sickness.

The skin may be regarded as the most peripheral outpost of the immune system; in its capacity as an environmental barrier, it initiates an immune response to foreign antigens or neoantigens, in order to remove potential toxins and damaged epithelium, destroy infective organisms and prevent cutaneous malignancy. Lymphocytes in normal skin are essentially exclusively of T-cell type.

The skin immune system, also known as the skin-associated lymphoid tissue (SALT), comprises of the following:

- Recirculating lymphocytes that home to the skin.

- Antigen-presenting CD1+ HLA-DR+ Langerhans' cells of monocyte-macrophage lineage, which circulate between the epidermis and the regional lymph nodes.

- Dermal APCs including perivascular factor XIIIa+ dermal dendritic cells and CD1a+ Langerhans'-like cells, keratinocytes, which produce a wide range of immunoregulatory and growth regulatory cytokines.

- High endothelial post-capillary venules, which may be induced to express adhesion molecules for leukocytes.

VARIOUS TYPES OF ALLERGIC REACTION

- Anaphylaxis: Immediate weal-and-flare prick test response, Allergic urticaria, Allergic angio-oedema, some transient erythemas and a component of atopic dermatitis.

- Arthus reaction and immune complex diseases: Serum sickness, several forms of cutaneous vasculitis, especially necrotizing or leukocytoclastic lesions and Immune-complex-induced glomerulonephritis.

- Cytotoxic reactions and autoantibodies: Bullous diseases, discoid and systemic lupus erythematosus, antibodies to epidermis as in (a) generalized eczema (b) bone-marrow graft and Antibodies to stratum corneum.

- Autoallergies.

- Delayed hypersensitivity: Allergic contact dermatitis, photo-allergy, interactions and skin responsiveness to bacteria, fungi, viruses, protozoa, granulomatous lesions, for example to beryllium and zirconium, insect bites, homograft rejection, and abnormal delayed hypersensitivity in atopic dermatitis.

CUTANEOUS ALLERGY

In the skin, there are two important but different allergic reactions.

- One as in urticaria, the causative antigen reaches the skin through ingestion, inhalation or injection of protein substances and the reacting antibodies circulate in the serum. Allergic reaction takes place in the dermis - *Dermal reaction.* In this type of allergy, Prausnitz- Kustner-passive transfer reaction is positive and only the intradermal (injection or scratch) tests show reactivity. The response is weal formation, which occurs in few minutes.

- The second type of allergic cutaneous reaction is *Epidermal reaction*, as seen in allergic dermatitis or eczema. Causative substances reach the skin by contact. Intradermal allergic tests are negative; on the contrary patch tests show reactivity. Prausnitz-Kustner-reaction is also negative. Sensitizers vary from simple substances (chromate and nickel) to complex chemicals (plastics) or even bacterial products (streptococci, fungi).

UNDERSTANDING MIASMS

It is essential to have a sound understanding of miasm to study various skin diseases.

The Miasmatic theory of chronic diseases propounded by Hahnemann has become the most controversial in the history of homeopathy.

It has polarized the homeopathic profession; at one extreme we find a group who holds that the theory is a delusion, at the other end is the group who affirms all that Hahnemann, Allen, Roberts, Kent wrote on the subject amounts to a priceless pearl given only to intuitive minds and that lesser minds should accept the theory on faith.

I personally feel that if Hahnemann were alive, then he himself would have preferred his theory and clarification of miasms to be examined objectively under the light of modern science.

PHENOMENOLOGICAL APPROACH

When we study the therapeutics of skin, we include skin and its appendages, viz. hair, nail. Like any other disease, the signs and symptoms of the patient should be analyzed into:

Location

- Epidermis, dermis, hair follicles, sweat glands, sebaceous glands.

Sensations

- Itching, burning, tingling, formication.

Modalities

- Hot application, cold application, rubbing, scratching.

Concomitants

- Symtpoms that have only time relationship with the chief complaint but no patho-physiological relationship, e.g. irritable at trifles with allergic rashes, impatient at trifles with post herpetic neuralgia, mania of cleanliness with dandruff, increased frequency of urination with itching, strong desire to vomit accompanied by urticaria.

The next step would be to classify the disease nosologically, e.g. skin can be affected primarily or it could be a local manifestation of systemic disease viz. viral exanthemata, Diabetes mellitus, Hodgkin's disease, SLE, etc.

Also many times one gets the skin symptoms, which only come in alternations, e.g. the psora tries to throw eruptions out on the skin and its appendages with its characteristic discharge clinically known as *Primary Psora*. Whenever these eruptions come out the internal trouble is relieved and the patient feels better. The appearance of boils and reappearance of eruptions and discharges under treatment is a reliable index of good action of a well-selected remedy.

When these peripheral extensions / expressions of primary psora are blocked through suppressive measures, the road is clear for progressive internalization of trouble with increasing involvement of more vital organs. This is to say, various other systems, e.g. metabolism, nutrition; Central Nervous System, Cardio Vascular System, etc. get affected. The symptomatology is known as *Secondary Psoric* expression. There is minimal structural alteration of a reversible type with maximum functional disturbance.

Hypersensitivity reactions that follow vaccination are a typical manifestation of psoric miasm. At this junction I would like to clarify that even though the phenomenon of alteration (or alternating states) is characteristic of psoric miasm, the expression of the state that follows alternation may be of any miasm depending on the pathology of that particular disease, e.g. scabies alternating with asthma.

The phenomenon of alternation between the two is characteristic of psoric miasm. But the expression of the two States is as follows (1) Scabies is classified under *tubercular miasm* (infection) (2) Asthma (aggravated in damp weather with greenish offensive expectoration) is classified under *sycotic miasm*.

Similarly whenever any skin lesion, irrespective of its nosological classification is suppressed by any agent – physical, chemical drugs (Homeopathic, Ayurvedic, Allopathic, Unani, etc.) the manifestation that follows could be classified from psora to sycosis to tubercular to syphilis e.g. suppression of exanthemata leading to encephalitis typical of tubercular miasm.

For simplicity, I have classified the diseases according to the Hahnemannian miasmatic evolution of sickness. The most important thing to remember in this classification is that no sickness is ever under a fixed miasm.

The miasmatic background changes (Psora to Sycosis to Tubercular to Syphilis) as the disease evolves from functional to structural changes.

Taking acne vulgaris as an example, one sees that to start with there is only a slight papule with itching, so characteristic of psora; followed by slight induration (sycotic), which is followed by pain and purulent discharge (tubercular); then rupture with necrosis (syphilis).

Skin eruptions with glandular involvement will necessarily have syphilitic or tubercular element to conform to the glandular involvement.

In ichthyosis (fishy skin), we find all the chronic miasms and where we find them all present, we usually find an incurable skin disease especially if hereditary. In ichthyosis we see the dryness of psora, the squamae of syphilis and often the moles and warty eruption of sycosis.

All miasms are present in erysipelas, carcinoma, epithelioma, and lupus.

In nevus or congenital markings of the skin we have all the miasms as in elephantiasis.

I repeat: All skin diseases are multimiasmatic!!

Chapter-9

Healthy Skin

A healthy skin is a source of pleasure, not only to its owner but also to the one who looks at it. To possess a nice skin is to have great social and economic advantage. Besides the positive health of the skin is an insurance against disease, the ideal of every individual as well as every medical man.

The normal healthy skin is clear, smooth, supple, elastic, uniformly pigmented without wrinkles and does not sap; the stratum corneum (horny layer) is thin, transluscent and invisibly casts off, the pores are hardly visible, secreting an imperceptible amount of sebum and sweat (except in summer, in hot environments and when exertion takes place) and there is no E/O active bacterial or fungal growth. This tone and glossiness is noticeably absent in the skin of the sedentary town worker.

The integument being the external covering of the human body is put to great stress and strain by the external environments involving factors like climatic changes, dust, irritants, non-pathogenic and pathogenic microorganisms, etc. Hair and nails grow constantly. Sebum is daily washed off. These agents have to be controlled.

The following factors are important in keeping the skin healthy:

Diet

- It should be balanced and digestible. A fair amount of animal proteins and vitamins are essential. The daily diet should contain liberal helpings of meat, fish, eggs, milk and its products, butter, green vegetables and fruits. Concentrated starchy food should be avoided. "Sattvik" diet is the answer. Spices, condiments, tea, coffee and alcohol should be consumed as little as possible. They produce a sense of heat hence, predisposing to allergic conditions and dermatoses. Occasional fasting is good for health. Keep your digestion healthy. Gluttons and dyspeptics tend to be greasy, flushed, sallow, pasty and pimply. They later, tend to develop seborrheic dermatoses. Besides, over-eating results in obesity, which produces side effects.

Fresh cool air, exercises and mild sun

- They stimulate the skin and thereby the thyroid, adrenals and sympathetic system on which are dependent the wellbeing and vitality of the skin and the body. Intertrigo and tinea are rare in individuals who indulge in regular exercise in cool, fresh surroundings. Exercise in fresh, cool air is very stimulating. Yogic exercises are beneficial because they exercise and relax the musculature and in a scientific manner. Hyperhidrosis and maceration due to scorching heat are responsible for several tropical conditions. The strong sun produces degenerative changes and even neoplasms especially in white people. An umbrella, solar hat and sun protective agents are useful aids.

Clothing

- The clothing and footwear should not contain sensitizers. They should not be tight fitting. Nylon clothes should be avoided especially in summers because they interfere with absorption and evaporation of sweat. The chemicals deposited by unevaporated sweat can cause contact dermatitis. The same applies to footwear (especially of rubber and plastic), spectacle-frames, furs, artificial jewellery, etc.

Bathing

- In tropical countries, daily bathing with clean and cool water is essential in the summer. In cold weather, one should bathe in warm water as often as possible, clean the various body folds, genitalia and feet properly. The skin should be thoroughly dried after washing. A hot bath followed by a cold one is stimulating to the skin and vital organs. To begin with the difference in between the two baths should not be great but in course of time, as a person gets used to the difference, he will greatly enjoy such baths, which benefit. These baths can be recommended in cases of chilblains, thermal urticarias and certain selected cases of atopic dermatitis.

Soap

- A simple, least alkaline soap is the best. For dry skin use superfatted soaps. It can be prepared by melting finely shredded soap in hot olive or coconut oil over a water-bath stirring it till a homogeneous mixture is formed and then allowing the mixture to cool and set to form a cake. Medicated soaps are the least useful as medication, and can be great sensitizers.

Oil

- Coconut, mustard and olive oil are better than medicated and perfumed oils. In cold, dry weather, apply vaseline or milk cream on the exposed parts before retiring to bed. A good substitute for oil is butter, ghee or lanoline. Ghee and butter are very useful for chapped lips, hands and feet. In India, 'Upvatnas' are popular with the fair sex for giving the required transluscence, opacity and glow to the skin. They consist of milk cream, gram flour and lemon juice.

Shaving

- Do not shave too finely by stretching the skin.
- Shave in one direction.
- Use clean, sterilized and sharp instruments and avoid repeated shaving over the same parts.

- The beard should be properly softened with soap or shaving cream before shaving. After shaving, rub in a little cream to lubricate the degreased skin. Strongly alkaline or sensitizing shaving soap, cream, after shave lotions should be avoided. The electric razor avoids trauma and use of alkaline soap.

Cosmetics

- Chemicals in cosmetics may harm the skin, cause blockage of pores and invisible, slow degeneration. Whenever one desires to change one brand for another in cosmetics, it is advisable to do a patch test.

Chapter-10

Care of the Hair

Washing

- Savlon (P), Cetavlon (P) and Selsun suspension (P) are useful in controlling dandruff.
- Sometimes beaten egg white is employed to give glossiness to the hair. Indigenous plant products like 'ritha' and 'amla' are used for washing the hair because they are cheap and effective. Greasy hair need frequent washing and less oil application. Dry hair requires less frequent washing and a good oil massage.

Combing and Brushing

- No force should be used and it should be done less frequently since it tends to irritate the scalp and often injures and atrophies the hair.

Singeing of Hair

- There are no advantages of over cutting for split ends and has no curative effect.

Dyeing of Hair

- Vegetable dyes (henna, chamomile) are safest in comparison to metallic dyes (bismuth, silver, lead) and chemical dyes (para-tolyendiamine, paraphenylenediamine, etc.). Patch test to the dye must be applied before its use.

Permanent waving and straightening of wavy hair in Negroes.

There are two methods of permanent waving:

1. The cold method

Hair is curled by means of curlers and softened with a reducing agent like ammonium thioglycolate so that it can conform to the undulations made by the curler. Later, undulations are fixed with a neutralizer or an oxidizing agent.

2. The hot method

The hair is first softened by an alkaline sulphate solution and these undulations are made by rods and the application of heat (electrical, steam or chemicals). The hair is shampooed before any of the two techniques of permanent waving are employed. Burning of the scalp by direct heat or chemical irritation and sensitization are some of the risks of permanent waving. Due precautions should be taken; patch tests should precede the use of chemicals.

Hair O rnaments

- Pins, clips and nets rarely cause dermatitis. Nickel and plastic materials should be used with caution to prevent irritation.

Chapter-11

Significance of Diet and Home Remedies in Dermatological Conditions

Skin is the mirror of the body. Any internal disorder usually manifests firsts at the level of the skin. Hence one has to pay most care to maintain proper skin care. One of the modality for healthy skin is to eat the right food for proper and normal skin. Certain diets over a period of years in our practice have been very useful for certain disorders.

GENERAL AIDS

- Excess intake of improper food must be controlled, better if avoided totally.
- Since teenage is the time when food temptations cannot be resisted, diversions like exercise, sports and games must be encouraged. This will have an added benefit as exercise is of great help in the treatment of acne.
- Quick lime rich in calcium improves overall resistance to infections.
- 'Neem' (Azadirachta indica) water is taken routinely as a medicine by some to protect the body against infection.

- Onion decoction or garlic soup is popular to build up body resistance against infection.

- A small piece of 'Chireta' (Swerata chirata) boiled in water, a teaspoonful of anise seed, a teaspoonful of 'Ajwain' (Bishop's seed) and a few cardamoms, this decoction taken on empty stomach in the morning, daily for a fortnight, is very useful to improve resistance and prevent boils.

- 'Jaljira' (decoction of cumin seeds), coconut water, carrot seeds infusion, barley water, etc. are some of the common beverages that by causing increased urination help in cooling the system.

- Lemon juice is natures most powerful antiseptic. Use it externally on sores, corn and dandruff.

- For clearing the complexion, use cucumber juice with water. Place the slices of cucumber over the face where needed.

- In general 16 ounces of prune juice, 1-gallon apple juice each day for 3 days also helps to clear the complexion.

- For rough skin eat silicon rich foods such as oats and wheat bran. Eat oatmeal and rub face and arms with oat water. Wheat bran makes the skin smooth. Make a thin paste of wheat bran and apply to face, neck and arms.

- For scars rub cocoa butter on the scar. It has to be done consistently, 2 times daily.

- Slices of pumpkin if rubbed on the face, hands and feet remove black patches, freckle and brighten the complexion.

- Raw turmeric if taken daily in the morning gives brightness to the complexion and makes it soft and smooth.

- A lemon-milk preparation is employed for whitening and softening the skin, hands and face.

- Raw papaya fruit if applied as a cosmetic removes freckles, black spots and makes the skin smooth and delicate.

SOME HINTS FOR A CLEAR SKIN AND TO IMPROVE THE COMPLEXION

- A special skin cleaning powder is a mixture of green gram, Bengal gram and fenugreek seeds. Equal proportions of green gram and Bengal gram with a fistful of fenugreek seeds is powdered and preserved. When needed the powder is mixed with plain water or starch water.

- White radish and carrot juice not only give a plenty of vitamin A but also act as a diuretic, flushing out toxins from the body.

- Curd is the most ideal to massage the skin as it tones up dry and oily skin. The mildly acidic lactic acid in curd acts as an antiseptic and astringent and the cream in the curd soothing to the skin.

- A glass of limejuice has enough vitamin C to meet the daily requirement of this particular vitamin.

- Cut a lime into two. Take one half and gently massage the face. Squeeze the other half into a cup of water and drink it with a crystal of rock salt. Do it every day for six to eight weeks to see a remarkable improvement in the appearance of your skin. This helps to remove the greasiness of the skin and lighten colour.

- For blackheads make a fine paste of turmeric rhizome with a few mustard seeds. This paste is touched on the blackheads and left overnight. In the morning the face is washed clean with gram flour. The blackheads soften and fall off.

- Following are some of the hints to help the complexion glow with health.

  - A tablespoon of honey either alone or with limejuice daily helps to improve the skin colour.

  - Be liberal in your fluid intake.

  - Carrots, lime, cucumber, onion, fenugreek and coconuts improve skin nutrition. Take them in plenty and as far as possible fresh, in any convenient combination to enhance skin colour.

- One 'amla' (gooseberry) daily helps to improve the skin colour.

- For active young people a bit of fresh butter daily in the morning is one of the best prescriptions for a healthy smooth skin.

ALLERGIC DERMATOSES (URTICARIA, ALLERGIC AND ATOPIC ECZEMA)

The single factor eliminative diet and a diet diary are two useful measures. In the former we start the patient on one foodstuff, like boiled milk. If the disease persists, he is given to start with, boiled rice and sugar. It is rarely that a patient is sensitive to both rice and milk. If the allergy is due to dietetic factors, the disease should be controlled with the diet alone. After the disease has been controlled on boiled milk or rice, every three days, one more foodstuff is added, starting with essential ones like wheat (chapattis and bread), fats (butter and ghee), mutton, eggs, peas, carrots, bananas, potatoes, lentils, till either an allergic attack develops, meaning that the patient is sensitive to the last added foodstuff, or the normal diet is reached. Usually patients are sensitive to protein diets or vegetables and fruits, or to the synthetic chemicals used for preserving food; starch, fats and minerals make poor allergens.

Diet diary

A specimen chart is maintained for a month or two depending upon the case. Every foodstuff taken during the day is marked by a cross (x), and at the bottom of the column, the patient puts down whether he felt better or worse, or suffered from an acute flare up the cause can be discovered.

Allergies (Urticaria)

• Five drops of castor oil in half of any fruit or vegetable or even plain water can be taken on empty stomach. This is very beneficial for allergies of the intestinal tract, skin and nasal passages.

- Fresh juices like carrot juice; carrot juice with beet and cucumber juices are useful in the treatment of allergies.
- The patient should take two teaspoons of turmeric powder mixed with a cup of water daily. This is very valuable in urticaria.
- About 7gm of mint and 25gm of brown sugar should be boiled together in 175ml of water and drunk. This relieves the itching.
- Foods which should be eliminated from the diet are tea, coffee, cola drinks, chocolates, sugar and its products, refined cereals, meat, fish, chicken, tobacco, milk, cheese, butter, salted pickled foods, and foods containing any chemical additives, preservatives and flavorings.
- Five drops of castor oil added to half a cup of any fruit or vegetable juice, or plain water, and taken on empty stomach early in the morning, is beneficial for allergies of the skin.
- One or two bananas a day are useful for those who are allergic to certain foods and who constantly suffer from skin rashes.
- To reduce severe itching, apply ice on the affected part.
- The herb rauwolfia is beneficial in relieving itching in urticaria. One gram of the powdered root can be taken with a cup of water daily.
- An equal quantity of alum and red ocher should be ground together and the powder rubbed on the weals.

Boils

- A thorough cleansing of the system is essential for the treatment of boils. An exclusive diet of fresh juicy fruits with proper regulation of the bowels helps to a great extent.
- The use of garlic or onion has proved very effective. The juice of garlic and onion may be applied externally to the boils to help ripen them and also to break them and evacuate the pus.
- Half a cup of fresh juice of bitter gourd (karela), mixed with half teaspoon of limejuice should be taken sip by sip, on an empty stomach daily for few days in treating this condition.

- Betel leaf is a valuable remedy for boils. A leaf is gently warmed till it gets softened. It is then coated with a layer of castor oil. The oiled leaf should be spread over the inflamed part. It should be replaced every few hour's. After a few applications the boil will rupture, draining all the purulent matter. The application can be made at night and removed in the morning.
- The seeds of black cumin ground in water and made into a paste can be applied to the boils with beneficial results.
- The application of turmeric powder to the boils speeds up the healing process.
- Warm moist compresses applied three to four times a day over the tender area helps to ripen the boil and helps in its easy drainage.

Chronic Erythroderma, Pemphigus and Leprosy

- Extra proteins and minerals should be added to the diet to keep up one's body strength and make up for the loss of these from the skin in the form of scales and serum, particularly so in the first two dermatoses.

Corns and Callosities

- A paste made by grinding 3-4 liquorices sticks and mixing it with sesame oil or mustard oil will prove very effective if applied over the affected area.
- A slice of fresh lemon tied over the hardened skin overnight is a valuable remedy for corns.
- The application of papaya juice over the corns is also helpful.
- The milky juice of green figs is beneficial for corns of long duration.
- A paste made of chalk and water applied over the affected area is also helpful.
- A light diet containing of vitamins and minerals in the form of fruits and vegetables is recommended.

- Grate white cabbage. Add hot water so that it is comfortable to your feet. Soak it in for 10-20 minutes.
- Soak your feet in warm water for about 15 minutes. Then cut a small piece of lemon peel and place the inside of it against the corn, tying it on, and let it stay there all night. Do this for three nights and the corn should lift out.

Dandruff

- Use of fenugreek (methi) seeds is one of the most important remedies in the treatment of dandruff. Two tablespoons of these seeds are soaked overnight in water and ground into a fine paste with curds the next morning. This paste is applied all over the scalp and left for half an hour. The hair is then washed with soap nut (aritha) or 'shikakai' powder.
- The use of a teaspoon of fresh limejuice for the last rinse, while washing the hair, is another useful remedy.
- Massage hot oil mixed with cedar vinegar in hot water over the scalp. Leave it overnight and rinse off with an egg shampoo the next morning.
- Put a few drops of limejuice in coconut oil and massage your hair with it to get rid of dandruff.
- Tops and roots of beets should be boiled in water and this water should be massaged into the scalp with the fingertips every night. White beet is the best for treating dandruff.
- The use of curds kept over 2-3 days, limejuice, cider vinegar and 'amla' (Emblica officinalis) juice also helps to disperse dandruff.
- Boil a handful of willow leaves. Strain and wash your hair and scalp in it. Put a little concoction aside and dampen the scalp a little everyday.

Disseminated and Acute Eczema

- Restricted salt and light diet. In endogenous eczema and urticaria bland vegetarian diet with restricted tea, coffee and alcohol (Sattvik is helpful). It should be continued for at least 4 – 12 weeks.

Eczema

- Muskmelon should be taken three times a day for at least forty days. The juice of the fruit is also useful for local application in acute and chronic cases of eczema.

- The pulp and the skin of mango should be simmered in a cup of water for half an hour. This should then be strained and applied as a lotion to the affected areas several times daily.

- Raw vegetable juices, especially carrot juice in combination with spinach juice is helpful in the treatment of eczema.

- Safflower oil is beneficial. Two tablespoons should be taken daily.

- Two tablespoons of molasses should be taken twice daily in a glass of milk. Improvement will be noticed within two weeks time.

- The patient should take a diet consisting of seeds, nuts, grains, vegetables and fruits. He should avoid tea, coffee, alcoholic beverages, all condiments, sugar, white flour products, denatured cereals and highly flavored dishes.

- Two or three cloves of garlic if chewed daily gives prompt relief.

- The green leaves of finger millet are valuable in chronic eczema. The fresh juice of these leaves should be applied over the affected areas.

- Sunbathing early in the morning is very beneficial. A light mudpack applied over the sites of eczema is also useful. In cases of acute eczema, cold compresses or cold wet fermentations are beneficial.

- Certain liquids have been found useful as washing lotions for cleaning the affected parts. This includes water in which 'neem' (Azadirachta indica) leaves have been boiled, rice starch water, which has been obtained by decanting cooked rice.

The suggested diet for eczema is as follows

5.00 a.m.

• Juice of one lemon in a glass of warm water.

7.30 a.m.

• Fresh fruits, especially melon (musk melon) and a glass of orange juice. Plenty of water should be taken in between the meals.

9.30 a.m.

• Fresh green vegetables (salads) and a glass of carrot juice.

11.30 a.m.

• Fresh vegetables, vegetable salad, a glass of carrot juice and 'palak' (spinach) juice mixed together.

2.30 p.m.

• Fresh fruits especially musk melon, a glass of fruit juice.

4.00 p.m.

• A large glassful of juice of 'palak' (spinach) and carrots (mixed).

7.00 p.m.

• Vegetable salads and fresh fruits.

This should be followed in the first week. In the second week, salt free boiled or steamed vegetables; curd and milk, sprouted grains and wheat bread (rotis) can be added to the meals. It is essential that all these should be salt free.

In chronic cases, the diet regulation must be followed for atleast two months.

HAIR LOSS

• 'Amla' (Emblica officinalis) oil, prepared by boiling the dry pieces of 'amla' (Emblica officinalis) in coconut oil, is a valuable hair tonic for enriching hair growth.

- Lettuce is useful in preventing hair loss. A mixture of lettuce and spinach juice can help the growth of hair.

- Juice of embylic myrobalan mixed with coconut oil after boiling may be applied on the head to prevent further loss of hair.

- The juice of alfalfa in combination with equal quantities of lettuce and carrot juices will promote the hair growth to a remarkable extent.

- Mustard oil, boiled with 'heena' (Lowsoni inermis) leaves is useful for healthy growth of hair. 'Heena' (Lowsoni inermis) leaves may be boiled in mustard oil and are burnt. The oil is then filtered. A regular massage with this oil will produce abundant hair.

- The seeds of lime and black pepper ground together in fine paste help in the treatment of patchy baldness.

- Onion has been found very effective in patchy baldness. The affected parts should be rubbed with onions till it is red. It should be rubbed with honey afterwards.

- Another useful remedy for falling hair is olive oil. The procedure is to heat the oil and allow it to cool, gently massage it into the roots and leave it all night. Next morning apply egg and wash off.

- The use of white radish with salt and black pepper every noon for six months regularly will improve the skin texture and make the hair long.

HEAD LICE

- Cinnamon applied externally as a hair wash helps to get rid of hair lice.

- A non-herbal treatment to get rid of nits is to mix kerosene and water in equal parts and apply to the parts.

- Rosemary oil is also thought to be useful in the treatment of head lice.

- The betel leaf juice if applied as paste on the hair roots at night before retiring to bed kills instantaneously all lice on the head.

IMPETIGO

- The treatment of impetigo is essentially constitutional and it should consist of proper diet, correct hygiene and fresh air.
- Avoid tea, coffee, and all condiments and highly flavored dishes as well as sugar, white flour products, denatured cereals and tinned or bottled foods.
- A few chopped pieces of turnip (salgum), after through cleansing, should be immersed in rice starch (kangi) or any natural vinegar for about six hours and this should then be eaten by the patient.
- Garlic crushed and spread over the irritated areas is useful in relieving the constant itching. One or two cloves of garlic should be chewed for better results.

LEUCODERMA

- The seeds of psoralea should be steeped in a juice of ginger for three days. The fluid should be renewed every day. The husk may be removed, dried in the shade and powered. One gram of this powder should be taken every day with one cup of fresh milk for forty days. The ground seeds should be applied to the white spots.
- The patient may embark upon a well balanced diet of seeds, nuts, grains, vegetables and fruits. This diet may be supplemented with cold pressed vegetable oils, honey and yeast. The patient should avoid tea, coffee, alcoholic beverages, all condiments and sugar.
- Red clay should be mixed with ginger juice in a ratio of 1:1 and applied over the white spots once a day.
- About 35 grams of radish seeds should be powdered in two teaspoons of vinegar and applied on the white patches.

- Turmeric mixed with mustard oil is also useful in leucoderma. About 500 grams of turmeric should be pounded and soaked in 8 liters of water at night. It may be boiled in the morning till only one litre is left and mixed with 500 ml of mustard oil. This mixture should be heated till only the oil is left. The mixture should be applied to the white patches every morning and evening for a few months.

PREMATURE GRAYING OF HAIR

- Use of Indian gooseberry is a leading home remedy for the prevention of graying of hair. The fruit, cut into pieces, should be dried and boiled in coconut oil till the solid matter becomes charred dust. Application of this dark colored oil is very useful in preventing premature graying of hair.

- Amarantha (chaule) is another effective remedy for hair disorders. Application of the fresh juice of Amarantha (chaule) leaves helps the hair to retain the normal black colour.

- Liberal intake of curry leaves also helps premature graying of hair.

- The butter made from cow's milk helps preventing premature graying of hair. It may be taken orally as well as applied externally.

- A sufficient quantity of yogurt, yeast and calcium is an excellent remedy for premature graying of hair.

PRICKLY HEAT

- A liberal intake of dilute lime juice, butter milk or lassi, coconut water, beverages with sandal syrup, water flavored with 'khus' grass roots etc., are supposed to decrease overall body heat and prevent skin flare-ups due to prickly heat.

- Sandalwood paste is cooling. The dry sandalwood powder mixed with rose water can be applied over the parts where sweating is excessive.

- Grated coconut is ground well with a teaspoonful of cumin. From the ground paste the milk is extracted and applied over the whole body followed by a cold bath.

- The inside soft pulp of 'targola' (palm-fruit) when massaged on the body is also an effective cure for prickly heat.

PSORIASIS

- Bitter gourd is a valuable remedy for psoriasis. A cup of fresh juice of this vegetable, mixed with a teaspoon of limejuice, should be taken on empty stomach daily for four to six months.

- Buttermilk should be taken in ample quantities. The application of buttermilk compresses over the affected parts will also be useful in treating the condition.

- All animal fats, including milk, butter, eggs, refined or processed foods, white sugar, condiments, tea and coffee should be avoided. The patient should adopt a well balanced diet consisting of seeds, nuts, grains, vegetables and fruits.

- The thickest and greenest outer cabbage leaves are most effective. The leaves should be thoroughly washed in warm water and dried with a towel. The leaves should be flattened, softened and smoothened out by rolling them with a rolling pin after removing the thick veins. They should be warmed and then applied smoothly to the affected part in an overlapping manner. A pad of soft woolen cloth should be put over them. The whole compress should then be secured with an elastic bandage.

- Cashew nut oil can be applied beneficially over the affected area.

- The patient should take vitamin E in therapeutic doses of 400 mg a day. It will help to reduce itching and scab formation.

- Juices of citrus foods should be avoided.

- The oil of avocado (kulu naspati) should be applied gently to the affected areas.

- The oil extracted from the outer layer of cashew nut has also been found valuable in the treatment of psoriasis.

PYODERMA

- Restrict sweets, stogy, concentrated starches and mangoes etc.

RINGWORM

- An ideal cure for ringworm is to apply carbonate of soda and strong vinegar on the affected area.

- Another remedy involves cutting the hair from the affected area and rubbing in turpentine. Finally the affected area is washed off with carbolic soap.

- An all fruit diet should be taken for the first 3-4 days. One should take fresh juicy fruits like apple, orange, papaya, pineapple and pomegranate during this period. Fruits, salt free, raw or steamed vegetables accompanied with whole-wheat chapattis may be taken after the all fruit diet. After a few days curds and milk may be added to the diet.

- Wash the skin thoroughly with hot water. Then apply a paste made from mustard seeds over the affected areas. This has proved to be very effective.

- A few slices of raw papaya should be rubbed on the ringworm patches twice daily. A paste made from dry seeds of papaya can also be applied beneficially on the ringworm patches.

- Castor oil rubbed liberally on the scalp is a valuable remedy for ringworm of the head. Noticeable improvement will take place within 2-3 days.

- Carrot juice (150 ml) and spinach juice (100 ml) in combination has proved beneficial.

SCABIES

- The oldest and the most effective of the treatment is the application of a paste, prepared by mixing two teaspoons of sublimed Sulphur with eight tablespoons of coconut oil. The whole body should be soaked for 20 minutes in a warm-bath using plenty of soap. Particular attention should be paid to the itching areas, scrubbing them thoroughly. After the bath, the Sulphur paste should be rubbed well over the entire skin surface, below the chin line, but particularly over the involved areas. This should be done for three successive nights, wearing the same underclothing during this period. About 10 or 12 hour's after the last application, a hot soap bath should be taken and a clean underclothing should be worn.

- Fresh juice of apricot leaves should be extracted and applied with beneficial results.

- Application of the juice of mint over the affected areas has also proved valuable.

- The flour of unroasted Bengal gram is a very effective cleansing agent.

WARTS

- Castor oil should be applied generously over the parts every night. The treatment should be continued for several months.

- Milky juice of figs (angeer), extracted from the fresh, barely ripe fruits, should be applied on the warts several times a day, for two weeks.

- Raw potato should be cut and rubbed on the affected areas several times daily for at least two weeks.

- The juice of the herb marigold (saldbarh) applied over the warts has shown beneficial results. The sap from the stem is also effective in the removal of the warts.

WHITLOW

- The finger should be lightly bandaged with a cloth soaked in milk cream. Continuously wetting the bandaged cloth with a little milk cream once in a few hours will completely dry up the infection.

- Thoroughly mix castor oil in limewater to get a thick emulsion. A complete cure is usual after a few applications of this emulsion on the inflamed finger.

- For early whitlow continuous wetting with the juice of onion is another home remedy.

- Apply a paste of betel leaf with a small pinch of quick lime on the inflamed finger and tie it up with a cloth. Take care not to wet the finger.

Chapter-12

Dermatoses Caused Due to Physical Agents

DERMATOSIS DUE TO MECHANICAL INJURIES TO THE SKIN

CALLUS & CALLOSITIES

Definition

In both the conditions there is a circumscribed hyperkeratosis of the skin due to repeated friction (resulting in callosity) or/and frequent intermittent pressure on the part (resulting in callus).

Etiology & Incidence

It is seen most often in people wearing ill-fitting shoes, or in those having orthopedic problems of the foot or in those habitually sitting with their foot tucked under their body or in those involved in certain kinds of sports or occupations.

Calluses on the edges of the weight-bearing area of the sole are often due to shoes that are too loose.

Callosities can also result from clothing, e.g. in those wearing trusses or in nuns wearing head-dresses that press on the rim of the auricle. It is also seen in cases of an anatomical abnormality of the varus or valgus position of the heel, resulting in excessive loads applied to the plantar skin, where the callosities occur.

Also, recently, studies have revealed an autosomal dominant inherited disposition to formation of callosities.

Pathology

There is epidermal hyperplasia, with thickening of the stratum corneum, and occasional parakeratosis over the dermal papillae and expansion of the granular layer. The underlying dermis may show an increase in dermal collagen and fibrosis around neurovascular bundles.

Clinical Features

There is a diffuse area of hyperkeratosis of a waxy color, and an almost even thickness, affecting the palms and soles, especially over (the skin overlying the metacarpo-phalangeal joints) or under the bony protuberances of the joints (the metatarsal heads being the most frequently affected).

It tends to disappear gradually over a period of time, when the pressure is removed.

Trusses, especially if ill-fitting, may cause circumscribed patches of hyperkeratosis and pigmentation. The head-dresses of nuns pressing on the rim of the auricle sometimes cause a callosity, with inflammatory changes in the underlying cartilage. Pressure from calipers or reinforced shoes may cause calluses in the disabled.

Differential Diagnosis

- It differs from a corn since it has no central core and has a more diffuse thickening of the skin.
- Granuloma annulare occasionally resembles callosity, but can be distinguished by biopsy.
- Various forms of keratoderma can resemble callosities, but these do not occur selectively over sites of excessive compression, and so are easily differentiated.

Treatment

- Padding should be done to relieve the pressure.
- Paring of the thickened callus can be done in a few obstinate cases.

CORNS

Synonym

Clavus; Heloma (In Greek, 'helus' is a stone wedge).

Definition

A corn is a sharply demarcated, circumscribed, horny, conical thickening occuring over a bony prominence, especially on the hands or the feet. Its base can be felt on the surface of the skin and its apex points inward and presses on subjacent structures, causing pain.

Etiology

They can arise out of a bony deformity (like bony prominences, a prominent condylar projection, malunion of a fracture, a short first metatarsal, or a toe deformity) or due to wearing ill-fitting or high-heeled shoes.

The soft corn usually occurs when tight shoes press the condyle of a metatarsal or phalanx against the base of a phalanx on the adjacent toe.

Pathology

Here there is a thick parakeratotic plug set in a cup-shaped depression of the epidermis, usually with loss of the granular cell layer.

Types

- Hard corns, which occur on the dorsal surfaces of the toes or on the soles. Its surface is shiny and polished, and when the upper layers are shaved off, a core is noted in the thickest part of the lesion. This is the part that causes the dull boring or sharp lancinating pain due to pressure on the underlying sensory nerves.

- Soft corns occur between the toes and are softened by the macerating action of sweat.

Clinical Features

A corn is smaller, usually very painful, and may have a glassy centre. They can occur within an area of callus, and are seen especially at sites of friction or pressure, and when these causative factors are removed, they may spontaneously disappear. Frequently a bony spur or exostosis is present beneath both hard and soft corns of long duration, and unless this exostosis is removed cure is unlikely.

The most frequent site where the hard corns occur is over the metatarsal heads and the interphalangeal joints and tips of the toe, although the sides of the arches and heel can be involved.

The soft interdigital corn usually occurs between the fourth and fifth toes, and is typically very painful, and it becomes soft, soggy, and macerated due to perspiration and so it appears white. Exostosis in the soft corn is seen usually at the metatarsal-phalangeal joint, causing pressure on the adjacent toe. A small sinus may be present in a few cases, and secondary bacterial infection can then present as cellulitis.

Diagnosis

Besides clinical examination, diagnosis is established after checking on what shoes the patient wears regularly. Also check for any orthoses, palpate for bony prominences, and examine the gait and alignment of the feet. Pressure studies (pedobarographs) can be helpful in evaluating foot biomechanics.

Differential Diagnosis

- Plantar corns must be differentiated from viral warts, especially when the latter has a zone of reactive hyperkeratosis around it. Corns are generally more painful when pressed vertical to the skin surface, whereas warts are tender when squeezed laterally between the finger and thumb. Paring off the surface keratin of the lesion will reveal either the pathognomonic elongated dermal papillae of the wart with its blood vessels, or the clear horny core of the corn.

- Parakeratosis plantaris discreta is a sharply marginated, cone-shaped, rubbery lesion that commonly occurs beneath the metatarsal heads. Multiple lesions may occur, and is a painful condition seen more frequently in women.

- Keratosis punctata of the palmar creases may be seen in the creases of the digits of the feet where it may be mistaken for a corn.

Treatment

- Wearing the right kind of footwear, addition of metatarsal pads and inlays, and other such appropriate corrective steps should be taken.

- Soak the feet in hot water and par the surface with the help of a pumice stone. For soft corns, the use of a toe separator (felt, foam, or silicone) can provide rapid relief.

FRICTION BLISTERS

In this condition there is the formation of vesicles or bullae at sites of pressure and frequent friction, and it is made worse by heat and moisture. The frictional force and the number of times an object moves across the skin determine the likelihood of blister development.

For friction blisters to occur, the stratum corneum must be strong enough not to be rubbed away. It is thus more frequently seen on the palm, sole, heel, or dorsum of the fingers, where the skin is thick. The size of the bulla depends on the site of the trauma.

HOMEOPATHIC APPROACH FOR CORNS AND CALLUSES

The first step in the treatment of corns and calluses requires removal of the source of chronic trauma, for instance, ill-fitting shoes can be discarded, and arch supports can be inserted where necessary and metatarsal bars can be added to the sole of shoes.

On rare occasions orthopedic procedures are required in order to repair underlying bony abnormalities. Surgical excision of corns and calluses is to be avoided since it does not get at the cause of the disease and the resultant scarring may only complicate it.

Introduction

Corns arise not only from tight fitting footwear and deformities of bony arch of foot but also from a certain disposition with some persons, who have tendency to develop recurrent corns.

Here I would like to stress that even though the cause is external, it is only the judicious use of internal remedy, which will cure the case permanently.

Causation

Since the most important cause of the corn is tight fitting footwear, patients should be advised to wear comfortable footwear preferably a sandal. Also wearing of narrow pointed shoes is strictly prohibited.

Foot deformities must be corrected by exercise advised by orthopedic surgeon or by expert physiotherapist.

The following points should be noted for case taking

Causation

Wearing tight shoes with repeated shoe bite (Arn, All-c, Paeonia)

Previous treatment

It is essential to know whether the patient had attempted to cauterize the corn or callosity with the help of following:

- Acetic acid.
- Caustic potash.
- Fluoric acid.
- Silver nitrate.
- Burning with help of incense stick (agarbatti).
- Manual removal of corns with the help of pedicurist or surgeon (Arn.).

Location

Palms or soles.

Characteristic

Flat, soft, or hard.

Whether corns are associated

- With or without inflammation.
- With or without itching.
- With or without bleeding.
- With or without suppuration.
- Tender or non tender.

Important characteristic sensation should always be inquired, e.g.,

- Burning.
- Pulsating.
- Stinging.
- Stitching.

This is very important when the corn is isolated.

It is strongly advised not to recommend any local application for treatment of corns. For example:

- Application of lime.
- Application of homeopathic mother tincture.
- Application of allopathic tubes or bandages.

Instead bathing the feet in warm water and applying Arnica ointment may obtain relief.

Treatment Review

As clearly demonstrated pathologically, corns represents a conical, painful, hyperkeratosis appearing on the soles and over the toe joints. Because of body's weight and shoes, hyperkeratosis of a corn gets pushed into the skin causing a pressure on nerve ending which produces pain. This clearly demonstrates a dominant sycotic maism with a mechanical exciting cause example trauma due to tight footwear; hence the drug selected should preferably have a sycotic base and also should act on the nerve ending.

Patients usually consult us for

- Painful tender corns, or
- Recurrence.

Some Important Homeopathic Remedies

Pimpinella saxifraga, sempervivum tectorum and Wiesbeden aqua are some of the rare remedies that have been very useful to me in the treatment of corns. For corns on the toes, I have found Adrenalinum and Lac vaccinum defloratum very useful.

ACUTE PAINFUL CORNS

Agaricus muscaris: Painful corns, burning, sore and stinging.

Antimonium crudum: Corns inflamed, large, and heavy; placed on sides close to the toes. Thickened skin of the soles and feet. Inflamed corn with great sensitiveness of soles on walking painful when touched. Aching, stitching pains in corns on soles and balls of toes. Fine pricking in soles < walking on stone pavement.

Arnica montana: Corns on heels and toes. Sensitive and sore. Very painful, stinging, stitching, smarting and tearing pain.

Borax veneta: Inflamed painful corns with burning and stinging especially in wet weather.

Bovista lycoperdon: Corns are painful, pressing, sore, stinging and shooting pains.

Bryonia alba: Slightest touch pains very severely, smarting, burning, sore, stinging, tearing pains. Soles sore with lameness and every spot is painful on pressure.

Camphora officinalis: Corns with skin parchment like sore, painful corns which are very sensitive. Soreness especially in toe joints and corns.

Carbo animalis: Numerous corns appear and become very painful to touch. Sensitive corns with stinging pains.

Hepar sulphur: Inflamed corns, pricking and sticking in affected parts. Great sensitiveness to slightest touch.

Ignatia amara: Corns painful as is sore. Stinging, tearing and burning in soles and joints of toes.

Ranunculus bulbosus: Corns are sensitive to touch, and tend to smart and burn. Hard excrescences. Horny skin.

Ranunculus scleratus: Acute painful corns on ball of 1st and 2nd left toes/ right big toe. Sensitive to touch and pressure smart and burn; very painful when letting leg hang down, they also throb and especially painful by flexing toes. Better by extending toes and wearing thick-soled boot. Numbness in corns. Knocking toes against any things so are to cause boot to grate against corns, causes great pain and burning.

Silicea terra: Inflamed corns with stitching and burning pains, soreness of soles. Stitches in the corns, jerking up the feet. Sore, stinging, tearing, pressing pains in inflamed corns. Icy coldness and sweaty feet.

Sulphur: Corns and callosities caused from pressure. If a shoe presses anywhere on the skin, a great corn on bunion develops. Burning, aching, tearing and stitching pain in inflamed corns. Aggravation by warmth of bed.

Thuja occidentalis: Suppurating corns with sore, tearing, stinging and burning pains.

RECURRENT CORNS

Ferrum picricum: Corns with yellow discoloration. Multiple corns, which are very painful.

Graphites: Rough, hard, dry, unhealthy skin. Burning, pressing, sore, stinging pain in the corns on toes. Corns with deep cracks.

Lycopodium clavatum: Corns are very sensitive with tearing pain. Skin becomes thick and indurated. Inflammation with stitching and soreness. Painful callosities on the soles; toes and fingers contracted.

Natrium muriaticum: Boring, tearing and stitching pains, < walking and standing.

Phosphorus: Corns bleed, they heal and break out again. Boring pains with aching. Stinging on walking. Corns on toes.

Sulphur: Corns and callosities from pressure. Desquamation, exfoliation of skin after local medication. Burning, aching, tearing and stitching pain.

REPERTORY

Acet-ac, agar, alum-p, am-c, anac-oc, ant-c, arn, bar-c, borx, bry, calc, calc-caust, calc-s, calc-sil, carb-an, caust, cench, chin, chin-b, coloc, cur, elae, ferr-pic, graph, hep, hydr, hyper, ign, kali-ar, lyc, lyss, med, nat-c, nat- m, nit-ac, nux-v, petr, ph-ac, phos, pimp, plb, psor, rad, ran-b, ran-s, rhod, rhus-t, rumx, sal-ac, sang, sars, sep, sil, staph, sul-ac, sulph, symph, ter, wies, thuj.

Corns and Callosities

- **Aching:** ant-c, lyc, sep, sil, sul-ac, sulph.
- **Boring:** borx, calc, caust, hep, kali-c, nat-c, nat-m, phos, puls, ran-s, rhod, sep, sil, spig, thuj.
- **Burning:** agar, alum, am-c, ant-c, arg-met, bar-c, bar-s, borx, bry, calc, calc-s, carb-v, caust, cench, graph, hep, ign, lith-c, lyc, mag-s, meph, nat-c, nat-m, nit-ac, nux-v, petr, ph-ac, phos, puls, ran-b, ran-s, rhus-t, sang, sep, sil, spig, staph, sulph, thuj.
- **Cracks deep:** cist, graph.
- **Drawing:** lyc, nat-c, sep.
- **Formation** of, tendency to: lyc, sil.
- **Hanging down** off: ran-s.
- **Horny:** ant-c, graph, ran-b, sulph.
- **Inflamed:** ant-c, borx, hep, calc, lyc, nit-ac, phos, puls, sil, sep, staph, sulph, rhus-t.
- **Jerking:** anac, cocc, dros, mag-m, nux-v, phos, puls, rhus-t, sep, sul-ac, sulph.
- **Numbness:** ran-s.
- **Painful:** agar, alum, alum-p, ambr, ant-c, arn, asc-t, aster, bar-c, bar-s, bov, bry, calad, calc, calc-s, caust, cench, chin-b, hep, ign, iod, kali-ars, kali-c, lach, lith-c, lyc, lyss, mag-m, med, meph, nat-c, nat-m, nit-ac, nux v, phos, puls, ran-b, ran-s, rhus-t, sep, sil, spig, sul-i, sulph.
- **Pinching:** bar-c
- **Pressing:** agar, anac, ant-c, arg-met, bov, bry, calc, calc-s, carb-v, caust, graph, ign, iod, lyc, ph-ac, phos, sep, sil, staph sulph, ruta, verat.
- **Pulsating:** calc, kali-c, lyc, sep, sil, sulph.
- **Pressure,** slight, from: ant-c.
- **Senstive, sore:** aesc, agar, ambr, am-c, ant-c, arn, bar-c, bar-s, bov, bry, bufo, calc, calc-s, calc-sil, camph, carb-an, fl-ac, graph, hep, ign, kali-c, lith-c, lyc, mag-s, med, nat-c, nat-m, nat-p, nit-ac nux-v, petr, phos, puls, ran-b, ran-s, rhus-t, sep, sil, spig, staph, sul-ac, sulph, thuj, verat.

- **Shooting:** alum, am-c, arn, bov, bry, calc, caust, cocc, hep, ign, kali-c, lyc, nat- m, nat-c, nux-v, rhus-t, sep, sil, sul-ac, sulph.
- **Smarting, soreness:** agar, ambr, ant-c, bry, arn, calc, camph, caust, fl-ac, graph, hep, ign, kali-c, lyc, mag-s, nat-m, nux-v, phos, ph-ac, puls, rhus-t, sep, sil, staph, sul-ac, verat.
- **Sticking, Stitching, Stinging:** agar, alum, alum-p, ant-c, am-c, arn, arum-t, ars, bar-c, bar-s, borx, bov, bry, calad, calc, calc-s, calc-sil, carb-an, carb-ac, carb-v, caust, cocc, graph, hep, ign, kali-c, lyc, mag-m, mag-s, nat-c, nat-m, nat-p, nit-ac, petr, ph-ac, phos, ptel, puls, ran-b, ran-s, rhod, rhus-t, rumx, sep, sel, sil, spig, staph, sul-ac, sulph, thuj, verat.
- - Night: ars, nat-m, sulph.
- - Walking: phos.
- - Weather, in rainy: borx.
- - Sitting, while: verat.
- - Suppurating: thuj.
- **Tearing:** am-c, arn, ars, bry, calc, cals-s, cocc, kali-c, lyc, mag-m, sep, sil, sul-ac, sulph, thuj.
- **Tender:** med.
- **Throbbing:** calc-c, kali-c, lyc, sep, sil, sulph.
- **Weather,** during rainy: borx.

Skin, hard

- **Callosities, like:** am-c, ant-c, bar-c, borx, dulc, fl-ac, graph, lach, led, lyc, ran-b, rhus-t, sep, sil, sulph, thuj.
- **Parchment, like:** acon, aeth, ars, camph, chin, cop, crot-h, dig, dulc, kali-c, led, lith-c, lyc, mag-c, op, phos, rhus-t, sars, sil, squil.
- **Desquamating,** Peeling off: am-c, ant-c, borx, dulc, graph, lach, ran-b, rhus-t, sep, sil, sulph.
- **Thickening,** with: alum, am-c, anac, ant-c, ars, borx, calc, choc, cic, clem, dulc, graph, hydr-ac, kali-c, lach, lyc, par, phos, psor, ran-b, rhus-t, sep, sil, sulph, thiosin, thuj, verat.

Location

- **Upper Limbs:** ant-c, borx, calc-f, graph, merc-i-r, nat-m, sil, sulph, thuj.
- **Hands:** phos.
- **Horny, on hands:** am-c, graph, kali-ar, rhus-t, sil, sulph.
- - With deep cracks: cist, graph.
- **Feet:** ant-c, bar-c, calc, caust, graph, lyc, ran-b, rhus-t, sep, sil, sulph.
- - Balls of: ant-c.
- - Skin thickened at edges: lac-d.
- **Soles:** ant-c, ars, bar-c, calc, lyc, plb, sil, sulph, tub.
- - Large horny places, close to toes: ant-c.
- - Tender: alum, bar-c, lyc, med, nat-s, sil.
- **Heels:** arn, lyc, phos.
- **Toes:** acet-ac, anac, ant-c, arn, chin-b, coloc, graph, nat-m, nux-v, phos, ran-s, ter.
- - Left toe, violent pains: aster.
- - Right little toe (on), violent burning preventing sleep after dinner: graph.
- - Between 2nd and 3rd of left toe: psor.
- - Burning alternating right and left: aphis.
- - Nervous debility, with: cur.
- - Numbness, with: ran-s.
- - Shooting: bov.
- - Smarting: ran-b.
- - Sore pain in lung disease: graph.
- - Soreness: calc, camph, fl-ac, lith-c, nux-v, rhus-t.
- - Sticking: calad.
- - Stitching jerking up feet: sil.
- - Tender: med.
- - Tenderness more in left little toe, had to remove shoe: chinin-ar.
- - Touch, sensitive to: ran-b.

PRESSURE ULCER

Synonym

Decubitus ulcer, bedsore, pressure sore.

Definition & Etiology

This condition presents as a localized area of tissue damage, resulting either from direct and prolonged pressure on the skin causing ischaemia of the underlying structures (of the skin, fat, and muscles), or from shearing forces causing mechanical stress to the tissues (shearing forces are exerted when the head of the bed is raised on a patient who is lying supine, resulting in damage of the blood vessels in fat and fascia due to the gravitational force), or due to both causes occuring simultaneously.

Pathology

In the initial stages, there is erythema, with dilatation of the superficial dermal venules and papillary capillaries, a mild perivascular inflammatory infiltrate and degenerative changes in occasional sweat coils and ducts. There is formation of platelet thrombi in many of the superficial vessels with extravasation of red cells. There is a resultant degeneration of the eccrine glands, with evident fat necrosis.

Then there is epidermal atrophy, subepidermal blister formation, tissue eosinophilia, intra and extravascular fibrin and necrosis of hair follicles.

Then there is the formation of ulceration, with loss of the epidermal layer first, and then a full-thickness destruction of the skin. In a chronic case of ulcer, there is fibrosis with isolated collections of capillaries and no residual appendages.

Clinical Features

It tends to occur especially in the chronically debilitated persons who are unable to change their position in bed. The bony prominences of the body are the most frequently affected sites. Nearly all pressure ulcers develop over one of the following sites sacral bone, greater trochanter, ischial tuberosity, tuberosity of the calcaneus, lateral malleolus and point of the shoulder.

It usually begins with erythema at the pressure point, sometimes accompanied by induration, temperature elevation and pain. The erythema at this stage is reversible when the pressure is relieved. Repeated pressure may result in brownish discoloration due to extravasation of red blood cells and deposition of haemosiderin. Then there is a blister formation and/or minor ulceration.

In a short time there is formation of a 'punched-out' ulcer at the site. Necrosis of the part with a grayish pseudomembrane is seen in the ulcer, especially if is left untreated. Then gradually there is a deeper degree of damage, involving the subcutaneous tissues, producing a thick black eschar. Removal of this necrotic tissue may reveal tendons, ligaments and muscle. In such patients, there is a high risk of septicaemia and other systemic complications, such as renal and amyloid disease.

Then there is deep fistula formation due to resultant osteomyelitis.

Complications

Potential complications of pressure ulcers include sepsis, local infection, osteomyelitis, pyoarthrosis, fistulas, anemia, electrolyte imbalance and squamous cell carcinoma.

Treatment

- The aim is to relieve the pressure on the affected parts by frequent change of position, meticulous nursing care (especially in a prone position), and the use of specialized pressure-relieving beds, mattresses and cushions, air-filled products, liquid-filled flotation devices or foam products.
- Other measures include ulcer care, managing bacterial

colonization and infection, operative repair if necessary, continual education, ensuring adequate nutrition, managing pain, and providing psychosocial support.

- Wounds should be cleaned initially and at each dressing change by a nontraumatic technique. Selection of a dressing should ensure that the ulcer tissue remains moist and the surrounding skin dry.

- Nutrition should receive special attention and a positive nitrogen balance achieved. For those with poor appetite, or unable to take sufficient solid food by mouth, frequent sip feeds of protein supplement or, occasionally, nasogastric tubal feeding may be required. Anemia, zinc and ascorbic acid deficiency must be corrected.

- Any serious underlying disease should be assessed and treated appropriately.

- The blood urea and serum albumin should be checked regularly.

HOMEOPATHIC APPROACH
FOR BEDSORES

Bedsore is a very troublesome affair. It usually occurs in old people who are bed ridden for days together and are lying in one position for a long time and also have a reduced immune status, e.g. old people suffering from paralysis, prolonged bed rest due to fracture of bones of lower extremities.

Examination of bedsore is a very important aspect for prescribing the correct homeopathic medicine. Examine the location of the sore, its margins, edges and base. Look out for any discharge and if present its type. Inquire from the patient regarding the type of pain and its modalities and any other accompanying symptoms.

For successful management of bedsores careful nursing and dressing care are very important. The bed should always be kept dry. Water bed or air bed is advisable. Regular cleaning of the wound and dressing with Calendula and Echinacea ointments is very helpful for faster healing. Allopathic physicians prescribe a lot of ointments which are many times also prescribed by homeopaths. But this only retards the cure, a correctly indicated and potentized homeopathic remedy will cure the bed sore must faster.

The most important homeopathic remedy that I have used so far is Arnica montana.

SOME IMPORTANT HOMEOPATHIC REMEDIES FOR BEDSORES AND PRESSURE SORES

Alcoholus: Skin appears smutty or yellowish-gray, soft and flabby. Skin becomes dry and hard. Tormenting eruption, exceedingly itching, rough, scaly patches. Skin does not heal readily. Large indolent, blue-looking bed sores. Varicose ulcers. In bed sore, saturate a cloth and apply locally.

Allium cepa: Very good remedy for ulcers or sores due to shoe bites or constant pressure. The ulcer or shoe bite is very close to the nails with inflammation of the surrounding lymphatics. Burning, stitching and sore pains. Ulcer is very sensitive to touch and painful on pressure and better by exposure to cold air. Left sided affection.

Aristolochia clematitis: Bed sore around the right hip. It is a good antiseptic remedy like Echinacea. Poorly healing wounds, infected wounds. Blisters from friction.

Arnica montana: Sore lame bruised feeling all over the body and especially on the bedsore. Bed feels too hard, toss about to find a soft spot. Skin- cracked, dry, excoriated. Dirty looking skin, inflamed and indurated. Sore is painful to touch, bruised, smarting and stinging. Easy suppuration. The areola is usually the painful and inflamed part. Foreign bodies within the bedsores can be easily emitted (Hep-s., Lob., Sil). Local lymph nodes are enlarged. Bedsores develop very rapidly. Petechial hemorrhages and ecchymosis present along with the bedsores. Mentally the patient develops indifference to everything, sleeps while answering the question. Stuporous condition in later stage.

Arsenicum album: Debilitated, prostrated, exhausted and chilly patients. Bedsore is extremely painful especially burning, shooting and smarting pains. Burning pain in the bedsore > warm applications. Proud flesh in bedsore (Sep., Sil.). Phagadenic ulcers, surrounded by pimplês. Inflamed and indurated bedsore turning gangrenous. Very foul odor. Discharge bloody, copious, offensive, ichorous; sometimes with maggots (Merc., Sabad., Sil., Sulph.). Ulcer appears black with burning around the margins on touch. Septic state with cellulitis. Itching around the ulcer which is > warm application; scratches until bleeds.

Baptisia tinctoria: Bed sore associated with typhoid fever. Foul odor from body. Dark spots appear on body. Intermittent pulse.

Borax veneta: Very good remedy for pressure sores and shoe bites (All-c.). Burning, sore pain. Ulcers towards the heel with foul smelling discharges. Sores associated with stomatitis. The pains are worse in evening.

Carbo vegetabilis: Bed sore has a bluish areola, bleeds easily on touch, turns gangrenous and has a burning pain on touch, but can occasionally be painless. Worse by warmth in any form. Skin appears blackish, bluish or mottled. Ecchymosis all over the body. Discharges are scanty, offensive and corrosive (Ars. – copious discharge). Bed sores are superficial with lot of proud flesh. Perspiration has a very offensive odor. Want open air or draft of air. Sluggish dull more useful in old people. Bed sore resembles that of Lachesis. The patient feels extremely weak like Arsenicum alb., but not restless as Arsenicum alb.

Carbolicum acidum: Bed sores due to neurological problems. Rapid formation of bed sores. Itching vesicles around the bed sores with extreme burning pains. Discharges are offensive and burning. Marked weakness associated with any condition. Malignant and septic conditions.

Chamomilla: Bed sores in children (Med., Rhus-t., Sep.,

Sulph.). Ulcers extremely painful and sensitive, better by cold applications. Burning, smarting, stinging, stitching pains worse at night. Discharges are corrosive and gelatinous. Suppurative tendency. Patient is oversensitive to all external impressions.

Comocladia dentata: Affection of sacro-iliac region. Throbbing pains in the bedsore worse by heat, night and better in open air. Bedsore with red discoloration and surrounded by pimples. Deep ulcers with hard edges. Discharges are offensive, bloody and green. Erysipelatous inflammation around the bedsore. Red stripes on the affected skin. Bedsore accompanied with swollen face and projecting eyes. Mentally patient becomes dull and indifferent with sleepiness.

Crotalus horridus: Degeneration of blood. Bed sores due to neurological problem. Bed sore near the hips. Extremely painful with soreness. Wounds have a tendency to heal slowly.

Echinacea angustifolia: Locally used for dressing in the ratio of 2:8, i.e. 2 drops of the mother tincture mixed with 8 drops of Normal Saline. Patient gives an H /O injury in form of blows, falls. Sore, bruised feeling. Excessive suppuration and inflammation of the affected part. Septic condition with excessive suppurative process all over body. Blackness of external parts. Wound may appear bluish. Emaciated patients with low grade septicemia. Frequent pulse. Mentally confused, dull, stupefaction and slow. Mental exertion aggravates the patient.

Fluoricum acidum: Bed sores on parts which does not sweat. Deep ulcers extending to the bones. Necrosis of the skin and deeper structures. Painful varicose veins. Hard, horny skin and eruptions (Ant-c., Graph.) around the bed sore. Bedsores worse by warmth in any form and better by cold applications and open air. Itching around the bed sores. Red edges with vesicles. Extreme burning pains, feels as if vapors were being emitted from pores. Patient has a tendency to uncover feet at night in bed (Med., Puls., Sulph.).

Hydrastis canadensis: Hydrastis is especially active in old, easily-tired people, cachectic individuals, with great debility, emaciation and prostration. Especially indicated in cancer and cancerous states. There is a general tendency to profuse perspiration and unhealthy skin. Bedsores around ankles. There is a network of blood vessels around the bedsore. The ulcers can be deep or superficial, have a shining base, but are extremely painful with burning and stinging pains and bleed on touch. The ulcers are elevated with indurated margins. Phagadenic ulcers with proud flesh. The discharge from the ulcer is thick, yellowish, ropy and offensive. The patient feels worse by any kind of warmth and washing. Patient moans with the pain. Tongue white, swollen, large, flabby, slimy; shows imprint of teeth (Merc.); as if scalded; stomatitis. Ulceration of tongue, fissures toward the edges. Concomitantly patient has a torpid and tender liver and can also have bronchitis with characteristic expectoration. Mentally the patient is depressed; sure of death, and desires it.

Insulinum: Bed sores in diabetic patients. Associated with enlarged liver and dyspepsia.

Lachesis mutus: Bed sores around sacrum and hips. Varicose veins are usually seen around the affected parts. Bed sores have bluish areola, dirty base and fetid odor. They may look gangrenous. There is burning when touched, worse night, more around margins. Wound appears quite deep with gnawing pain. Pimples around bed sore. Skin appears blue and mottled. Bed sores are extremely sensitive to touch and pressure, cannot tolerate even touch of clothes around the bed sore. Bed sore with black edges. Tendency to severe suppuration and septicemic condition. Wounds have a tendency to heal very slowly and sometimes they heal and open up again. Hemorrhages are dark and black. Patients have a flushed face and left sided affections.

Muriaticum acidum: Bed sores and ulcers occur easily especially of mucous membranes. They are extremely sensitive usually suppurate and have very offensive discharges. Skin is extremely cold and ulcers may appear black. Patients do not like the bed sore to be cleaned and dressed due to sensitivity. Bed sore with typhoid fever. Generalized weakness accompanies all diseases;

patient slips to foot end of bed. Patient has a fetid breath, dry tongue, feeble pulse, watery diarrhea and edema around ankles. Marked aversion to open air. Septicemic condition.

Nitricum acidum: Bed sores around the toes. They bleed very easily on touch. Dirty looking deep ulcers with dirty thin, brownish, watery discharge. Stinging pains in the bed sores. Extremely painful and sensitive to touch (Hep.). Bed sores look extremely unhealthy. Patient is chilly and is worse by draft of cold air. Lean, thin people with marked sensation of weakness.

Nux moschata: Bed sores accompanied with extreme dryness and coldness of skin; skin has an inability to perspire. Skin has a mottled appearance with bluish spots. Ulcers have a foul and offensive discharge and they bleed freely.

Paeonia officinalis: Tendency to develop bed sores. Chronic bed sores on the lower parts of the body. Ulcers below coccyx and around sacrum. Very sensitive and painful ulcers accompanied with itching and worse in open air.

Plumbum metallicum: Bed sores develop due to neurological problems. Skin appears wrinkled, shriveled and drawn over the bones. Wounds turn gangrenous. Small wounds get easily inflamed and suppurate. Dry, burning ulcers. Anesthesia or hyperesthesia of the affected parts.

Pyrogenium: Skin appears blue, cold and moist. Burning pains especially around the bed sores. Indolent ulcers. Septicemic condition. Soreness of the body, bed feels too hard. Tingling in the right little toe as if frost bite.

BUNIONS

Patients suffering from bunions come to a physician only when they are inflamed and painful, as bunions are painless. It is always important to remember that the patient's habit of sitting should be changed because it is the pressure and friction, which is the important cause. If there is any associated bone deformity it has to be corrected surgically.

It is very essential to inquire about sitting habits of the patient and the type of footwear.

HOMEOPATHIC APPROACH OF BUNION

It is a circumscribed swelling consisting of a callus covering a fibromatous growth. A bunion is nature's protection against constant pressure and friction.

Sites: Metatarso-phalangeal joint – first and fifth and in deformed feet that have been confined to ill-fitting shoes. They look ugly, but are generally painless.

Some Important Homeopathic Remedies for Bunions

Agaricus muscarius: Bunions are extremely sensitive and painful. Burning itching and redness < winter, and draft of air. Bunion is prone to develop ulcer. Sensation in the bunion is as if pierced by needles of ice.

Benzoicum acidum: Great toe is affected. Bunion of the affected part due to constant friction, burning sensation < open air and cold, > heat. Uric acid diathesis. Pain in bunion alternates with urinary symptoms.

Graphites: Rough horny, dry bunion. Foul odor, which comes out with bunion sensation < heat. Bleeding and cracking with thin, gluey, offensive discharge.

Paeonia officinalis: Extremely sensitive (touch, pressure, friction). Shooting and splitting type of pain is there in bunions.

REPERTORY

Agar, am-c, benz-ac, graph, hyper, kali-chl, kali-i, kali-n, paeon, ph-ac, phos, plb, rhod, sil, sulph, verat, zinc.

–**Excruciating, painful:** hyper.

- **Frost bite, after:** calc.

- **Soles:** calc.

- **Toe, big, on:** agar, benz-ac, borx, hyper, iod, kali-i, rhod, sang, sars, sil, verat-v.

- **Little toe and ball of foot on, with stinging pain on walking:** zinc.

CRACKS IN SKIN

It is seen mostly on hands and feet in dry weather, particularly in the dry cold of the Indian winter, which dries up the integument, roughens and cracks it because of its diminished elasticity. If the cracking is severe, fissures may be produced. The hands are further predisposed to cracking by poor general health, avitaminosis and frequent washing with soap and water. Cracking itself is uncomfortable; besides it predisposes to secondary infection and pyoderma.

TREATMENT

1.   Lubricating the parts with Nivea cream or pure fat (ghee). These soften the integument and help it to retain moisture.
2.   Avoiding frequent washing with soap water.
3.   Improving general health.
4.   Protection from dry climate by proper clothing, gloves, air conditioning, etc.

HOMEOPATHIC APPROACH TO CRACKS, CHAPS, FISSURES AND RHAGADES

It is essential on the part of a homeopath to inquire in detail about the general health of the patient, as avitaminosis and poor general health predisposes the person to develop cracking. Also since cracks are prone to secondary infection and so patient's general condition should always be taken care of.

Too frequent washing of hands with soap and water should be prevented. The affected parts should be kept moist by applying a mixture of half ounce of calendula extract in one and half ounce of olive oil to be applied three to four times a day.

Tendency to develop cracks indicates dominant syphilitic maism. For repertorial reference rubrics like fissures, rhagades, chaps, cuts, cracks, etc. should be used.

Some Important Homeopathic Remedies

Alumina: Dry, rough, cracked skin. Chapped and dry, tettery skin, which itches or becomes moist especially in the evening. Symptoms recur periodically at every new or full moon. Intolerable itching when getting warm in bed, must scratch till it bleeds; then becomes painful; cracks, especially in winter. Developments of cracks are caused especially after frequent washing of skin.

Anthracokali: Chronic cracks, mainly found on nostrils, hands and feet. Cracks are prone to ulcerations, itching < at night.

Arsenicum sulphuratum flavum: Dry, cracked, itching > steam or hot water.

Baryta carbonica: Hot and dry. Itching, pricking and burning in the cracks, which is not better by scratching or rubbing. In fact, scratching can < the problem. The cracks do not heal readily. Associated with cracks are cold, foul perspiration and multiple warts on the skin.

Cactus grandiflorus: Dry, scaly skin with much itching < evening > rest. The affected part is icy cold to touch.

Calcarea carbonica: Cracks < washing, < by winter. Cold spots on the skin. Even small wounds don't heal rapidly. Unhealthy, readily ulcerating, flaccid skin.

Carboneum sulphuratum: Cracks < winter. Chronic skin diseases with much itching. Anesthesia, burning, itching, ulcers small wounds fester.

Cistus canadensis: Hard thick dry cracked skin, cracks of mercuro-syphilitic origin with hardening of the surrounding skin. Tendency to cracks in scrofulous diathesis. It is especially indicated in persons who lift heavy objects with their hand as a result of which there is hardening of the skin with subsequent development of deep oblique cracks. Location - hands and tips of the fingers. There is much itching, so much so, that the person cannot sleep.

Cundurango: Cracks about muco-cutaneous junctions. Painful cracks in the corner of the mouth. Tendency to develop cracks in the individuals with syphilitic and cancerous diathesis.

Graphites: Cracks in nipples, mouth, between the toes, anus, etc. Foul, acrid foot sweat chafes the toes. Unhealthy, rough, dry, hard skin, every little injury suppurates. Cracks deep, bloody, painful < in winter.

Hepar sulphur: Chapped skin and deep cracks of hand and feet, which are very sensitive. Cracks suppurate easily and give off a foul/sour odor. Dry and cracked condition of the axillae especially left side, much itching < when body becomes heated. Stinging, burning pains, generally worse in the cold. Cracks of the skin after use of mercury or its compounds.

Lycopodium clavatum: Cracks due to frequent washing, cracks are present on fingers, toes, palms, soles and heels. The palms are dry and hot; soles moist and cold. There is a sensation of soreness in cracks from which oozes a watery fluid. The cracks are associated with urinary, gastric, hepatic disorders. Violent itching; fissured eruptions.

Malandrinum: Dry, rough unhealthy skin has occurred after vaccination. Deep rhagades on the palms and soles, which are worse in cold weather and < by washing with any kind of soap.

Mercurius iodatus flavus: Troublesome itching associated with cracks. The cracks are painful with some pricking pain; < night, < pressure. There is intolerable itching at night.

Mercurius iodatus ruber: Small multiple cracks chiefly involving skin of the palms. Sore to touch and prone to suppuration and also they tend to ulcerate easily. Discharge from the cracks is yellow, sticky and offensive.

Natrium muriaticum: Cracks in between toes, around the nails, knuckles and heels. Also affects flexures of the skin. Violent itching with raw and sore sensation. Tendency to develop cracks after excessive consumption of salt.

Nitricum acidum: Cracks are found on hands and also on various muco-cutaneous junctions. Deep, sensitive to touch, bleed easily < cold weather, wetting the skin, < after washing, use of mercurial compounds. Cracks are prone to suppuration and ulceration. Discharge is purulent, bloody, and offensive. Splinter like pains in the cracks which is worse by cold, > by heat and by covering at night. Tendencies to formation of crack in patients with a syphilitic miasm, as the predisposing cause.

Petroleum: Cracks at angles of the mouth, folds of the skin, nipples, finger tips, heels, and palms. < Winter, washing. Sensation of burning and itching in the cracks, the patient scratches violently till it bleeds. The area around the crack is hard, rough and thickened.

Pix liquida: Back of the hands are affected with violent itching at night. When scratched, leads to bleeding.

Sarsaparilla officinalis: Sides of the finger, sides of the toes, thumb, feet. < by washing. Peculiar burning < at night. It is especially indicated in persons with gouty diathesis or person who had suppressed gonorrhea. Cracks may also be caused after administration of vaccines.

Silicea terra: Cracks on hands, around the nails, first finger, between the toes, etc. Cracks are painful and sensitive when exposed to cold weather. Patient feels better when the affected part is covered. Cracks tend to suppurate very easily. Itching in cracks only during daytime and evening. The tips of the finger are dry; tendency to develop cracks in the patient with (1) scrofulous diathesis, (2) after improper vaccination, (3) after injury.

Sulphur: Cracks on hands, between fingers and toes, arms, near and around the joints, feet, and heels. Itching and burning sensation, which is worse at night, warmth of the bed, and from washing. Even though the patient is hot, he develops cracks in the winter. Cracks bleed, ulcerate and suppurate, sensitive to touch and painful. Discharge is offensive, thick, and acrid. Pain < heat, < night. Psoric constitutions and who have suppressed eruptions in the past by strong ointments or those who have indulged in excess vaccinations.

Xerophyllum: Rough, cracked like leather, intense itching, stitching and burning.

X-ray: Cracks on hands, feet, knees, extensor surfaces of joints. Skin is dry, cracked with much itching, which is worse in the bed, in the evening and at night. Itching is better in the open air. There is much swelling of the part, which is sensitive to touch. It antidotes abuse of Sulphur.

REPERTORY

Aesc, aloe, alum, alum-sil, am-c, ant-c, arn, aur, bad, bals-p, bar-c, bar-s, benz-ac, bry, cadm-s, calc, calc-s, calc-sil, carb-an, carb-v, carbn-s, caust, cham, com, corn-a, cund, cycl, graph, hep, hydr, iris, kali-c, kali-s, kali-sil, kreos, lach, lyc, mag-c, mag-p, mang, merc, nat-c, nat-m, nit-ac, olnd, osm, paeon, petr, phos, psor, puls, rhus-t, ruta, sars, sep, sil, sulph, teucr, viol-t, zinc, zinc-p

- **Air, exposed to if:** alum.
- **Burning:** petr, sars, zinc.
- **Deep, bloody:** merc, nit-ac, petr, psor, puls, sars, sulph.
- **Delicate skin, on, parts covered with:** sil.
- **Discharges, serious fluid:** com.
- **Fetid:** merc.
- **Herpetic, chapping:** alum, aur, bry, cadm-s, calc, cycl, graph, hep, kali-c, kreos, lach, lyc, mag-c, mang, merc, nat-c, nat-m, nit-ac, petr, puls, rhus-t, ruta, sars, sep, sil, sulph, viol-t, zinc.
- **Humid:** aloe.
- **Ichorous fluid, irritating surrounding parts:** cund.
- **Itching:** merc, petr.

- **Mercurial:** hep, nit-ac, sulph.
- **New skin cracks and burns:** sars.
- **Orifices at:** sulph.
- **Painful:** graph, mang, zinc.
- **Painful and bleeding:** merc.
- **Sequelae of itch:** calc.
- **Small:** merc-i-r.
- **Sleeplessness:** pix.
- **Summer agg.:** cocc.
- **Ulcerated:** bry, merc.
- **Washing or working in water, after:** alum, ant-c, bry, calc, calc-s, cham, hep, kali-c, lyc, merc, nit-ac, puls, rhus-t, sars, sep, sulph, zinc.
- **Winter, in:** alum, calc, calc-s, carbn-s, graph, petr, psor, sep, sulph
- **Wounds, cuts:** Arn, led, merc, nat-c, ph-ac, sil, staph, sulph, sul-ac.
- **Yellow:** merc.

Location

- **Head:** graph, mag-c, petr, ruta.
- **Eye, cracks, canthi in:** alum, alum-p, ant-c, borx, calc-s, cist, graph, iod, lyc, merc, mez, nat-m, nit-ac, petr, phos, plat, sep, sil, staph, sulph, zinc.
- - Outer: graph, nat-m, sulph, zinc.
- **Eyelids:** alum, arn, bar-c, bry, calc, carb-v, caust, coloc, croc, euphr, iod, kali-c, lyc, nat-m, nit-ac, nux-v, phos, sep, sil, staph, sulph.
- - Tarsi: graph.
- **Ears:** calc, chel, mag-c, sep.
- - Behind the ears: chel, graph, hep, hydr, lyc, petr, sep, sulph.
- - Ear; eruptions, cracked and desquamating a substance like powdered starch: com.
- **Nose:** ant-c, arum-t, bell, carb-an, caust, graph, merc, nit-ac, petr.

- - Corners: graph, merc.
- - Nostrils: ant-c, anthraco, aur, aur-m, graph, nit-ac, petr.
- - Septum: merc.
- - Tip: alum, carb-a.
- - Wings: aur-m, caust, hep, merc, sil, syc, thuj.
- **Face:** arum-t, bufo, calc, cench, choc, graph, kali-c, lach, merc, nicc, nit-ac, petr, psor, sil, sulph.
- **Lips:** agar, ail, aloe, alum, alum-p, am-c, am-m, ant-t, apis, arn, ars, ars-s-f, arum-t, aur, aur-ar, aur-s, bar-c, bar-s, bell, bov, bry, calc, calc-s, calc-sil, caps, carb-ac, carb-an, carb-v, carbn-s, caust, cench, cham, chel, chin, chinin-ar, cimic, cist, colch, con, cop, cor-r, croc, cupr, dros, fl-ac, gink-b, graph, guare, ham, hell, hep, hydrog, hyos, ign, iris, jatr-c, kali-ar, kali-bi, kali-c, kali-i, kali-p, kali-s, kali-sil, kalm, kreos, lach, lyc, luna, mag-m, mang, meny, merc, merc-c, mez, mur-ac, nat-c, nat-m, nit-ac, nux-v, nat-ar, nicc, ol-an, par, petr, ph-ac, phos, plat, plb, ptel, puls, rhus-t, sabad, sel, sep, sil, spig, squil, staph, stram, sulph, syph, sabin, tab, tarax, ter, tub-m, tub-r, verat, zinc, zinc-p.
- - Coryza, during: staph.
- - Lower lip: anag, apis, arag, borx, bry, cham, cimic, graph, mez, nat-c, nit-ac, nux-v, plat, puls, phos, sep, sulph, zinc.
- - - Middle of: agar, am-c, aur, calc, cham, chin, dros, graph, haliae-lc, hep, nat-c, nat-m, nux-v, ph-ac, phos, puls, sep.
- - Upper lip: agar, androc, bar-c, calc, hell, kali-c, nat-c, nat-m, tarax, zinc.
- - - Middle of: calc, chin, hell, hep, mag-m, nat-c, nat- m, nux-v, ph-ac, phos, sel, sep, tarax.
- **Mouth:** ambr, bism, bufo, cocc, lach, merc-c, ph-ac, phos.
- - Corners of: am-c, ambr, ant-c, apis, arum-t, calc, caust, cinnb, cund, eup-per, gink-b, graph, hell, hydrog, ind, iod, merc, merc-c, mez, nat-ar, nat-m, nit-ac, psor, rhus-t, sep, sil, sulph, syph, thala, v-a-b, zinc.

- - Right: kreos, lyc.

- - Gums: plat.

- - Tongue: ail, anan, apis, ars, ars-i, ars-s-f, arum-t, arund, atro, aur-met, aur-ar, aur-s, bapt, bar-c, bar-i, bar-m, bar-s, bell, benz-ac, bor-ac, borx, bry, bufo, calad, calc, calc-f, calc-i, calc-p, calc-s, camph, carb-ac, carb-v, carbn-s, cham, chel, chin, chinin-ar, chlorp, cic, clem, cob, crot-h, cupr, cur, fl-ac, hell, hyos, iod, kali-bi, kali-c, kali-i, lach, leon, lyc, mag-m, merc, mez, mur-ac, nat-ar, nat-m, nit-ac, nux-v, ph-ac, phos, phyt, plat, plb, plb-act, podo, puls, pyrog, raja-s, ran-s, raph, rhus-t, rhus-v, sacch, sec, semp, sin-n, spig, stram, sulph, syph, tub, verat, zinc, zinc-p.

- **Shoulder**: arn, valer.

- **Wrist joint**: sulph.

- **Hands**: aesc, alum, alum-sil, am-c, anan, apis, arn, aur, calc, calc-sil, calen, carb-ac, cench, graph, ham, hep, hydr, kali-c, kali-sil, kreos, lyc, mag-c, merc, nat-c, nat-m, petr, prim-o, psor, puls, rhus-t, sars, sep, sil, sul-ac, sulph, zinc.

- - Palms: alum, cist, graph, kreos, merc-i-r, petr.

- - Back of hands: cist, kreos, nat-c, petr, rhus-t.

- **Fingers**: calc, hep, merc, nat-m, nit-ac, petr, sars.

- - Between: ars, aur-m, graph, zinc.

- - Finger joints: sulph.

- - Nails, about the: ant-c, nat-m, sil.

- - Tips: bar-c, alum, aur, bell, graph, merc, petr, sars, sil.

- - Thumb: sars.

- **Lower limbs**: alum, aur-met, bar-c, calc, chin, coff, croc, hep, merc, nat-c, nat-m, petr., plat, puls, ruta, sars, sulph, valer, verat, zinc.

- **Heels**: graph.

- **Toes**: lach.

- - Between: graph, lach.

- - Under: sabad.

MACERATION

Prolonged moisture produces two effects:

- Maceration
- Paronychia.

The former is seen in flexures like the interdigital spaces, the groins and axillae during the monsoon where it results in intertrigo. Interdigital maceration is common in people who wear shoes for long hours. Paronychia due to maceration is frequently seen in domestic servants, washermen, housewives, cooks and barmen.

Macerated skin predisposes to monilia, tinea and streptococcal infection. In the case of patients confined to bed continuous pressure and maceration ressults in necrosis of the tissues as is seen in bedsores. The treatment of all these conditions consists in correcting the basic causes and keeping the affected part dry.

HOMEOPATHIC APPROACH TO MACERATED SKIN

Maceration of the skin usually takes place in the folds of the skin e.g. axilla, groin, in between toes and fingers. Hence one should refer the rubric – Skin folds, flexors, where the following drugs have got marked affinity ars, calc-c, carb-v, graph, hep, lyc, merc, nat-m, ol-an, petr, psor, puls, sel, sep, sil, sulph.

The macerated skin is highly prone to develop secondary infection; hence every care should be taken to clean the affected part either with Calendula or Echinacea diluted with water in 1:10 ratio. Also since moisture aggravates the condition, the affected part should be kept dry.

Simple maceration is an example of psoric miasm but when secondary infection occurs with formation of pus, it represents tubercular maism. If the macerated skin leads to ulceration and necrosis it indicates syphilitic maism. The importance lies in prescribing appropriate anti-miasmatic remedy.

Some Important Homeopathic Remedies

Carbo vegetabilis: Burning in macerated skin < night, < in bed. Skin is raw, ulcerated with an offensive odor with tendency to suppuration and ulcer formation. It is specifically indicated in old broken down constitution with chronic illnesses who are bed ridden. Burning > heat.

Graphites: Itching at folds < at night. Burning sensation. Thin, sticky, acrid offensive and gluey discharge, which oozes from the skin. The affected part burns after scratching and there is tendency to form cracks and fissures. When skin is cleaned with warm water it aggravates. > In open air.

Mercurius solubilis: Itching in macerated skin > scratching, < night in bed, on getting warm. After scratching there is burning and skin becomes rough and secretes a thin fluid with small vesicle formation. Bleeding after scratching. Dirty parts with offensive odor; prone to suppuration and ulceration. Burning < scratching, warmth.

Natrium muriaticum: Oily, greasy, dirty looking withered sensation of rawness and soreness. Near the edges of hair on the genitals and groin excessive itching with secretion of acrid, thin discharge with formation of cracks. Crusts form on the scratched areas. < Warm room, sun, > open air, < eating salt itching.

Petroleum: Dirty, hard rough, thickened skin especially in folds of skin. Deep painful cracks in affected part. Violent itching; scratches until it bleeds, parts become cold after scratching. < Winter; > warm air and dry weather.

Psorinum: Inactive skin with want of perspiration. Dirty, unwashed look of the skin. Itching < warmth of bed. Scratches until it bleeds. Offensive odor from parts on scratching < before midnight, < open air. The maceration of skin may be as a consequence of skin disease suppressed by antibiotics.

Chapter-13

Dermatoses Due to Physical Agents Like Cold, Heat and Light

COLD INJURIES

Due to exposure to excessive cold, there is intense vasoconstriction, and this is further reinforced by the passage of cold blood through the vasomotor center of the brain. Vasoconstriction provokes tissue anoxia. Decreased muscular activity further diminishes the blood supply. In severe cases where there is ice crystal formation in the blood vessels, necrosis ensues.

CHILBLAINS

Synonym

Erythema pernio.

Definition

It is a recurrent, localized erythema and swelling caused by exposure to cold. Blistering and ulcerations may develop in severe cases.

Etiology & Incidence

People with poor peripheral circulation and sometimes with poor general health, are the victims. It is more common among females than males.

Clinical Features

It occurs especially on the fingers and toes, and less frequently on the hands, feet, ears, and face. The patient may be unaware of the injury at first, but later there is burning, tenderness, itching and redness, which brings it to their attention. The area becomes dusky or bluish-red (which reduces on pressure) and is cold to touch. The extremities may become cyanotic and clammy due to excessive sweating. It usually subsides completely in summer. Itchy swelling also develops and occasionally these ulcerate.

Differential Diagnosis

* It is distinguished from lupus erythematosus, which may even complicate chilblains. In LE of the hands, bluish red slightly infiltrated and scaly lesions develop on the back of fingers, accompanied by typical lesions on face.

* When one comes across chronic whitlows and erosions on fingers the possibility of chilblains must be considered.

TREATMENT

Affected parts should be cleaned in water and massaged gently with warm oil every day. Care should be taken to protect it against further injury and exposure to cold or dampness. If the feet are affected, woolen socks should be worn at night during the cold months. Electric pads may be used to warm the parts. The patient is strongly advised to stop smoking.

FROSTBITE

Synonym

Congelation.

Definition

Frostbite is when there is freezing of the soft tissue with local deprivation of blood supply.

Clinical Features

The ears, nose, cheeks, fingers, and toes are most often affected. Any part of the body getting wet, strong winds and poor general health predispose to frost bite. Cold temperatures lead to contraction of the arterioles, later to dilatation of the capillaries and last of all, to the freezing of the parts.

The affected part first appears cold and bluish red. Then as freezing sets in, it becomes white, waxy and numb. There is erythema, edema, vesicles and bullae, superficial gangrene, deep gangrene, and injury to muscles, tendons, periosteum, and nerves.

On thawing, the part becomes swollen, bluish red and painful, with necrosis of the frozen tissue and blood vessels. The latter results in thrombosis and gangrene.

Treatment

- Gradual warming of the part is necessary in the early stages of the condition. Do not apply direct heat. Wrap the affected part in warm and sterile gauze. Rapid rewarming in a water bath between 100 and 101 degrees F is the treatment of choice for all frostbite cases. When the skin flushes and is pliable, thawing is complete.
- Supportive measures like bed rest, a high protein and a high calorie diet should be given, with appropriate wound care and avoidance of further trauma to the part. Do not rub or massage the part.

- Recovery may take months, and on recovery, gradual exercise to restore the function.

- Every care should be taken by a homeopath to prevent secondary infection and vascular thrombosis in the affected part. Hence, after the initial relief obtained by the short acting remedy, a deep acting constitutional remedy is to be prescribed, preferably snake venom, which acts as an anti-coagulant. Kindly refer the therapeutics of chilblains.

ACROCYANOSIS

Definition

This is a condition where there is persistent cyanosis, with coldness and hyperhidrosis of the affected parts.

Etiology

It is thought to be due to arteriolar spasm with dilatation of venules in the skin, but there is no known cause for its occurance. It is seen to occur especially in young women, who are emotionally sensitive, with rather unstable vasomotor systems. Acrocyanosis may also be seen in elderly patients with cardiac disease and in neurological disorders such as stroke, poliomyelitis and multiple sclerosis.

Clinical Features

The hands and feet are more often involved, and less commonly, the tip of the nose and the ears may be involved in people with a poor peripheral circulation.

On exposure to cold, the part becomes cold, white and insensitive. Cyanosis increases as the temperature decreases and the color of the part changes to a dusky red or bluish hue, accompanied by over-sweating of the part.

Treatment

- Limbs must be kept warm, through indirect heat or warm applications.
- Smoking, coffee, and tea should be avoided.

ERYTHROCYANOSIS CRURUM

In this condition the circulatory disturbance (arteriolar spasm with dilatation of venules) affects the legs and thighs of young girls and women. There is unilateral, cold, dusky red or bluish pink swelling over the outer side of the lower parts of the legs.

The affected parts are cold to touch with a dull ache in them. The patient may present with a history of cramps in the legs at night. Small tender nodules may be found on palpation, which may break down to form small, often multiple ulcers, as in erythema induratum.

Atypical varieties are common, presenting either as cinnabar red spots, bullae, indurations, or lichenoid papules.

Treatment

The treatment consists of exercising the affected parts, keeping them warm with proper clothing – gloves, thick stockings and footwear, and a good nourishing diet.

LIVEDO RETICULARIS

It is a skin condition where there is a blotchy, mottled or reticulated pink or bluish red discoloration of the skin, on the extremities, especially the feet and legs. In a few cases the thighs, trunk, and forearms may be affected. It gives a marbled discoloration to the skin, with white areas in the center of the mottled pattern. The lesions are often asymptomatic, though in a few cases coldness, numbness, tingling or a dull ache may be present. Only in a few cases there is formation of cutaneous nodules and ulceration, and these are termed as necrotizing livedo reticularis.

Etiology

Young girls are particularly affected with this condition in countries with a cold climate, probably due to patchy arteriolar vasospasm in the skin. It can also be a secondary manifestation in patients with hepatitis C, polyarteritis nodosa, polycythemia vera, lupus erythematosus, dermatomyositis, hypercalcemia, mycosis fungoides, pancreatitis, scleroderma, syphilis, rheumatic fever, thrombocytopenic purpura and tuberculosis.

HOMEOPATHIC APPROACH TO CHILBLAINS AND FROSTBITE

There is enough scope of homeopathic drugs in the treatment of chilblains. Here once again questions pertaining to general health are quite essential because poor general health sometimes predisposes the individual to develop chilblains. Also, poor peripheral circulation can lead to formation of chilblains; hence homeopathic drugs acting on vasomotor system, skin with tendency to ulceration should be included in the therapeutics of chilblains. The above pathology indicates dominant syphilitic maism. The following are the most common symptoms encountered itching, burning, and ulceration.

The following points should be noted during history taking:

- Site: Most commonly fingers and toes.
- Thermal modalities.
- Causative factor and other associated symptoms.
- The description of ulcers with its discharge.

The hands and feet must be kept warm with gloves and woollen stockings. Sudden changes of temperature, like exposing parts of the body to cold and then warming them near a fire, act badly on the malady.

Locally *Rhus venenata.* mother tincture should be applied to give immediate relief.

SOME IMPORTANT HOMEOPATHIC REMEDIES

Abrotanum: There is sensation of itching in the lesion (Agar, Petr.). The other characteristic symptoms of the skin are:

- Loose and flabby skin.
- Skin becomes purplish after suppression of eruptions.
- This is specially indicated in persons with tendency towards marasmus.
- Patient in general is worse by cold air, worse wet weather.

Agaricus muscarius: Burning, itching, redness and swelling as from frostbite. Itching changes place on scratching. Pricking as from needles.

< Cold air, freezing air, open air, stormy weather, alcohol.

Toes itch and burn; are red and swollen as if frostbitten. Feet cold like ice up to ankles.

Borax venenata: Chilblains > open air. Wilted wrinkled skin. Unhealthy skin; slight injury suppurates.

Calendula officinalis: Tendency to develop chilblains after injury with formation of ulcer with excessive secretion of pus. The surrounding part is red. Ulcers, irritable inflamed, sloughing, painful as if beaten. Pain in chilblains < night.

Cantharis vesicatoria: Burning pain in the chilblains > by cold application, burning when touched. Tendency for the chilblain to develop into ulcers and finally leading to gangrene.

Carbo animalis: Frostbite, inflammation burning. Chilblains < evening, in bed, from cold. Chilblain associated with glandular enlargement. Tendency to from ulcers, which bleed very easily.

Fragaria vesca: Chilblains associated with urticaria. Especially tendency to develop chilblains in hot weather.

Hepar sulphur: Extremely sensitive to cold air. Deep cracks with chilblains. > Warm application, warms wraps, and heat. < Cold air, winter, cold application. Easy suppuration developing in chilblains.

Lachesis mutus: Chilblains with bluish-red or bluish-black discoloration around it. Chilblains tend to develop ulceration leading to gangrene. Severe burning sensation worse at night and during sleep. Very sensitive to touch, bleeds easily and copiously. There is severe excoriation of the affected part.

Ledum palustre: Dryness of skin with want of perspiration. Itching chilblains < after scratching. Sensation of burning after scratching. Burning worse in open air.

Muriaticum acidum: Chilblains burn at the margins and covered with scurf. Voluptuous itching sensation in chilblains.

Nitricum acidum: Dryness, severe pricking, shooting, burning pain, <open air, cold application, < nights, cold weather. Tendency to from multiple cracks surrounding the chilblains, which are very sensitive and painful to touch.

Petroleum: Itching chilblains with chapped hands and feet. Slightest injury on the chilblains tends to suppurate. Severe excoriation of the affected part. Itching sensation and from it moist discharge comes out which is very acrid. In general there is aggravation of symptoms from warmth of bed.

Psorinum: Itching, smarting, burning pain after scratching. Rough thick scaly skin with offensive odor from the affected part. Cracks break out easily on various parts of the skin.

Pulsatilla pratensis: Itching with burning < in the evening at night, warmth of bed, scratching. Especially indicated when the chilblains turn blue. Tendency to develop ulcers from chilblains.

Rhus venenata: Chilblain with severe burning sensation. Affected part looks red, indurated, swollen. Formation of deep, corroding phagedenic ulcers with offensive discharge. Itching < warmth, > cold (locally apply for instant relief).

Sulphur: Voluptuous itching, burning sensation < open air, wind, washing. Chilblains alternate with various other bodily complaints. Skin is dry rough, chapped. Offensive odor of skin < night in bed, < scratching, and washing.

Tamus communis: Chilblains and chapped hands. It takes away black and blue marks that come after bruises and dryness. It dissolves coagulated blood. It removes pain when it is applied locally on painful parts.

Terebinthiniae oleum: Skin is warm and moist with presence of erythema around chilblains.

Thyroidinum: Crust with chilblains. Suppuration within the lesions. Early peeling of skin. Bluish blackish discoloration of skin. Skin gets desquamated quite freely.

REPERTORY

Abrot, acon, agar, all-c, alum, alumn, aloe, ant-c, apis, arn, ars, asar, aur, bad, bell, borx, bufo, bry, cadm, calc, calen, canth, camph, carb-an, carb-v, cham, chin, colch, cop, croc, crot-t, cyc!, ferr-p, frag, hep, ham, hyos, ign, kali-ar, kali-c, kali-chl, kalm, lach, led, lyc, mag-c, merc, mur-ac, nit-ac, nux-m, nux-v, op, petr, plan, phos, ph-ac, puls, rheum, rhus-t, ruta, sep, sil, staph, sulph, sul-ac, tam, ter, thyr, thuj, verat-v, zinc.

- **Blue:** arn, bad, bell, kali-c, kali-s, kalm, puls.
- **Bleeding, rhagades:** nux v.
- **Burning:** carb-an, sulph.
- **Crawling in:** arn, colch, nux-v, rhus-t, sep.
- **Inflamed:** ars, bell, cham, hep, lyc, nit-ac, nux-v, phos, puls, rhus-t, staph, sulph.
- - From the slightest degree of cold: nit-ac.
- - With bluish red swelling and rhagades: puls.
- **Itching:** abrot, agar, petr, zinc.
- **Irritable subjects with delicate skin, great redness of parts affected by cold:** nit-ac.
- **Painful:** arn, ars, aur, bell, chin, hep, lyc, mag-c, nit-ac, nux-v, petr, phos, ph-ac, puls, sep.
- **Pulsating:** nux-v.

- **Suppurating:** calc-s, hep, sil.
- **Throbbing in summer:** nux-v.
- **Vesicles or bullae, with:** ant-c, bell, carb-an, chin, cycl, mag-c, nit-ac, phos, rhus-t, sep, sulph.

Location

- **Ear** (Refer to Ears, itching, meatus, burning or Ears, discolouration redness, chilblains): agar, alum, arn, ars, arund, bad, bry, calc, calc-p, carb-an, carb-v, caust, corn, lach, lyc, mur-ac, nat-p, nit-ac, nux-v, petr, phos, puls, stry, sulph, shuj, zinc.
- **Nose, frost bitten:** agar.
- **Easily:** zinc.
- **Face** (Look in Face, itching, frost bitten, as if or Face, burning, frost bitten, as if): agar, arg-met.
- **hands:** agar, aloe, arg-met, cic, croc, kali-chl, nit-ac, op, petr, puls, stann, sul-ac, sulph, zinc.
- **fingers:** agar, berb, carb-an, lyc, nit-ac, nux-v, petr, puls, sul-ac, sulph.
- **feet:** abrot, agar, alumn, am-c, anac, ant-c, aur, bad, bell, berb, borx, bry, bufo, cadm, carb-an, carb-v, cham, chin, colch, croc, crot-h, cycl, hep, hyos, ign, kali-chl, kali-n, lyc, merc, mur-ac, naja, nit-ac, nux-m, nux-v, op, petr, ph-ac, phos, puls, ran-b, rhus-t, sep, stann, staph, sul-ac, sulph, thuj, zinc.
- **bunions after frostbite:** calc.
- **cracked:** merc, nux-v, and petr.
- **inflammation:** lach, merc, nit-ac, petr.
- **purple:** lach, merc, puls, sulph.
- **suppurating:** lach, sil, sulph.
- **swollen:** merc.
- **heel, swollen, red:** petr.
- **toes:** agar, alum, ambr, aur-met, aur-ar, borx, carb-an, croc, hydrog, kali-c, nit-ac, nux-v, petr, phos, puls, rhod.
- **bluish:** kali-c.
- **pain in the fifth toe, as from chilblain:** aloe.

HEAT INJURIES

Our body requires and can tolerate heat upto a certain extent, beyond which, there is a resulting injury, in the form of burns or scalds, to the part.

BURNS

A burn is an injury caused by transfer of energy into tissue with a resulting disruption in its functional integrity.

The source of the energy may be thermal, chemical, electrical or radiation

Pathophysiology

The pathophysiological reaction to a burn injury is complex and varies with the cause. In thermal injuries, the changes in the burn wound are mainly caused by the direct effects of heat but superimposed on these are changes associated with an acute inflammatory process. It is these latter changes that account for the widespread and devastating effects of major burns on the entire homeostatic functions of the body.

The local response to a sudden increase in body surface temperature is the dilatation of blood vessels in an attempt to dissipate heat. A further increase in tissue temperature triggers an inflammatory response.

The key cells in the postburn inflammatory response are the polymorphonuclear leukocyte (PMN), mast cell and endothelial cells. These cell types together with platelets represent the prime target sites responsible for the mediation, progression and resolution of the inflammatory response.

Activation of complement and coagulation cascades with the release of histamine from mast cells results in a short phase of vasodilatation and plasma protein leakage from postcapillary venules resulting in local edema formation. Intracellular proteases released as a result of cell damage activate kallikrein, which is responsible for transforming kininogen to kinin. Kinins have several effects, including vasodilatation, pain stimulation and leukocyte migration. A delayed phase of leukocyte and platelet margination then results in the release of prostaglandins, prostacyclins, thromboxanes, leukotrienes and lipoxins, which is accompanied by a substantial increase in microvascular permeability and changes in vasomotor permeabilities. The prolonged post-traumatic phase of vasodilatation and antiplatelet aggregation is regulated through endothelial cells via two different mediators, prostaglandin I and nitric oxide. Hypercoagulability of the lymph and the plasma has been observed 2-3h after injury and correlates with the finding of increased levels of kinins in lymph.

Treatment

The general line of treatment includes the following:

The rationalization of the care of burns patients requires effective prehospital management, transportation and assessment/ triage in a hospital emergency department. The importance of education/communication at this level cannot be overestimated. Subsequent, safe transfer of a stable patient to a specialized burns unit initiates the next phase of treatment. Several recent texts give excellent comprehensive accounts of total burn care.

Stop the burning process

• The patient must be removed from the source of injury and the ongoing damage halted. Patients sustaining chemical injuries should have clothing removed, as quickly as possible and copious irrigation with water is the key to first aid. In chemical burns, the tissue damage is very much a function of the concentration of the agent and the duration of exposure, therefore in the otherwise fit patient, copious irrigation at the scene of the accident is preferable, rather than immediate transfer to an emergency centre. It is essential to be aware of the possible dangers of handling contaminated clothing, and appropriate protective clothing including gloves and eye protection should be available for the emergency services.

Primary survey

- The primary survey is the rapid assessment of the patient to ensure immediate survival. Attention is focused on airway, breathing, circulation and cervical spine immobilization. It is important to establish that there is a pulse. In a large burn, this may be more meaningful than blood pressure measurement in establishing that there is a circulation.

Secondary assessement

- The secondary assessment involves a thorough head-to-toe examination of the patient. A rapid check is made of the patient's head, neck, thorax, abdomen, upper and lower limbs to ensure that no other life-threatening injuries are present and that, if they are, the appropriate measures may be taken. It is also appropriate at this time to ascertain, if possible, any relevant past medical history, medications or allergies and to establish the mechanism and time of injury.

Assessment of the depth and the area of the burn

Fluid resuscitation

- The goal of resuscitation is to maintain vital organ function while avoiding the complications of inadequate or excessive fluid infusion. Excessive volumes of intravenous fluid can increase tissue edema formation and compromise tissue oxygenation. This is particularly a problem with pulmonary and/or cerebral oedema. Inadequate fluid resuscitation can cause diminished perfusion of the renal and mesenteric vascular beds, which can lead to organ failure.
- The *hypovolemic shock* that follows burn injury is due to a shift of fluid from the vascular to the extravascular compartment. The more extensive the burn, the more extensive the shift of fluid. This fluid shift is a progressive phenomenon, which is maximal within hours of the burn and can persist for several days after the burn. As a simple guide, all patients who have burns in excess of 10% body surface area (BSA)

should be commenced on intravenous resuscitation. The intravenous fluid infusion has to be regulated to give in the first 24h.

- Adults 2-4ml Hartmann's solution/kg body weight/% BSA burn.
- Children 3-4ml Hartmann's solution/kg body weight/% BSA burn.

The intravenous fluid rate is adjusted to give one-half of the estimated volume in the first 8h post-burn. The remaining half of the estimated resuscitation volume should be administered over the subsequent 16h of the first day post-burn.

Urine output

- It is the single best indicator of fluid resuscitation in the uncomplicated burn.

Garstrointestinal tract decompression

- It is important to be aware that the patient may require surgery and general anesthesia. The patient should be given nil by mouth until seen and assessed by a burns physician.

Immediate Wound Care

- **Pain relief.**
- **Escharotomy.**
- **Monitoring reponse to fluid resuscitation.**
- **Surgical intervention.**

Prognosis

Superficial partial thickness burns will heal without scarring, although there may be some loss of pigment, which is usually temporary. Deeper burns are associated with scarring and there is a high incidence of hypertrophic scarring especially in the deeper, partial thickness burns that have been allowed to heal conservatively. Hypertrophic scars go through a phase of many months when they can be intensely pruritic and this can be a significant problem for children. Pressure garments and silicon gel and elastomers are used in the management of hypertrophic scars.

Occasionally, the scarring can result in functional problems that require surgical intervention. Aesthetic problems related to scarring and contracture with deformity also require combined approaches of splinting and surgical intervention, which may need to be repeated over a considerable period of time.

THERMAL BURNS

It is a dermatitis resulting from the action of excessive heat on the skin. The changes in the skin resulting from dry heat or scalding are classified into four types:

First degree burn

- Active congestion of the superficial blood vessels, causing an erythema that may be followed by peeling (epidermal desquamation) e.g. sunburn. The pain and increased surface heat may be severe, and it is common to have some constitutional reaction if the involved area is large.

Second degree burn

- It is of two types
- Superficial: There is transudation of serum from the capillaries, which causes edema of the superficial tissues. Serum accumulation beneath the outer layers of the epidermis gives rise to the formation of vesicles and blebs. Here complete recovery without scar formation results.
- Deep: It is pale and anesthetic. Injury to the reticular dermis comprimises blood flow and destroys appendages thus resulting in scarring. The healing takes over one month.

Third degree burn

- There is loss of tissue of the full thickness of the skin and at times even involves the subcutaneous tissue. Here there is epithelium available for regeneration. An ulcer is produced, which heals with scar formation. It requires grafting for closure.

Fourth degree burn

There is destruction of the entire skin and subcutaneous fat with the underlying tendon. It requires grafting for closure. The constitutional symptoms depends on the severity of the burns i.e. the size of the involved surface, the depth of the burn and particularly the location of the lesion. The more the vascularity of the area the more severe are the symptoms.

Symptoms of shock may appear within 24 hours after a burn, followed by toxemia and symptoms of wound infection.

Prognosis

It is poor if large surface areas of the skin is involved and is very grave if more that 2/3 of the body surface has been affected.

Treatment

- Prompt application of cold applications.
- Vesicles and blebs of second degree burns should not be opened but should be protected from injury. If they become very tense the fluid should be drained under strict aseptic precautions.

ELECTRICAL BURNS

Two types:

1. Contact burn small and deep causing necrosis of underlying tissues.
2. Flash burn usually cover a large area.

HOMEOPATHIC APPROACH TO BURNS

This is one of the most common injuries that one comes across in the homeopathic practice and thus its therapeutics should be properly learnt. First of all we should know where to look for

'Burns' in the repertory, and what are the common types of burns that one can encounter.

The commonest burn we encounter in our private practice is the one acquired after drinking something hot – hot soup, hot tea, etc. The second very common type of burn we encounter in India is the one got during the Diwali season from bursting firecrackers, where the sparks of the crackers goes into the eyes and produces burns. One can also get an accidental injury resulting in burns on the skin.

After systemic examination of the patient and trying to give all the other auxillary modes of treatment, the homeopathic treatment of burns is through local application. There are certain remedies that one can apply *locally* and it will give excellent results.

• Most important is an ointment made from *Picricum acidum* or simply *Picricum acidum* mother tincture, diluted 9:1, where 9 drops of saline and one drop of Picricum acidum is mixed, and applied to the wound. Why I prefer Picricum acidum in severe burning pains after a burn injury is because of the following – When you try to mix *Nitric acidum* upon *Carbolic acidum,* you get formation of fine yellow scales, which are soluble in water or alcohol, which becomes a brilliant yellow color. Now when you use Picricum acidum to reduce the pain, it acts like a local anesthetic agent. It also limits the tendency to suppuration on account of its strong antiseptic properties and the power it possesses to coagulate albuminous discharges. Healing takes place rapidly and the resultant scar formation is smooth and it shows very little tendency to formation of keloid at a later stage. To me Picricum acidum is best indicated in superficial burns and scalds with vesication of the skin, and hence should be applied as follows – After careful removal of the clothing, the wound should be cleaned as thoroughly as possible with the solution of Picricum acidum mother tincture.

• Also, adding two drops of *Urtica urens* mother tincture onto a gauze piece will quickly relieve the pain of the burn and helps in healing.

F- 11

- Sometimes to prevent infection, when there is suppuration of the wound, I use *Calendula officinalis* mother tincture as a local application instead of *Urtica urens* mother tincture.

For *internal medication,* let us first examine the *rubrics.*

- In the chapter of 'Eye' you will see 'Inflammation, burns from'. Here *Cantharis vesicatoria* is an important remedy.

- In the chapter of the 'Mouth' you should look for 'burns on the tongue and lips', and here *Hamamelis virginiana* is an important remedy.

- In the chapter of 'Generalities', there is a general rubric of 'Burns', where there are more than about 75-80 remedies.

- There are certain types of burns where the patient may complain of a severe burning pain, but they are better by warm applications. In such conditions, Margeret Tyler has mentioned two very beautiful remedies – *Arsenicum album* and *Ledum palustre,* which are very useful.

- If the burns are due to Radium, then remedies like *Radium bromatum* and *Phosphorus* are important.

- If the burns are due to radiation or X-rays, then remedies like *Calcarea fluorica, Phosphorus, Radium bromatum* and *X-ray* come into picture.

- When a patient is really never well since his last burn, remedies like *Carbolicum acidum* and *Causticum* play an important role.

- Also, there are many mental rubrics that we can use for the selection of a correct similimum, like delirium after burns, unconsciousness after burns, or mild wildness after burns.

In my practice, *constitutional remedies* that have been really very useful are *Causticum, Fluoricum acidum, Calcarea fluorica, Sulphuricum acidum* and *Picricum acidum.* You have to try and differentiate each individual remedy to find out which remedy is more suitable to the patient. One should give a lot of importance to the *characteristic modalities.*

In tissue salts, *Kalium muriaticum* is an important remedy for first-degree burns. There is a formation of blisters with a whitish or greyish exudation. If the burn leads to suppuration, *Calcarea sulphurica* is a good remedy.

At times when lighting a cigarette or a matchstick, one can burn his or her finger, which one then tends to put in cold water. In such cases, *Apis mellifica* 6C is a useful remedy, but in cases where the part becomes extremely red and hot, then *Belladonna* 6C has helped me in my practice.

In cases of *second-degree burns,* where there is formation of vesicles and there is intense itching, restlessness and the patient is thirsty, *Rhus toxicodendron* is an important remedy. Another remedy that is equally useful is *Cantharis vesicatoria.* The difference between the two remedies is that Cantharis vesicatoria has an intense burning thirst and vesicles are quite big, while in Rhus toxicodendron the vesicles are tiny and the patient is not as thirsty as Cantharis vesicatoria.

In *third-degree burns*, there is an accompanying severe shock and dehydration. Here remedies like *Arsenic album* are useful. In cases of septicemia with severe burns, remedies like *Echinacea angustifolia* have to be thought of.

Very rarely when you find the involvement of fine nerves with the burn, and burning pain is better by cold application, and there is an excrutiating intense pain, with pus formation and a septic state developing, *Hypericum perfoliatum* is one more remedy that can help in case of burns.

Calendula officinalis is also an important remedy since it promotes the granulation tissue, prevents disfiguring keloid formation, favors cicatrization with least possible amount of suppuration and prevents delirium and exhaustion from the loss of blood.

In the end I can only say is that the most important duty of every homeopathic physician is to help to remove the pain. The homeopathic remedies often work very rapidly to relieve the intense pain of the burn.

Hahnemann always used to recommend the use of warm water or warm application to the burn because of its homeopathicity. I have very often seen in my practice that the patient becomes almost addicted to cold applications, even in a minor burn. The patient often desires ice-cold application for hours after the burns, but if following an initial cold application, a short period if warmth or heat is applied, the pain intensifies for some time and then disappears. For more advanced, second and third degree burns, this technique is not appropriate.

The next important duty of the homeopath is to prevent infections and avoid healing of burns by keloid formation.

LIGHT INJURIES

This section covers disorders that involve abnormal sensitivity to ultraviolet (UBV and UBA) and sometimes to visible sunlight. There are resultant sunburns and solar erythema, blister and scar formation, freckles, itchy papular, eczematous or urticarial eruptions.

SUNBURN & SOLAR ERYTHEMA

Sunburn is a normal cutaneous erythematous reaction to sunlight in the presence of an excess of UBV exposure (especially between 10 am to 2 pm). The erythema is followed by tenderness, and in severe cases there is blister formation, that may become confluent. The sites most often involved are the face and the limbs. In a few cases, chills, fever, nausea, tachycardia and hypotension may be present. Desquamation follows within a week's time at the site of the sunburn.

Prevention & Treatment

Avoiding exposure to the sun at the peak hours of UBV intensity. Also, wearing of hats and loose, full-sleeved, cotton clothing is advised. Use of an effective sunscreen lotion with the sun protection factor (SPF) of 15 and above is recommended, atleast 20 minutes before going out in the sun.

FRECKLE

Synonym

Ephelis.

Etiology

It is genetically determined, and blondes and redheads are especially susceptible to getting it.

Clinical Features

These are small, brown macules, occuring in crops on the sun-exposed areas of the face, neck, shoulders, and back of hands. They are most prominent during the summer months due to exposure to the sun, and reduce in the winter months. They start to appear around the age of 5 years.

Histopathology

There is an increased production of the melanin pigment by a normal number of melanocytes.

Differential Diagnosis

- Lentigo simplex is a benign hyperpigmented macule appearing at any age and on any part of the body. It is not related to exposure to the sun.
- In cases of solar lentigo, there are sharply demarcated brown macules on the back of the hands and face, with the distinguishing feature being that it appears at a later age, and the histological features show elongated rete ridges, which appear club-shaped.

Photoaging

Here there is development of uneven pigmentation, with poorly demarcated hyperpigmented and white atrophic macules, due to chronic sun exposure. This condition is genetically determined and is most commonly seen in the blue-eyed, fair-complexioned people, who do not tan. This condition can very often lead to malignancy and has to be thus examined frequently.

PHOTOSENSITIVITY

These include skin reactions that are chemical or drug induced, metabolic, idiopathic and photo-exacerbated.

Chemically Induced Photosensitivity

Here the injury results from interaction of the photosensitizing agent on the skin (derived either through external application or through internally administered drugs) with ultraviolet or visible radiation, leading to release of reactive oxygen species and subsequently inflammatory mediators. Here, only a short exposure to sunlight can cause marked erythema, edema and blister formation of the exposed part (within 48 hours), without prior allergic sensitization. This is termed as 'phototoxicity'.

In contrast, photoallergy is a type IV delayed hypersensitive response, a true allergic reaction with worsening erythema and an eczematous rash, within a few days after exposure to sunlight, produced either due to internal administration of drugs or by external applications. Thus, photoallergy occurs only in sensitized persons, and has a delayed onset of upto 14 days, and it shows histologic features of contact dermatitis.

Metabolic Photosensitivity

Here there is an inborn error in the metabolism, such as the porphyrias, resulting in the production of endogenous photosensitizers. Sun-induced tense blisters are seen on the back of the hands, which are slow to heal, producing atrophic scars, milia and hyperpigmentation. The skin becomes sensitive and fragile with a tendency to easy erosions.

Idiopathic Photosensitivity

Here there is no known cause for the photosensitivity reactions.

Polymorphic light eruption

It is the commonest type, where there are itchy, papular eruptions on some sun-exposed areas, developing within 1-4 days of sun exposure, and persisting for upto a week's time. It is especially common in young women. In a few cases papulovesicular, eczematous, erythematous and plaque-like lesions (especially in the elderly) are also seen. The sites involved are the face, upper chest, neck, shoulders and upper limbs.

Actinic prurigo

This chronic and persistent disorder, seen especially in Native Americans, begins in childhood with an eczematous eruption, which is especially marked on the areas exposed to the sun. These begin as small papules or papulovesicles, which form crusts, and are extremely itchy. In children, the face, sparing the forehead, is especially affected. Additionally, there is cheilitis and an associated prurigo nodule formation on the limbs.

Hydroa vacciniforme

It is a chronic and rare photodermatitis seen in children. Here there is development of crops of vesicles on the face following exposure to the sun, preceded by fever and malaise. These lesions rupture within a few days, become centrally necrotic and heal leaving depressed smallpox like scars. The sites most often involved are the nose, cheeks, ears, and extensor arms and hands. In a few cases conjunctivitis, corneal ulceration and opacity may occur.

Solar urticaria

This condition is seen in adults, especially females aged between 20-40 years. Here, typical urticarial lesions (weals) develop within a few minutes after exposure to sunlight (UBV rays), and these tend to resolve within 1-2 hours.

Chronic actinic dermatitis

Here there is a persistent, chronic, eczematous eruption in the absence of exposure to known photosensitizers. The lesions consist of edematous, scaling, thickened patches and plaques, which can become confluent. Marked depigmentation can also be seen. It is known to affect middle-aged or elderly men, who may not realize that their condition gets worse by exposure to light, since it persists in all seasons. Diagnosis is established by phototesting and histological examination.

Photo-exacerbated Photosensitivity

Here skin conditions that tend to worsen by exposure to the sun are listed. Some of them are hereditary disorders where there is an increased sensitivity to ultraviolet rays – like xeroderma pigmentosum and Cockayne's disease. In others there is an acquired sensitivity to the ultraviolet light – like pemphigus foliaceus, psoriasis, eczema, erythema multiforme, herpes simplex, lupus erythematosus, dermatomyositis, Darier's disease, albinism, piebaldism, vitiligo, porphyrias, and pellagra.

HOMEOPATHIC APPROACH TO PHOTODERMATITIS AND SUNSTROKE

Homeopathic drugs having aggravation from exposure to sun are considered here.

For pigmentary disorder after exposure to the sun, Tuberculinum bovinum should be considered.

ACUTE SUNSTROKE

Aconitum napellus: Skin dry with absence of sweat. Skin may be very hot or very cold to touch. There is a sensation of itching, which is better by taking stimulants. The three characteristic symptoms that justify Aconite 1. Great anxiety. 2. Agonizing fever. 3. Restlessness.

The other symptoms are hot head, red and hot cheeks, intense thirst and burning hot palms. The patient feels better in open air and by fanning.

Amylenum nitrosum: Typical features of sun stroke. Flushing heat and drenching sweat. Throbbing sensation in the head, surging of blood to the head with fiery red face. < Heat, in a closed room, > open air, drinking cold water.

Antimonium crudum: The overall look of the antimonium crudum skin is unhealthy. It is full of various types of eruptions. Whenever a person is exposed to the sun, he develops small acne like eruptions, which are red in colour and give an appearance of insect bites. There is a sensation of itching and the skin feels sore when scratched. Also the solar dermatitis of Ant-c. may come up due to suppression of eruptions or ulcers in the past. The solar dermatitis is commonly associated with gastric derangement and there is a tendency for the patient to develop (1) pimples, (2) vesicles (3) corns, (4) urticaria, etc.

Arnica montana: Dry, red, oedematous skin. Red spots on the extremities, on exposure to the sun. There is intense pricking or itching which moves from place to place after scratching. There is a tendency for the patient to develop acne or crops of boils.

Belladonna: Hot, dry and scarlet red, smooth and shiny skin. Fever and headache may accompany it. On exposure to sun, the patient may develop the following complaints throbbing, hammering headache, < temples < motion. Redness of conjunctiva with photophobia. Dry hot mouth, great thirst for cold water.

Cactus grandiflorus: On exposure to sun there is a troublesome itching as of a fleabite. The other concomitants symptoms being compressive dull pain in the head, face red and bloated.

Camphora officinalis: Skin becomes dry, hot, parchment like on solar exposure. It can occur after suppression of eruptions. Typical head symptoms develop as a concomitant to solar dermatitis. They are – throbbing pain in the occipital region, head feels knotted up. The ear lobes are red and hot to touch. There is a sensation of coldness with burning thirst.

Carbo vegetabilis: Burning sensation in various areas of the skin with an itching sensation. The skin becomes raw and sore when scratched. The other concomitant symptoms could be :

- Cold sweat on the forehead.
- Head hot with cold extremities.
- Compressive heavy headache < occiput.
- Face cold with cold sweat.
- Rancid loud eructations with increased flatulence.
- Burning sensation in various places.

Gelsemium sempervirens: On exposure to the sun there is an extreme red discolouration of the face and neck. The skin is hot and dry. There is a sensation of itching all over the body. The other concomitant symptoms are :

- Dull heavy pain over the occiput to over the eyes.
- Blood rushes to the head.
- Heavy drooping eyelids with diplopia.
- Face dusky red, tongue heavy and numb.
- Thirstlessness.
- Cold hands and feet.
- Gastric and nervous complaints.

Glonoinum: On exposure to the sun, the patient develops itching all over, especially on the extremities. The other concomitants are as follows:

- Violent pulsations, ebullitions, blood rushes upwards.
- Eyes protrude, look wild.
- Flushed hot face.
- Violent palpitations with profuse perspiration especially on face and chest.

Ilex paraguaiensis: It is said to be a prophylactic against sunstroke.

Natrium carbonicum: Dry, rough skin, cracked in places. The skin has a tendency to sweat easily. On exposure to sun, there is a sensation of itching all over the body as from fleas. Solar dermatitis is associated with both gastric and nervous symptoms. Other concomitant symptoms are:

- Vertigo and headache from slightest exposure to sun.
- Weak digestion < slightest error in diet.
- Weak ankles.

Opium: There is absolute dryness of skin. On exposure to sun, it turns red. There is a sensation of itching with formation of red blotches after scratching. There is a sensation of heat all over the body with hot sweat. The other concomitants are:

- Drowsy, stuporous condition, internal dryness.
- Rush of blood to head with throbbing arteries.
- Ill effects of suppressed discharges.
- Ailments from exposure to sun.

Veratrum album: On exposure to sun, patient develops bluish eruptions and rash over the body especially on face and hands. The skin is cold to touch. Other concomitants are:

- Ill effects of suppressed exanthemata.
- Sensation of a lump of ice under vertex.
- Craving for ice water.
- Violent retching with cutting colic.
- Cramps in limbs with rapid prostration.

Veratrum viride: On exposure to sun, itching of different parts of body. There is a burning sensation, which follows scratching. The skin maybe cold and moist or hot and burning to touch. Other concomitants are:

- Vertigo with nausea and sudden prostration.
- Eyes blood shot.
- Face flushed, livid and turgid.
- Very thirsty but drinks little.
- Slow heavy breathing.

CHRONIC EFFECTS OF SUNSTROKE

Natrium carbonicum: Refer Therapeutics of Solar Dermatitis.

Lachesis mutus: Intense itching almost driving to distraction mostly at night but also paroxysms in daytime; often changing to a severe, burning, stinging sensation. The skin is dry and burning. There may be a tendency for the patient to develop multiple swellings with a purplish hue. There may be presence of purpuric spots. The other characteristic symptoms are as follows:

- Mentally the patient is loquacious, suspicious and jealous.
- There is a sensation of heat in the vertex with flushes.
- There is a tendency to hemorrhages in various parts of the body.
- The symptoms develop in sleep and patient wakes up from symptoms; at any time at day or night.
- Sensation of choking in the throat.

FOR BAD EFFECTS OF SUNBURN

Bufo rana: Blisters on palm and soles. Bullae bursts, leaves raw surface with ichorous discharge. Itching and burning. Patches of skin lose sensation.

Cantharis vesicatoria: Burning, scalding with rawness and smarting, better by cold applications followed by inflammation, bleb formation, eruption with mealy scales.

Chapter-14

Pruritus

Introduction

The Hindustani equivalent for pruritus is 'Kharash' or 'Khujli'.

It is a sensation exclusive to the skin and may be defined as the sensation that produces the desire to scratch. It is a symptom, and scratch marks are its sign.

Pathophysiology

The exact mode in which pruritus is produced still remains obscure.

It has been suggested that these sensations arise in fine unmyelinated C nerve fibre endings in the sub epidermal area and are then transmitted via the lateral spinothalamic tract to the thalamus and sensory cortex. That is why comatose patients itch and people scratch in dreams. Central itch mechanisms are as important as peripheral cutaneous mediators.

Pathophysiology of pruritus still eludes satisfactory explanation and understanding. Histamine, kinins and certain proteases (and enzymes) whether introduced from outside or liberated as a consequence of antigen-antibody reaction evoke pruritus.

Etiology

Physical and Physiological

- Rough clothing, wool next to skin, tight clothes.
- Heat, cold, dryness, humidity. Hot and cold baths also produce itching.
- An unclean body, dirt and dust accumulations in the absence of frequent bathing.
- Hot, spicy food and alcohol cause cutaneous flushing.

Pruritic Dermatoses (skin disease)

- Winter itch.
- Animal parasites: scabies, pediculosis, insect bites, flees, bugs, mosquitoes, etc.
- Ringworm.
- Dermatitis and eczema.
- Urticaria, angioneurotic edema.
- Lichen planus.
- Neurodermatitis – localized and disseminated.
- Prurigo simplex, nodularis, atopic.
- Psoriasis patients itch in tropical climate.
- Mycosis fungoides and reticuloses.
- Erythrodermal.
- Prickly heat.
- Dermatitis herpetiformis.
- Local stasis, Schamberg's disease.

Local irritation by discharges, etc.

Systemic disorders producing itching, but perhaps no skin lesion

- Hepatic diseases (especially obstructive), hepatitis C (with or without evidence of jaundice or liver failure).

- Renal failure (uremic pruritus).
- Hypothyroidism and hyperthyroidism.
- Iron deficiency anemia.
- Intestinal parasites – intestinal worms, trichiniasis, onchocerciasis.
- Polycythemia vera.
- Malignant lymphoma (especially Hodgkin's disease), leukemias, myeloma, internal malignancies, carcinoid.
- Multiple sclerosis.
- Neuropsychiatric diseases (anorexia nervosa).
- Diabetes, myxedema.
- Drugs – morphia, cocaine, barbiturates.
- Senility.
- Pregnancy and oral contraceptives.
- Internal malignancy.

Psychogenic

- Neurasthenia.
- Neurodermatitis.
- Acarophobia.
- Prurigo.

Clinical Features

It is a very annoying condition inferring with daily activities thus causing social problems.

The intensity of itching excited by a stimulus varies with the sensitivity of the skin and the mind, from person to person. Tramps, for instance, hardly feel mosquito bites, people with morbid minds, on the other hand, may start scratching at a mere suggestion.

The skin and nervous system are closely related because of their common origin in embryo; for this reason mental stress cannot only start itching but also complicate several skin disorders, especially pruritus.

Threshold of pruritus is lowered in thin-skinned individuals under emotional stress and loneliness. People prone to sense of heat are more prone to pruritus.

Itching may be elicited by many normally occurring stimuli such as light touch, temperature change and emotional stress. Chemical, mechanical, thermal and electrical stimuli may also elicit itching.

Consequences of Itching

Local

- Scratch marks.
- Broken hair.
- Excoriations.
- Polished nails.
- May be secondary pyoderma.
- Eczematization and even ulceration.
- Lichenification.
- Pigmentation and even depigmentation.

General

- Interference with physical and social activities.
- Irritability.
- Insomnia.
- Exhaustion and wasting.

Treatment

The treatment in general consists of:

- Eliminating the cause.
- Removing exciting factors. The patients must be properly clothed; avoid sudden changes of temperature; indulge in luke warm baths; take simple blend food, avoid excess of tea, coffee and alcohol. The bowels must be kept open.
- Reassurance.

The details of various skin dermatoses where itching is a principle symptom are mentioned under the respective conditions. Here we shall study certain conditions that do not fall under any specific category.

WINTER PRURITUS

Other names given to this condition are asteatotic eczema, eczema craquele, pruritus hiemalis and xerotic eczema.

It implies itching in the cold winter months in certain individuals; the itching disappears with the onset of the warm weather; other known causes of pruritis are absent. It is characterized by generalized body pruritus that is usually more severe on the arms and shins. The skin is dry, and fine flakes are often generalized, but the condition tends to spare the face, scalp, groin and axillae. The pretibial areas are particularly susceptible and may exhibit fine cracks in the eczematous areas that resemble cracks in old porcelain dishes (eczema craquele).

Itching occurs mostly on undressing. Exposure to cold weather is the precipitating cause, though dry skin, a run-down condition; the use of strong alkaline soaps, a very cold or very hot bath and woolen clothes tend to cause pruritus. Frequent and lengthy bathing with plenty of soap during wintertime is the most frequent cause. This is especially prevalent in elderly persons, whose skin has decreased rate of repair of the epidermal water barrier. Low humidity in overheated rooms during cold water contributes to this condition.

Treatment

The treatment consists in correcting the exciting and predisposing causes. It consists of educating the patient regarding the factors responsible, using soap only in the axilla and the inguinal area, and lubrication of the skin immediately after bathing with bath oils, clothing the body suitably and improving the general health.

F- 12

SUMMER PRURITUS

It is a fairly common compliant during the summer months in the hotter parts of tropical countries. In Northern India, it is seen in between the months of April and August, but it occurs in the worst form during the monsoon. Dry heat frequently causes pruritis, but the other more common causes are profuse perspiration, which results in clothes sticking to the body; dusty environment; uncleanliness; heat spots and prickly heat. Common in people who are overweight and overclothed for the climate.

Treatment

The treatment should lay emphasis on correcting the responsible causes, improving the general health of the patient, and encouraging him to use thin clothing, to live and work in cool hygienic environments. Air-conditioning, if possible, is very helpful. A talcum dusting powder massage is also beneficial. For an extreme case, a holiday at a cool hill station is the answer.

SENILE PRURITUS

Strictly speaking, the term implies generalized itching in elderly people, usually past the age of 50 or 60, with senile, atrophic, dry skin; itching is precipitated by rough or woolen clothing, sudden changes in temperature, baths, etc. The other known causes of pruritis and itching dermatoses are absent. Though itching becomes generalized sooner or later, to begin with, it may be confined to the trunk or the lower extremities. The course is usually progressive and the outlook is rather poor.

Treatment

• Massage with olive oil, Nivea cream (P) or pure animal fat like butter or ghee, olive oil and Calendula mixture in a 1:6 ratio.

• Protection from exciting physical causes.

PRURITUS ANI

It may occur as such, or be associated with pruritus vulvae and scrotum. It is often centered in the anal or the genital area.

It is a fairly common complaint seen as simple pruritus with a sodden anal skin, but sooner or later, sequelae of pruritus like excoriations, pyoderma, lichenification and eczematization develop to complicate matters. Pruritus ani is commoner in males than females, common in Asiatic countries because of heat and perspiration causing maceration, frequent gastrointestinal disorders, hot spicy food and the high incidence of intestinal worms, etc.

Anal neurodermatitis is characterized by paroxysms of violent itching where the patient may tear at the affected area until bleeding is induced.

Fissures and white sodden epidermis characterize mycotic pruritus ani.

Etiology

Local (inside anus)

- Threadworms.
- Fissure in ano, hemorrhoids, polyp, and fistula.
- Moist anus due to improper cleansing after bowel movements.
- Chronic constipation or diarrhea.
- Hot spicy or sensitizing foods.
- Use of cathartics

Anatomical factors

- Leakage of rectal mucus onto perineal skin

Skin diseases

- Tinea, monilial infection, intertrigo.
- Condylomalata and acuminatum.
- Seborrheic dermatitis.

- Psoriasis, eczema.
- Pediculoses.
- Lichen sclerosis et atrophious.
- Contact dermatitis to toilet paper, enemas.

Systemic

- Diabetes.
- Use of antibiotics and other drugs.
- Achlorhydria.
- Reticuloses.
- Senility.

Psychogenic – Neurodermatitis

- Spread of pruritus from vulval region in conditions like diabetes, leucorrhea or pelvic tumors.

Diagnosis

Patient must be subjected to a thorough examination and investigation to establish the cause. Firstly, cutaneous diseases and the possibility of pruritus having spread from neighbouring areas must be ruled out. If both these causes are absent, the GIT must be completely investigated by history taking, repeated stool examination, a rectal swab, a proctoscopic examination etc. Only when no etiological factor is identified, may primary psychogenic causes be considered as producing the neurodermatitis.

Treatment

- Reassurance.
- Meticulous toilet care should be followed no matter what the cause of the itching. After defecation, the anal area should be cleansed with soft cellulose tissue paper, and whenever possible washed with mild soap and water. Cleansing with wet toilet tissue is advisable in all cases.
- Eradication of causes – the diet should be simple, light and

wholesome. All indigestible foodstuffs, chillies, condiments, curries and alcohol must be withheld. Anal region should be lubricated with oil at bath time.

- The affected area must be kept clean, cool and dry. Underwear should be cotton and loose.

PRURITUS OF THE SCROTUM AND PENIS

The scrotum of an adult is relatively immune to dermatophyte infection, but is a favorite site for circumscribed neurodermatitis. It is fairly common complaint in young or middle aged persons in tropical countries.

Lichenification may result, be extreme, and persists for many years.

Etiology

PRURITUS ON PENIS

- Glycosuria.
- Hepes progenitalis.
- Pediculoses, scabies.
- Contact dermatitis due to contraceptives, pessaries etc.
- Irritation by vaginal discharges.
- Prostatic affections.
- Neurodermatitis.
- Spread of itching from neighbouring areas, other cutaneous diseases, etc.

PRURITUS ON SCROTUM

- Scabies, pediculoses.
- Contact dermatitis due to contraceptives, irritation by vaginal discharges etc.

- Excessive sweating.
- Intertrigo starts at the junction of the penis with the scrotum.
- Chaffing by underwear, loin cloth or suspendory bandage.
- Tinea cruris.
- Nutritional deficiency.
- Use of broad-spectrum antibiotics.
- Neurodermatitis.
- Spread of itching from neighbouring areas and other cutaneous diseases including sebaceous cysts.

Treatment

Treatment is similar to that employed in pruritus vulvae and ani.

PRURITUS VULVAE

It is also a common cause for pruritus of different causes. It is a counter part of pruritus scroti, and the same mechanisms may be responsible.

Itching may either be confined to the vulval skin or include the vaginal walls and urethral orifice. Excoriations, lichenification, eczematization and pyoderma soon complicate simple pruritus. It is common in married women, 30-35 years of age. Occasionally it occurs in children and adolescents.

Etiology

Cutaneous diseases of the vulval region

- Scabies.
- Pediculoses.
- Tinea.
- Contact dermatitis due to contraceptives, douches, pessaries, medicated sanitary pads, toilet paper and local medicaments.
- Lichen planus.

- Psoriasis.
- Herpes progenitalis.
- Intertrigo, infective eczema, seborrheic dermatitis.
- Lichen sclerosus et atrophicus, leukoplakia.
- Senile vulvitis and kraurosis vulvae.
- Filariasis – elephantiasis and schistosomiasis.
- Lymphogranuloma venereum causing esthiomene.
- Fox Fordyce's disease.

Local causes in the vaginal and urinary tract

- Vaginal discharge – monilial or trichomonas infection.
- Cystitis, vaginitis and cervicitis.
- Acid urine and urinary incontinence.
- Urethral stones.
- Pregnancy and pelvic congestion.

Spread from neighbouring areas

- Anus – threadworms and pruritus ani (other causes).
- Thighs – tinea, intertrigo, etc.

Systemic disorders

- Diabetes.
- Drug eruptions, especially antibiotics.
- Achlorhydria.
- Senility.
- Liver disease.
- Malignancy.
- Reticulosis.

Psychogenic

- Neurodermatitis due to sexual frustration, perversion sex, guilt, fear of venereal disease.

Diagnosis

A complete examination should be made of the skin of the vulval region for cutaneous disease and also of the urogenital tract, the anus and the neighbouring regions.

Routine investigations include examination of urine for sugar and acidity; of stools for ova and vaginal discharge for infective flora. Though mental and emotional factors are responsible for a great deal of chronic pruritus vulvae (both primarily and secondarily), physical organic causes must first be excluded. The help of a psychoanalyst and a social worker may prove useful in tracking down the psychogenic causes.

Prognosis

Pruritus vulvae can be most distressing; in a small percentage of cases, it becomes an obstinate complaint.

Treatment

The basic principles of treatment are almost the same as those applied in general pruritus and pruritus ani. They consist of

- Reassurance, particularly about the absence of cancer and other contagious diseases.
- Keeping the affected part clean, dry and lubricated.

PRURITUS IN PREGNANCY

Besides, the usual causes of pruritus, there is a small group of dermatoses, characterized by pruritic papules and urticarial plagues that occur predominantly, if not exclusively during pregnancies, clearing up on delivery and recurrence with subsequent pregnancies. These conditions now number nine and of these four stand out as distinct entities either because their mechanism of production is now elucidated (Herpes gestatious, pruritus gravidarum, auto-immune progesterone dermatitis of pregnancy) or because of unique clinical and laboratory findings (impetigo herpetiformis).

HOMEOPATHIC APPROACH TO PRURITUS

Some Important Therapeutic Hints

- Pruritus vulvae washing the affected area 4-5 times a day with mentha piperata mother tincture diluted in water is adviced.

- Senile pruritus Baryta aceticum and Fagopyrum esculentum are important drugs to be kept in mind.

- Pruritus due to renal failure Hippuricum acidum is an important drug found useful in practice.

- Pruritus due to herpes of the genitalia herpes virus type I should be potentized and be used in the 30th potency.

Some Important Homeopathic Remedies

Aethusa cynapium: Pimples on vulva – itching < warmth or patient becoming warm.

Aloe socotrina: Itching and burning in anus preventing sleep. Itching of prepuce and legs. Itching of the urethral orifice; pruritus vaginae; itching in eyelids, anus, scrotum and shoulders. Rough skin all over the body.

Alumina: Intolerable itching over whole body, especially when getting warm in bed, scratches till the skin bleeds, which is then painful; itching piles, with burning excoriation and great sensitiveness; itching, throbbing and stitches in vagina.

Ambra grisea: Voluptuous itching on scrotum; severe itching on pudenda, must rub parts, swelling of labia; pruritus vulva during pregnancy.

Ammonium carbonicum: Violent itching of skin, after scratching burning blisters appear; itching and stinging of skin keep him awake; though lessened by scratching; itching and burning at anus; itching at genitals.

Antimonium crudum: Itching of skin, feels sore as if scratched; itching of penis, of tip of glans; biting, itching, as from salt on left side of scrotum.

Antimonium tartaricum: Violent itching of pudenda, pustules on external genitals.

Argentum metallicum: Intolerable itching as from crawling, on head and body, unchanged by scratching, even motion of skin is almost unbearable; pruritus scroti.

Argentum nitricum: Itching smarting mostly on thighs and axillae, when warm in bed; skin brown, tense and hard.

Arsenicum album: Itching with burning or an eruption emitting watery fluid like sweat and attended with much constitutional weakness; chronic cases; senile pruritus in broken down constitutions < from cold applications > from warmth; itching of genital organs.

Caladium seguinum: Pruritus vulvae during pregnancy and after miscarriage; pruritus vaginae induces onanism, with mucus discharge and pimples around parts; violent itching on external genitals compelled her to scratch in spite of punishment, reduced her in mind and body; violent itching on scrotum, < at night, dry and scaly, violent corrosive itching, burning, must touch parts, but cannot scratch there, no swelling, but much heat, in face frequent sensation as if a fly were crawling there > from cold water.

Calcarea carbonica: Itching and stitches in internal or external vulva < towards evening or after going to bed; severe itching on various parts of body in bed; violent irritation about chest, back, neck and shoulders, in calves of legs, followed by a reddish rash < at night.

Cantharis vesicatoria: Pruritus vulvae, especially from masturbation, itching intense; pruritis, with strong sexual desire, during climaxis; itching changing place; as from fleas.

Causticum: Itching over whole body at various parts, on tips and wings of nose, face, scrotum, back, arms, palms, dorsum of feet, preventing sleep; itching of orifice of urethra, scrotum, skin of penis.

Chelidonium majus: Itching of skin, crawling and itching in rectum and on perineum; sticking and itching in anus; itching and creeping in scrotum and glans.

Coffea cruda: Voluptuous itching, would like to scratch, but parts are too sensitive, the least itching prevents sleep.

Collinsonia canadensis: Pruritus vulvae with hemorrhoids, obstinate constipation during dysmenorrhea or in pregnancy < when lying down, parts swollen and bulging, itching intolerable, making her almost delirious > by bathing in cold water.

Conium maculatum: Violent itching of pudenda and even within vagina day and night < just after menstruation; erratic itching of all parts of body, as from fleas.

Croton tiglium: Frequent corrosive itching on glans and scrotum < while walking; intense itching of female genitals, < at night > by very gentle scratching; eruptions on body itch very much, cannot bear severe scratching but a mere rub suffices to allay the itching.

Cuprum aceticum and Cuprum arsenicosum: Skin sensitive to contact with clothing; itching especially of arms and legs < undressing at night and in bed, with slight relief only from scratching of coarse rubbing; sleep disturbed and unrefreshing; pruritus ani; scrotum constantly moist.

Dolichos pruriens: Intolerable itching all over body in pregnant women < at night preventing sleep and from scratching, no perceptible eruption on skin, constipation, and jaundice. Itching without eruption, first on feet every winter higher up, after 7 years reaches upto abdomen.

Euphorbium officinarum: Itching of mons veneris; burning, itching in different parts which induces scratching.

Ferrum metallicum: Pruritus recti, he cannot sleep at night; worms creep out of anus at night.

Fluoricum acidum: Itching within and around anus, on perineum.

Graphites: Pruritus ani; with moisture and tendency to form little vesicles; itching in vulva, < just before menses (Con. after menses), especially for persons inclined to obesity; continuous itching < at night, nothing visible upon skin before scratching, which causes nodules and long welts.

Hamamelis virginiana: Itching at anus, which feels sore, as if raw; pruritus of female parts; soreness and smarting on small spots, not very sensitive to touch.

Helonias dioica: Excessive pruritus vulvae, which is puffed, hot red and itching terribly; labia swollen and covered with a curdy, white deposit like aphthae; leucorrhea of bad odor, easily changing to flow of blood.

Hepar sulphur: Itching of penis and at fraenum preputic; smarting itching of vulva, little pimples around ulcer, with leucorrhea; burning itching of body, with white vesicles after scratching; unhealthy skin, slight injuries suppurate.

Hydrastis canadensis: Pruritus vulvae with profuse leucorrhea and sexual excitement.

Ignatia amara: Itching of skin of a fine pricking character resembling flea bites and changing from one place to another; itching > gentle scratching, < getting heated in open air.

Iodium: Papules that are very apt to run together or around which the skin is brownish and scaly; irresistible nocturnal itching, compelling one to scratch and thus causing insomnia, cachectic appearance emaciation and dyspepsia.

Kalium carbonicum: Furious itching in the region of mons veneris; burning itching herpes. Moist after scratching (Kali-br.).

Kreosotum: Itching towards evening so violent as to drive one almost wild; soreness and smarting between labia and vulva, offensive discharges.

Lachesis mutus: Itching at anus, < after sleep; burning itching of whole body with yellow or purplish blisters.

Lac caninum: Slight excoriation and itching of the external labia, feels at times as if caused by something alive in it, crawling about and itching terribly; same sensation on shoulders and neck, occasionally on hands, < towards evening < when warm.

Ledum palustre: Violent itching on dorsum of ankles and feet, especially at night < after scratching; itching rash on wrist joint, all of them much < in warmth of bed.

Lilium tigrinum: Pruritus most marked after menses (Con.); voluptuous itching in vagina with fullness in parts; stinging in left ovarian region.

Lycopodium clavatum: Diurnal itching (Nat-m.), biting itching when becoming warm during day; itching eruption at anus, painful to touch; itching of inner surface of prepuce.

Magnesium muriaticum: Itching on genitals and scrotum, extending to anus, formication over whole body < while sitting > exercise and motion.

Mercurius solubilis: Moist, itch-like eruption on hand, with rhagades, < at night; when warm in bed, zoster with itching and tendency to suppurate.

Mezereum: Inveterate cases with unbearable nocturnal itching burning, especially in parts where there is very little fat deposited < evening and from warmth; general coldness and twitching of the subcutaneous muscles; burning sensation changes place after scratching.

Muriaticum acidum: Itching of scrotum not relieved by scratching; organs weak, penis relaxed.

Natrium muriaticum: Diurnal itching (Lyc.); itching, soreness and moisture between scrotum and thighs, pus like smegma on glans; itching and crawling sensation at the corona glandis; leucorrhea causes itching with yellow complexion; itching of female external parts, with falling off the hair; itching of skin but no rash (Dolichos pruriens) after violent exercise.

Natrium sulphuricum: Itching < undressing, between scrotum and right thigh, small scabs, itching better by scratching, also on forehead, scalp, neck, chest, sycosis.

Nitricum acidum: History of syphilis or psora, skin around anus dry and cracked, with tendency to bleed from scratching; and fissure; falling off of the hair from genitals; itching, swelling, and burning of vulva and vagina; itching of shins, bleeding when scratched, small scales form; skin dark, dirty.

Oleander: Itching of skin when undressing (Nat-s.); after stool itching and burning in rectum and anus; skin sensitive all over, the mere friction of the clothing makes it sore, raw and painful.

Opium: Redness and itching of skin very troublesome all over, fine pricking, rarely sensitive to touch.

Petroleum: Itching humid herpes on scrotum between scrotum and thighs, on perineum, soreness and moisture on female genitals, with violent itching; itching herpes, followed by ulcers.

Platinum metallicum: Furious itching inside of uterus, pruritus vulvae, voluptuous tingling with anxiety and palpitation of heart (Coff.), sensation of soreness, tingling, smarting, itching, burning, with inclination to scratch on different parts of the body.

Psorinum: Pruritus from amenorrhea, with phthisis, during pregnancy, pimples, itching violently about nipples, oozing a fluid; itching between fingers; heat and itching of soles; body itches intolerably < in bed and from warmth; scratches until it bleeds, which relieves.

Pulsatilla pratensis: Itching and burning on inner and upper side of prepuce; itching < at night from pastry or pork, < from delayed menses > from cold water, pruritus senilis.

Rhododendron chrysanthum: Itching and sweat on scrotum, soreness between scrotum and thighs.

Rumex crispus: Itching < by cold > warmth, more formication than burning, chiefly < when undressing < by every exposure to cold air < uncovering. Intense itching especially lower extremities.

Silicea terra: Prurigo formicans, during night itching sensation as if ants were crawling over the skin; itching humid spots on genitals, mostly on scrotum, sweat on scrotum; itching at pudendum; itching of soles, driving to despair.

Staphysagria: Pruritus genitalium in newly married people, with frequent urging to urinate; voluptuous itching of scrotum; stinging itching vulva.

Sulphur: Voluptuous itching burning < evenings and in bed; chronic cases with itching, burning, stinging at anus < after scratching.

Tarentula hispanica: Intense pruritus of vulva and vagina < nights, with dryness and heat of the parts.

Teucrium marum verum: Cannot sleep on account of the intense itching of the anus, causing him to toss and roll at night.

Zincum metallicum: Crawling in skin of whole body, < only by rubbing, frequent violent itching as from fleabites especially on back and abdomen, < at night, excessive itching during menses, inducing masturbation with fidgety lower extremities (Canth-masturbation); itching in bends of joints; sudden itching here and there, in bed at night, goes off by contact.

REPERTORY

For repertory refer the chapter on 'Dermatitis and eczema' and under respective conditions where itching is a principle symptom.

■

Chapter-15

Dermatitis and Eczema

Introduction

Both the terms 'dermatitis' and 'eczema' can be used interchangeably, since in both the conditions the various types of lesions have similar morphological and histopathological features.

Definition

'Eczema' or 'dermatitis' is defined as an inflammation of the epidermis and the superficial layer of the dermis, caused by a wide range of external and internal factors, resulting in redness, itching, swelling, scaling, oozing and formation of clustered papulo-vesicles.

Incidence

Eczema is one of the most commonly seen skin disorders by a practicing physician, where the lesions tend to disseminate and spread rapidly and distantly from its point of origin.

'Atopic eczema' is seen most frequently in infants and young children, where the lesions are especially seen on the hands and around the mouth. This condition is seen very rarely in the elderly age group.

Other eczematous lesions seen most commonly in children are – lichen striatus, juvenile plantar dermatosis, pompholyx, seborrheic dermatitis of infancy, and napkin dermatitis. Pompholyx is rarely seen in the elderly group.

Discoid eczema is a condition seen especially in the elderly males, especially in the winter season. Also, asteatotic eczema of the legs is another condition seen most frequently in this age group.

Contact dermatitis becomes less common with advancing age.

Histopathology

In the 'acute stages' of this condition one finds interstitial epidermal edema (called as spongiosis), which leads to stretching and eventual rupture of the intercellular attachments, with the formation of microvesicles. There is also a variable infiltration of the epidermis and superficial dermis by lymphocytes.

In the 'subacute stage', there is less of spongiosis, and more of thickening of the stratum malpighii (termed as acanthosis), and parakeratosis, with the formation of a horny layer.

In the 'chronic stage', there is marked acanthosis, with elongation and broadening of rete ridges, and hyperkeratosis. There is then more of lichenification.

Vascular dilatation in the dermis is marked in all stages, where especially the papillary vessels are involved. In chronic stages with lichenification, the vessels may become tortuous.

Pathogenesis

The pathogenesis of eczematous cases is usually not very clearly understood as yet, especially for the endogenous variety.

There has been some understanding of the contact dermatitis; where, in the chronic irritant types, there seems to be a disturbed barrier function and increased epidermal cell turnover leading to lichenification; whereas, in the acute irritant contact dermatitis, there is an inflammatory reaction, with release of inflammatory mediators and cytokines.

Classification

This disease condition of the skin can be divided into two major types, depending on the cause. The first one is 'Exogenous eczemas' where there is a definite external or environmental trigger factor for the condition, and where genetic influence plays a minor role. The second is the 'Endogenous eczemas', where the eczema results not from some exogenous factor, but occurs due to some constitutional or genetic factors, where there are internal precipitating factors or processes responsible for the condition.

Though these two form the two major types of this condition, in a few cases one can observe that both internal and external factors may be responsible.

A few conditions under each of the main types are:

- Exogenous Eczema
    - Contact dermatitis.
    - Infectious eczematoid.
- Endogenous Eczema
    - Atopic dermatitis.
    - Seborrheic dermatitis.
    - Discoid eczema.
    - Pompholyx.
    - Gravitational eczema.
    - Lichen simplex chronicus dermatitis.

CONTACT DERMATITIS

Introduction

Contact dermatitis is an inflammatory response of the skin to an antigen or irritant, which causes a lot of itching and discomfort to the patient. It is the one of the most common skin conditions seen among those working in factories.

Incidence

This condition can affect individuals of all ages, though it is most commonly seen in adults. The allergic variety of contact dermatitis is seen especially in the elderly age group, where there is more frequent use of topical medication; and in infants, due to the use of diapers.

Etiopathogenesis

The causes of contact dermatitis are classified according to the mechanism of response.

ALLERGIC CONTACT DERMATITIS

This is a cell-mediated, Type IV, delayed hypersensitivity reaction, which results from specific antigens penetrating the epidermal layer of the skin. The antigen combines with a protein mediator and travels to the dermis, where the T lymphocyte becomes sensitized. On the next presentation of the antigen, the allergic reaction takes place.

- Contributing factors include genetics, concentration and duration of exposure, and the presence of other skin diseases.

- The most common allergens are Adhesive of bindi, airborne contact allergens (pollens, cement, wood dust, etc.), cosmetics, deodorants and perfumes, elastic garments, ethylenediamine (dyes, medications), formaldehyde, kum-kum, leather and rubber used in footwear, nickel and cobalt (present in the various metal alloys used, e.g. hair clips, bands, earrings, bangles, rings, necklaces, strap of the watch, etc.), paraphenylenediamine (hair dyes, photographic chemicals), plants of the Toxicodendron genus (e.g., poison ivy, poison oak, poison sumac), potassium dichromate (cements, household cleansers), and thiram (fungicides).

IRRITANT CONTACT DERMATITIS (ICD)

Irritant contact dermatitis occurs as a result of a direct local cytotoxic effect of an irritant on the cells of the epidermis, with a subsequent inflammatory response in the dermis. It is caused by non-immune mechanisms as opposed to allergic contact dermatitis.

Chemicals (like acids, alkalis, cleansers, soaps, detergents, organic solvents, phenols, and oxidants), plants (like chillies, citrus fruits, garlic and tobacco), and certain medications (like benzoyl peroxide and retinoic acid) are all also known to cause it. The severity of the reaction is related to the amount and the duration of exposure to the irritant.

PHOTODERMATITIS

This condition is caused by an interaction between a certain chemical substance (topically applied or systemically given) and solar radiation (ultraviolet or visible light).

This results in the transformation of the substance into:

- Allergens, which means that the person is already sensitized to the substance. This is termed as 'photoallergic contact dermatitis' (immunological); OR

- Irritants, which affects a majority of people, where there is no sensitization involved. This is termed as 'phototoxic' (non-immunological).

Medicines (especially sulphonamides, phenothiazines, several NSAID's tetracycline, quinine, and some sunscreen agents), dyes, tars (especially tar products used in wood preservation), cadmium sulphate (used in tattoos), musk perfumes, and plants [especially the Rutaceae (Rue and citrus fruits) family, Moraceae (fig) family, Umbelliferae (parsnip, celery) family, and Leguminosae family] are known to cause photodermatitis after exposure to light.

Histopathology

The changes are similar to the ones explained earlier, in addition to which the following points can be noted.

'Primary irritant dermatitis' occurs due to direct injury to the skin, due to exposure to specific irritants and is known to usually produce some discomfort immediately following the exposure or contact.

'Allergic contact dermatitis' only tends to affect individuals who are already previously sensitized to a contactant. It is a delayed hypersensitivity reaction, where the symptoms are manifested after a few hours, during which time the cellular immune reaction takes place.

Clinical Features

The symptoms of all the types of contact dermatitis are almost the same, though the inflammatory response can be categorized into acute, subacute and chronic phases.

- In 'acute' contact dermatitis, clear fluid filled vesicles or bullae appear on a bright red and edematous skin. As the lesions break, the skin becomes exudative and discharges a clear fluid, which then leads to crust formation.

- 'Subacute' contact dermatitis is characterized by less edema, more scaling, and the formation of papules.

- In 'chronic' contact dermatitis there is minimal edema, marked scaling, lichenification (thickening of skin with prominent marking), fissuring and hyperpigmentation.

The differentiation of the various types of contact dermatitis usually occurs in terms of the history, site and type of exposure to the contactant.

ALLERGIC CONTACT DERMATITIS

Acute cases of 'allergic contact dermatitis' develop lesions with intense itching, erythema and swelling within 1-4 day's time of exposure to the allergen. The area where the lesions occur the most is probably the site of the causative allergic exposure. In chronic cases of allergic dermatitis, the skin becomes dry, scaly and thick; later on followed by lichenification and fissuring.

IRRITANT CONTACT DERMATITIS

When the causative factor includes mild irritants, there is prolonged or repeated exposure required before an inflammation is noted. Whereas in cases where strong irritants like strong acids and alkalis are the causative factors, there is an immediate reaction, which can be similar to a thermal burn. There can be redness, stinging, smarting, burning, or sensations of dryness and tightness, and chapping. Irritants may also penetrate skin via appendageal structures and cause folliculitis and other types of reaction.

Although the nature, concentration and duration of contact with the irritant chemical are of primary importance, mechanical, thermal, climatic and constitutional factors are important modifying and/or enhancing factors in many irritant responses.

Two common varieties of contact dermatitis are:

• Housewife's eczema caused by prolonged and repeated contact with soaps, detergents, water and a few vegetables (chillies, garlic, etc.). The hands are most often affected, especially the fingers and its webs. Preventive measure consists in using gloves to avoid direct contact with irritant.

• Diaper dermatitis occurs in infants due to prolonged occlusion of the pores of the skin due to use of non-absorbable plastic diapers. Additionally the ammonia caused by the action of certain microorganisms on the urine tends to cause more irritation of the part locally, which is then followed by secondary fungal or bacterial infections. The lesions occur most often on the thighs, buttocks and genitalia. Preventive and therapeutic measure consists in avoiding plastic diapers, and being careful to keep the part open, at regular intervals, to improve air circulation for better healing.

PHOTODERMATITIS

'Photodermatitis' can be diagnosed by the presence of lesions limited to the sun-exposed areas of the body. Here burning and pruritus are the main complaints.

Photo-allergic reactions can resemble sunburn, but usually simulate allergic contact dermatitis. The dermatitis is localized to exposed areas of the skin, usually with a distinct margin at the collar. The area below the chin is usually spared. The most distinctive sign is the exempt 'Wilkinson's triangle' behind the earlobe.

Phototoxic reactions resemble sunburn and are often quite severe, with erythema, oedema and bulla formation. It may be strictly limited to the area of contact, or diffuse if caused by volatile or airborne agents. Phototoxic reactions may develop as long as a week after exposure to chemicals retained in the skin.

The intensity of response to phototoxic and photo-allergic agents depends upon a number of factors, which include:

- Nature and concentration of the substance applied.
- Duration of exposure to the substance.
- Percutaneous absorption.
- Intensity and wavelength of the radiation.
- Duration of radiation exposure.
- Radiation absorption in the skin, depending on the thickness of stratum corneum as well as the amount and distribution of melanin.
- Extraneous matter and secretions on the skin.
- Humidity.

Differential Diagnosis

- Seborrheic dermatitis occurs with scaling on the scalp, eyebrows, around the alae nasi and ears, in the axillae, inguinal and anal regions.
- Psoriasis can mimic a dry scaling contact dermatitis.
- Cellulitis, erysipelas and angio-oedema of the eyelids can mimic an acute contact dermatitis.
- Dermatomyositis may be differentiated from allergic contact dermatitis by the violet hue and slightly darker shade, and the additional characteristic changes on the fingers.
- Atopic dermatitis can at times be difficult to differentiate from

allergic and irritant dermatitis; and they are also known to coexist. Dermatitis of the hands may be the first sign of atopic dermatitis in a young adult, precipitated by exposure to irritants at home or work. The finding of ichthyotic skin, wrinkled palms and a history of dermatitis in childhood or in first-degree relatives may help to establish the diagnosis.

- Tinea may have the same appearance as dermatitis, and mycological examination of scrapings should be performed, especially in cases of an unilateral hand dermatosis.

- Mycotic infections involve the hairy part of the axillae, which is usually spared in contact dermatitis.

- Papular drug eruptions or scabies may sometimes be difficult to distinguish from nickel or textile contact dermatitis.

- Generalized erythroderma may be the result of a chronic contact dermatitis maintained by continued exposure to allergens in the environment, even in hospital departments, for example contact with formaldehyde-disinfected mattresses, or bed linen impregnated with topical medicaments.

Diagnosis

- 'Patch test' done may be of some benefit to identify the contact allergen. Here a series of suspected contact allergens in standard concentration are applied over the upper back with adhesive tape and the result is read after 48 hours. The interpretation of the test is as follows:

–	Negative Reaction.
?	Doubtful reaction – Macular erythema.
+	Weak reaction – Erythema, infiltration, papules.
++	Strong reaction – Oedema, vesicles.
+++	Extreme reaction – Ulcerations, bullous lesions.
IR	Irritant reaction.

- Biopsy Pathological findings include intercellular edema and bullae.

Complications

- Secondary bacterial infections can occur.
- There can be generalized eruption secondary to autosensitization.

Prognosis

- Most contact dermatitis will resolve without intervention in 4-6 weeks if further exposure is prevented.
- Long-term success in treatment is poor if the offending agent is not identified.

INFECTIOUS ECZEMATOID DERMATITIS

Synonym

Infective eczema; Microbial eczema.

Definition & Introduction

Infective eczema is eczema which is caused by an allergic reaction to microorganisms or their products, and which clears when the organisms are eradicated.

This should be distinguished from 'infected eczema' in which eczema due to some other cause is complicated by secondary bacterial or viral invasion of the broken skin. In practice, however, the two conditions can coexist, and the distinction can be difficult.

Patches of eczema that occasionally develop around lesions of molluscum contagiosum provide a good example of infectious eczematoid dermatitis, because the pearly papules are the initiating event, and eczema can develop in the surrounding skin some days later, even when the lesions have not been scratched or traumatized. The eczema generally clears when the molluscum lesions subside. Similarly, one can also see eczematous skin occurring around infected wounds.

Histopathology

There is spongiosis with acanthosis, hyperkeratosis and patchy parakeratosis. The inflamed dermis shows polymorphonuclear and lymphocytic infiltration, which invades the epidermis to a variable extent. In some stages, subcorneal pustulation may be conspicuous.

Clinical Features

This condition usually presents as an area of advancing erythema, occasionally with microvesicles. It is seen especially around discharging wounds or ulcers, or moist skin lesions of other types. It usually occurs on the legs and can present as chronic folliculitis. It is also common in patients with venous leg ulcers, but care must be taken to distinguish it from contact dermatitis due to the application of topical medicaments.

Differential Diagnosis

- Infected eczema shows marked erythema, exudation and crust formation. There can be accumulation of layers of somewhat greasy, moist scales, beneath which the surface is raw and red. The margin is characteristically sharply defined with small pustules at the advancing edge. In cases where a flexure is involved, there is formation of a deep and persistent fissure.

- Microbial eczema of the feet is a condition that predominantly involves the interdigital spaces on the dorsum of the medial toes. It occurs in patients who maintain a poor standard of hygiene, or in those who wear a closed shoe inspite of perspiring a lot from their feet.

- Tinea pedis can become eczematous due to the over-growth of Gram-negative organisms.

Diagnosis

The presence of an increased level of C-reactive protein in the blood may offer a useful clue to diagnosis and differentiation of this condition from infected eczematous cases.

ATOPIC DERMATITIS

Introduction

The word 'atopy' literally means 'out of place', and it represents an inherited tendency in a person that predisposes him to develop atopic dermatitis, asthma or hay fever.

Definition

Atopic dermatitis (also termed as 'Atopic eczema') is a chronic or chronically relapsing, inflammatory, pruritic skin condition of unknown etiology. The condition is a very distressful one, characterized by very itchy papules or vesicles, which become excoriated and lichenified, with raised serum IgE levels. It usually begins in infancy, and is associated with personal and/or family history of other atopic condition, and a typical distribution and morphology.

Incidence

This condition is seen in both sexes equally, but females are known to have a poor prognosis.

Approximately 60% of patients will have their first outbreak by age 1 and 90% by age 5. The onset of atopic dermatitis in adolescence or later is uncommon and should prompt consideration of another diagnosis.

Etiology & Pathophysiology

The etiology of this condition is as yet not known for sure, except that there is a defect in the cell-mediated immunity, especially an imbalance of cytokines, with defect in the neutrophil and monocyte chemotaxis. There is also a strong hereditary component to this condition, and is thus seen in families with a strong positive history of asthma, allergic rhinitis, and atopic dermatitis.

A few risk factors known to precipitate this condition are:

- Chemicals and contact with solvents, detergents, deodorants, cosmetics and soaps.

- Dryness of skin caused by excessive bathing, swimming, or hand washing.
- Emotional stress. Patients suffering from atopy usually appear calm, but have a lot of suppressed emotions like anger and anxiety; this conflict causes a lot of internal turmoil and tends to form a trigger factor for this condition.
- Excessive or prolonged heat (hot showers or baths, overdressing, use of electric blankets or heating pads, and exposure to high humidity).
- Exposure to cold weather.
- Exposure to tobacco smoke.
- Food allergy.
- Irritating clothes, like woolen clothes, or loose synthetic clothes that constantly rub and irritate the skin.
- Sweating is known to aggravate this condition.

Histopathology

In infancy, early lesions show acanthosis, spongiosis, oedema of the dermis, and marked infiltration with lymphocytes, histiocytes, plasma cells and eosinophils. In later age groups, there is more of lichenification, with excessive eosinophils in the dermis, and with an increase in the number of Langerhans' cells. Though there is marked eosinophilia in the tissues as well as in peripheral blood in many cases of atopic dermatitis, it is of no help in determining the role of allergy in producing the symptoms.

Clinical Features

It is usually the parent who gets their infant, usually between 2-6 months of age, to the clinic for a rash that doesn't seem to go away. The rash seems to come and go but doesn't seem to be cured. The infant has a dry skin since birth, with severe itching, redness, and macular erythema, papules or papulovesicles as the presenting complaint; there is no fever or any other constitutional symptom along with this condition.

The presentation of the condition depends on the stage of the disease:

- In the 'acute phase', there can be erosions with serous exudate or intensely itchy papules and vesicles on an erythematous base.

- The 'subacute phase' is characterized by scaling, excoriated papules or plaques over erythematous skin.

- 'Chronic eczema' is recognized by the presence of dry skin, with crust formation, lichenification, pigmentary changes (increased or decreased), and excoriated papules and nodules.

- As a result of scratching these lesions, may become secondarily infected. Infected lesions will present with the characteristic yellow crusting or an erythematous surrounding.

- Also in a few cases the nails may be involved where there is coarse pitting and ridging.

Site

- **In infants:** The pruritic, papulovesicular, oozing, atopic, symmetric lesions occur especially on the cheeks, forehead, scalp, trunk, hands, flexures and the extensor surfaces. The diaper area is usually spared. In a few cases of severe scalp involvement, there can be alopecia.

- **In children:** Here itchy lichenified lesions occur symmetrically, especially on the cubital and popliteal fossae, sides of the neck, wrists and ankles. In a few cases, generalized eruptions can also occur.

- **In adults:** The lichenified lesions occur especially on the flexor areas of the arms, legs and neck, and also on the face, upper chest, nipples, and genital areas.

Other manifestations that occur along with atopic dermatitis are:

- Asthma and allergic rhinitis, which occur in about 40-50% of the cases. The age of onset is later than that of the eczema. The asthma and eczema keep fluctuating together, either alternately or usually quite independently, suggesting an allergic cause for both.

- Dry skin is seen pretty commonly with atopic conditions, and it is usually associated with ichthyosis vulgaris (where there are hyperlinear palms and soles and polygonal fish-like scales on the lower limbs) or keratosis pilaris (where there is formation of asymptomatic horny follicular papules on the extensor surfaces of the upper arms, buttocks and anterior thighs).

- Hand and foot dermatitis may be the only manifestation in adults and adolescents. There are often fissures on the palms, soles and fingers.

- Facial erythema, perioral pallor, infraorbital fold, increased palmar linear markings, pityriasis alba (hypopigmented asymptomatic areas on face and shoulders), alopecia areata and pilaris are other associated features seen in this condition.

- Drug reactions of the anaphylactic type are more common in atopic persons because of the increased propensity to produce IgE after natural exposure to antigens.

Diagnosis

- The diagnosis is made on the basis of the clinical history and physical examination.

- Serum IgE levels are elevated in about 80% of the cases.

- **Biopsy:** Pathological findings include a thickened and hyperkeratoid epidermis with the dermis showing perivascular inflammation.

Differential Diagnosis

- Scabies always needs to be excluded, and can especially cause confusion when superimposed on pre-existing atopic dermatitis.

- Seborrheic dermatitis (especially in the first few months of life).

- Contact dermatitis.

- Exfoliative dermatitis.

- Immunodeficiency states should also be considered in infants in whom the disease is unusually severe, when there are recurrent systemic or ear infections, and if there is failure to thrive, malabsorption or petechiae.

- In adults, flexural eczema may be a consequence of secondary dissemination of other types of eczema, for example in nickel allergy.
- Photosensitivity rashes.
- Psoriasis.

Treatment

The management of atopic dermatitis usually lies in terms of its prevention. The physician is expected to make the proper diagnosis, educate the patient about skin care, and treat the acute exacerbations and complications appropriately. He should educate the patient and his relatives (in case if a child or an infant is the patient) about the common trigger factors of the condition and the necessity to avoid them.

- Bathing should be kept to a minimum. Patients should be instructed to take short baths or showers in lukewarm water, use a mild soap and that too only in the axilla, groin and feet region. In the winter, bathing on alternate days is recommended.
- Liberal use of a good skin moisturizer after bath is necessary for lubrication, especially in winter.
- Minimizing contact with cosmetics, deodorants, detergents, solvents, or other known triggers should also be stressed.
- Avoid contact of skin with irritating agents like wool and perfumes. Wear the right kind of cotton clothing to minimize sweating.
- Humidify the house.
- Adults with this condition need to try and reduce the stress they are facing, if possible.

Complications

- Due to intense itching and frequent scratching and cracks in the skin, secondary bacterial (staphylococci or streptococci) and viral infection is pretty common, which presents as fever, surrounding erythema or yellow crusting of the lesions.

- Acute generalized infections with herpes simplex (eczema herpeticum) and vaccinia (eczema vaccinatum) viruses are seen in atopic patients. The condition may present itself as widespread multiple grouped vesicles or papulovesicles with high fever.

- Widespread molluscum contagiosum is also common.

- Conditions like AIDS can aggravate or cause a relapse of the atopic dermatitis.

- Eye: Conjunctival irritation, keratoconjunctivitis, the Dennie-Morgan fold of skin under the lower eyelids, keratoconus (conical cornea), retinal detachment, and bilateral cataract (especially in individuals between 15-25 years of age).

- Exfoliative dermatitis: Eczema may be the underlying disorder in this diffuse, warm, erythematous dermatitis that affects the entire body. Hospital admission is usually required.

- Cartilaginous pseudocyst of the external auricle, and olecranon and pretibial bursitis are also common in children with atopic dermatitis.

- Atrophy or striae if fluorinated corticosteroids are used on the face or in skin folds to treat this condition.

- Systemic absorption of steroids may occur if large areas of the skin are treated, particularly if high-potency medications and occlusion are combined.

Prognosis

Patience and care to avoid risk factors is needed in treating this disorder. Most of the cases improve spontaneously through childhood, though some of them relapse during adolescence. The prognosis is poor in those cases where there is a strong family history of an atopic disorder. The personality of the child and its parents, and the environmental factors around him, serve an important guide to judging the prognosis of the case.

30-50% of the cases of atopic eczema in the infant subsequently end in asthma or hay fever, whereas in adults, it results in chronic hand or foot dermatitis, eyelid dermatitis or lichen simplex chronicus.

SEBORRHEIC DERMATITIS

Synonym

Pityrosporal dermatitis; dermatitis of the sebaceous areas.

Definition

This is a chronic dermatitis, which is difficult to define exactly, but it has a distinctive morphology (red, sharply marginated papulosquamous lesions covered with greasy scales) and a typical distribution in areas with a rich supply of sebaceous glands, especially the scalp, face and upper trunk.

'Dandruff' (Pityriasis capitis), which is a visible desquamation from the scalp surface, appears to be the precursor or mild form of seborrheic dermatitis. This may gradually progress into a red, irritated skin with marked increase in the scaling of the scalp, and thus become a true seborrheic dermatitis.

Etiology

The yeast Malassezia ovale (Pityrosporum ovale), which is normally present on the skin, is increased in the scales of seborrheic dermatitis, and is thus supposed to be the cause of it.

Incidence

This condition is more commonly seen in males than in females. It can occur in all ages, even in infants below 2 months of age.

It is also seen to occur with increasing frequency in patients suffering from early HIV infection, possibly due to the enhanced growth of yeasts secondary to immunosuppression.

It is also seen to occur secondarily in patients suffering from Parkinsonism.

Histopathology

The histology is not diagnostic, but generally shows features of both psoriasis and chronic dermatitis. Most of the cells of the stratum corneum are parakeratotic, with a slight to moderate acanthosis, and mild spongiosis (which distinguishes it from psoriasis). The dermis shows a mild chronic inflammatory infiltrate. There is an increase in production of keratinocytes, with marked epidermal proliferation and desquamation.

Malassezia ovale yeast, with marked follicular involvement of the skin is more characteristic of seborrheic dermatitis in an immuno-suppressed (AIDS) individual.

Clinical Features

Most forms of seborrheic dermatitis share certain distinctive characteristics. They commonly originate in hairy skin, and involve the scalp, face, upper trunk, and the flexures. In rare cases, it can be generalized, occuring all over the body. The lesions tend to be dull or yellowish red in color and covered with greasy scales. Pruritus is minimal, and chronicity of the lesion or recurrence is very common.

Scalp

Dandruff is usually the earliest manifestation of seborrheic dermatitis on the scalp. Gradually there is perifollicular redness and scaling evident, which spreads to form sharply marginated patches, which either remain discrete or tend to coalesce together. There can be loss of hair occurring with this condition. There is redness and sticky scale and crust formation behind the ears (in the retroauricular folds), which can spread to involve surrounding areas. There can also be infection of the external ear canal along with this.

Face

The medial half of the eyebrows, eyelids, glabella, and nasolabial folds are especially affected. Inflammation of the eyelids with whitish scale formation is common. In extensive or chronic cases there are yellow crusts, with destruction of lash follicles, and small ulcers, which heal with scar formation.

Trunk

The commonest pattern of seborrheic dermatitis seen in males are petal-shaped lesions on the front of the chest and in the interscapular region. The initial lesion appears as a small, reddish-brown follicular papule, covered by a greasy scale. These then spread and tend to coalesce to form a particular circular pattern.

Another pattern is a generalized erythematosquamous eruption, somewhat similar to, but more extensive than, pityriasis rosea, which involves the trunk, neck and extends right upto the hairline.

Flexures

The most commonly involved flexures are the axillae, groins, and the area in the breast fold, and in a few cases the anogenital and umbilical region may also be involved. Here the condition appears like an intertrigo, with diffuse, sharply marginated erythema and greasy scaling, with crusted fissures at the folds. There is usually increased perspiration in these parts and is thus more prone to secondary infection if left untreated. In chronic cases the skin becomes thickened and erythematous.

Complication

Increased susceptibility of the seborrheic skin to bacterial infection and to physical and chemical injury results in a high incidence of contact dermatitis and other skin infections.

Diagnosis

In a classical case the diagnosis is easy, but in some cases the diagnosis can be difficult, partly because of the lack of well-defined diagnostic criteria.

- Psoriasis is most often confused with seborrheic dermatitis, especially in cases where the lesions are present only on the scalp. The differentiating feature is that the psoriatic lesions are usually thicker and bright pink in color with a silvery scale. Also psoriatic changes of the nails should be looked for, and a family history of psoriasis should be checked for.

- Lichen simplex can appear similar to seborrheic dermatitis, but here the thickened plaques are often much more irritable than that seen in seborrheic dermatitis.

- Pityriasis rosea must be distinguished from the pityriasiform type of seborrheic dermatitis, in which the lesions are more widely distributed, and in which there is no herald patch.

- Ringworm infections, pityriasis versicolor and candidiasis should be ruled out in cases of lesions occurring only at the flexures, by performing a microscopic examination of the scrapings from the advancing margin.

- Contact dermatitis needs to be ruled out with the help of a patch test.

- Biopsy may be required to rule out pemphigus.

DISCOID OR NUMMULAR ECZEMA

Definition

This type of endogenous eczema presents itself as pruritic, circular or oval lesions, with closely set papulovesicles on an erythematous base. They have a clearly demarcated edge, which is its characteristic feature.

Etiology & Incidence

There is no particular cause traced in this condition, except that in quite a few cases it is seen to erupt after a sort of physical or chemical trauma to the part; or it is also seen to occur at the site of an old injury or scar.

It is rarely seen in children, and is seen to occur more frequently in individuals with a dry skin. Discoid eczema is also associated to stress and excessive alcohol consumption.

Histopathology

Spongiotic vesicles and a predominantly lympho-histiocytic infiltrate is seen in the dermis, with presence of eosinophils in the superficial layers. The intense intercellular edema leads to a reduction in the number of desmosomes between the cells of the basal layer, whereas those in the stratum spinosum are mostly preserved.

Clinical Features

The lesion consists of an oval or coin-shaped plaque of closely set, thin-walled vesicles or papulovesicles, which seem to arise very rapidly due the confluence of tiny papules. There is an erythematous base below and around the vesicles. The hands, forearms, feet, legs and trunk are especially involved.

It can be either of an acute variety (with dull red, oozing and crusted lesions); OR of the chronic variety (where there is less of vesicle formation, and more of dry scaling and hyperpigmentation, with central clearing of vesicles and their peripheral extension). The lesions in the acute phase are especially very itchy and irritable.

This pruritic skin condition tends to be a chronic one, with acute exacerbations; or there is recurrence occurring especially during the winter.

Differential Diagnosis

- Ringworm needs to be ruled out due to the annular lesions. In discoid eczema, the edge of the lesion is broader, more vesicular and more vivid in colour than those seen in ringworm, where scaling of the edge is characteristic. The superficial scraping of the skin will confirm the diagnosis.

- Psoriasis has drier lesions, with intense scaling, and mild pruritus.

- It is differentiated from contact eczema due to its well-demarcated edge and also since here the levels of IgE are in the normal range.

Treatment

Patients are only asked to avoid contact with irritants as a precautionary measure.

POMPHOLYX

Synonym

Dyshidrotic eczema.

Definition

It is a vesicular eczema with chronic and recurrent lesions affecting especially the palms and soles. Here the oedema fluid accumulates to form visible vesicles or bullae. Because of the thick epidermis in these sites, the blisters tend to become larger than in other body areas before they burst.

This condition was also called dyshidrotic eczema, due to its supposed (though false) connection with sweat-gland activity, since it is known to get worse in the hot weather.

Etiology

Studies have revealed a hereditary predisposition to this disorder. Stress is also known to play a role in causing and being a result of this skin disorder.

Histopathology

Fully formed lesions show the changes of acute eczema modified by the thick, overlying epidermis. The subsequent course is that of a subsiding eczema, with hyperkeratosis and epidermal shedding.

Clinical Features

Pompholyx is seen to especially affect adults before 40 years of age, but rarely in children below 10 years of age. There is sudden onset of crops of clear, deep-seated, sago-like, usually symmetrical vesicles, with intense itching. There is no redness of the part, but a sensation of heat and prickling of palms, before the attacks. The vesicles can coalesce and present as large bullae, especially on the feet. The eruptions tend to subside spontaneously within a few weeks, though scratching can make them worse. The symptoms are known to be worse during the summer months.

Complications

There can be secondary infection with pustule formation and lymphangitis complicating the symptoms in certain patients.

In cases of recurrent attacks, dystrophic changes in the nails can take place, with irregular transverse ridging and pitting, thickening and discoloration.

Diagnosis

- A circumscribed, asymmetrical lesion of scaling and vesiculation can also occur due to a fungal infection, which needs to be ruled out by checking the scrapings.

- Contact dermatitis needs to be ruled out, especially in cases where there are asymmetrical lesions, with the help of a careful history and a patch test.

- Repeated attacks of pompholyx may produce hyperkeratotic lesions that mimic psoriasis vulgaris.

GRAVITATIONAL ECZEMA

Synonym

Venous eczema; Stasis eczema.

Definition

Gravitational eczema is a condition that results from venous hypertension, usually in the lower leg, and it often occurs as a late result of a previous deep vein thrombosis.

It was misnamed wrongly in the earlier days as 'stasis eczema', since it is associated with an increased perfusion of the tissues rather than stasis.

Histopathogenesis

Venous hypertension, when transmitted to the capillaries, results in widened endothelial pores through which fibrinogen escapes and forms deposition of fibrin around the capillaries. Reduced oxygenation of the tissues and skin around the medial malleolus is thought to be responsible for the eczema.

Clinical Features

This condition especially affects middle-aged or elderly females, and the eczematous lesions here develop suddenly or insidiously, usually on the lower legs, with pruritus, oozing, dilatation or varicosity of the superficial veins, oedema, purpura, pigmentation or haemosiderosis, and ulceration. Dilated venules with purple papules around the dorsum of the foot or ankle are common.

Complications

In quite a few cases there results secondary contact dermatitis, as a result of infection and rubbing.

Differential Diagnosis

- Atopic dermatitis in children or young adults can appear as lichenified patches around the ankle or behind the knees.

- Contact dermatitis of the lower legs is usually due to topical medicaments, and may complicate other forms of eczema, insect bites or leg ulcers.

- Psoriasis may present as a single, irritable plaque on the leg, but is usually identified by its characteristic scale and circumscribed edge.

Treatment

The patient should be asked to rest with elevation of legs for at least several hours each day and regular use of firm and supportive elastic bandages or stockings.

LICHEN SIMPLEX CHRONICUS
DERMATITIS

Synonym

Neurodermatitis.

Definition

Lichenification is a pattern of cutaneous response to repeated rubbing or scratching.

Incidence

This condition is seen especially in females, usually after puberty. The individuals suffering from it are usually described as stable but anxious individuals, whose reactions to stress are relieved by ritualized behaviour such as rubbing. Aggression and hostility related to anxiety caused by emotional disturbance may lead to itching.

Histology

Acanthosis and hyperkeratosis is characteristic of this disorder. The rete ridges are lengthened. Spongiosis is sometimes present, and small areas of para-keratosis are occasionally seen. There is hyperplasia of all components of the epidermis.

Clinical Features

This condition is caused due to a vicious circle involving an itch-scratch-itch response. The initial stimulus could be something as benign as an insect bite or some small trauma or infection. There is then constant rubbing and scratching, which causes lichenification and a reduced threshold for the itch. Thus the vicious circle sets in. The behaviour takes the form of rubbing with either the hands or knuckles and in extreme cases sometimes with the use of an instrument such as a hairbrush, a pen or some other domestic implement. The actions may not be conscious ones and may proceed without continuous conscious control. However, in some cases patients subject themselves to frenetic, prolonged spasms of uncontrollable self-damage.

Regular rubbing and pressure on the skin produces the characteristic thickened, coarsely grained nodules, or well-marginated plaques with occasional scaling and hyperpigmentation. The usual sites involved are those within easy reach, especially on the nape and sides of the neck, elbows, arms, thighs, legs, and ankles. These areas may be in varying stages of evolution, from early papules with surface excoriations to chronic areas that present as plaques with pigment changes, described as 'dermatological worry beads'.

Treatment

The patient must be educated not to scratch or rub the affected area inadvertently. The maladaptive response of itch-scratch-itch can be treated successfully with behaviour therapy to break the vicious cycle.

HOMEOPATHIC APPROACH TO DERMATITIS AND ECZEMA

The outlook rests mainly on correct elicitation and the complete eradication of the cause or causes. It is regrettable that potential sensitizers are sold so freely in the market and advertised as panaceas in the lay press. The skin is a superficial subject and so it is easily accessible to over-treatment and ill treatment.

Dermatitis and eczema are, as a rule, curable conditions. Eczemas are non-infective except when they are impetignized and of the infective variety. They do not leave scars. The point needs reassurance of these points.

It must be remembered that epidermis is an ectodermal structure and so, takes time to heal. Patience must be the watchword; energetic treatment is to be strongly discouraged. Once warned, the patient will readily cooperate.

Acute eczema heals readily, in about 1-4 weeks with treatment. Chronic eczema, in which anatomical and functional changes set in, takes time to disappear. Disseminated and generalized eczema is not only slow to heal, but are accompanied by ill health. Infantile and atopic eczema are troublesome and uncomfortable. The former lasts till the age of two unless it develops into atopic eczema, which may continue till the age of twenty-five or even through life. Spontaneous remissions and exacerbations mark its course. Climatic extremes, psychogenic stresses and poor health, aggravate dermatitis and eczema. The cure of these conditions is retarded in tropical countries, by heat, humidity and the prevalent unhygienic conditions.

Treatment

It consists of :

- Reassuring the patient and his relatives about the disease being curable, non-infectious and non-scarring. A patient with chronic eczema naturally worries about the nature of his illness, the expense of treatment and loss of income because of his inability to work. Hence reassurance of on all these accounts is very important in winning his confidence and thus his co-operation in treatment. Tactful bedside psychotherapy pays dividends in all cases.

- Elimination of predisposing, exciting and complicating causes. In one individual, more than a single cause may be at play. Where it is impossible to remove a known cause from a patient's environment, attempts should be made to desensitize or hyposensitize him. To prevent recurrence, advice should be given to the point regarding exposure to causes. Improving the general state of nutrition is also important.

- Correction of environment:

    - Moderate atmospheric temperature and humidity help recovery, whereas heat, sweating, high humidity (especially in rainy season), dust and unhygienic surroundings have an untoward influence. Poverty and backwardness of the people are great obstacles especially when the climate is extreme. A change to a moderate climate should be recommended to a point suffering from chronic eczema.

- Rest to the affected part may be recommended; bed rest becomes necessary in generalized eczema. With rest, healing is accelerated; that is why hospitalization is so beneficial for chronic, resistant cases.

- Diet should be simple; salt and fluids should be cut down. Sattvik (vegetarian food without spices and beverages like tea, coffee, and alcohol) is helpful in bad cases. In acute disseminated eczema, it is advisable to put the point on light food for a few days to help the body to get rid of toxic substances. In allergic eczema, eliminative diets may be tried.

- The protection of the affected part is desirable; more so, in exogenous eczema where a cotton bandage or a glove or a mask ensures complete protection from offending agents. Cotton wool must never be employed in bandaging, it retain heat, thereby worsening the eczema.

- Patients should be asked to refrain from scratching as far as possible. In difficult cases, particularly in infantile and atopic cases, physical restraint with splints and bandages may be necessary.

Some Important Homeopathic Remedies and Some Therapeutic Hints

Arsenicum album: The Arsenic skin eruption is usually dry, seldom moist, combined with severe burning of skin. Itching is not so prominent. There is aggravation from scratching and cold. The skin bleeds easily and is covered with crusts. Open air and radiated heat are unpleasant to the patient. Arsenicum seems to be especially valuable in degenerative processes, so often caused by eczemas of the aged and in suitable forms of diabetic eczemas.

Graphites: Graphites has often been found to be an excellent eczema remedy. Its domain is the chronic form, but often one must have much patience till its action becomes evident. Its type is the slow, thickest, indolent and gluttonous patient, women have delayed and weak menses. It is strange that these people do not perspire; but the women have much 'flying heat'. Eczemas behind the ears and on occiput, often very moist with tough, yellow crusts, and that is characteristic. Callosities on hands and feet reminds one of Graphites. An aggravation of all symptoms in the evening is often marked.

Antimonium crudum: It is the opposite of Graphites in many ways; perspiration is one of its characteristics. Its eczema is usually moist, begins with purulent pustules in face. Impetigo in children is one of its great fields of action. The tongue is usually coated with bad, flat taste mornings. Chronic digestive disturbances, the patient is very tired and lazy, may have severe horny calluses, especially on the feet; deformed nails.

Calcarea carbonica: It has lately played a prominent role in dermatology. In itching eczemas it has often acted splendidly but again in other cases which seemed to be the same. It failed. Perhaps in these cases there was no Calcium type as in the others. I have found that Calcium type fat, phlegmatic, easily perspiring patient, women who menstruate too early and profusely, respond often very well to Calcarea carbonica. Important is, that though skin getting wet is not tolerated, there is a craving for water. Cold, moist feet fit well into the picture. Warmth relieves. In children's eczema Calcarea often acts well. I generally try to learn whether or not patients have had eczema or milk crust in younger years, which indicate circumscribed eczema on the hands of young girls which resists all other therapy respond well to Calcarea carbonica. Natrium muriaticum must not be forgotten here, as it often exactly suits these cases.

Baryta carbonica: Baryta carbonica is for children as well as for the aged is well indicated in many instances, and especially in backward children.

Petroleum: It has the chronic eczemas in the fall and winter with cracked skin, which does not heal well.

Sepia officinalis: Sepia is pre-eminent in eczemas in the climateric or at its end, if they also have small, very itchy vesicles on the fingers worse from water. Of course, there should be other Sepia symptoms too. During summer one must be sure that it is not a case of mycosis from athlete's feet. In such cases anti-parastic treatment must be instituted and a constitutional remedy should be given, like Calcarea or Silicea.

Lycopodium clavatum: It is a valuable remedy in eczema Itching severely, bleeding from scratching; disturbed digestion. Bulimia satisfied by a few bites; flatulency not relieved by passing of gases. I mention these symptoms because they are the opposite of Carbo vegetabilis, which is also efficient in the treatment of chronic leg ulcers of older people. Often it is advisable to alternate with Calcarea fluorica.

Thuja occidentalis: Thuja can be used in facial seborrheic eczema, especially if there exists also an oily condition of the hair. There are women who distinctly show the Thuja type.

Croton tiglium: Croton tig. is especially for eczema of scrotum with terrible itching.

Silicea terra: It is a constitutional remedy, which should be tried repeatedly in many cases.

Berberis vulgaris: It is useful in eczema with much uric acid, often accompanied by troubles of joints and bladder.

Nitricum acidum: It is for itching and eczema, rhagades and moist conditions.

All these remedies have this in common. They are especially valuable in chronic cases from disturbed metabolism, or when they are constitutionally indicated. For acute eczema with redness and swelling of skin, vesicle formation, the following briefly mentioned remedies must be compared.

Belladonna: The when skin is tightly drawn and hot; during infectious diseases and intestinal disturbances.

Apis mellifica: It has oedema of skin, stitching pains; no thirst.

Rhus toxicodendron: Acute blisters on skin, intensely itching and burning. Often after colds and change of weather.

Cantharis vesicatoria: In Cantharis ves. acute eczema is preceded or soon followed by bladder troubles.

Not to be forgotten Formic acid therapy (internally, or preferably hypodermically or intravenously in medium aqueous potencies).

CHRONIC ECZEMA

Aethiops antimonialis: Typically affects persons with scrofulous and syphilitic diathesis who are prone to easy suppuration. The lesions are characterized by formation of thick crusts with pus beneath the discharge, which is extremely acrid. Eczema in individuals after abuse of mercury.

Alnus rubra: Eczema associated with gastric disturbances situated especially on the fingers, characterized by crusts and pustules with disagreeable odour. Eczema that tends to ulcerate easily, angry looking eczema associated with glandular enlargement.

Aethusa cynapium: Eczema in children especially during dentition. It typically affects the area around the joints with itching and burning sensation > local application of heat. Skin is cold and covered with cold, clammy sweat. Lymphatic glands swell like strings of beads. Eruption itches when exposed to heat.

Alumina : Scalp, nails. Eruptions are humid, scabby, and scurfy with gnawing, itching sensation. Scratching leads to bleeding, < evenings, < alternate days, < heat of bed, < full and new moon, < eating potatoes, > open air. Dry skin even in hot weather. Skin feels as if white of egg had dried on its surface. Eczema, that appear periodically, especially in winter.

Ammonium carbonicum: Bends of extremities, excoriation between thighs above genitals and in the arms. Eczema in individuals with scrofulous diathesis who dislike washing. < Wet applications. Violent itching after scratching, burning blisters appear. Desquamation of skin over the palms.

Ammonium muriaticum: Hands, wrists, shoulders, tips of fingers. Eczema associated with desquamation of the skin, with a fine brown exfoliation. Itching > applying cold water, in the evening, bleeds easily on touch and friction. Eczema is < during menses. Individuals who are fat, indolent, lax muscles and who are prone to frequent gastric upset like vomiting and diarrhea. Eruptions bleed on scratching. Skin symptoms alternate with asthma.

Anacardium occidentale: Fingers, eyelids, face, scrotum, chest, around neck. Vesicles turn fast into pustules. Multiple vesicles which later confluent and discharge a yellow transparent fluid, hardening to a crust. The discharge is acrid and excoriating. The eruption tends to spread from left to right. Itching < scratching, eczema in individual with neurotic personality of nervous, hysterical women.

Anthrakokali: Hands, tibia, shoulder, dorsum of feet, scrotum. Papule like eruption with a vesicular tendency. Itching < during the night and disappearing in the daytime. Eruptions decrease with appearance of the full moon. The skin has got tendency to develop cracks and ulceration. Eczema in individuals with bilious affection and intense thirst.

Antimonium crudum: Face, genital, extremities, neck, chest, back. Eczema in individuals who are gluttons in their eating habits and frequently suffer from gastric troubles. Suppurating, yellow crusted eruption, painful to touch and easily detached; green serous pus oozes out from beneath. The thick, hard, yellow crust, irritating the surrounding parts, itching violently < from application of poultices, bathing, working in water, alcohol and in the sun.

Antimonium tartaricum: Impetiginous eczema, vesicles surrounded by a red areola, with itching, chiefly above nose, neck and shoulder and back of the ears; the eruptions leave a bluish red mark. It is indicated in individual who has ailments from ill effects of vaccination.

Apis mellifica: Eruptions sting and burn like bee stings, sensitive to touch, chiefly in circumscribed spots all over body, causing itching and restlessness < by heat, > exposure to air. The skin is dry and hot alternating with gushes of sweat. Eczema developing in individual after suppressed eruptions.

Arsenicum album: Scalp, face, extremities, genitals, margins of hair. They are dry and scaly or with vesicles, having fetid and acrid discharge. Sensation of itching and burning < at night, < cold air, scratching, > warm application.

Arsenicum iodatum: Beard. Eczema in individuals with tuberculous, scrofulous or syphilitic diathesis. Small vesicles, which burst and discharge an acrid fluid with severe itching and burning. < Night, application of cold. < Washing.

Asterias rubens: Eczema on thighs, legs, ankles, and insteps. Vesicles break and form small ulcers, which spread superficially. It typically affects individuals with cancerous, scrofulous and sycotic diathesis. Eczema is typically left sided.

Baryta carbonica: Moist vesicular eruption with formation of thick crust, itching, burning, causes the hair fall out; skin is humid and sore.

Eczemas of fat, dwarfish children with swollen lymphatics, enlarged tonsils who take cold easily.

Berberis vulgaris: Anus and hands. Eczemas in individual with arthritic, nephritic and urinary complaints. Eruptions that leave a brown stain. Severe itching, burning, smarting. < Scratching, > cold application. Circumscribed pigmentation following eczematous eruptions.

Berberis aquifolium: Scalp and extends to face and neck. Dry eczema in individuals with chronic catarrhal affections. Itching of the scalp followed by severe scaling.

Borax venenata: Fingers, toes, and nails. Sensation of itching and stinging. Appearance of skin is dry, wrinkled and wilted. Eczemas tend to ulcerate with slightest friction.

Bovista lycoperdon: Back of hands (Baker's and Grocer's itch) mouth, nostrils, bends of elbows and knees. When skin is irritate by repeated washing. Eruptions moist, vesicular with formation of thick crusts or scabs, with pus beneath. Itching not better by scratching, < warmth. Skin is flabby to feel. Blunt instruments leave a deep impression on the skin.

Bromium: Covers entire scalp like scab, dirty looking offensive discharge. Scalp is tender to touch. Profuse moist eruptions in armpit and perineum.

Caladium seguinum: Burning vesicular eczema on chest, forearm and vulva. Eczema alternates with asthma. Sweat is so sweet that it attracts flies.

Calcarea carbonica: Occiput and then spread to the face. Neck, around navel, flexures of extremities, scalp. Thick large yellow scab with thick bland pus under the crust; itching not very intense, but on awakening from sleep person is apt to scratch his head till it bleeds. Eruptions < by water. Eruptions are associated with cold feet as if damp stockings on them, chalky stool; skin inclined to ulcerate.

Calcarea sulphurica: Scalp and extremities with formation of greenish, brownish or yellowish scab. Severe itching followed by scratching and bleeding < warm application, > cold application. Skin is unhealthy and prone to abscesses and carbuncles. The discharge is yellow, thick and lumpy.

Cantharis vesicatoria: Scalp, genitals, extremities. Begin in a small spot and spreads so as to involve a large surface, with a watery discharge underneath the scalp. There is intense burning with itching < warmth > cold application. Typically affects right side. Associated with urinary complaints.

Causticum: Nape of neck, around the nipple, around the mouth. Itching < at night, evening, open air with formation of thick crust that tends to ulcerate. > Heat, warmth of bed. Indicated in cases where eruptions are suppressed by local application of mercury or Sulphur.

Chelidonium majus: Ankle and foot. Chronic eczema characterized by formation of vesicles, pustules and scabs with excessive itching > eating. Also lips and above nose are affected where it develops painful vesicles and pustules which later turn into crust. It usually affects the right side and is suited for those individuals who suffer from bilious and pulmonary disturbance.

Chrysarobinum: Ears, eyes, legs, and thighs. Dry scaly eruptions with scabs and pus from the vesicles, a foul smelling discharge with crust formation, tending to become confluent and to give the appearance of a single crust covering the entire area. Violent itching which leads to burning < warmth.

Cicuta virosa: Scalp, chin, upper lip. Whitish scurf with oozing from purulent eruptions which later become confluent and starts drying down to hard lemon crust, like dried honey. There is no itching whatsoever with eczema. Suppression of eczema leads to disease of the brain.

Clematis erecta: Occiput, nape of neck, face, lower legs. Itch violently with profuse desquamation, vesicles and pustules. Easily corrode the skin and ultimately develops flat eating ulcer with thick crust. Eruptions moist during increasing moon dry during waning moon. < When washed in cold water. Eczema develops after suppressed gonorrhea with glandular enlargement.

Comocladia dentata: Extremities, around the eyes. Presence of redness all over the skin with formation of multiple pustules. Eczemas that recur periodically. Itching < warmth, < night, > scratching, > open air.

Conium maculatum: Face, arms, mons veneris. Moist vesicle with bluish sticky discharge forming hard crust. Itching < by scratching. Eczema developing in old person after being overheated.

Copaiva officinalis: Small vesicles, itching, pricking with severe inflammation of parts. Denuding of epithelium.

Croton tiglium: Face, genitals, eyelids, soles, temples, vertex. Small vesicles, pustules, blisters, which get clustered or may burst too. Violent itching, burning < after eating, < night, > gentle rubbing, > after sleep.

Curare: Face and behind ears, scrofulous children; presence of small vesicles on scrotum with serous exudation forming squamous scab, with intense itching < evening and night.

Dulcamara: Scalp, cheeks, forehead, chin, extremities. Itching vesicles that pass into suppuration and become covered with a thick brown or yellowish crust. The discharge coarsens the skin causing loss of hair. Itching followed by scratching and bleeding. Itching of the skin diminishes after formation of crust, but remains sensitive to contact and bleeds after scratching; the eczema tends to become worse before menses.

Euphorbia lathyris: Starts on the face and spreads all over the body, they are characterized by itching, burning and smarting sensation. When eczema is scratched, it forms deep ragged ulcers. < By touch, cold air, > sweet oil application.

Graphites: Folds of the skin, vertex, scalp, ears, extremities, around anus. Eczema – humid, scurfy with formation of dirty crust which oozes, foul acrid gluey discharge; it matts the hair together and leads to formation of deep rhagades with ulceration. Eruptions bleed easily on scratching. Extreme dryness of skin with inability to perspire. Eczema of fat, blonde women with scanty menses < heat, > cold.

Hepar sulphur: Scalp, genitals, folds of scrotun and thighs. There is presence of foul moist eruption, which tends to ulcertate; they are sore and very sensitive to touch. Itch violently on rising in the morning. There is presence of thin, acrid, offensive discharge from the eczema. Eczema in individuals with coldness of palms and soles.

Hydrastis canadensis: Margin of hair, in front of head. < Coming from cold into warm room, oozes after washing; itching when warm; scalp and face with thick crust which upon removal, expose red, raw patches. Eczema in individuals with tendency to profuse perspiration and unhealthy skin.

Juglans cinerea: Lower extremities, sacrum and hands. Itching associated with burning and redness. Eczema simplex on upper chest with presence of itching and pricking when heated especially by over-exertion. Eczema associated with dyspepsia and bronchial irritation and scrofulous swelling. Itching on arms > scratching.

Juglans regia: Behind ears of children. Vesicular eruptions with itching associated with burning vesicles, tend to be on cracked surface. Greenish discharge that stiffens the linen, large blood boils on shoulders and in hepatic region that are very painful. Itching with restless sleep with dreams and erections.

Kalium arsenicosum: Produces dry, scaly eczema especially affecting bends of arms and knees. Presence of severe itching < warmth, < walking, < undressing. Eczema developing in individuals with malignant disease.

Kalium bichromicum: Starts on ears and spreads over the ear with formation of greenish crust that oozes thick whitish matter. Eruptions tend to ulcerate. Eczema developing in individuals with suppressed catarrh. Eczema, gastric complaints and rheumatism alternates with each other. Sensation of itching < from heat and hot weather.

Kalium bromatum: Chest, shoulder, legs. Moist eruption, which at a later stage, turns into pustules and finally leads to scaling.

Kalium carbonicum: Abdomen and around nipples. Sensation as from burning of mustard plaster in the eczema. Eruptions dry at first, but when scratched, exude moisture.

Kalium muriaticum: Eczema develops after vaccination with oozing from inflamed skin. Whitish opaque mucopurulent discharge. Eczema from suppressed gastric and menstrual disorder.

Kalium sulphuricum: Abundant desquamation, scaling of epithelium leaving the base, moist and sticky. The discharge is yellow and sticky. Violent itching and burning sensation > application of very hot water.

Lappa arctium: Head and face. Moist eruptions oozing foul discharges. Formation of grayish, white crust with destruction of the hair in the surrounding part. Tendency to form boils.

Ledum palustre: Chronic alcoholics. Dry eczema with sensation of lice crawling over the surface. Eruption only on covered parts. Sensation of itching < heat, night, motion.

Lycopodium clavatum: Starts on back of head, hands. Thick crusts which bleed easily, oozing of fetid moisture. Violent itching < 4-8 p.m., from getting heated, < poultices. > Cold air, uncovering parts. Eczema associated with urinary, gastric and hepatic disorders. Tendency to develop blood boils and abscesses.

Manganum aceticum: Chronic eczema with amenorrhea, < menses or menopause, perspiration. Itching > scratching. Itching on palms, with red spots, lips sore. Rhagades in bends of joints, with soreness. Deep cracks in bend of elbows, etc. Burning in small red spots on chest, arms, hands and feet accompanied by rheumatism.

Mercurius solubilis: Moist eczema. Eruptions are humid, fetid, thick, yellowish discharge or crusts form on scalp. Vesicular and pustular eruption. These eruptions are surrounded by irregular margins. Itching is worse by warmth of bed with pain from scratching and tendency to bleed. Excessive odors. Viscid perspiration, worse at night. Complaints increase with sweat and rest. All associated with a great deal of weariness and prostration.

Mercurius dulcis: Eczema over whole body – the eruptions are of round copper coloured spots; in center are dry papules. Inflammation with plastic exudates. Skin is flabby and ill nourished with swollen glands.

Mezereum: Those parts of the skin that are deficient in fat. Intolerable itching compelling patient to scratch and has to change position. Vesicles are full of serous exudation, especially on nose and back. Itching is < in bed, from touch, burning and change of position after scratching. Scurf like fish scales on back, chest, thighs and scalp. Scabs thick, lamellated, like rupia, blood secretion beneath, they look like chalk and spread to brows. Nape and throat. Honey like crust above mouth and cheeks, worse from undressing. Eruptions ulcerate and form thick scabs under which purulent matter exudes. There is marked thirst and scrofulous tendency.

Muriaticum acidum: Eczema on back of hands and face. Papular and vesicular eruptions with violent itching. Blood boils pricking when touched. Ulcers, painful, deep, putrid, covered with scurf, on lower legs, with burning at their circumference. < Damp weather, before midnight. There is marked restlessness, frequently changes the position, but soon grows weak and very debilitated.

Natrium arsenicosum: Squamous eruptions thin, white and when removed leaves the skin slightly reddened; if scales remain they cause itching; worse when warm and from exercise.

Natrium carbonicum: Eczema solaris. Inclination to perspire easily. Great debility caused by summer heat. Skin is dry, rough, cracked with itching like fleas over whole body. Fingertips, knuckles and toes; dorsum of hands. Soles of feet raw and sore vesicular eruptions in patches and circles. < Summer heat, sun, mental exertion, least draught.

Natrium muriaticum: Affects the margins of the hairy scalp; flexures of skin, knuckles, skin behind ears, mouth and eyelids. Persons with oily/dry, harsh, unhealthy skin who are always < at seashore. Eczema in a person with habit of eating too much salt, raw red inflamed eczema. Eczema oozes a corrosive fluid more so at 10 a.m., in warmth and during exercise. Discharge decreases when lying down.

Natrium sulphuricum: Moist eczema with much oozing of fluids. Secretions more watery than sticky. Vesicular eczema, thin watery discharge exuding from stiff, swollen fingers. The palms are raw and sore with fine blisters. Itching < when undressing.

Nitricum acidum: Anus, vertex, temples, genitals, auditory meatus. Eczema of anus with long lasting pain in rectum after stool. Eruptions bleed easily when scratched and there is splinter like pain. Adapted to persons with gouty diathesis and persons who crave sweets.

Oleander: Very sensitive skin with violent itching eruptions, bleeding and oozing. There is absence of sweating. Vesicular eruption on scalp in children. Humid scaly eruption on back part of head and behind ears with itching. Itching as from lice. The symptoms are first better but later become worse from scratching.

Petroleum: Occiput, scrotum, perineum, thighs, back of hands, webs of toes. Inflamed skin heals with difficulty. Skin symptoms are always worse in winter. Yellow-green thick crusts on face and neck, discharges profuse, excoriating. Pain as of slight burn in denuded area. Itching, moist sore places or cracks in skin. < Touch, contact of clothing, scratching. < Bathing, cold air, before and during thunderstorm, warmth of bed. A/F suppressed eruptions. < night (especially eruptions or itching on scrotum). Great sensibility of surface of skin. Dreadful irritation all over body, very intense in vagina, anus and perineum preventing sleep.

Phytolacca decandra: Skin becomes shrunken, hot and dry, pale, papular and pustular lesions. Erythematous blotches, irregular, slightly raised pale red ending in dark red or purple spots. Itching, < by scratching, too sore to allow any scratching. < Damp weather, night, > warmth, dry weather. Aching, soreness, restlessness, prostration are marked associated symptoms with glandular affections.

Pilocarpus microphyllus: Dry eczema. Persistent dryness of skin. Excessive perspiration from all parts of the body. Unilateral sweat. It is a powerful glandular stimulant.

Plumbum metallicum: Rough, dry, scaly, feels dry and cool. Serous infiltration and puffy looking yellow or pale bluish skin. Skin wrinkled, shriveled and drawn over bones. The patient is sensitive to open air, to touch, especially on arms and eyelids.

Primula obconica: Moist eczema of face. Papular eruption on chin. Eczema on arms, wrists, forearms, hands, papular and excoriated. Eruptions between fingers, purple blotches on back of hands. Small papules on a raised base. Cracking over joints and fingers. Skin symptoms accompanied by febrile symptoms. Great itching, worse at night, red and swollen like erysipelas.

Psorinum: Eczematous eruptions after severe exertion accompanied by sensation of tension and swelling. Behind ears, on scalp, bends of elbows and armpits; accompanied by abscesses affecting bones; humid eruption on face. Raw, red oozing scabs around ears. Intolerable itching with offensive discharge from eczema around ears. Eruptions - small vesicles quickly filling with a yellow lymph, painful sore to touch. Crusty eruptions all over the dirty looking skin. < Cold weather, change of weather in hot sunshine, from cold, dread of least cold air or draft. > Heat, warm clothing, summer. Psoric constitutions subject to glandular and skin affection with tendency to diarrhea.

Ranunculus bulbosus: Vesicular and pustular eruptions with thickening of skin and formation of hard, honey scales. Vesicular eruption on face appears as from a burn, smarts as if scalded, vesiculation followed by scabbing and this by a renewal of vesicles, attended by burning and itching. Coarse itching in hollow of hand. Crawling in skin of fingers. < Open air, atmosphere changes, wet stormy weather, cold air.

Rhus toxicodendron: Genitals. Fine vesicular, crusty, eczematous eruptions. Burning eczematous eruptions with tendency to form scales. Itching is worse in the hairy parts. Moist eruptions on head beginning with small yellow vesicles with red areolae forming thick horny crusts and scabs that eat off the hair. < Change of weather, wet weather, winter.

Rhus venenata: Vesicular eruptions with intense itching > application of hot water, < night. Dry eruption on back of hands during winter, which disappears in spring.

Ruta graveolens: Palms, hands, feet with unbearable itching. Itching < after eating meat.

Sarsaparilla officinalis: Emaciated shriveled skin which lies in folds. The base of the eruption is inflamed, crusts get separated in open air and the adjoining skin gets chapped. < Summer, spring, abuse of mercury, evening in bed, morning when rising.

Sepia officinalis: Face, vertex, occiput, bends of joints. During pregnancy and lactation. Itching vesicles and pustules with soreness of skin. Eruptions dry or moist and discharges copious offensive, pus like fluid, which when dry, cracks and exfoliates. Itching vesicles and pustules with soreness of skin. Itching changes to burning when scratched. < Open air, > warm room.

Silicea terra: Behind ears, scrotum, hand scalp and neck. Itching burning offensive eruptions ending in scales discharging pus. Skin is sensitive to cold > warm wrapping. Unhealthy skin, every injury suppurates. Painful pustular eruptions forming ulcers on forehead, occiput, sternum and spine. Itching over whole body which is of a crawling or shooting kind < at night.

REPERTORY

Aeth, alum, alum-p, alum-sil, alumn, am-c, am-m, anac, ant-c, arg-n, ars, ars-i, ars-s-f, ars-s-r, astac, aur, aur-ar, aur-m, aur-s, bar-m, bell, berb-a, borx, bov, brom, bry, calad, calc, calc-s, calc-sil, canth, carb-ac, carb-v, carbn-s, carc, caust, cere-b, chin, cic, clem, cod, com, cop, crot-t, cur, cycl, dulc, fago, ferr-s, fl-ac, graph, hep, hydr, iodof, iris, jug-c, jug-r, kali-ar, kali-bi, kali-c, kali-chl, kali-m, kali-s, kali-sil, kreos, lach, lappa, led, lith-c, lyc, med, merc, merc-c, merc-i-r, mez, napthin, nat-m, nat-p, nat-s, nit-ac, olnd, osm, petr, ph-ac, phos, phyt, pip-m, pix, prim-o, prim-r, psor, pyrog, rad-br, ran-b, rhus-d, rhus-t, rhus-v, polyg-xyz, sanic, sars, sep, sil, skook, solid, staph, sul-i, sulph, tarent, tell, thuj, thyr, tub, vac, vinc, viol-t, zinc, xero, x-ray.

- **Acidity,** with: nat-p, vinc, zinc.

- **Acute form:** acon, anac, bell, canth, chin-s, crot-t, mez, rhus-t, sep, vac.

- **Alternating** with internal affections: graph.

- **Anaemia,** with: calc-p.

- **Bleeds** easily and is covered with thick crusts, with fetid secretion beneath: lyc.

- **Burning:** ars, canth, merc, rhus-t, sulph.

  - Burning, worse from touch, rubbing and evening and during night: merc.

- **Children of** (infantile): alum, am-c, ant-c, ant-t, ars, bar-c, bell, brom, calc, calc-p, caust, crot-t, cur, dulc, graph, hep, jac-c, lyc, mez, nat-m, nit-ac, oleand, petr, psor, rhus-t, sars, sil, sulph
  - Dry: calc-s, dulc, frax, viol-t.
- **Complexion,** sallow: lac-d.
- **Creamy** secretion: nat-p.
- **Crusts,** thick: staph, tell.
  - Crusts, thick, oozing, offensive: rhus-t.
- **Digestive** affections, with: lyc.
- **Discharge,**
  - Corrosive: ars, clem, graph, merc-iod, nat-m, sulph.
  - Honey coloured: nat-p.
  - Yellow acrid, oozes from under crusts: staph.
  - Yellow, slimy, sometimes sticky or watery: kali-s.
- **Dry:** Ars, bar-c, calc, canth, fl-ac, kali-c, lyc, sep, sil, sulph.
  - Chronic, irritable, occasional exacerbation with eruption of distinct vesicles: kali-ar.
  - Crusty: calc-p.
  - Dry at first, exuding moisture when scratched: kali-c.
- **Drunkards,** of: led.
- **Eating** too much salt, from: nat-m.
- **Excoriated:** ars, canth, clem, graph, hep, merc, nat-m, rhus, sulph.
- **Exertion,** after any severe, accompanied by sensation of tension and swelling on fingers, dorsum of hands, nape of neck and towards ears: psor.
- **Exudation** dries into hard, lemon, coloured scales: cic.
- **Fetid:** ars, graph, hep, lappa, lyc, merc, psor, rhus, sep, sil, staph, sulph, vinc.
- **Fever,** with: acon, bell, dulc, petr, phos.
- **Figurata:** ars, calc, clem, con, dulc, graph, lyc, merc, thuja, sulph.

- Tendency to spread: merc.

- With gastric complaints: iris.

- After abuse of mercury, in psoric constitution: clem..

- **Gleet, with:** kali-m.

- **Headache,** produced by suppression: mez.

- **Hypertrophic skin,** dark red corrosive fluid, dries into thick crusts: calc.

- **Impetigenoides:** ant-c, ant-t, anthraco, carb-v, con, dulc, graph, hep, jug-c, kali-bi, mez, oleand, petr, rhus, sars, sulph, ust.

- **Inflammatory,** early stage: canth.

- **Intertrigo:** petr.

- **Itching:** ars, calc, canth, caust, crot-t, dulc, hep, merc, mez, phyt, psor, rhus, sep, sil, staph, sulph, vinc.

  - Night: iris.

  - Scabby, singly or in clusters, looking like herpes: syph.

  - When she gets warm: kali-ar.

  - Without: cic.

- **Mercurial:** acon, bell, dig, cinch, hep, nit-ac, sulph.

- **Moist:** brom, calc, clem, dulc, graph, hep, kali-br, kali-m, lyc, merc.

  - Moist, at times dry, forming yellow crusts: merc, mez, nat-m, phyt, rhus, sep, sil, staph, sulph, vinc.

  - Moist, itching, terribly, worse washing in cold water, from warmth of bed and from wet poultices: clem.

  - Moist, oozing from inflamed skin: kali-m.

  - Moist, oozing profusely, secretions more watery than viscid: nat-s.

  - Moist, sore after scratching: petr.

- **Morning,** worse in, itches, burns, smarts: hep.

- **Pigmentation** in circumscribed areas, following: berb.

- **Pimples** form scales: carb-s.
- **Pustular** (impetigo): ang, arg-n, calc, calc-p, carb-ac, carb-s, caust, cic, con, crot-t, jug, kali-bi, kali-i, merc, mez, nat-m, rhus-t, sil, sulph.
    - Chronic: cinnb.
- **Raw fluid** destroying hair: nat-m
- **Redness,** small blisters, intense itching: anac.
- **Recurrent:** com.
- **Right side** on, most: caust.
- **Rubrum:** acon, alum, anac, apis, bell, bov, calc, canth, carb-v, crot-t, dulc, lyc, mez, rhus-t, sulph.
- **Scabida:** anthraco, dulc, lyc, sulph.
- **Scales,** thick and honey combed: hep.
- **Scales** thick, hard from which pus exudes on pressure: mez.
- **Scratch** the more they, greater the urgency to scratch: rhus-t.
    - Scratching one place itching ceases but appears at another: staph.
- **Seashore,** ocean, voyage, excess of salt, worse: nat-m.
- **Scurfy:** kreos.
    - Scurfy, discharging corrosive fluid, which eats hair, worse in edges of hair: nat-m.
- **Small,** thin, white scurfs on surface: merc.
- **Smarting,** burning when touched: canth.
- **Smarts** as if scalded: ran-b.
- **Scrofulosa inveterate:** iod.
- **Scrofulous:** dulc, tell.
- **Severe and stubborn** of sweating parts of body, exposed to fumes of poison: merc-c.
- **Solaris:** acon, arum-m, bell, camph, canth, clem, hyos, nat-c, mur-ac.

- **Strumous** persons: aethi-a, ars-i, calc, calc-i, calc-p, caust, cist, crot-t, hep, merc-c, rumx, sep, sil, tub.
- **Sun,** exposure, from: mur-ac.
- **Squamosum,** in conjunctivitis scrofulous: kali-bi.
- **Stinging:** merc.
- **Suppressed:** cupr-act, kali-s.
    - Suppressed in epilepsy: kali-m.
    - Suppressed following vaccination: amm-c.
    - Suppressed or deranged uterus functions, from: kali-m.
    - Suppressed, head of agg.: mez.
- **Thickening** of skin and hard horny scales: ran-b.
- **Tingling:** rhus-t.
    - When she gets warm: kali-ar.
- **Urinary,** gastric, hepatic disorders with: lyc.
- **Urine,** suppressed, agg.: solid.
- **Ulcer** large surrounded by smaller ones, some healing, some healed: phos.
- **Vaccination** after, with itching: mez, rhus-t.
    - Cured by vaccination in two children: vario.
    - From bad vaccine lymph: kali-m.
- **Vesicles,** small in neighborhood of joints, itch, dried up rapidly and frequently recurred: phos.
    - Small vesicles, smaller and flatter than mercurial eczema: cop.
- **Washing** agg.: ars-i.
- **Watery** vesicles: canth.
- **Weeping** after taking cold, worse in warmth of room, after having been in cold air, itching when warm, worse washing: hydros.
- **White** secretions: kali-m.
- **Winter**, every, for a number of years: merc.

- Of twelve years standing: phos.

- **Yellow** crusts and inflamed surroundings after scratching: merc.

Location

- **Head:** Agar, ant-t, ars, astac, ars-i, ars-s-f, arum-t, bad, berb, barm, berb-a, brom, calc, calc-ar, calc-p, calc-s, calc-sil, carb-s, caust, cic, cocc, clem, dulc, fl-ac, graph, hep, hydr, iris, kali-ar, kali-bi, kali-m, kali-s, kali-sil, kreos, lyc, meli, merc, mez, nat-m, nat-p, nat-s, olnd, petr, phyt, psor, rhus-t, sars, sel, sep, sil, staph, sul-i, sulph, tell, tub, ust, viol-t, vinc, viol-o.

  - Margin of hair: hydr, kali-sil .

  - Ear to ear, posteriorly from: kali-sil, nat-m, nit-ac, petr, sulph.

  - Forehead: hydr, nit-ac, sulph.

  - Occiput: caust, lyc, petr, sil, staph, sulph, tell.

  - Temples, around: alum.

- **Eye,** about the eyes: bry, kali-sil, sep.

  - Eyebrows, eczema: kali-sil.

  - Eyelids, on: bry, clem, rhus-t, graph, hep, sep, tell, thuj, tub.

  - Margins of lids: Bac.

- **Ear:** Ars, arund, bov, calc, chrysar, graph, hep, jug-r, kali-bi, kali-s, psor, kali-m, mez, lyc, olnd, petr, psor, rhus-t, sanic, scrophul, sep, staph, sulph, tell, tub.

  - About the ears: Ars, bov, chrysar, clem, crot-t, graph, hep, kali-m, mez, olnd, petr, psor, rhus-t, sanic, scroph-n, tell.

  - Behind the ears, eczema: Aur-m, calc, graph, lyc, olnd, psor, scroph-n, stront-n, sulph, tell, tub.

  - Meatus: Borx, graph, kreos, nit-ac, petr, psor.

- **Face:** alum, ambr, anac, ars, alum-p, ars-i, bar-c, bar-s, borx, bell, bry, calc, calc-s, carb-an, carb-v, caust, cic, clem, con, corn, crot-t, cur, cycl, calc-ar, calc-sil, dulc, ferr-i, fl-ac, graph, hep, hyper, iris, kali-ar, kali-sil, kreos, lach, led, lyc, lac-d, lec, merc, merc-i-r, mez, mur-ac, merc-pr-r, nat-m, nat-s, petr, phos, ph-ac, psor, ran-b, rhus-t, sars, sep, sil, staph, sulph, sulph-ac, sulph-i, syph, vinc, viol-t.

- Beard of: ars-i.

- Bleeding: alum, ars, dulc, hep, lyc, merc, petr, psor, sep, sulph.

- Burning: cic, viol-t.

- Chin: borx, cic, graph, kali-sil, merc-i-r, phos, rhus-t, sep.

- Ear spreading from: ars.

- Forehead: nat-p.

- Honey, like dried: ant-c, cic, mez..

- Infants, in: dulc.

- **Lips:** kali-sil.

- **Margins** of hair: sulph.

- **Moist:** graph, kali-sil, lyc, petr, psor, rhus-t.

- **Mouth,** around: ant-c, mez, mur-ac, nat-m.

  - Corners around: graph, hep, lyc, rhus-t, sil.

- **Nose:** ant-c, caust, cist, kali-sil, rhus-t, sep, sulph.

  - Fissure of right wing: thuj.

  - Nursing mothers, in: sep.

  - Occiput, spreading from: lyc, sil.

  - Washing agg.: Ars-i.

- **Abdomen and Rectum:**

  - Anus, about: nit-ac.

  - Epigastrium: ars.

  - Perineum: petr.

  - Rectum and anus: nat-m, nit-ac, berb.

  - Umbilicus, around: scroph-n, sulph.

- **Genitalia,** male: arg-n, ars, chel, graph, hep, lyc, nat-m, nit-c, petr, rhus-t, sep, sulph, thuj.

  - On scrotum: calc, crot-t, graph, nat-m, petr.

F- 16

- Rubrum: chel.
- **Genitalia,** female: caust, dulc, petr, borx, rhus-t.
  - Vulva, labia: rhus-t.
- **Neck** and throat: anac, aur-i, caust, lyc, petr, sep, sil, sulph, psor.
- **Chest:** anac, ars, aur-i, calc, calc-s, carb-v, cycl, graph, hep, kali-s, petr, psor, staph, sulph.
  - Axilla: Carb-an, hep, jug-r, lyc, merc, nat-m, petr, psor, sep.
  - Mammae: Anac, caust, dulc.
  - Nipples: Graph, sars, sulph.
- **Back:** arn, merc, sil.
- **Cervical region**: anac, aur-i, lyc, psor, sil.
- **Extremities:** arn, ars, ars-i, kali-br, merc, psor, graph, tarent.
- **Joints:** led, phos.
- **Flexor of joints:** aeth, am-c, caust, graph, hep, kali-ar, manc, nat-m, psor, sep, sulph.
  - Upper limb: canth, graph, hell, merc, mez, phos, psor, sil.
  - Shoulder: petr.
  - Elbow: brom.
    - Bend of: cupr, graph, kali-ar, mez, psor.
- **Forearm:** aur-i, graph, merc, mez, sil, thuj.
- **Wrist:** jug-c, mez, psor.
- **Hand:** anag, ars, bar-c, berb, borx, bov, calc, canth, clem, graph, hep, hyper, jug-c, kreos, lyc, maland, merc, mez, nit-ac, petr, plb, phos, rhus-v, sabal, sanic, sel, sep, sil, still.
  - Back of: graph, jug-c, kreos, merc, mez, nat-c, phos, sep.
  - Swelling hand with: psor.
- **Fingers:** borx, calc, kreos, lyc, sil, staph.
  - Accompanied by falling out of nails: borx.
  - Painful: arn.
- **Lower** limb: anil, apis, arn, ars, bov, chel, jug-r, kali-br, merc, petr, psor, rhus-t.
- **Thigh:** graph, petr, rhus-t.
  - Between: nat-m, petr.

- **Knee:** anil, arn, rhus-t.
  - Hollow of: graph.
- **Leg:** apis, ars, carb-v, graph, kali-br, lach, led, lyc, merc, nat-m, petr, rhus-t, sars, sulph.
  - Calf: graph.
  - Ankle: nat-p, psor.
- **Foot,** back of: merc, psor.
- **Toes,** eczema, accompanied by falling out of nails: borx.

Chapter-16

Diseases Due to Viral Infection

Introduction

Viruses are the smallest infectious agents (18-300 nm in diameter one nm = one millionth part of a millimeter). A virus particle, or virion, consists of a length of nucleic acid, either RNA or DNA, but never both, within a protein shell, the capsid. The genetic information is sufficient to encode proteins involved in viral replication and production of the protective coat, but requires host-cell ribosomes for translation. This absolute dependence on the host is the distinguishing feature of viruses.

Histopathogenesis

For a virus to produce infection, it must gain entry into a susceptible cell within an appropriate host. Many viruses, in particular those producing systemic infection, enter the body via mucous membranes after inhalation, ingestion or contact.

Attachment to the cell surface by means of a receptor is followed by entry of the virion into the cell, by pinocytosis or phagocytosis. Viruses differ in the range and type of cells which they can infect; host specificity and tissue tropism are hallmarks of viral infections. Poliovirus, for example, can infect neurones and is called a neurotropic virus, and human papilloma viruses (HPV) have a tropism for epithelial cells. A cell in which a particular virus can replicate is described as permissive for that virus. After entry into the cell, pre-existing cell enzymes remove or damage the capsid sufficiently for the nucleic acid to emerge.

The next stage depends on the nature of the virus. In relatively simple ones, like enteroviruses, the RNA acts as a messenger, is infectious on its own and is immediately translatable by host ribosomes into viral proteins. More complex RNA viruses, such as influenza, have non-infectious RNA, sometimes called 'negative-strand' RNA, which has to be transcribed into messenger RNA (mRNA) by a polymerase enzyme carried in the virus itself. RNA tumour viruses contain a 'reverse transcriptase' enzyme which synthesizes DNA from the viral RNA template. DNA viruses are generally more complex and are able to transcribe mRNA from their DNA using either cell polymerase, for example adenoviruses, or viral polymerase, for example vaccinia. At the same time, replication of the viral nucleic acid also occurs.

A variety of proteins, regulatory, enzymic and structural, are produced and these, together with the products of cell damage, probably contribute to the local and general response to the infection.

The surface proteins of the virion have special affinity for specific receptor sites on the host cell. Proteins also contain the viral antigens that stimulate the host's immune responses during infection. Viruses possess the property of hemagglutination. Interferon, a protein produced by the cell after infection with a virus, interferes with the replication of the other viruses. Inactivated virus and also a few other substances (foreign nucleic acids and other synthetic polynucleotides) also induce synthesis of interferon.

Any of the following events may occur following presence of virus within a cell:

- **Destruction:** During this process the cell itself may be destroyed by a lytic virus infection, for example enterovirus and herpes simplex or damaged transiently, for example myxovirus. With time, an immune response develops against the virus particles and processed viral proteins, which can lead to containment and clearance of the infection.

- Stimulation and multiplication: Some viruses infect cells which apparently remain normal and may multiply while virus replication continues within, i.e. persistent infections. When persistently infected cells produce no infectious virus because the replication cycle is arrested, the virus is said to be latent. From time to time, a latent virus can become active-reactivation-new virions are produced and other cells are infected. This process can result in clinical signs and symptoms as in the case of cold sores (reactivated herpes simplex) and shingles (reactivated varicella-zoster).

- Stimulation of the cells to proliferate: Other viruses cause cell proliferation, for example poxviruses and human papillomaviruses.

Skin is one of the principal target organs for viral attack. Rashes (exanthemata) are characteristic of many acute systemic viral infection, where virions in the blood invade the endothelium of the capillaries and venules of the dermis. Viral rash may also be related to antigen-antibody reaction and the circulation of immune complexes. The rash may be an outward sign of the centralization of circulating virus by antibody. Hemorrhagic rashes may be due to disseminated intravascular coagulation precipitated by the circulating virus antibodies and immune complexes.

In some instances where the primary process of invasion is in the epidermis intracellular inclusions and the formation of multinucleate giant cells characterize the skin lesions.

Skin probably offers a peculiarly sensitive situation for some viral growth because of its lower temperature.

Classification

In dermatological practice, the following group of viruses appear important:

DNA viruses	RNA viruses
I. Herpes viruses	I. Picorna viruses
Varicella	Coxsackie
Herpes zoster	Herpengina
Epstein-Barr Virus	Rubella
AIDS	
Herpes simplex	
II. Pox viruses	III. Echo viruses
Variola, Vaccina	Hand – Foot – Mouth
	Disease (HFMD)
Molluscum contagiosum	
Orf Milker's nodes	
IV. Papoviruses	
Warts	

HERPES

The term 'Herpes' signifies a group of vesicles on an inflammatory base like a bunch of grapes. The herpesvirus group consists of relatively large DNA viruses. Their replication is intranuclear and produces typical intranuclear inclusions detectable in stained preparations.

The viruses under this group are:

- Herpes virus hominis (herpes simplex virus (HSV) types 1 and 2 (alpha).

- Herpes virus varicellae (varicella-zoster virus- beta).

- Human cytomegalo virus (beta).

- Epstein-Barr virus (gamma).

- Human herpes virus 6 (beta).

- Human herpes virus 7 (beta).

- Human herpes virus 8 (gamma)

It is important here to mention that in infection by members of the herpes virus group there is absence of virus elimination following clinical recovery. The virus thus persists throughout the person's life as a latent infection in the cells for which the strain is specific. Under certain conditions, especially immune suppression, the virus may become reactivated and produce an acute infective episode with cellular damage.

HERPES SIMPLEX

Etiology

It is caused by herpes virus hominis and is one of the commonest infections of humans throughout the world.

There are two major antigenic types:

1. Type 1- Classically associated with facial infections.

2. Type 2 - Associated with genital infections

After primary infection, the virus persists in sensory nerve ganglia. No viral proteins are produced during the latent phase and therefore remains undetected by host defence mechanisms. From this state of latency, the virus may travel peripherally along the nerve fiber. If it replicates in the skin or mucous membrane, it may cause recurrent disease. In asymptomatic individuals, especially in the months following the first episode of disease, the virus can be shed in saliva and genital secretions, although the amount shed from active lesions is 100-1000 times greater.

Spread is by direct contact with, or droplets from, infected secretions. Transmission was most frequent during periods of asymptomatic shedding.

Following conditions are known to excite the disease:

- Trauma facilitates transfer of the virus to fully keratinized skin. The source may be endogenous (autoinoculation), for example to the finger especially in nail biters or thumb suckers. Examples of exogenous inoculation are lesions of the hand in health-care workers and others; facial lesions contracted during contact sports, and infection of a breastfeeding mother's nipples from the infected mouth of her baby. Even sunburn may stimulate reactivation of the virus.

- **Stress:** For instance, a psychogenic stress, fever, particularly malaria, pneumonia, meningitis, etc.
- General illness and debility.
- **Immunological abnormalities:** Where immunity is deficient (either congenitally or due to disease or drugs) there is higher incidence of the infection and the course may be prolonged and atypical.

Cell-mediated and humoral immune responses follow primary infection, the latter being more important. They do not fully protect against re-infection or recurrent disease. The acquisition of HSV at a new site in a patient previously infected at a different site is referred to as a non-primary, first-episode infection. Initial (non-primary) genital herpes tends to be less severe in patients who have had previous oral infection.

A maternal primary genital infection at the time of birth, before the maternal immune response has taken place, is transmitted to the infant in about 50% of cases and the neonatal infection may be severe and fatal. Primary infection earlier in the third trimester may cause fetal growth retardation and prematurity. However, serious morbidity is rare if non-primary, first-episode or recurrent genital infection occurs during pregnancy or at delivery, presumably because the fetus in those situations is protected by maternal antibody.

The virus of herpes is ubiquitous; it is more prevalent in the temperate climate and the cold season. This accounts for the layman's name of 'Cold Spots'.

Development of carcinoma may be related to HSV-2 infection of the cervix.

Histopathology

In the cutaneous lesions, the cytoplasm of the infected epithelial cells becomes oedematous and the cells swell, producing the so-called 'ballooning de-generation'. Thick-walled vesicles are formed by the combination of intra- and intercellular oedema. The dermis, and later the epidermis, are infiltrated with polymorphonuclear leukocytes. Specific changes occur in the cell nuclei and different stages in the process of the development of the intranuclear inclusions can usually be seen in a single section. In addition, giant cells containing two to 15 or more nuclei are almost invariably present in cutaneous and corneal epithelium. The cytological changes are essentially the same in all organs and foci of necrosis surrounded by a zone of inflammation are characteristically found in brain and liver when these organs are involved. Viral particles can be identified ultrastructurally, mainly in the cell nucleus, and with detailed examination, HSV types 1 and 2 can be distinguished.

Clinical Features

Primary infection

Primary infection may be subclinical, but when clinical lesions develop, the severity is generally greater than in recurrences. Genital primary disease is more commonly symptomatic than oral.

Herpes starts with a sensation of burning or itching. Exposure to cold, sun etc., is known to precipitate the attack. Pinhead sized, superficial vesicles rapidly develop, grouped together on erythematous merciless. Their contents soon become opaque. They may rupture and become crusted, or dry up to leave faint, reddish stains. There are usually negligible constitutional symptoms. The course of herpes is about 7 to 14 days. There is usually no scarring except when secondary infection occurs. Occasionally, hyperpigmentation or depigmentation may follow.

Herpetic gingivostomatitis

It is the most common clinical manifestation of primary infection by type 1 virus. Most cases occur in children between 1 and 5 years of age. After an incubation period of approximately 5 days, the stomatitis begins with fever, which may be high, malaise, restlessness and excessive dribbling. Drinking and eating are very painful and the breath is foul. The gums are swollen, inflamed and bleed easily. Vesicles presenting as white plaques are present on the tongue, pharynx, palate and buccal mucous membranes. The plaques develop into ulcers with a yellowish pseudomembrane. The regional lymph nodes are enlarged and tender. The fever subsides after 3-5 days and recovery is usually complete in 2 weeks.

Differential diagnosis is with streptococcal infections, diphtheria, thrush, aphthosis, Coxsackie infections including herpangina, Behçet's syndrome and the Stevens-Johnson syndrome.

Herpes genitalis

It implies herpes simplex lesions on the genitalia. It is transmitted sexually. In the male, the lesions are on the glans, prepuce or the body of the penis; in the female on the labia, vaginal wall and cervix.

Penile ulceration from herpetic infection is the most frequent type of genital ulceration seen. The ulcers, which may be preceded by a general malaise, are most frequent on the glans, prepuce and shaft of the penis. They are sore or painful and last for 2-3 weeks if untreated. In male homosexuals, herpes simplex is common in the perianal area and may extend into the rectum. In HIV-infected individuals, ulceration may become chronic.

In the female, similar lesions occur on the external genitalia and mucosae of the vulva, vagina and cervix. Pain and dysuria are common. Infection of the cervix may progress to a severe ulcerative cervicitis.

The eruption on the genitalia is painful, and may cause a constitutional upset. Genital herpetic eruptions rupture early producing erosions, which at times are in a circinate patern. The common predisposing causes of recurrent genital herpes are phimosis, lack of personal hygiene, discharge per vaginum, and sexual neurosis. Furthermore recurrent herpes progenitalis is responsible for syphilophobia in some cases.

Keratoconjunctivitis

It causes a severe and often purulent conjunctivitis with opacity and superficial ulceration of the cornea. The eyelids are grossly edematous and there may be vesicles on the surrounding skin. There is enlargement and tenderness of the pre-auricular gland.

Inoculation herpes simplex

After an incubation period of 5-7 days of direct inoculation of the virus into an abrasion or into normal skin, indurated papules, large bullae or irregularly scattered vesicles develop. The regional nodes are enlarged but fever and constitutional symptoms are usually mild. Herpetic whitlow is a condition where inoculation of the fingertips results in painful, deep vesicles, which coalesce to give a honeycombed appearance or to form a large bulla. The condition is easily confused with pyogenic infections. On the face of the adult male the appearance of herpes may be deceptive; it may take the form of a folliculitis, but satellite umbilicated vesicles soon suggest the correct diagnosis.

Complications

Eczema herpeticum, pharyngitis, headache and meningism, radiculoneuropathy, seen occasionally in primary anogenital infection in women, and especially in perianal disease in homosexual men, sacral paraesthesia, urinary retention, constipation and, in men, impotence, disseminated or systemic infection in the immunodeficient and in those neonates not protected by maternally acquired antibody are commonly known complications.

Recurrent Infection

After the initial infection, whether symptomatic or inapparent, there may be no further clinical manifestations throughout life. Recurrences occur in 30-50% of cases of oral herpes, but are more frequent after genital herpes infection, developing in 95% of those with type 2 HSV compared with 50% in individuals with type 1 infection.

Recurrent herpes implies relapsing type of herpes simplex occurring on the same site – usually perioral and genitalia.

Recurrences may be triggered by minor trauma, by other infections including febrile illnesses but also trivial, non-febrile, upper respiratory tract infections, by ultraviolet radiation, by trigeminal neuralgia and especially after intracranial operations for that disease, by other neural surgery, by dental surgery. Some women have more recurrences in the pre-menstrual period. Emotional stress is blamed in some cases possibly related to the effect on immune function. However, in many cases no reason for the eruption is evident.

Recurrent infections differ from primary infections in the smaller size of the vesicles and their close grouping and in the usual absence of constitutional symptoms.

DIAGNOSIS

Diagnosis of infection by culture of the virus from vesicle fluid usually requires only 1-5 days. Seroconversion or a rise in antibody titre (e.g. complement-fixation test) can distinguish primary infections. Recurrences tend to produce little change in antibody titre; measurement of antibody is therefore not helpful in the diagnosis of recurrent HSV. For a more rapid diagnosis, viral antigen may be detectable by immunofluorescence in scrapings from lesions or the virus seen by electron microscopy in vesicle fluid. The detection of HSV DNA in the cerebrospinal fluid by PCR has become the diagnostic method of choice for herpes encephalitis and aseptic meningitis.

Prognosis

In an individual attack of herpes the prognosis is good, in the sense that the lesions heal up nicely and no scarring results. Only in recurrent herpes, is the treatment rather unsatisfactory and the malady can become a nuisance especially in herpes progenitalis.

HERPES ZOSTER AND VARICELLA (CHICKEN POX)

Synonym

Shingles

Zoster (zoster = a girdle, a reference to its segmental distribution)

The same virus, herpes virus varicellae, sometimes referred to as varicella-zoster virus (VZV) causes varicella and zoster. Varicella is the primary infection with a viraemic stage, after which the virus persists in nerve ganglion cells (posterior root ganglion), usually sensory. Zoster is the result of reactivation of this residual latent virus.

Etiology

Herpes zoster is uncommon in childhood and the incidence increases with age. The sexes are equally affected. Zoster patients are infectious, both from virus in the lesions and, in some instances, the nasopharynx. In susceptible contacts of zoster, chicken pox can occur.

Varicella occurs throughout the world and is transmitted by droplet infection from the nasopharynx. Patients are infectious to others from about 2 days before to 5 days after the onset of the rash. Vesicle fluid contains a large amount of virus, but its importance in transmission is not known. Dry scabs are not infectious. Varicella confers lasting immunity and second attacks are uncommon, especially in immunologically healthy subjects, but clinical reinfection with a mild varicella-like illness occurs occasionally.

Histopathology

In varicella following an initial period of replication in the oropharynx a viraemia causes widespread dissemination. In the skin, in varicella, cells of the Malpighian layer show ballooning of their cytoplasm by intracellular oedema, and distinctive nuclear changes comprising eosinophilic inclusions and marginated chromatin. Some nuclei develop additional nuclear membranes which divide the nucleus into small compartments. The multinucleate giant cells with up to 15 nuclei, which are a characteristic feature of infections with herpes virus varicellae and herpes virus hominis, are produced mainly by cell fusion. Intracellular oedema combined with intercellular oedema forms the vesicle, the roof of which consists of the upper Malpighian and horny layers. A mild inflammatory reaction in the dermis later extends to the epidermis and the proportion of polymorphonuclear cells increases with ulceration.

In zoster, as well as skin lesions, there are inflammatory changes in the posterior nerve roots and ganglia and sometimes these involve the anterior horn. Virus particles have been seen in ganglion cells and Schwann cells in the affected nerve bundles. Zoster can cause some destruction of nerve fibres in the middle and lower dermis, detectable with silver-impregnation techniques. Partial denervation may persist for over a year and characteristically does so in patients with post herpetic neuralgia. Corresponding fibres in the spinal cord degenerate and there may be scarring in the region of the ganglion.

Clinical Features

VARICELLA

The incubation period is usually 14-17 days (range 9-23 days). After a day or two of fever and malaise, often slight or absent in children, an inconstant and fleeting scarlatiniform or morbilliform erythema is followed by the development of papules which very rapidly become tense, clear, unilocular vesicles. Within a few hours the contents become turbid and the pustules are surrounded by red areolae. In 2-4 days a dry crust forms and soon separates, to leave a shallow, pink depression which, in the absence of secondary infection, heals without scarring. The vesicles appear in three to five crops over 2-4 days. They are most numerous on the trunk, then on the face and scalp and on the limbs. Their distribution is centripetal, and on the limbs the eruption is more profuse on thighs and upper arms than on lower legs and forearms. A characteristic feature is the presence of lesions at different stages in each site. The total number of lesions is very variable they may be few or profuse. The distribution may be modified by pre-existing inflammatory changes at the sites of which lesions may appear in increased density. The vesicles in such areas tend to be at the same stage and are often small, but may occasionally be bullous. In exceptional cases of normal distribution the lesions are larger and umbilicated or varioloid. Vesicles are common in the mouth, especially on the palate, and are occasionally seen on other mucous membranes, including the conjunctiva. On the anal mucosa they may be followed by painful ulcers.

Fever is variable in severity and duration and roughly parallels the extent of the eruption. It may be trivial or may reach 40 or 41°C for 4 or 5 days. Constitutional symptoms tend to be proportionate to the fever. In some patients pruritus is troublesome. Hemorrhagic varicella, in which a very extensive eruption of hemorrhagic vesicles is accompanied by high fever and severe constitutional symptoms, is rare in the previously healthy patient. It is relatively more common in some tropical regions in which malnutrition may be a factor, but most cases now seen in temperate regions occur in immunocompromised patients.

ZOSTER

The sites of predeliction are the trunk (intercostal nerves), neck (cervical) and face (trigeminal distribution).

Severe pain, sharply localized to the same area but may be more diffuse, is the first manifestation of zoster. It may be accompanied by fever, headache, malaise, tenderness and local increased sensitivity of the skin (hyperaesthesia) localized to areas of one or more dorsal roots.

The time between the start of the pain and the onset of the eruption averages 1.4 days in trigeminal zoster and 3.2 days in thoracic disease. Sometimes, the rash may develop suddenly without any premonitory symptoms. Closely grouped red papules, rapidly

F- 17

becoming vesicular and then pustular, develop in a continuous or interrupted band in the area of one, occasionally two and, rarely, more contiguous dermatomes. Mucous membranes within the affected dermatomes are also involved. New vesicles continue to appear for several days. Towards the end of this period, the lesions rupture or dry up to form crusts. When the crust separates in about a week's time, there is temporary pigmentation and faint scarring. The latter is marked when there is secondary infection and ulceration. The lymph nodes draining the affected area are enlarged and tender. The pain and the constitutional symptoms subside gradually as the eruption disappears. In uncomplicated cases recovery is complete in 2-3 weeks in children and young adults, and 3-4 weeks

'Zoster sine eruptione' is a condition where the pain is not followed by an eruption. Involvement of the first root of the trigeminal nerve gives rise to lesions on the eyes – herpes ophthalmicus.

Variations in the zoster syndrome depend on which dorsal root are involved, on the intensity of its involvement and on the extension of the inflammatory changes into the motor root and anterior horn cells. Visceral involvement may be responsible for abdominal pain, pleural pain or temporary electrocardiographic abnormalities with or without precordial pain.

Complications

VARICELLA

- These are rare in otherwise healthy children, are less infrequent in neonates and adults and are common in the immunosuppressed. Relatively short courses of oral steroid treatment in children and adults may permit the development of severe and potentially fatal chicken pox.

- Encephalitis in the otherwise healthy patient occurs in less than one per 1000 cases and complete recovery occurs in 80% is common. Other neurological complications are very rare. The other main systemic complications are varicella pneumonia and hepatitis.

- Secondary infection is seldom a serious problem in temperate climates, but under tropical conditions may be severe and may be complicated by septicaemia.

- Cutaneous gangrene ('varicella gangrenosa') may follow secondary infection, but rarely extensive local gangrene may occur in the absence of bacterial involvement, and sometimes during a mild attack of varicella.

- Thrombocytopenic purpura, beginning on the fifth to 10th day and usually recovering spontaneously after 3 or 4 months, occasionally follows otherwise benign varicella.

- Rhabdomyolysis has been reported in association with varicella.

- Viral arthritis during varicella has been reported, although bacterial arthritis also occurs.

- Reye's syndrome has been associated with preceding varicella.

- Stevens-Johnson syndrome occurring as a consequence of varicella infection has been reported.

ZOSTER

Motor involvement

It is commoner in older patients and in those with malignancy, and in cranial nerve compared with spinal nerve involvement. The motor weakness usually follows the pain and the eruption, by a few days to a few weeks, but occasionally precedes or accompanies them.

Trigeminal nerve zoster

In ophthalmic nerve zoster, the eye is affected in two-thirds of cases, especially when vesicles on the side of the nose indicate involvement of the nasociliary nerve (Hutchinson's sign). Ocular complications include uveitis, keratitis, conjunctivitis, conjunctival oedema (chemosis), ocular muscle palsies, proptosis, scleritis (which may be acute or delayed for 2-3 months), retinal vascular occlusion, and ulceration, scarring and even necrosis of the lid. Involvement of the ciliary ganglia may give rise to Argyll-Robertson pupil. Zoster of the maxillary division of the trigeminal nerve produces vesicles on the uvula and tonsillar area, whilst with involvement of the mandibular division, the vesicles appear on the anterior part of the tongue, the floor of the mouth and the buccal mucous membrane. In orofacial zoster, toothache may be the presenting symptom.

Herpes zoster oticus

The facial nerve, mainly a motor nerve, has vestigial sensory fibres supplying the external ear (including pinna and meatus) and the tonsillar fossa and adjacent soft palate. Classical sensory nerve zoster in these fibres causes pain and vesicles in part or all of that distribution, though the skin involvement may be minimal and limited to the external auditory meatus. To what extent other neural elements are actually infected is debated, but swelling of the infected sensory fibres in their course through the confined spaces of the facial canal and the internal auditory meatus, leading to compression of adjacent neural structures, can explain the commonly associated features. Thus, pressure on the facial nerve motor fibres adds facial palsy, which with the ear pain and associated vesicles completes the classical triad of the Ramsay-Hunt syndrome; compression of the vestibulocochlear nerve may cause sensorineural hearing loss, dizziness and vertigo; and involvement of the nervus intermedius or its geniculate ganglion would impair taste sensation from the anterior two-thirds of the tongue and alter lacrimation.

Post herpetic neuralgia

The commonest and most intractable sequel of zoster is post-herpetic neuralgia, generally defined as persistence or recurrence of pain more than a month after the onset of zoster, but better considered after 3 months. It occurs in about 30% of patients over 40 and is most frequent when the trigeminal nerve is involved. The pain has two main forms, a continuous burning pain with hyperaesthesia, and a spasmodic shooting type, but a pruritic 'crawling' paraesthesia may also occur. Allodynia, pain caused by normally innocuous stimuli, is often the most distressing symptom and occurs in 90% of people with post-herpetic neuralgia. The neuralgia varies in intensity from inconvenient to profoundly disabling.

Other Complications

1. Scar sarcoid and other granulomas have been reported in healed zoster scars.
2. Bacterial infection of damaged skin.
3. Encephalitis or meningoencephalitis. This is more common in the elderly, the immunosuppressed and in association with disseminated zoster.
4. Acute retinal necrosis syndrome. This rare complication follows an attack of shingles affecting the ophthalmic nerve or an unrelated dermatome.
5. Guillain-Barré syndrome and transverse myelitis have also been noted occasionally following zoster.

Diagnosis

The distinctive features of varicella are the centripetal distribution, the polymorphism in each affected site and the rapid progression of the individual lesion from vesicle to crust.

Typical zoster presents few difficulties once the eruption has developed and can be confused only with zosteriform herpes simplex. This diagnosis should be excluded virologically in apparently recurrent zoster.

HOMEOPATHIC APPROACH TO HERPES

Herpes is primarily a virus infection. That is why it should be classified under the tubercular miasm. However, if one closely observes the evolutionary pattern of herpes, then one can appreciate its multi-miasmatic nature, viz:

1. Burning sensation prior to development of eruption – psoric stage.

2. Formation of vesicles – sycotic stage.

3. Transformation of vesicles to pustules – tubercular stage.

4. Rupture of pustules forming thick scabs with ulceration – syphilitic stage.

It is extremely essential on the part of the homeopath to clearly state in the history at what stage the patient presented initially.

Herpes is known to occur with many systemic conditions:

(a) Fever – malaria, pneumonia, meningitis.

(b) Injury.

(c) Psychogenic stress, which is the common exciting factor.

Exposure to cold and lack of personal hygiene are also to be considered in the history. History of adultery or sexual indulgence should be ruled out in herpes progenitalis. They should be advised to keep proper personal hygiene of the genitals.

Recurrent herpes is one of the trickiest problems. Increase the general resistance of the patient by giving the indicated constitutional medicine preferably a nosode. Eliminate precipitating causes like chronic rhinitis, phimosis, debility, anxiety, stress, etc.

I have found encouraging results with the use of RNA and DNA potentised and used in cases of recurrent herpes infection. The reader is advised to read the provings in detail before prescribing, from a scientific paper written by Dr. Maurice Jenaer.

In cases of herpes zoster one has to be careful of a rare complication of meningo-encephalitis. In post herpetic neuralgia, drugs like Variolinum and DNA should be thought of.

The pattern of arriving at the prescription are:

(i)   Location.

(ii   Sensation e.g. burning, pricking, cutting.

(iii) Pattern of eruption – vesicles, pustules, and crusts.

(iv) Nature of discharge.

(v) Thermal and time modalities.

(vi) Exciting and causative factors if any.

(vii) Past and family history to decide the fundamental cause.

(viii)Patient as a person, i.e. General and mental symptoms.

For post herpetic neuralgia I have found Box jellyfish as a very useful remedy. Also local application of Plantago major mother tincture at the site is extremely useful. Some of the worst cases of post herpetic neuralgia have been successfully treated where the guiding symptoms were stitching pain better by pressure. Herpetic eruptions especially Herpes Zoster associated with any gastric problems have been successfully in my practice using Iris versicolor.

Locally on the lesions, mixture consisting of Calendula and water in the ratio of 1:2 should be applied as it reduces the irritation as well as prevents secondary bacterial infection.

At the site of post herpetic neuralgia, Hypericum perforatum mother tincture should be applied to give a soothing sensation to the patient.

Some Important Homeopathic Remedies

Aethiops mineralis: Herpes after abuse of mercury. Especially adapted to persons of scrophulous and syphilitic diathesis, who are prone to easy suppuration.

Agaricus muscarius: Herpetic eruptions are characterized by burning, itching and redness with swelling. The burning pain is worse whenever the patient is exposed to cold air or cold application.

Alnus rubra: Chronic herpes. The fingers are covered with pustules, which cause formation of a crust. Eruptions of skin alternate with disease condition of the mucus membranes.

Arsenicum album: Lips, face, intercostal region, right side of face, neck or torso. The eruptions are confluent with intense burning sensation in the blister. < Night, cold or open air, after midnight. >

Warmth. Associated with herpes the patient feels very thirsty and gets prostrated very easily.

Apis mellifica: Shingles on the face, especially on the left side of the face. The skin is red or pink with severe burning pains. Marked swelling of the face and especially so about the eyes. > Cold applications.

Borax venenata: Herpes on the cheeks, around chin and on the nates. Tiny vesicles which when rupture exude hot, excoriating, watery fluid. Burning sensation is < warm room and > cold air, fan. Post herpetically the skin becomes wrinkled and wilted.

Bovista lycoperdon: Hard lentil sized eruptions on chest and foot. The vesicles are moist like small red pimples. The discharge from the eruption is sticky and watery forming thick crusts or scabs with pus underneath. Itching and burning sensation < getting warm, after scratching, hot weather, full moon, on washing.

Calcarea carbonica: Herpes with burning and jerking pains, which are < cold, night. Herpes with thick corrosive scabs, which have yellow pus underneath. Suppressed herpes causes central nervous system disorders.

Capsicum annuum: Face, forehead, breasts. Stinging, burning pain as if cayenne pepper were spread on the affected part which is worse from scratching, uncovering and changing position. Intense itching on the scalp as if due to vermin, which causes great restlessness and is worse from scratching.

Carbo vegetabilis: Moist herpetic eruptions on face, chin, about lips and mouth and on the knees. Fugitive itching when getting warm in bed. Scratching leads to burning. Itching < after eating pork or butter tendency to hot perspiration.

Carboneum oxygenisatum: Vesiculation along course of nerves associated with anesthesia.

Carboneum sulphuratum: Chronic herpes. Dorsum of left hand. Herpes phlyctenoides with vesicles on a red inflamed and swollen base. Vesicles contain an opaque yellowish fluid which either forms thick scales or discharges, excoriates and causes violent itching which is better in open air < on bathing, < warm damp weather.

Causticum: Shoulders, neck, around nipples and chin, face, prepuce. There is itching burning pain, which is worse in open air, in clear fine weather and is better in damp weather and from walking.

Chrysarobinum: Vesicular lesions, which are associated with a foul smelling discharge and crust formation. The lesions tend to coalesce and give the appearance of a single large scab. Thighs, legs, ears and skin around the eyes and ears.

Cistus canadensis: Face, ears and various parts of the body. Patient has an itching as if ants are running through the whole body, which is worse at night. Herpes on a mercurio-syphilitic base. Zoster like eruptions on back.

Clematis erecta: Herpetic eruptions, which are moist during increasing and dry during decreasing, moon. Herpetic eruptions coming up after suppression of gonorrhea. Chronic constitutional herpes. Scaly herpes with yellow corrosive watery discharge. There is a tendency of the vesicles to rupture and ulcerate. Gnawing, itching severely in the skin that is not better by scratching and is worse from washing in cold water, from warmth of bed at night and from wet poultices.

Comocladia dentata: Face, arms and legs with tormenting itching and burning which is better in open air, by scratching and worse by warmth, touch, night.

Conium maculatum: Herpes which appears suddenly beginning as a small spot and spreading over the whole part of the arm. The skin is red, swollen, corrugated and oozes blood or lymph from broken places. These form crusts under which the exudation still continues. Herpetic eruptions forming scales as large as the hand on various parts of the body. There is intense itching and an irresistible desire to scratch especially in the evening. Adapted to persons of a scrofulous and cancerous diathesis with induration of glands. Patient complains of stinging like fleabites but always a single sting at a time.

Croton tiglium: Herpes alternating with summer diarrhea. Vesicular and pustular herpes with redness of skin, burning, stinging which is worse after eating, from touch, > by rubbing gently. The vesicles become confluent and form large brown scabs. Itching followed by painful burning which is better by very gentle scratching.

Dolichos pruriens: Arms, legs, axilla. The eruptions of axilla spread forward to the sternum and backwards to the spine. Left scapula extending to chest, gums. Itching, burning < on scratching and at night preventing sleep. > Cold bathing post herpetic neuralgia.

Dulcamara: Hands, arms, face, genitals. In persons who are sensitive to cold season and persons of rheumatic diathesis. Moist suppurating herpes with red areolae which bleed when scratched. The eruptions are associated with fetid perspiration. Herpes with glandular enlargement. Itching, tearing pains that are aggravated by application of cold water, at night, damp cold weather, around menstrual period and is better by moving about.

Eucalyptus globulus: Herpetic eruptions that are associated with glandular enlargement and later develops foul indolent ulcers.

Graphites: Joints, behind ears, groins, neck. Herpes in obese females with delayed and scanty menses. Herpes appearing at climacteric. Large blisters from umbilicus to spine mainly affecting left side. Large blisters which break open and ooze a watery sticky fluid. Itching as though foreign matter would pass out of the skin. Circular herpes, feels hard to touch and is wrinkled. Itching < at night, during and after menses, > wrapping up, > open air.

Hepar sulphur: Face, hands, genitals, bends of knees and elbows. Herpes after abuse of mercury. Herpes zoster from spine forwards especially the left side. The eruption is the seat of acute neuralgic pains that are worse at night. Vesicles on an inflamed base associated with splinter like pains, severe itching and scratching. There is marked aggravation at night, from cold, from touch and the patient feels better in damp weather and from wrapping up warmly. Herpes circinatus. Especially suited to persons with a sour body odor.

Iris versicolor: Herpes zoster associated with gastric derangement. Right side of body especially abdomen. Itching pain < at night. Severe burning in herpes outbreak and life long neuralgia.

Kalium bichromicum: Herpes after exposure to cold; herpes with respiratory disorders. At first, there is violent itching over the whole surface, then there is pustule formation mostly over the extremities. The scabs smart and burn < hot weather, < undressing, > cold weather.

Kalium carbonicum: Face. In persons with dry sensitive skin, where there is burning, stitching pain as if from a mustard plaster associated with itching which is better after scratching. The eruption is dry at first but when scratched exudes moisture. Itching is worse from cold air and better when getting warm. Adapted to persons of tubercular diathesis and who have had eruptions suppressed in childhood.

Kalmia latifolia: Post herpetic neuralgia. Pains shift rapidly, shooting outwards along the course of the nerves. The skin is stiff, dry. Adapted to person of a rheumatic diathesis. Location - More often on the right side. Face, shoulder, trunk, extending down the affected limb.

Kreosotum: Dorsal and palmar surfaces of hands, fingers, joints, on the ears, elbows, knuckles and malleoli. Herpes is moist and itches violently. The itching is < in the evening and in open air to such an extent as to drive the patient wild, > warmth.

Lachesis mutus: The eruption consists of large vesicles, at first yellow in colour and then turning dark with much pain. Deep red or purple eruptions leaving a purplish scar after healing. The eruptions come on every spring and fall and are worse from acids. Old reddish herpes with thick scurf affecting the whiskers. The vesicles later break and leave an excoriated surface that burns when touched. Herpes of the face that reappears after suppression. Herpes zoster after external application of Rhus tox. characterized by hemorrhagic pustules in-groups near the spine and spreading to the mid axillary line. Location – begins under left scapula and extends to the flank. < Heat, night, disturbing sleep.

Ledum palustre: Face and forehead. Violently itching dry herpes. < Evenings, before midnight, open air. > Cold application, rest. Adapted to persons of rheumatic diathesis who have a lack of internal heat yet is intolerant of external heat.

Lithium carbonicum: Herpes of hands. Rough, harsh, dry skin with much itching and burning.

Lycopodium clavatum: Nape of neck, axillae, arms, thighs, tibiae, calves of legs. Scaly furfuraceous herpes, which is yellow at the base in persons with unhealthy humid skin. Insensible yellow brown shrivelled herpes or moist suppurating herpes full of deep rhagades with violent itching as from lice. Itching < pressure, touch, eating cabbage, oysters, drinking wine. > Uncovering. Herpes associated with urinary, gastric or hepatic disorders.

Magnesium carbonicum: Chest, calves of legs, about mouth. Itching vesicles on hands and fingers. Violent itching over whole body > scratching sensation of formication at night.

Manganum: Forearm. Lancinating pains < touch, > while lying on a feather bed. Itching < when sweating, > scratching.

Mercurius solubilis: Right side. Right forearm, wrist and hand. Herpes prepucialis of right side extending across the abdomen. Itching, which changes to burning on scratching and shooting pains < night, heat of bed, lying on painful side, > cold damp weather, and open air. Herpetic eruptions, which are surrounded by small pimples. Herpes with a tendency to suppurate especially in persons with profuse sweat and gastric disturbance. Eroding or spreading vesicles with burning of the eruption when touched; humid and large scabs on edges.

Mezereum: Following the intercostal or supraorbital nerves with severe neuralgia; itching after scratching turns into burning.

Neuralgic pains come and go suddenly, leaving the part numb. Post herpetic neuralgia and burning with great coldness of the body. Herpes tends to ulcerate and forms thick scabs under which purulent matter exudes; tearing off these scabs causes great pain and retards healing. Itching intolerable < warm bath, heat of bed, night. Itching changes place on scratching. > Local heat. Coldness after scratching. Cold feeling, as though cold air was blowing in the eye. Herpes after suppressed eruptions; vaccination and abuse of mercury. Other location - About lips and gums, spreads over whole right face.

Natrium carbonicum: Herpes circinatus; herpes iris. Spreading and suppurating herpes on outside of hands, around nose and mouth; on tips. Herpes with yellow rings. Vesicles with shooting pains and itching > gentle rubbing.

Natrium muriaticum: Skin about the mouth; on arms and eyes, chest, nape of neck, genitals, bends of elbows and knees; knuckles. Herpes labialis during fever. Herpes circinatus with burning spots. Gnawing, itching, shooting pains which are < from heat, sun, at seashore, < eating too much salt; > open air, while sweating.

Natrium sulphuricum: Herpes associated with bilious complaints. Vesicles with watery yellow fluid with itching vesicular eruptions around mouth and chin. Itching and swelling of fingers in bakers. < Undressing, damp houses, basement, < eating plants or fruits growing near water.

Nitricum acidum: Whiskers, between fingers, on alae nasi, on outer side of the thigh. Itching < undressing, change of weather, contact, open air. Post herpetic neuralgia where the pain is sticking like a splinter. Appearance of skin – dry, cracked, fissured with blackish discoloration.

Petroleum: Nape of neck, chest, scrotum, inner side of thigh, perineum, knees and ankles. Herpes zoster when external hard pressure is not painful, but a soft touch, the contact of the shirt, is unbearable. Itching herpes followed by crust, cracks, ulcers. Patient scratches till the skin bleeds and becomes cold. < Cold air, perspiring > warmth, warm air.

Psorinum: Bends of joints especially elbows and knees. Herpetic eruptions after suppression of itch. Itching intolerable < when getting warm before midnight and open air.

Prunus spinosa: Shingles with tightness and stitching pains. Herpes zoster combined with angina pectoris. Location: Chest and torso. Face and orbit, especially on the right side.

Ranunculus bulbosus: Left sided especially chest and flank. Along the course of supraorbital or intercostal nerves, fingers and palms. Sharp, stitching pains which are worse from touch, motion, change of temperature and on entering a cold place, > warm application. The vesicles are filled with a thin, acrid fluid and are found in clusters. Herpes in drunkards. Herpes zoster; bluish vesicles; dark blue, in groups or along course of nerves and burning, shooting pains and forming hard, horny scurfs.

Rhus toxicodendron: Left scapula, right side face, hairy parts. Itching, burning neuralgic pains. Restless with pain and itching. Itching alternates with pains in chest and dysenteric stools. < Sweating, night, after midnight, < winter, > warmth, hot bathing, constantly moving.

Sarsaparilla officinalis: Genitals, upper lip, hands, left leg, calves. Herpes which follow hot weather and vaccinations. Herpetic ulcers, extending in a circular form, forming no crusts, red granulated bases, white borders. The lesion oozes red serous fluid.

Sepia officinalis: Herpes circinatus in isolated spots on upper part of body. Lips, mouth, nose, on neck, behind ears, in the bends of elbows and knees. Lesions are quite painful and often prevent sleep. Periodic outbreaks of herpes zoster. Dry scaly desquamation after drying up of vesicles. Intolerable itching, which turns to burning when scratched. Itching is worse during menses, pregnancy, lactation < cold weather, menses. Especially adapted to females with yellow complexion and uterine complaints.

Silicea terra: Dry herpes affecting the chin. Eruptions are inclined to suppurate.

Staphysagria: Bends of joints, hands, thighs and legs. Dry crusty herpes in-patients with easily suppurating skin. Chilly creeping feeling in affected parts < rubbing, contact. Itching > scratching, but reappears at a different location. Itching associated with tingling as from insects.

Sulphur: Herpes miliaris, phlyctenoides, circinatus and squamous. Dry scaly herpes on nape of neck and ankles. Moist herpes with small white vesicles in-groups, forming scabs over the whole face, especially above nose and about eyes. There is burning pain after scratching. The patient is always worse from washing, bathing, getting warm in bed. Herpes after suppressed eruptions. Location: Flank of abdomen, circling both backwards and forwards.

Thuja occidentalis: Herpes all over the body with violent itching and burning. Eruptions only on covered parts, burning violently when scratched and are < worse from cold water, evening, night < heat of bed. > Gentle rubbing. Adapted to persons of hydrogenoid or lymphatic constitution. Herpes after vaccination. Red pimples become confluent resulting in large blisters. Very sensitive to slightest touch. Location – Face, chest, buttocks. Left sides shingles, breast, arms, and abdomen.

Tellurium metallicum: Herpes circinatus in intersecting rings. Minute itching vesicles on lower limbs or on single parts of scrotum, perineum. Itching and pricking as from bugs. < At night, cool air, sweating. Vesicles are filled with a watery, excoriating fluid smelling like fish brine.

Variolinum: Herpes zoster with sensation of bugs crawling under the skin. Neuralgia persisting after disappearance of herpes. It is an excellent remedy for post herpetic neuralgia. Shingles with pustular eruptions.

Xerophyllum: Flexures of knees. Vesication and itching associated with stinging and burning.

Zincum metallicum: Back and hands with burning pains. Herpes with formication and tingling felt as if between skin and flesh. Dry herpes all over whole body with herpetic ulcers.

Neuralgia following herpes zoster with burning, jerking and itching
< evenings, > touch.

REPERTORY

Acet-ac, acon, aeth, agar, ail, alum, alum-p, alum-sil, am-c,
ambr, anac, anan, anthraco, apis, ars, ars-i, ars-s-f, aster, aur, aur-
ar, aur-i, aur-s, bar-c, bar-m, bar-s, bell, berb, berb-a, borx, bov,
bry, bufo, cadm-s, calad, calc, calc-f, calc-i, calc-s, calc-sil, caps,
carb-an, carb-v, carbn-s, caust. chel, chrys-ac, cic, cist, clem, cocc,
coloc, com, con, crot-h, crot-t, cupr, cycl, dol, dulc, equis-a, ery-m,
gink-b, graph, grat, hell, hep, hydrog, hyos, ictod, iod, iris, jug-c,
jug-r, kali-ar, kali-bi, kali-c, kali-chl, kali-i, kali-m, kali-n, kali-p,
kali-s, kalm, kreos, lac-c, lac-d, lach, led, lyc, mag-c, mag-m, manc,
mang, merc, mez, mosch, mur-ac, nat-ar, nat-c, nat-m, nat-p, nat-s,
nit-ac, nux-v, olnd, par, petr, ph-ac, phos, plb, psor, puls, ran-b,
ran-s, rhus-t, rhus-v, rob, rumx, ruta, sabad, sarr sars, sep, sil, sol-
o, spig, spong, squil, stann, staph, sul-ac, sul-i, sulph, tarax, tell,
teucr, thuj, ulm-c, valer, vario, viol-t, zinc, zinc-p.

- **Alternating** with chest affections and dysenteric stools: rhus-t.
- **Right side:** iris.
- **Barbers itch:** nat-ar, nat-s.
- **Bleeding:** anac, aeth, dulc, lyc.
- **Biting,** itching: psor.
- **Blotches red** after scratching: ip.
- **Body,** all over: dulc, psor, ran-b.
- **Bran,** like: psor.
- **Brown,** thick red, border: dulc.
- **Burning:** agar, alum, alum-p, ambr, am-c, anac, ars, aur, aur-i,
  bar-c, bell, borx, bry, calad, calc, caps, carb-an, carb-v, caust,
  cic, clem, cocc, con, dulc, hell, hep, kali-c, kali-n, kali-sil, kreos,
  lach, led, lyc, mang, merc, mez, nat-c, nat-m, olnd, par, petr,
  ph-ac, phos, plb, psor, puls, ran-b, rhus-t, sabad, sars, sep, sil,
  spig, spong, squil, staph, stram, sulph, teucr, thuj, verat, viol-t,
  zinc.

- Excessive: mosch.
- **Chapping:** alum, aur-met, bry, cadm, cadm-s, calc, cycl, graph, hep, kali-c, kreos, lach, lyc, mag-c, mang, merc, nat-c, nat-m, nit-ac, petr, puls, rhus-t, ruta, sars, sep, sil, sulph, viol-t, zinc.
- **Chronic:** agn, anthraci, clem.
    - Constitutional: clem.
- **Circinate:** anac, anag, ars-s-f, bar-c, calc, chlor, chrys-ac, clem, dulc, equis-a, eup-per, graph, hell, hep, iod, mag-c, nat-c, nat-m, phos, phyt, sep, spong, sulph, tell, thuj, tub.
    - Isolated Spots, in: sep.
    - On back: all-s.
    - On single parts: tell.
    - Pustular: hippoz.
    - Spring, every: sep.
    - Suppressed: ars.
- **Clusters:** dulc.
- **Constipation,** with: carb-ac.
- **Cracking:** cadm-s.
- **Cold water** agg.: clem, dulc, sulph.
- **Corrosive:** alum, alum-p, am-c, bar-c, calc, carb-v, caust, chel, clem, con, graph, hell, hep, kali-c, kali-sil, lach, lyc, mag-c, mang, merc, mur-ac, nit-ac, nux-v, olnd, par, petr, ph-ac, phos, plb, rhus-t, sep, sil, squill, staph, tarax, viol-t..
- **Crusty:** alum, alum-p, ambr, am-c, anac, ars, aur-met, aur-m, bar-c, bell, bov, bufo, calc, cal-sil, caps, carb-an, carb-v, cic, clem, con, cupr, dulc, graph, hell, hep, kali-c, kali-sil, kreos, lach, led, lyc, mag-c, merc, mez, mur-ac, nat-m, nit-ac, nux-v, olnd, par, petr, ph-ac, phos, plb, puls, ran-b, rhus-t, sars, sep, sil, squil, staph, sulph, thuja, verat, viol-t, zinc.
- **Crusty,** itching: guaj, rhus-t.
    - Thick crusts: clem, lyc, sulph.

- **Dry:** alum, alum-sil, anac, ars, bar-c, bov, bry, cact, calc, calc-sil, carb-v, caust, clem, cocc, cupr, dol, dulc, fl-ac, graph, hep, hyos, kali-i, kreos, led, lyc, mang, mag-c, med, merc, nat-c, nat-m, nit-ac, par, petr, phos, ph-ac, psor, rhus-t, sars, sep, sil, stann, staph, sulph, teucr, thuj, valer, verat, viol-t, zinc.

    - Especially in bends of knees: psor.

    - Over the whole body: zinc.

    - Scaly, without itching: cact.

    - Violently itching, burning in open air: led.

    - With scabs on joints: staph.

    - With white scales and behind ears: marr-vg.

- Excoriating: caps, clem, grat, nat-m.

    - Worse evening and in open air, better by warmth: kreos.

    - Fevers, in: carb-v, nat-m, rhus-t.

    - Exudate: sil.

    - Exudes, acid purulent fluid: clem.

    - Exudes of Lupus: kali-bi.

    - Exuding sticky matter: graph.

- Furfuraceous: calc, dulc, merc-s, mur-ac, phos.

- Glands covered, with: dulc, graph.

- Glandular swelling, with: dulc.

- Gray: ars.

- Heat, worse from, which causes burning: con.

- Impetiginous: ars, bapt, cinch, merc, psor, rhus-t.

- Indolent: lyc, mag-c, psor.

- Itching: agar, alum, alum-p, alum-sil, ambr, am-c, anac, ant-t, ars, aur-i, bar-c, bell, borx, bry, calad, calc, calc-sil, caps, carb-an, carb-s, carb-v, caust, chel, cic, clem, cocc, con, cupr, dulc, elaps, graph, guare, hep, jug-r, kali-ar, kali-c, kali-i, kali-sil, kreos, lach, led, lyc, mag-c, mag-m, mang, merc, mez, nat-c, nat-m, nit-ac, nux-v, olnd, par, petr, ph-ac, phos, plb, puls, ran-

b, ran-s, rhus-t, sabad, sars, sep, sil, spig, spong, squil, stann, staph, sulph, tarax, thuj, valer, verat, viol-t, zinc.
- Burning: ars, psor.
- Burning after scratching: lac-d.
- Crusty: thuj.
- Hollow of knees, in: ars.
- Menses, before: carb-v.
- Old, at time of menses: carb-v.
- Pain: nit-ac.
- Prevents sleep till late: staph.
- Warmth of bed and after washing: clem.
- **Jerking,** pain, with: calc, caust, cupr, lyc, puls, rhus-t, sep, sil, staph.
  - Itching and burning, with: rhus-t.
  - With meal dust, humid: psor.
- **Mealy:** am-c, ars, aur-met, borx, bry, calc, cocc, culx, dulc, graph, kreos, led, lyc, merc, mur-ac, phos, sep, sil, sulph, thuj, verat.
- **Menses during:** gink-b, petr.
- **Mercurial:** aur-met, mosch, nit-ac.
- **Moist:** alum, am-c, anan, ars, bar-c, bell, borx, bry, cact, cadm, calc, carb-an, carb-v, caust, cic, cist, clem, con, dulc, graph, grat, hell, hep, kali-c, kreos, lach, led, lyc, merc, mez, nat-c, nat-m, nit-ac, olnd, petr, ph-ac, phos, psor, ran-b, rhus-t, ruta, sep, sil, squil, staph, sulph, sulph-ac, tarax, tell, thuj, viol-t.
  - Moist red: clem.
  - Moist with large scales on edge: merc.
- **Neuralgia, post-herpetic:** kalm.
- **Old, tettery, itch** when menses appear: carb-v.
- **Patches:** ant-c, caust, con, crot-h, graph, hyos, lyc, merc, mur-ac, nat-c, nat-m, nit-ac, petr, phos, sabad, sars, sep, sil, sulph, zinc.

- Brown: sep.
- **Phlyctenoides:** acon, ars, borx, calc, canth, carb-s, clem, merc, phos, ran-s, rhus, sarr, sol, sulph, tell.
    - Phlyctenoids over dorsal surface of hand: carb-s.
    - Pricking: nit-ac.
    - Pale red: dulc.
- **Pimples or pustules** surrounding, spreads by coalescing: hep.
- **Red:** am-c, ars, bry, cic, clem, dulc, kreos, lach, led, lyc, mag-c, mag-s, merc, olnd, petr, ph-ac, staph, tax, tell .
- **Round,** scaly, small: dulc.
- **Scabby:** sulph.
    - Forming scabs as large as hand: con.
- Scaly: agar, anac, anan, ars, aur-met, bell, borx, cact, cadm, calc, cic, clem, con, cupr, dulc, graph, hep, hyos, kali-c, kreos, lach, led, lyss, mag-c.
    - Joints, herpes: dulc, kreos, staph.

Location

- **Eye:**
    - Herpes zoster opthalmicus: ars, canth, crot-t, graph, merc, puls, ran-b, rhus-t.
    - About the eyes: alum, bry, caust, con, kreos, lach, olnd, spong, sulph.
    - Cornea: graph, hep, ign, ran-b.
    - Lids: bry, com, graph, kreos, psor, rhus-t, sep, sulph, tarent, tub.
- **Ear:** am-m, caust, cist, graph, kreos, mag-m, olnd, phos, ptel, sep, teucr.
    - About the ears, vesicles: olnd.
    - Behind the ears: am-m, bufo, caust, cist, con, graph, mag-m, mez, sep, teucr.

- Scabby: kali-i.
- Front of the ear, in: olnd.
- Lobes, on: caust, cist, sep, teucr.
- Meatus: merc.
- **Face:** agar, alum, am-c, am-m, anac, anan, androc, arn, ars, bar-c, bar-s, bell, bry, bufo, calc, calc-f, calc-s, calc-sil, caps, carb-an, carb-v, carbn-s, caust, chel, cic, coloc, con, crot-t, dulc, elaps, gink-b, graph, hep, kali-ar, kali-bi, kali-c, kali-i, kali-s, kali-sil, kreos, lach, led, lyc, merc, nat-ar, nat-c, nat-m, nat-s, nicc, nit-ac, petr, ph-ac, phos, psor, rhus-t, sabad, sarr, sep, sil, spong, sulph, tarent, thuja.
- Burning and itching, with: mez.
- Cheeks: alum, am-c, ambr, anac, ant-t, borx, carbn-s, caust, chel, con, dulc, graph, hep, kali-i, kreos, lach, merc, nat-m, nicc, ph-ac, sars, sil, spong, staph, stront-c, thuj.
- Chin: am-c, borx, carb-v, chel, dulc, nat-m, nux-v, ph-ac, sars, sil .
- Circinatus: anag, bar-c, calc, cinnb, clem, dulc, graph, hell, kali-chl, lith-c, lyc, med, nat-c, nat-m, phos, sep, sulph, tarent, tell, tub.
- Cough, with spasmodic: arn.
- Forehead: bad, bar-c, borx, caps, dulc, tarent.
- Lips, about: agar, anac, ars, asc-t, borx, calc-f, canth, carb-v, caust, chel, choc, conv, crot-t, dulc, graph, hep, hyos, ip, kali-p, lac-c, lach, med, nat-ar, nat-c, nat-m, nicc, par, petr, ph-ac, rhus-t, sars, sep, sil, spong, sulph, tub, urt-u.

    - Upper: agar, carc, gink-b, sars.

    - Right, painful: med.

    - Above: phos.

- Mealy: ars, bry, cic, kreos, lyc, merc, nit-ac, sulph, thuj.
- neuralgia, with facial: kalm.

- scurfy: anac, anan, calc, graph, kreos, led, lyc, phos, rhus-t, sep, sulph.

- mouth, around: am-c, anac, ars, borx, cic, con, hep, kreos, mag-c, med, nat-c, nat-m, par, petr, phos, rhus-t, sep, sulph.

  - Corners: carb-v, choc, lyc, med, ph-ac, phos, sep, sulph.

  - Below: calc-f, nat-m.

  - Tongue, on: nat-m, zinc.

- **Nose:** Aeth, aloe, aur-met, calc, carc, chel, conv, gink-b, graph, led, lyc, nat-c, nat-m, nit-ac, ph-ac, phys, rhus-t, sep, sil, spig, sulph.

  - Itching: nit-ac.

  - Across nose: sep, sulph.

  - Saddle, like a: sulph.

  - Nostrils: phys.

  - Tip of: aeth.

  - Wings of: nit-ac.

  - Menses, during, beginning of menses at: gink-b.

  - Whiskers: agar, calc, lach, nat-m, nit-ac, sil.

- **Chest:** ars, graph, hep, lyc, mag-c, petr, staph, syph.

  - Zona: dol, graph, lach, mez, rhus-t, staph, thuj.

- **Back:** all-s, ars, lach, lyc, nat-c, sep, zinc.

  - Zoster: cist, lach, merc, rhus-t.

  - Cervical region: ars, carb-an, caust, clem, con, graph, hyos, kali-n, lac-d, lyc, nat-m, petr, psor, sep, sulph.

  - Itching: caust.

  - Moist: carb-an, caust, nat-m, sep.

- **Extremities:** alum, borx, caust, com, con, cupr, dulc, graph, led, lyc, manc, mang, merc, mur-ac, nat-m, nicc, nux-v, petr, psor, sars, sec, sep, staph, thuj, zinc.

  - Upper limbs: alum, borx, bov, calc, caust, con, cupr, dol, dulc, graph, kali-c, kreos, lyc, mag-s, manc, mang, merc, nat-c, nat-m, nux-v, phos, psor, sars, sec, sep, sil.

    - Crusty: con, thuj.

    - Furfuraceous: merc, phos.

    - Joints, on the: calc, merc.

- **Shoulder:** kali-ar.

- **Upper arm:** kali-c, mang, nat-m, sulph.

- **Elbow:** borx, cact, cupr, hep, kreos, phos, psor, sep, staph, thuj.

- **Forearm:** alum, con, mag-s, mang, merc, nat-m, sulph.

- **Wrist:** ip, merc, psor.

- **Hand:** borx, bov, calc, cist, con, dulc, graph, kreos, merc, mez, nat-c, nat-m, ran-b, sars, sep, staph, verat, zinc.

    - Back of: carbn-s, graph, lyc, nat-c, petr, sep, thuj.

    - Palm: aur, kreos, psor, ran-b, sep.

    - Between the fingers: ambr, graph, merc, nit-ac.

    - Between index finger and thumb: ambr.

- **Fingers:** ambr, caust, cist, graph, kreos, merc, nit-a, psor, ran-b, thuj, zinc.

- **Lower limbs:** alum, borx, caust, clem, com, graph, kali-c, lach, led, lyco, merc, mur-ac, nat-m, nicc, petr, sars, sep, sil, staph, tell, zinc.

- **Nates:** borx, caust, kreos, nat-c, nicc.

- **Hip:** nat-c, nicc, sep.

- **Thigh:** clem, graph, kali-c, lyc, merc, mur-ac, nat-c, nat-m, nit-ac, petr, sars, sep, staph, zinc.

- **Knee:** ars, carb-v, dulc, graph, kreos, merc, nat-c, nat-m, petr, phos, psor, sulph.

    - Hollow of: ars, calc, con, graph, kreos, led, nat-c, nat-m, petr, phos, psor, sulph.

- **Leg:** ars, calc, calc-p, com, graph, kali-c, lach, lyc, lyss, mag-c, merc, nat-m, petr, sars, sep, staph, zinc.

- **Calf:** cycl, lyc, sars.
- **Ankle:** cact, cycl, kreos, nat-c, nat-m, petr, sulph.
- **Feet:** alum, mez, nat-m, petr, sulph.
- **Toes:** alum.
  - Toes, between: alum, graph.

MEASLES

Synonym

Morbilli.

Etiology

Measles virus initially replicates in the naso-pharynx and upper respiratory tract before disseminating widely throughout the body.

During the prodromal period there is lymphoid hyperplasia and a wide distribution of multinucleate giant cells or syncytia with up to 100 nuclei. In uncomplicated infections these disappear as the rash emerges. The prodromal rash appears to be the result of viraemia with lodgement of antigen and virus in the capillaries. Cells in the Koplik's spots also contain viral nucleocapsids. The conspicuous macular eruption on the fourth day is the result of the CMI response against this material. If the response is defective as in leukaemia, especially when cytotoxic drugs are used, there may be no rash but progressive viral replication to produce a giant-cell pneumonia or a fatal encephalopathy. Shortly after the rash appears, measles virus causes a transient depression of the T-cell-mediated immune responses, which is an important feature of the infection.

Clinical Features

After an incubation period of about 10 days, the prodromal symptoms of fever, malaise and upper respiratory catarrh begin acutely. The conjunctivae are injected and there may be photophobia. From the second day, Koplik's spots are usually present on the buccal mucous membrane opposite the premolar teeth-bluish white spots with bright-red areolae. Fever, catarrh and cough increase for 3-5 days. The exanthema characteristically develops on the fourth day on the forehead and behind the ears, and spreads within 24 hrs. to the rest of the face, the trunk and the limbs. The rash is at first macular but soon forms dull red papules which tend to coalesce in irregularly concentric patterns but may be more diffusely confluent. From the sixth to the 10th day the rash fades, to leave some brownish staining and fine desquamation.In very severe forms it may be hemorrhagic. An extensive bullous eruption may develop during the acute stage of measles. In some cases this eruption has the features of Stevens-Johnson syndrome, but in others it resembles epidermal necrolysis. It is possible that in some suspected cases drugs were responsible, but in others the eruption appears to have been directly related to the virus infection. It is sometimes inappropriately referred to as measles phemphigoid.

Complications are more common in young children, the malnourished and the chronically ill. Bronchopneumonia, enteritis and otitis media are less frequent now. The most serious complication is encephalitis.

Diagnosis

The features of other infective exanthems are considered in this chapter. Drug eruptions should not cause confusion as the upper respiratory catarrh and conjunctival suffusion are absent. Specific measles antibodies are usually detectable 3 or 4 days after the appearance of the rash, and maximum titres are reached 2-4 weeks later. Virus isolation is not easy but viral antigen can be detected by immuno-fluorescence in cell smears prepared from nasopharyngeal aspirates taken early during the illness.

HOMEOPATHIC APPROACH TO MEASLES

It is a disease, which in my practice has given me undue stress as after the introduction of measles vaccine in India we find only 15-20% of the cases matching to the textbook picture of the disease.

Majority of them are atypical presentations that can be easily misdiagnosed to be enteric fever, malaria, influenza and streptococcal sore throat. Only a thorough history taking and proper clinical examination can minimize the risk of misdiagnosing measles.

When you see a full-fledged case of measles the symptoms will match very closely to Pulsatilla, but remember that all the patients do not improve with Pulsatilla. Hence one has to study the case very minutely in order to differentiate closely related remedies.

Selection of the remedies has to be on the totality of symptoms at that particular time. As majority of the patients, children or adults, present with fever or symptome of upper respiratory tract infection one has to study the chapters of Fever, Chill and Perspiration with all its concomitants thoroughly especially from the Boger-Boenninghausen Repertory.

I have very rarely used Morbillinum in my clinical practice and hence I shall not advocate its use by students and practioners as a specific remedy or a preventive remedy for measles.

I have repeatedly observed that once the rash comes up one should not repeat the remedy as repetition always invites complications.

Drugs like Bryonia alb., Camphor, Cuprum met., Sulphur and Zincum met. have been useful in my practise in cases where the eruptions fail to appear as either the patient is too weak to bring it out or due suppression from the indiscriminate use of antibiotics in the past.

In cases of Encephalitis or SSPE drugs like Hoitzia coccinea and Rajania subsamarata are extremely useful.

Some of the most obstinate cases of cough after measles have been treated successfully using drugs like Euphrasia, Eupatorium perfolatum and Sticta pulmonaria. In cases for asthma developing after measles Carbo veg. has been very useful.

Measles being predominantly tubercular miasm use of

Tuberculinum as an anti miasmatic drug is very important at the end of the attack. Here one may also use the current constitutional remedy for the same purpose.

VERRUCAE (WARTS)

Synonym

Warts (Hindustani equivalent is 'masse').

Introduction

HPVs (Human pappilloma virus) can infect and cause disease at any site in stratified squamous epithelium, either keratinizing (skin) or non-keratinizing (mucosa). The clinical problems encountered with such infections can be broadly divided into cutaneous warts, genital warts, oral warts and laryngeal warts.

Warts are a very common problem in practice, particularly among children. It can affect any part of the body. In countries with highly developed medical services, referral rates of warts to dermatology clinics have greatly increased in the last four decades.

Incubation Period

Common and plantar warts: The time of acquisition of the infection can seldom be ascertained. An estimated period ranges between a few weeks and more then a year.

Genital warts: Incubation period of 3 weeks to 8 months, average 2.8 months. Perinatally acquired HPV infection may not manifest as genital warts for up to 2 years.

Laryngeal warts: Only 57% of cases of laryngeal papilloma in children are diagnosed by 2 years of age.

Infectivity

In genital warts infectiviy is highest early in the course of the disease. Any sexual contact of a patient with genital warts is likely also to be infected. There is no reliable information on the infectivity of common and plantar warts, but experience suggests that it is substantially less. The infectivity of maternal genital HPV as regards laryngeal papilloma in the child seems low.

Modes of Trasmission

Warts are spread by direct or indirect contact. Impairment of the epithelial barrier function, by trauma (including mild abrasions), maceration or both, greatly predisposes to inoculation of virus, and is generally assumed to be required for infection, at least in fully keratinized skin, as in the following examples:

- Plantar warts are commonly acquired from swimming pool or shower-room floors, whose rough surfaces abrade moistened keratin from infected feet and help to inoculate virus into the softened skin of others.

- Common hand warts may spread widely round the nails in those who bite their nails or periungual skin, over habitually sucked fingers in young children, and to the lips and surrounding skin in both cases.

- Shaving may spread wart infection over the beard area.

- Occupational handlers of meat, fish and poultry have high incidences of hand warts, attributed to cutaneous injury and prolonged contact with wet flesh and water.

- Genital warts have a high infectivity. The thinner mucosal surface is presumably more susceptible to inoculation of virus than is thicker keratinized skin, but in addition lesions were noted to be commonest in sites subject to greatest coital friction in both sexes.

Histopathology

The characteristic histological feature of viral warts is vacuolation in cells in and below the granular layer, often with basophilic inclusion bodies composed of viral particles, and eosinophilic inclusions representing abnormal keratohyaline granules. This cytopathic effect may show detailed features typical of the HPV type involved and is almost always accompanied by epidermal acanthosis and often papillomatosis.

Clinical Features

COMMON WARTS

Common warts (excluding plantar warts) are due mainly to HPV 2. They range in size from less than 1mm to over 1cm in diameter, and by confluence can form large masses. They are characterized by firm papules with a rough, horny surface.

Site

Commonly situated on the backs of the hands and fingers.

Age

In children under 12 years of age. A single wart may persist unchanged for months or years, or large numbers may develop rapidly or after an interval. New warts may form at sites of trauma, though this Köbner isomorphic phenomenon is usually less marked than in plane warts. However, multiple warts around the nail folds are often seen in nail biters.

Common warts are usually symptomless, but may be tender on the palmar aspects of the fingers, when fissured or when growing beneath the nail plate. Warts around the nail folds or beneath the nail may disturb the nail growth, and warts on the eyelids may be associated with keratitis or conjunctivitis.

About 65% of warts disappear spontaneously within 2 years and tend to do so earlier in boys. Neither the patient's age nor the number of warts present influences the course. Regression of common warts is asymptomatic and occurs gradually over several weeks, usually without blackening. Malignant change is extremely rare.

PLANTAR WARTS

Site

As suggested by the name, they occur mainly on the soles of the feet. Most plantar warts are beneath pressure points, the heel or the metatarsal heads. In older girls and women they occur predominantly beneath the forefoot and toes. They are sometime found on the palms of the hand.

Appearance

A plantar wart at first appears as a small shining 'sago-grain' papule, but soon assumes the typical appearance of a sharply defined, rounded lesion, with a rough, keratotic surface surrounded by a smooth collar of thickened horn. If the surface is gently pared with a scalpel the abrupt separation between the wart tissue and the protective horny ring becomes more obvious, as the epithelial ridges of the plantar skin are not continued over the surface of the wart. If the paring is continued, small bleeding points, the tips of the elongated dermal papillae, are evident.

Mosaic wart is so described from the appearance presented by a plaque of closely grouped warts on the sole with a polygonal outline and a rough surface.

Pain is a common but variable symptom. It may be severe and disabling but may be absent, and many warts are discovered only on routine inspection. Mosaic warts are often painless.

The duration of plantar warts is very variable. Spontaneous regression occurs sooner in children than in adults and is delayed if hyperhidrosis or orthopaedic defects are present.

The number of warts present does not influence the prognosis, but mosaic warts tend to be persistent. Regression is occasionally clinically inflammatory, and often culminates in blackening from thrombosed blood before the lesion separates, but in many cases simply takes the form of apparent drying and gradual separation.

Differential Diagnosis

- Plantar warts are often confused with callosities or corns, with which they may indeed be associated.

- Callosities have a uniformly smooth surface across which the epidermal ridges continue without interruption. In cases of doubt the horny layer should be gently pared.

- Corns occur on pressure points on the toes, soles or interdigital skin. When the surface is scraped it shows the absence of papillomatous surface typical of plantar warts. Corns are most painful when pressed from the top as compared to the wart in which the pain is felt on pressure from the top as well as the sides.

PLANE WARTS

Site

The face and the backs of the hands and the shins are the sites of predilection. Children are most commonly affected.

Appearance

They are smooth, flat or slightly elevated and are usually skin-coloured or greyish-yellow, but may be pigmented. They are round or polygonal in shape and vary in size from 1 to 5 mm or more in diameter. Contiguous warts may coalesce and a linear arrangement in scratch marks is a characteristic feature.

Regression of plane warts is usually heralded by inflammation in the lesions, causing itch, erythema and swelling, such that previously unnoticed warts may become evident. Depigmented haloes may appear around the lesions. Resolution is usually complete within a month.

Differential Diagnosis

In differential diagnosis, lichen planus causes most difficulty. It is relatively less common in children, favours the flexor aspects of the forearms, is unusual on the face and is often itchy. The mucous membranes may be involved. The flat, polygonal papules are lilac-pink and smooth and may show Wickham's striae. In contrast, the surface of plane warts has a stippled appearance under the hand lens. The lesions in molluscum contagiosum are pearly in colour, look like solid vesicles, and when squeezed, cheese like material is demonstrated.

FILIFORM AND DIGITATE WARTS

Site

Commonly seen in males, on the face and neck, irregularly distributed, and often clustered. Digitate warts, often in small groups, also occur on the scalp in both sexes, where they are occasionally confused with epidermal naevi. Isolated warts on the limbs often assume filiform shape.

Appearance

The lesions are flesh coloured or somewhat darker, rounded or oval papules or nodules. The size of these varies from lentil seeds to split peas (somewhat bigger). Their verrucous surface is very typical; once seen it is seldom missed. On the scalp the wart may have a cauliflower like appearance. The warts do not itch but the subungal warts may be painful. Koebner's phenomenon represented by linear group of warts following innoculaton of virus into the scratch may be seen. In the beard region, they may take the form of finger like processes: filiform warts.

Differential Diagnosis

A single common wart should be distinguished from Butcher's or postmortem wart (tuberculosis cutis verrucosus), which is marked by induration around the periphery of the lesion. Verruca vulgaris should be distinguished from seborrheic warts, which are multiple, circumscribed, flat elevations covered with dark, greasy scales. They occur mainly on the trunk, forehead and temples.

ANOGENITAL WARTS

The term condyloma acuminatum (condyloma = knuckle; acuminatum = pointed), pl. condylomata acuminata, was originally used to emphasize the difference between ano-genital warts, which are usually protuberant, and the flatter syphilitic lesions, condylomata lata. It became an accepted term, mostly in the American literature, for viral anogenital warts.

With recent developments in the understanding of HPV disease, it is clear that the term is used variously to denote (i) the classical protuberant type of anogenital wart only; (ii) all clinically identifiable HPV disease of the anogenital region including flat warts on the external genitalia and cervical 'flat condylomas'; (iii) all clinical lesions due to the HPV types usually associated with genital warts, including those in extragenital sites, for example the mouth.

Site

The area of frenulum, corona and glans in men, and the posterior fourchette in women, correspond to the likely sites of greatest coital friction.

Appearance

They are often asymptomatic, but may cause discomfort, discharge or bleeding. The typical anogenital wart is soft, pink, elongated and sometimes filiform or pedunculated. The lesions are usually multiple especially on moist surfaces, and their growth can be enhanced during pregnancy, or in the presence of other local infections. Large malodorous masses may form on vulvar and perianal skin. This classical 'acuminate' (sometimes called papillomatous, or hyperplastic) form constitutes about two-thirds of anogenital warts.

Patients with genital warts frequently have other genital infections. These are mainly minor conditions such as candidiasis, trichomoniasis and non-specific genital infection. The duration of anogenital warts varies from a few weeks to many years.

F- 19

Recurrences can be expected in about 25% of cases, the interval varying from 2 months to 23 years.

Differential Diagnosis

Differentiation is from condylomata. In long standing cases, giant condyloma accuminatum of Buschke and squamous cell carcinoma must be excluded by microscopic examination. Genital warts are often acquired along with other venereal infections and as such tests for syphilis and gonorrhea should be carried out.

EPIDERMODYSPLASIA VERRUCIFORMIS

Invasion of viral warts in genetically predisposed persons, manifested by profuse coalescent eruptions of verruca plana type lesions, usually on the limbs.

HOMEOPATHIC APPROACH TO WARTS

Warts are something very peculiar. Some, specially, if they are numerous, sometime heal very rapidly, whereas others isolated warts, sometimes bid defiance to all treatment. This is one of the important manifestations of sycotic miasm.

The following points should be noted very carefully during case taking:

Causation

E.g.,
- After Gonorrhea: Thuja.
- After having consumed too much salt: Nitri spiritus dulcis.
- After abuse of mercury: Sarsaparilla.
- After syphilitic infection: Aurum met.
- After injury: Bellis perennis.

Previous Treatment

It is essential to know whether patient has attempted to cauterize with the help of the following:

- Acetic acid.
- Caustic potash.
- Fluoric acid.
- Silver nitrate.
- Burning with the help of Agarbatti (a perfume stick used in India).

If it is so then it should be antidoted as follows:

- Ailments after cauterization: Caust, Nit-ac, Thuj.
- Use of Acetic acid, Caustic Potash and Fluoric acid preferably in high potencies.
- For bad effects of Silver nitrate – Use Natrium mur. in high potencies.
- When Agarbatti is used, then to neutralize its ill effects, use Carbolicum acidum or Causticum.
- When electric cautery is used for cauterization, it should be antidoted with drugs like Carbolicum acidum, Causticum, Radium bromatum and X-ray.

Location

E.g.,
- Face
- Fingers
- Palms, etc.

Characteristic

- Flat
- Fleshy
- Hard
- Horny
- Pedunculated
- Smooth, etc.

Whether warts are associated:

- With or without inflammation.

- With or without itching.
- With or without bleeding.
- With or without suppuration.
- With or without ulceration.
- Tender or non-tender.

Important Characteristic Sensations

You should always enquire about e.g.:

- Burning.
- Pulsating.
- Stinging.
- Stitching.

This is very important when the wart is isolated.

The colour of the warts

Sometimes the colour of the wart also helps us to select remedy indirectly:

- Red: Calc Carb, Thuja.
- Brown: Sepia, Thuja.
- Greyish brown: Conium.

It is strongly advised not to recommend to the patient any local application for the treatment of warts, e.g. application of lime, homeopathic mother tinctures or remedies like Salicylic acid, Fluoric acid, for the following reasons:

- It is against the basic principle of homeopathy.
- Recurrence rate is very high.
- Since the cause lies within, it is futile to cure disease externally.

Treatment Review

- I have observed that majority of cases get cured, where only, constitutional remedies were prescribed and occasionally those remedies, which do not produce warts in its provings, have frequently cured the cases at the beginning should be on a constitutional background.

- Failing to respond to the above method a drug should be selected taking into account the local signs and symptoms. If this also fails then only one should take help of empirical or specific medicine.

- It is always wise to restudy the case at least three times before seeking these specific medicines.

- Ficus carica, Calcarea ovi testae and Calcarea calcinata are three good homeopathic remedies that I have found useful in my practise.

Some Important Homeopathic Drugs

Aceticum acidum: On touching the wart one feels a moist sensation. These flat warts are present in pale, lean, thin, anemic, debilitated persons with lax, flabby muscles. The skin is dry and hot to touch. There is excessive perspiration on the skin.

Alumina: Warts associated with chapped, dry skin. There is intolerable itching when getting warm in bed. The skin is dry, rough and cracked. The skin symptoms usually become worse in winter, full moon and new moon.

Anacardium orientale: Warts are found on palms of hands. The Anacardium patient is found mostly among the neurasthenics; such have a type of nervous dyspepsia, relieved by food; impaired memory, depression and irritability; diminution of senses.

Antimonium crudum: Hand – hard, horny, soft or smooth with stinging pain. A circle of ulcers surrounds warts. Warts develop in individuals who have suppresion of eruptions or ulcers and who are prone to pressure and friction; especially suited to individuals who have a tendency to grow fat. The other locations of warts are the neck and arms.

Argentum nitricum: Palate, near anus. Brownish and hard to touch. The wart tends to ulcerate easily. Tendency to develop warts in-patients with mental and digestive symptoms.

Baryta carbonica: Hands, fingers. Small warts with stinging pain, gradually due to friction warts get excoriated and start oozing. It typically affects patients who are dwarfish mentally and physically with a tendency to enlargement of glands with induration. There is a strong tendency to take cold.

Belladonna: Warts inflamed with burning pain. They are hot and tender to touch with characteristic throbbing pain.

Bovista lycoperdon: Upper limb. They are very painful due to the inflammation surrounding it. They also tend to suppurate easily.

Calcarea carbonica: Face, neck, upper extremities, male genitalia, canthi, fingers. They are black, fleshy, hard, horny, sometimes inflamed and painful. They are indented, round or become hollow. They tend to suppurate giving an odor of stale cheese. A circle of ulcers surrounds the warts. The skin is icy cold to touch with cold and profuse perspiration. Development of warts in-patients having a history of suppression of eruptions and perspiration. Development of warts in individuals with scrophulous diathesis with faulty development of bones. It has a typical physical constitution, i.e., fat, flabby, fair, perspiring, cold and moist.

Causticum: Nose, eyebrows, face, lips, near the nails, tips of fingers, upper limbs. They are large, horny, broad, flat and hard, moist and pedunculated, small and fleshy. They tend to bleed easily. They are also prone to easy suppuration. Warts after suppressed eruptions. The warts can be sensitive to touch.

Dulcamara: Face, hands, fingers, close to nails. Warts are smooth, hard, flat, fleshy, usually coming in crops. Worse from cold washing. The warts can be large and pedunculated.

Euphorbium officinarum: The warts are covered by erythema with fine bran like desquamation. There is a smarting and burning sensation in the warts.

Ferrum picricum: Multiple warts, especially on hands, usually pedunculated. There is a sensation as if warts are growing on the thumb.

Fluoricum acidum: Hands and fingers. They are flat and hard with presence of elevated red blotches, which resemble fleshy warts. The appearance of the skin is dry, harsh, with multiple cracks and itching.

Graphites: Female genitalia: cauliflower shaped. They discharge sticky exudation, which smells like old cheese or herring brine. The appearance of skin is dry, rough, irritable that breaks easily and exudes a gluey moisture which is worse in folds. Warts are present in persons who have tendency to develop erysipelas. The patient is extremely sensitive to cold. Digestive symptoms are important conconitant symptoms to warts.

Hepar sulphur: Truly indicated in syphilitic warts with burning, sore, stitching and stinging pain in warts. They tend to suppurate easily. Their discharge smells like old cheese. The warts are small in size and bleed easily.

Lachesis mutus: Hard, smooth, small warts with bluish, purple surrounding. The wart may appear small but it has strong tendency to bleed.

Lycopodium clavatum: Two types:

1. Isolated warts,

2. Warts in crops.

Warts are situated usually on face, tongue, male genitalia, upper limbs and fingers. Warts are associated with terrible itching. They are large, fagged, furrowed, splitted and pedunculated. They exude moisture, surrounded by a herpetic areola with desquamation. The warts have tendency to bleed easily.

Millefolium: Tendency to develop sycotic warts that bleed very easily.

Medorrhinum: Warts are small, pedunulated resembling small button mushrooms/filiform especially on thighs and other parts of the body. They emit offensive odor. The skin is cold to touch. It affects individuals who have poor resistance due to sycotic taint.

Natrium muriaticum: Palms, hands, knuckles. Cutting pain in wart, look of the skin is oily, dry, harsh, unhealthy or yellow. Tendency to develop warts in individual after cautery with silver nitrate.

Nitricum acidum: Female genitalia, anus, cervical region, inside nose, external throat, sternum, eyelids, canthi. They usually develop after abuse of mercury. The following are the characteristics - Moist, cauliflower like, hard/soft, rhagadic, large, indented, inflamed, Pricking pain < night, emit fetid discharge, and bleeds on touch.

Nitri spiritus dulcis: Warts after abuse of excessive salt.

Phosphoricum acidum: Mouth, male genitalia. They are hot to touch, large, jagged in appearance.

Psorinum: Canthi, around mouth, near male genitalia. There is a sensation of itching, < heat of bed. The appearance of skin is dirty, rough, scabby, and greasy. It breaks out in folds.

Ranunculus bulbosus: Produces cauliflower like warts especially situated on outer side of terminal phalanx of right thumb.

Rhus toxicodendron: Fingers, hands, upper limb. Warts are horny, rough, and knotty. Thickened epidemis forms hard crust, which peels off.

Sepia officinalis: Male genitalia, upper lip, fingers, face. They are small, flat, hard dark, sometimes brownish with a horny excrescences in center. There is sensation of itching. Appearance of skin blotched, raw, rough, hard or cracked. Tendency to form induration and warts from constant pressure.

Silicea terra: External throat, upper limb, back, forearm. They are large, fleshy and suppurating, painful to touch. Development of warts in individual with scrofulous diathesis. The patient is keenly sensitive to noise, pain and cold.

Staphysagria: Anus, tongue, male genitalia. They are moist pedunculated and are extremely sensitive to touch. Warts appear after abuse of mercury and suppressed eruption. Warts in syphilitic individual.

Sulphur: Face, near eyelids, on upper lip. Warts covered with thin epidermis. The appearance of skin is dry, rough, wrinkled, and scaly. Warts alternate with other complaints. Suppression of warts leads to asthma.

Thuja occidentalis: Back, cervical region, upper limb, face, nose, eyebrows, eyes, eyelids, external throat. They are broad, conical, flat, pedunculated, indented, in appearance. They are reddish in colour, bleed easily. The warts have a tendency to split from their edge or from the surface.

REPERTORY

Acet-ac, alum, am-c, ambr, anac, anag, anac, anan-c, ant-c, ant-t, arg-nit, ars, ars-br, aur-met, aur-ar, aur-m, aur-m-n, bar-c, bell, benz-ac, bov, borx, bufo, calc, calc-cn, calc-o-t, calc-s, carb-an, carb-v, carc, castm, castor-eq, caust, chel, chr-o, chr-ac, cinnb, cupr, colch, cub, cund, cupre-l, dulc, euphr, euph, ferr, ferr-ma, ferr-p, ferr-pic, fic-c, fl-ac, graph, hep, kali-ar, kali-br, kali-c, kali-chl, kali-m, kali-perm, lac-c, lach, limx, lyc, mag-s, med, merc-c, merc-i-f, merc-i-r, mill, nat-c, nat-m, nat-p, nat-s, nit-ac, nit-s-d, ox-ac, pall, petr, ph-ac, phos, pic-ac, phyt, psor, puls, ran-b, rhus-t, ruta, sabin, sars, semp, sep, sil, spig, staph, sulph, syph, thuj, x-ray

- **Black:** calc, hecla.
- **Bleeding:** ambr, caust, cinnb, hep, lyc, nat-c, nit-ac, ph-ac, phos, staph, rhus-t, thuj.
    - Washing from: nit-ac.
    - Easily, jagged, large: caust, nit-ac.
- **Broad:** caust, dulc.
- **Broad,** dry, moist: acet-ac..
- **Brown:** sep, thuj..
- **Burning:** am-c, ars, hep, lyc, petr, phos, rhus-t, sabin, sep, sulph, thuj.
- **Cauliflower like** on outer side of terminal phalanx of right thumb: ran-b.

- **Cold washing agg.:** dulc.
- **Conical:** ant-t, nat-m.
- **Cylindrical:** carc.
- **Cracked,** ragged with furfuraceous areola: lyc.
- **Drawing** in: con.
- **Dry:** fl-ac, sars, staph.
- **Fan shaped,** on genitals: thuj.
- **Fissured:** thuj.
- **Filiform:** med.
- **Flat:** acet-ac, berb, caust, dulc, fl-ac, lach, merc-i-r, merc-i-f, ruta, sep, thuj.
- **Flat, smooth,** sore: ruta.
- **Fleshy:** calc, carc, caust, dulc, sil, staph, thuj.
- **Girls,** young: sep, sulph, thuj.
- **Growing:** kali-c.
- **Granular:** arg-n, calc, nit-ac, staph, thuj.
- **Hard:** ant-c, calc, calc-sil, caust, dulc, fl-ac, lach, ran-b, sep, sil, sulph, thuj
- **Hollow,** becomes: calc.
- **Horny**: ant-c, calc, caust, dulc, graph, nat-c, nit-ac, ran-b, rhus-t, sep, sulph, thuj.
- **Horny,** broad: rhus-t.
- **Indented:** calc, euphr, lyc, nit-ac, ph-ac, rhus-t, sabin, sep, staph, thuj.
- **Inflamed:** am-c, bell, bov, calc, calc-sil, caust, hep, lyc, nat-c, nit-ac, rhus-t, sars, sep, sil, staph, sulph, thuj.
- **Isolated:** lyc, thuj.
- **Itching:** carb-an, euphr, graph, kali-c, kali-n, nit-ac, phos, psor, sabin, sep, sulph, thuj.
- **Jagged:** caust, nit-ac, lyc, ph-ac, rhus-t, sep, staph, thuj.

- **Large:** caust, dulc, kali-c, nat-c, nit-ac, ph-ac, rhus-t, sep, sil, thuj.
- **Hard,** dark color: sep.
    - Jagged: caust.
    - Jagged and pedunculated, exuding moisture and bleeds easily: lyc.
    - Seedy: thuj.
    - Smooth, fleshy on back of hands: dulc.
    - Soft: mag-s, dulc.
    - Suppurating, fleshy: sil.
- **Lupoid:** ferr-pic.
- **Mercury,** after abuse of: aur-met, nit-ac, staph.
- **Moist:** nit-ac, thuj, caust, rhus-t, lyc, ph-ac, psor, staph.
    - **Oozing:** nit-ac.
    - **Moist,** itching, flat, broad: thuj.
- **Old:** calc, caust, kali-c, nit-ac, rhus-t, sulph, thuj, rhod.
- **Painful:** am-c, ambr, bov, calc. calc-sil, caust, hep, kali-c, kali-s, kali-sil, lach, lyc,.nat-c, nat-m, nit-ac, petr, phos, rhus-t, ruta, sabin, sep, sil, sulph, thuj.
    - Sore pains: ruta.
    - Hard, stiff, shining: Sil.
    - Sticking: nit-ac, staph, thuj.
- **Pedunculated:** caust, nit-ac, dulc, lyc, med, nat-s, ph-ac, rhus-t, sabin, sil, staph, thuj.
- **Pricking:** nit-ac.
- **Pulsating:** calc, kali-c, lyc, petr, sep, sil, sulph.
- **Red:** calc, nat-s, thuj.
- **Round:** calc.
- **Ragged:** nat-c, ph-ac, rhus-t, thuj.
- **Rough,** seed warts: caust.

- **Salt,** having used too much: nit-s-d.
- **Scrofulous:** aur.
- **Seedy:** thuj.
- **Sensitive** to touch: caust, cupr, hep, nat-c, nat-m, staph, thuj.
- **Shooting:** bov.
- **Small:** bar-c, bar-s, berb, calc, carc, caust, dulc, ferr, ferr-p, hep, lach, nit-ac, rhus-t, sars, sep, sulph, thuj.
    - All over body: caust.
    - Many: calc, sars.
    - Pedunculated all over body: caust.
- **Smell like old cheese or herring brine:** calc, graph, hep, thuj.
- **Smooth:** ant-c, calc, dulc, ruta.
- **Soft:** am-c, ant-c, calc, calen, carc, nit-ac, nat-s, sil, thuj.
- **Sore:** nit-ac.
- **Spongy:** calc, lyc, nit-ac, staph, thuj.
- **Stinging:** am-c, ant-c, bar-c, bar-s, calc, calc-sil, caust, graph, hep, kali-sil, lyc, nit-ac, rhus-t, sep, sil, staph, sulph, thuj.
- **Stitching:** bov, hep, nit-ac.
- **Suppressed:** mang, merc, meny, nit-ac, staph, thuj.
- **Suppurating:** ars, bov, calc, calc-sil, caust, hep, kali-sil, nat-c, sil, thuj.
- **Sycotic:** alum, mill, nat-s.
- **Syphilitic:** aur, aur-ar, aur-m-n, aur-s, hep, merc, nit-ac, staph, thuj.
- **Sycotic, syphilitic:** nit-ac.
- **Tearing:** am-c.
- **Thick:** dulc.
- **Thin epidermis,** with: nit-ac.
- **Throbbing:** calc-c, kali-c, lyc, petr, sep, sil, sulph.
- **Ulcers,** become, warts: calc, hell.

- surrounded by a circle of ulcers, warts: ant-c, ars, calc, nat-c, phos.

Location

- **Generalized, all over body:** nat-s, sep.
- **Forehead:** castor-eq.
- **Eye:** arund, calc, cinn-b, merc, nit-ac, phos, staph, thuj.
    - Sclerotics: arund.
    - Canthi: calc, nit-ac, psor.
    - Cornea: ars.
    - Eyebrows: anan, caust, thuj.
    - Eyelids: caust, cinnb, nit-ac, sulph, thuj.
      -Right, lower: nit-ac.
      - Bleeding when touched: nit-ac.
    - Iris: cinnb, merc, staph, thuj.
- **Ear,** external ears, on: Bufo.
    - Wart like growth inflamed and ulcerated behind the ear: calc.
- **Nose:** caust, nit-ac, thuj.
    - Inside nose: nit-ac.
    - Tip of nose: caust.
    - On nose, finger tips, and eyebrows: caust.
- **Face:** calc, caust, dulc, kali-c, lyc, nit-ac, sep, sulph, thuj.
    - Chin: lyc, thuj.
    - Lips: caust, kali-s, nit-ac, thuj.
    - Mouth around: cund, psor.
    - Mouth: ph-ac.
    - Palate: arg-n.
    - Tongue: aur, aur-m, aur-m-n, kali-s, lyc, mang, mang-act, staph.
- **Throat:** arg-n, merc-c, nit-ac, thuj.

  Throat external : nit-ac, psil, sil, thuj.

- Side, left: carc.
- **Soft and smooth, on neck, arms, and hands:** ant-c.
- **Abdomen, brown warts:** thuj.
- **Rectum:** Arg-n, aur, aur-m, aur-s, benz-ac, caust, cinnb, euphr, jac-c, kali-br, lyc, merc, merc-d, mill, nat-s, nit-ac, petr, phos, sabin, sep, staph, sulph, syph, thuj.
  - Bleeding, copious: mill.
  - Cauliflower: sabin.
  - Itching: euphr.
  - Flat: euphr, sulph, thuj.
  - Sensitive, extremely: staph.
  - Sore: benz-ac, thuj.
  - Stitching: euphr, thuj.
  - Touch on: euphr.
- **Urethra, excrescences:** ter.
- **Fungoid growth:** calc, con, graph, lyc, thuj.
- **Male genitalia, condylomata:** alumn, apis, arg-n, aur, aur-m, aur-m-n, aur-s, calc, cinnb, euphr, fl-ac, hep, lyc, med, merc, merc-d, mill, nat-c, nit-ac, ph-ac, phos, psor, sabin, sars, sep, staph, thuj.
- **Anus, around, and:** nit-ac.
  - Bleed easily: calc, cinnb, med, mill, nit-ac, sulph, thuj.
  - Cheese, smelling like stale: calc, hep, sanic, thuj.
  - Fetid bleeding when touched: cinnb, nit-ac, thuj.
- **Glans:** Ant-t, aur-met, aur-m, aur-s, cinnb, kali-chl, kali-i, lac-c, lyc, med, nit-ac, ph-ac, psor, sabin, sep, staph, sulph, thuj.
  - Hot: ph-ac.
  - Itching: lyc, psor, sabin, staph, thuj.
- **Penis:** alumn, ant-t, apis, aur, aur-m, bell, calc, cinnb, euphr, hep, kali-i, lac-c, lyc, merc, merc-c, mill, nat-s, nit-ac, nux-v, ph-ac, psor, sabin, sanic, sep, staph, sulph, thuj.

- Bleeding: cinnb, nit-ac, sulph, thuj.
- Burning: apis, cinnb, nit-ac, ph-ac, psor, sabin, thuj.
- Butternut shaped, hard growth, on the dorsum of penis: sabin.
- Cauliflower like: lac-c, nit-ac.
- Fan shaped: cinnb, thuj.
- Itching: psor, sabin.
- Oozing: aur-m, cinnb, lyc, nit-ac, psor, thuj.
- Offensive: nit-ac.
- Soreness: euphr, nit-ac, ph-ac, sabin, thuj.
- Itching and: psor, sabin.
- **Prepuce:** aur, aur-m, aur-m-n, caust, cinnb, cub, lyc, med, merc, merc-c, nit-ac, ph-ac, psor, sabin, thuj .
  - Edge of, itching and burning: psor.
- **Frenum:** cinnb.
- **Scrotum:** aur, aur-m, sil, thuj.
  - Sensitive: nit-ac, staph .
  - Soft: calc, sep.
  - Sticking pain: nit-ac.
- **Female genitalia,** condylomata: Arg-n, aur-m, calc, cinnb, euphr, lyc, med, merc, nat-s, nit-ac, phos, sabin, sars, staph, thuj.
- **Cauliflower like:** kali-ar, nit-ac, phos.
- **Cervix:** calen, kali-ar.
  - Dry: lyc.
  - Itching: euphr, lyc, sabin.
  - Pedunculated: lyc.
  - Soft red fleshy: nat-s.
- **Uterus:** calc, calen, cub, graph, kreos, merc, nit-ac, sec, tarent, thuj.
- **Vagina:** nit-ac, phos, staph, tarent, thuj.
  - Bleed easily: phos.

- **Larynx:** arg-n, calc, hep, merc-c, nit-ac, thuj.
- **Vocal cords:** arg-n.
- **Chest:** carc.
- **Mammae on:** castor-eq.
- **Sternum on:** nit-ac.
- **Back:** bar-c, nit-ac, sil, thuj.
- **Cervical region:** ant-c, nit-ac, thuj.
- **Upper limbs:** ars, bar-c, bov, calc, carb-an, caust, dulc, kali-c, lyc, merc, nat-c, nat-m, nat-s, nit-ac, petr, phos, rhus-t, sep, sil, sulph, thuj.
- **Elbow** bend of: calc-f.
- **Forearm:** sil.
- **Wrist:** ferr-ma.
- **Hands:** anac, ant-c, bar-c, berb, bov, bufo, calc, calc-sil, carb-an, caust, dulc, ferr, ferr-ma, ferr-pic, fl-ac, kali-c, kali-chl, kali-m, lach, lyc, mag-s, nit-ac, ph-ac, phos, psor, rhus-t, ruta, sep, sil, sulph, thuj.
    - Back of hand: thuj .
    - Face, and hands: calc, carb-an, caust, dulc, kali-c.
    - Flat: berb, dulc, lach, ruta, sep.
    - Horny: ant-c, caust, sep, thuj.
    - Itching: sep.
    - Large: calc-sil, dulc.
- **Knuckles:** pall.
- **Palm:** anac, berb, borx, dulc, nat-c, nat-m, ruta.
  - Flat: dulc, nat-m, ruta.
  - Painful on pressure: nat-m.
- **Fingers:** ambr, bar-c, berb, calc, carb-an, caust, dulc, ferr, fl-ac, lac-c, lach, lyc, nat-m, nit-ac, petr, psor, ran-b, rhus-t, sang, sars, sep, sulph, thuj.

- **Joints:** sars.
- **Tips:** caust, dulc, nit-ac, thuj .
  - First: caust, thuj.
  - Horny: caust.
  - Second: berb, lach.
  - Third: nat-s.
  - Fourth: lac-c.
- **Nails,** close to: caust, dulc, fl-ac, graph, lyc, sep.
- **Thumb:** berb, calc-sil, lach, mur-ac, ran-b, thuj.
- **Lower limbs:** bar-c.
- **Nates:** con.
- **Thigh:** med.
- **Ankles:** ball.
- **Foot:** sulph .
- **Soles:** ant-c, calc, carc, con, lyc, nat-m, sep, sil, sulph .
  - Horny: ant-c .
- **Toes:** spig.
  - Sensitive: nat-c.
  - Sore: ambr, fl-ac, ruta.

MOLLUSCUM CONTAGIOSUM

Molluscum contagiosum virus (MCV) causes characteristic skin nodules, and is largely if not exclusively a human disease..

Incidence

The virus occurs throughout the world. The disease is common, but its incidence in most areas is not reliably known. Infection follows contact with infected persons or contaminated objects, but the importance of epidermal injury is unknown. The disease is rare under the age of 1 year, perhaps due to maternally transmitted immunity and a long incubation period. Otherwise the incidence seems to reflect exposure to others..

It is more common in the summer, though one may come across cases through out the year. Infections are commonly picked up at the gymnasia; swimming pools, playgrounds, etc. by school children.

Unusually widespread lesions have been reported in patients with sarcoidosis, those taking immuno-suppressive therapy, or with HIV disease suggesting that cell-mediated immunity is significant in control and elimination of the infection.

Histology

Acanthotic mass with a well-developed basal cell layer is seen. The prickle cells become round and show eosinophilic masses (inclusion bodies) with nuclei pushed to the periphery. The process becomes more and more marked as the epidermal cells reach the surface. There is slight round cell infiltration in the upper corium.

Clinical Features

Sites

The distribution of the lesions is influenced by the mode of infection, and by the type of clothing worn, and hence by the climate. In temperate regions they are commonly seen on the neck or on the trunk, particularly around the axillae, except in sexually transmitted infection, when the anogenital region is usually involved. In children in the tropics lesions are more common on the limbs.

The incubation period is variously estimated at 14 days to 6 months. The individual lesion is a shiny, pearly white, hemispherical, umbilicated papule, which may show a central pore. A molluscum contagiosum looks like a vesicle. When squeezed, cheesy material is ejected. It may be identified with a hand lens when less than 1mm in diameter. Enlarging slowly it may reach a diameter of 5-10mm in 6-12 weeks. Rarely, and usually when one or very few are present, a lesion may become considerably larger. Plaques composed of many small lesions ('aguminate' form) occur rarely. Lesions frequently spread and the number of lesions ultimately present is sometimes very large. After trauma, or spontaneously after several months, inflammatory changes result in suppuration, crusting and eventual destruction of the lesion.

The duration both of the individual lesion and of the attack is very variable and although most cases are self-limiting within 6-9 months, some persist for 3 or 4 years.

HOMEOPATHIC APPROACH TO MOLLUSCUM

1. Refer warts.
2. It should be remembered that lesions disappear spontaneously in many cases; hence claims for cure must be thoroughly scrutinized.
3. It is a highly contagious disease and hence the patient should avoid public places like swimming pools, playgrounds, gymnasia, etc.
4. Local applications of salicylic acid, podophyllum, etc. should be avoided at any cost.

Molluscum contagiosum indicates the presence of a tubercular miasm hence drugs like Bacillinum, Tuberculinum, should be used intercurrently. The secondary lesions resemble chicken pox, hence the use of Variolinum and DNA in obstinate and chronic cases.

Some Important Homeopathic Drugs

A few useful remedies for this condition are Calc, Dulc, Nat-m, Sil, Sulph, etc. For detailed therapeutics refer the therapeutics of warts.

■

Chapter-17

Superficial Bacterial Skin Infections

Introduction

Bacterial infections with their distinct morphological features should alert the physician of the existence of a potentially treatable and reversible condition. These cutaneous signs may be an indication of generalized systemic process or simply an isolated superficial event.

An important clinical implication about pyogenic bacterial infections is that if they cannot be neatly fitted into one of the primary types then it indicates the presence of an underlying skin disorder which needs to be treated along with the secondary bacterial infection.

The normal human skin is colonized by huge numbers of bacteria that live harmlessly as commensals on its surface and within its follicles. At times, overgrowth of some of these resident organisms may cause minor disease of the skin or its appendages. On other occasions, bacteria not normally found there may colonize the epidermis and lead rapidly to disease. Apart from the arrival of these frankly pathogenic organisms, a wide range of bacteria land more or less fortuitously on the skin, and linger briefly in small numbers before disappearing, unable to multiply and thrive in this relatively inhospitable environment.

When the skin is inflamed or otherwise abnormal, it is often difficult to determine whether an organism isolated from its surface is causing or contributing to the observed pathology. Bacteriology reports must be interpreted with caution in the light of the known capabilities of the organism isolated.

With respect to the causative organism the number of organisms in the inoculum is of considerable importance. Also within a given species there are also strain differences in virulence.

From the point of view of host defence, there are three aspects to be considered.

1. The nature and health of the epithelial surface including its ability to replicate and produce secretions.

2. The interactions between commensal organisms of the normal flora and the potential parasite.

3. The cellular and humoral factors acting within the body-both classical immune mechanisms and non-specific mechanisms.

Bacterial infections can be further categorized as those caused by:

1. Gram-positive organisms e.g. impetigo, ecthyma, cellulitis and erysipelas, inflammatory disease of the hair follicles, scalded skin syndrome, anthrax, listeriosis, gas gangrene, etc.

2. Gram-negative organisms meningoccal, gonococcal, chancroid, salmonella, brucellosis, etc.

3. Miscellaneous diseases as those caused by rickettsiae, mycoplasmas, chlamydiae and spirochetes.

In this chapter we shall discuss in details about the superficial bacterial and tropical infections.

PYODERMA

Pyoderma is a group name for pyococcal dermatoses. In tropical countries, pyoderma is a common problem, particularly in summer and the monsoon.

The most important pyogenic organisms are the staphylococcus aureus and the streptococcus pyogenes. Bacillus proteus, pseudomonas and coliform bacilli are other organisms, which are associated with pyodermas.

Pyodermas can be classified further depending on the locations of the lesion and the causative organisms as follows:

1.	Epidermal	Impetigo pityroides, streptococcal intertrigo. Impetigo contagiosa, pustular bacterias. Granuloma pyogenicum, pyoderma gangrenosum, infectious eczematoid, dermatitis, otitis externa.
2.	Sub-epidermal	Erysipelas.
3.	Follicular	Bockhart's impetigo, sycosis furunculoses, carbuncle, stye, marginal blepharitis.
4.	Sweat glands	Eccrine – Sudoripora suppurativa. Apocrine-Hiradenitis suppurativa.
5.	Dermis	Cellulitis.
6.	Subcutaneous fat	Panniculitis
7.	Blood vessels	Arteritis, capillaritis, vasculitis, and phlebitis.

IMPETIGO

Definition

It is a contagious superficial pyogenic infection of the skin. Two main clinical varieties known are non-bullous impetigo (or impetigo contagiosa of Tilbury Fox) and bullous impetigo.

IMPETIGO CONTAGIOSA

Etiology

The causative organisms are mainly pyogenic staphylococci, less so streptococcus pyogenes.

Incidence

It is relatively frequent throughout the world and is frequent in temperate climates. The peak seasonal incidences are seen in late summer. Preschool and young school age children are most often affected. In adults, males predominate.

Over-crowding, poor hygiene and existing skin disease, especially scabies, predispose to infection.

Impetiginization is the name given to the process where impetigo contagiosa occurs secondarily as a complicating factor in scabies, pediculoses, eczemas, seborrheic dermatitis and herpes simplex.

Infection is transmitted by contact with any individual carrying pyogenic organisms, directly or through towels, handkerchiefs etc. The sites of predilection are the exposed regions of the body, especially of the face and scalp though it can occur on any part of the body.

The incubation period is two to three days.

Clinical Features

In impetigo contagiosa, the initial lesion is a very thin-walled vesicle on an erythematous base. The vesicle ruptures so rapidly that it is seldom seen as such. The exuding serum dries to form yellowish brown - honey-colored crust. This characteristic crust is the most important diagnostic feature of impetigo contagiosa. The crust is usually thicker and dirtier in the streptococcal forms. Gradual irregular peripheral extension occurs without central healing, and multiple lesions, which are usually present, may coalesce. The crusts eventually dry and separate to leave erythema, which fades without scarring. In severe cases, there may be regional adenitis with fever and other constitutional symptoms. The face, especially around the nose and mouth, and the limbs are the sites most commonly affected, but involvement of the scalp is frequent in tinea capitis, and lesions may occur anywhere on the body, especially in children with atopic dermatitis or scabies. Involvement of the mucous membranes is rare. There is a tendency to spontaneous cure in 2-3 weeks but a prolonged course is common, particularly in the presence of underlying parasitic infestations or eczema, or in hot and humid climates. In heavily pigmented skin, temporary hypopigmentation or hyperpigmentation may follow the lesions.

BULLOUS IMPETIGO

Etiology

Bullous impetigo is a superficial cutaneous infection with S. aureus. The organism can generally be cultured from blister fluid.

Epidermolytic toxin has been recovered from the blister fluid of some cases and is accepted as the basis for the bulla formation. The toxin is produced commonly but not exclusively by staphylococci of phage group II.

Incidence

Bullous impetigo is usually sporadic, but clusters of cases may occur in families and other groups, and larger outbreaks are occasionally seen in insitutions. It is most frequent in the summer months. Bullous impetigo occurs at all ages. It is said to be commoner in childhood but adult cases are probably under-reported.

In the newborn, bullous impetigo may be especially widespread and was formerly called pemphigus neonatorum.

Clinical Features

In bullous impetigo, the bullae are less rapidly ruptured and become much larger; a diameter of 1-2cm is common but they may be of very considerable size, and persist for 2 or 3 days. The contents are at first clear, later cloudy. After rupture thin, flat, brownish crusts are formed. Central healing and peripheral extension may give rise to circinate lesions. Although the face is often affected, the lesions may occur anywhere, and may be widely and irregularly distributed, often favouring the sites of existing skin disease, especially miliaria or trivial injuries such as insect bites. The buccal mucous membrane may be involved. Commonly, rather few lesions are present, but the picture is very variable. Regional adenitis is rare.

ECTHYMA

In cachectic and debilitated individuals the impetigo lesions are rather deep, giving rise to epidermal necrosis, thereby producing shallow ulcers with dirty brown crusts and pus underneath. This condition is called Ecthyma.

Clinical Features

A hard crust of dried exudate, which increases in size soon, surmounts small bullae or pustules on an erythematous base, by peripheral accretion. The base may become indurated and a red oedematous areola is often present. The crust is removed with difficulty, to reveal a purulent irregular ulcer. Healing occurs after a few weeks, with scarring. The lesions are usually few but new lesions may develop by autoinoculation over a long period. The buttocks, thighs and legs are most commonly affected.

Streptococci may produce streptococci gangrene and fuso-spirochaetal infection may spread from the gingiva to produce extensive necrosis of the lips, mouth and face (Cancrum Oris-Noma).

PYODERMA GANGRENOSUM

It is a hypersensitive reaction. Necrosis of the skin associated with trauma, coccal infection, ulcerative colitis, rheumatoid arthritis and drug addiction (Fortwin-Behl). Ulceration, deep necrosis, boggy violaceous, undermined edge, surrounding red areola and rapid evolution are characteristic.

IMPETIGO NEONATORUM

It implies impetigo contagiosa of the newborn. The eruption is extensive and involves the limbs, trunk, face and neck. Palms and soles are spared. The bullae are tense and contain clear fluid; rupture produces a superficial raw surface with overlying epidermal tags. Crusting is not prominent. Fever, emaciation and collapse mark toxemia. Infected genital passages, infected nipple, attendants with infected wounds or throats, or from other impetigo cases in a maternity ward convey infection. The condition used to be dreaded in maternity hospitals because of its easy communicability and high mortality rate.

Pathology

In bullous impetigo, the epidermis splits just below the stratum granulosum forming large blisters. Neutrophils migrate through the spongiotic epidermis into the blister cavity, which may also contain cocci. Occasional acantholytic cells may be seen, perhaps due to the action of neutrophils. The upper dermis contains an inflammatory infiltrate of neutrophils and lymphocytes. Cases with positive pemphigus-like antibodies on direct or indirect immunofluorescence have been reported.

The histology is similar for non-bullous impetigo except that blister formation is slight and transient.

Complications

Infective complications are uncommon in the absence of systemic disease or malnutrition, although deeper infections like cellulitis occasionally occur with the streptococcal disease. Streptococcal impetigo accounts for the majority of cases of post-streptococcal acute glomerulonephritis (AGN). The latent period for development of nephritis after streptococcal pyoderma is 18-21 days.

Scarlet fever, urticaria and erythema multiforme may follow streptococcal impetigo.

Rheumatic fever is not a complication of streptococcal impetigo.

Differential Diagnosis

In persistent impetigo of the scalp, pediculosis must be suspected and a search should be made for nits and parasites.

Persistent impetigo like lesions on the body may be due to scabies and dermatitis herpetiformis. Intense nocturnal pruritus, burrows, and a typical distribution of lesions and characterize the former by a history which reveals that several members of the patient's family have been affected. Acarus and ova can also be demonstrated by skin shavings. Dermatitis herpetiformis is distinguished by the presence of chronic, symmetrical polymorphous lesions on the arms, scapula and lower back accompanied by itching.

Annular lesions need to be differentiated from tinea. In the latter, there are no bullae or honey-colored crusts. On the other hand, it shows an inflammatory border of papulo-vesicles accompanied by itching. Also impetigo is usually an acute condition while tinea is chronic.

In chronic crusted lesions, infective granulomas like syphilis, tuberculosis and leishmaniasis must be borne in mind. A chronic history, underlying infiltration and associated accompanying features, a biopsy and bacteriological examinations, help to distinguish them. Impetigo neonatorum is differentiated from syphilitic pemphigus by the presence in the latter of symmetrically distorted bullae on the hands, feet and face. The child is poorly developed and has a waxen appearance. Lesions develop within a few days of birth and there is no history of a septic source of infection. Serological tests for syphilis are positive, both in mother and the infant.

Prognosis

The disease usually lasts for 3 to 4 weeks. In some cases, particularly when it complicates other skin conditions, it may last for months. An average case can be cured in 6 to 10 days leaving behind no scars. Being a contagious disease, it can spread to other parts of the body and to other people.

HOMEOPATHIC APPROACH TO IMPETIGO

Dominant is the tubercular miasm. The suppurating tendency that one frequently observes in homeopathic practice is best seen in pyodermas and impetigo since they have a strong tendency to recur if inadequately treated, hence proper selection and administration of acute, chronic and intercurrent drugs should be undertaken.

1. After a detailed case taking, evaluate the present stage that is

    (a) Whether it is the first attack?

    (b) Whether the patient has recurrent attacks?

    (c) Whether in the past suppressive measures were taken?

    (d) Whether patient has come in early or late stage?

    The above facts help us to select the type of remedy that has to be administered.

2. It has to be remembered that patient with low susceptibility develops lesions deep enough, thereby producing epidermal necrosis and shallow ulcerations. Hence, the basic duty of a homeopath is to increase the susceptibility with the help of similimum so that suffering is at its minimum.

3. Whenever these lesions heal they usually leave behind a permanent scar, hence proper precautions should be taken to prevent the same.

4. Since streptococcus and staphylococcus are the commonest organisms responsible, drugs like streptococcinum and staphylococcinum should be kept in mind. I would also advise the student to read the provings of isopathic drug, e.g. Terramycin that in potentized form is an excellent drug for impetigo.

5. The affected part must be kept dry clean and covered. In children with extensive affection of the scalp, the hair must be shaved off.

6. The crusts are removed with a warm solution of Calendula and water mixed in the ratio of 1:2.

7. Being a contagious disease, it can spread to other parts of the body. Hence, patients especially children, should be advised strictly not to scratch the lesion.

Selection and Administration of Homeopathic Remedies

Enough clinical hints can be drawn by mere observation.

(a) Location e.g. face Viol-t.

(b) Type and character of crust e.g. hard, soft, red, bloody, yellowish, greenish crust.

(c) Discharge: Thin, thick, offensive, bloody, yellowish, greenish.

(d) Presence of itching with its characteristic modalities.

(e) Use of intercurrent remedies like nosodes e.g. Staphylococcinum, Sycotico, Ttuberculinum and Variolinum or certain rare remedies like Antimonium sulphuratum auratum, anthrakokali, Calc-m, Narcissus pseudonarcissus and Solanum oleraceum should be strongly considered.

In Repertorization also Look for Rubrics like

(a) HEAD - ERUPTIONS - impetigo.

(b) FACE - ERUPTIONS - eczema - accompanied by - impetigo.

(c) FACE - ERUPTIONS - impetigo.

(d) BACK - ERUPTIONS - impetigo.

(e) EXTREMITIES - ERUPTIONS - Foot - Back of - impetigo.

(f) SKIN - ERUPTIONS - impetigo.

Keeping at the back of the mind, the patient's conceptual image and the sectorial totality of impetigo, the drug is selected.

The selection of potency is based on the resemblance of the patient's symptoms with the materia medica and the stage of the disease.

There are cases, which are, recorded where only nosodes have helped to clear the picture or an acute remedy like viola-t has permanently cured the impetigo. This is obviously because of symptom similarity. There are no small or big remedies, acute or chronic remedies in the material medica. Any remedy if proved properly can turn out to be a very useful remedy just like a polycrest.

Some Commonly Indicated Homeopathic Remedies

Agnus castus: Impetigo with gastric disturbances situated especially on the fingers, characterized by crusts and pustules. Impetigo that tends to ulcerate easily, angry looking, impetigo associated with glandular enlargement.

Alumina: Impetigo on scalp. Eruptions are humid, scabby, and scurfy, with gnawing itching sensation. They bleed easily when scratched < evenings, < alternate days; from heat of bed; at full and new moon; from eating potatoes; > open air (Bar-c.). Dry skin even in hot weather. Impetigo that appears periodically, especially in winter, skin feels as if the white of egg had dried on its surface.

Ammonium carbonicum: Impetigo on bends of extremities; excoriation below the thighs and above the genitals < wet application. Violent itching, after scratching, burning, blisters appear. Impetigo in individuals with scrofulous diathesis who dislike washing.

Antimonium crudum: Impetigo on face, genitals, extremities, neck, chest and back. Impetigo in individuals who are gluttans in their eating habits and frequently suffers from gastric upsets. Suppurating, yellow crusted eruptions, painful to touch and easily detached – green serous pus oozes out from beneath. Thick, hard, yellow crusts, irritating the surrounding parts, itching violently < from application of poultices < bathing, working in water, alcohol and in the sun.

Antimonium sulphuratum auratum: Impetiginous eruptions, especially on hands and feet. Typical pustular lesions are accompanied by itching. As with other antimonys there is disordered digestion, pasty mouth and taste in the morning. Respiratory affections like chronic bronchitis may act as concomitant.

Antimonium tartaricum: Impetigo around the face, chiefly around the neck and shoulders, above the nose and behind ears with itching. Pustular eruptions like varioloids as large as peas, with red areola and which afterwards form a crust and leave a scar. The eruptions have a bluish red mark. It is indicated in individuals who have ailments from ill effects of vaccination.

Arsenicum album: Scalp and face, extremities, genitals, margins of hair. Black pustules filled with black blood and fetid pus. Painful sensation as from cutaneous ulceration < night, cold, touch, > from warmth. Eruptions bleed on scratching. Skin symptoms alternates with asthma.

Arsenicum iodatum: Face, especially beard. Small vesicles, which burst and discharge an acrid fluid with severe itching and burning, worse night; application of cold. Scratching till it bleeds. Impetigo in individuals with tuberculous, scrofulous or syphilitic diathesis.

Arum triphyllum: Impetigo affecting corners of mouth, face, fingers, and toes. Appearance is raw, red, and bloody.

Baryta carbonica: Old people and children who are fat, dwarfish, swollen lymphatics, enlarged tonsils, who take cold easily. Moist vesicular eruptions with formation of thick crust, itching, burning, causes the hair to fall out; skin is humid and sore.

Calcarea carbonica: Occiput and then spreads to face. On neck, around navel and flexures of extremities. On scalp, there is a thick, large, yellow scale with thick bland pus under the crust. Itching is not very intense but on awakening from sleep, person is apt to scratch his head till it bleeds. < By water. Impetigo during dentition. Impetigo associated with cold feet as if damp stockings on them; sweat of forehead, chalky stool. Skin inclined to ulcerate.

Calcarea muriatica: Scalp, especially in infants. Impetigo associated with glandular enlargements and gastric disturbances.

Causticum: Nape of neck, around nipple, around mouth. Itching < night, evening, open air, with formation of thick crusts that tend to ulcerate. > Heat, warmth of bed. Eruptions are suppressed by local application of mercury or Sulphur.

Cicuta virosa: Impetigo sparsa. Scalp, chin, upper lip and covered part of face. Eruptions which form thick yellow crusts, honey comb like crusts, which fall off and leave a bright red smooth surface. No itching whatsoever with impetigo. Suppression of impetigo leads to neurological diseases.

Conium maculatum: Impetigo affecting face, arms, mons veneris, seropurulent eruptions in the aged. Moist vesicles with bluish sticky discharge forming hard crusts. Itching < after scratching. Impetigo developing after being overheated. Impetigo in old, feeble persons with scrofulous diathesis.

Croton tiglium: Face, genitals, eyelids, soles, abdomen, temples, vertex. Pustular eruption upon an inflamed base with itching and stinging pain. Presence of small vesicles, which get cleared or may burst. Violent itching and burning after eating < at night > gentle scratching and after sleep.

Clematis erecta: Occiput, forehead, nape of neck, root and sides of the nose, face and lower lips. Tender to touch. The eruptions itch violently with profuse desquamation, vesicular and pustular. Easily corrode the skin and ultimately develops flat eating ulcers with thick crusts. Eruptions change character during the changes of moon < in bed; when washed with cold water and towards morning. Impetigo developing after suppression of gonorrhea with glandular enlargement.

Dulcamara: Scalp, forehead, cheeks, chin, extremities. Itching vesicles that pass into suppuration and become covered with thick brown or yellow crust. Discharge corrodes the skin and causes loss of hair. Itching of skin diminishes after formation of crusts but remains sensitive to contact and bleeds after scratching. Impetigo < before menses.

Euphorbia lathyris: Impetigo starts on face and spreads all over the body. The eruptions are characterized by itching, burning and smarting sensation < by touch, cold air > sweet oil application. When the impetigo is scratched it forms deep ragged ulcers.

Graphites: Folds of skin, vertex, scalp, ears, extremities, around anus. Scabby eruptions with excessive oozing around the mouth and nose or the whiskes; hair fall out. Foul acrid gluey discharge; it makes hair together and leads to formation of deep rhagades with ulceration. Eruptions bleed easily on scratching. Skin is dry and sensitive to cold. Eruptions < from heat > from cold. Impetigo of fat, blonde women with scanty menses and an inability to perspire.

Gunpowder: Contains nitre, sulphur and charcoal. Hence, it has symptoms that resemble that of Sulphur and Carbo veg. When the suppuration sets in impetigo with very offensive discharge and there are no indications of healing, this remedy should be thought of.

Hepar sulphur: Impetigo after mercurialism. Sites – scalp, genitals, folds of scrotum, thighs. Presence of foul, moist eruptions with tendency to ulcerate. They are very sore and sensitive to touch. Humid scales and pustules upon the head oozing a fetid substance; there is a presence of thin, acrid, offensive discharge. Impetigo in individuals with coldness of palms and soles.

Iris versicolor: Impetigo capitis. Pustular eruptions associated with gastric complaints, nausea and vomiting. Impetigo with nightly itching.

Juglans cinerea: Lower extremities, sacrum and hands. Presence of itching and pricking when heated. Itching with burning, redness. Impetigo associated with dyspepsia, bronchial irritation and scrofulous swelling.

Kalium bichromicum: Eruption starts on the ear and spreads over the ear with formation of greenish crusts that oozes whitish thick matter. Eruptions tend to ulcerate. Sensation of itching < from heat and hot weather. Impetigo, gastric complaints and rheumatism alternate with each other. Impetigo developing in individuals with suppressed catarrh. Itching which on scratching leads to peeling. Itching, burning, rawness in affected part. Symptoms < at night.

Kreosotum: Painless, pustular eruption all over the body. Violently itching, moist or scurfy impetigo on eyelids, face, joints, back of hands. Sticking pains. Mentally the patient is sad and weeping < in open air.

Lycopodium clavatum: Impetigo arising after abuse of mercury, eruption on the head, face and also on the hands. Itching and suppurating eruptions, which form thick crusts, that bleeds easily; oozing of fetid moisture. Violent itching < 4-8 p.m., getting overheated, from poultices; > cold air or uncovering the parts. Impetigo that is associated with urinary, hepatic and gastric disorder. Individuals with tendency to develop blood boils and abscesses.

Mercurius solubilis: An important remedy for impetigo, eruptions are humid, fetid with thick yellow discharge or yellow crust formation. Moist scabs with excoriation of scalp and destruction of hair. These eruptions are surrounded by irregular margins. Itching < from warmth of bed with pain from scratching and tendency to bleed. Excessive odorous viscid perspiration < at night. Complaints increase with perspiration and rest. Also associated with a great deal of weariness and prostration.

Mezereum: Impetigo affects those parts of the skin, which are deficient in fat. There is intolerable itching, compelling patient to scratch and change his position. Eruptions moist and full of serous exudation, especially on nose and back. Deep inflammation, redness of face. Ichor from scratched places, which excoriates other parts. Itching < in bed, touch, burning and change of position after scratching. Scurf like fish scales on back, chest, thigh, and scalp. Scabs thick, lamellated like rupia with blood secretion beneath. They look like chalk and spread to brows, nape and throat. Crusts above mouth and cheeks < from undressing. They ulcerate and form thick scabs under which purulent matter exudes. There is marked thirst and scrofulous tendency.

Natrium carbonicum: Inclination to perspire easily. The skin is dry, rough, cracked, itching as if fleas all over the body. Eruptions on fingertips knuckle and toes. Vesicular eruptions in patches and circles. Impetigo on dorsum of hands. The soles of feet are raw and sore < from summer, heat, mental exertion, change of weather, sun, and least draught. Great debility caused by summer heat.

Natrium muriaticum: Margins of hairy scalp, flexures of skin, knuckles, behind ears and covers mouth and eyelids. Persons with oily, harsh, unhealthy skin < at seashore, < eating too much salt. Raw red inflamed impetigo <10-11 a.m., warmth, exercise.

Nitricum acidum: Anus, vertex, temples, genitals, auditory meatus. Eruptions bleed easily when scratched and there is a pricking, splinter like pain. Impetigo of the arms with long lasting pain in rectum after stool. Pustular eruption on face with large red margins and heavy scales. Adapted to persons with gouty diathesis and persons who crave for sweets.

Rhus toxicodendron: Vesicular crusty impetiginous eruptions, more around the genitals, small pustules on a black base; greenish pus with violent itching at night. Itching is worse in the hairy parts. Humid eruptions with thick scales on face and head, destroying the hair. Burning eruptions with a tendency to scale formation. The eruptions alternate with dysentery. Impetigo < change of weather < during wet weather < winter. The skin is sensitive to cold air.

Rhus venenata: Vesicular eruptions with intense itching > application of hot water < night. Dry eruptions on back of hand during winter, which disappears in spring.

Sarsaparilla officinalis: Affects persons with emaciated shriveled skin, which lies in folds. Eruptions, which come in summer and spring; also after abuse of mercury. The base of eruption is inflamed. Crusts get separated in open air and the adjoining skin gets chapped.

Sepia officinalis: Face, vertex, occiput, bends of joints. Eruptions during pregnancy and lactation. Itching vesicles and pustules with soreness of skin. Eruption is dry or moist and discharging copious purulent matter which when dries, cracks and exfoliates. Itching < open-air, > warm room. Itching changes to burning when scratched.

Silicea terra: Acts on the skin behind ears, skin of scrotum, hands, scalp and neck. Itching and burning with offensive eruptions ending in scabs discharging pus. Violent itching of scalp. Moist scald head. Skin is sensitive to cold. Patient wants to wrap up warmly. Unhealthy skin – every injury suppurates.

Staphysagria: Impetigo with thick scabs that itch violently. The person changes the place of itching on scratching. Impetigo alternates with joint pains. Presence of early ulceration once the scabs are removed. Eruptions extremely sensitive to touch. Impetigo developing in individuals with ill effects of anger and insults, sexual excess and abuse of mercury.

Sulphur: Dry, thick, yellow scabs on scalp with profuse discharge, great itching, which is relieved by scratching. Purulent eruptions on elbows.

Thuja occidentalis: Eruptions all over the body; itching and shooting especially at night. Pustular eruptions about the knee; better from gentle rubbing.

Viola tricolor: Good for acute cases. Pustular eruptions and scabs upon face with burning and itching and discharging fetid pus; worse at night. There is a sensation as of tension of the integument of face. The patient has horribly offensive smelling urine-like discharge like that of cat's urine.

REPERTORY

Kent's Repertory gives impetigo directly under the chapter skin under eruptions impetigo. Many other rubrics should be considered e.g.

- **Skin, eruptions, crusty.**
- **Skin, eruptions, discharging moist.**
- **Skin, eruptions, suppurating.**
- **Skin, eruptions, pustules.**
- **Skin, eruptions.**

  - Impetigo: aln, alum, am-c, ang, ant-c, ant-t, anthraco, apis, arg-n, ars, ars-i, arum-t, bac, bar-c, bor-ac, calc, calc-m, calc-p, calc-s, carb-ac, carb-ac, carb-v, carbn-s, caust, cic, cinnb, clem, con, crot-t, dulc, graph, hep, hydr, iris, jug-c, jug-r, kali-bi, kali-i, kreos, lact, lyc, maland, merc, mez, nat-c, nat-m, nit-ac, olnd, ph-ac, phos, psor, rhus-t, rhus-v, sars, sep, sil, staph, staph, sulph, tarent, thuj, tub, vario, viol-t.

  - Blisters: ail, all-c, alum, alum-sil, am-c, anac, ant-c, ars, ars-s-f, aur, aur-ar, aur-s, borx, bry, bufo, canth, carb-an, carbn-s, caust, cham, clem, crot-h, dulc, graph, hep, kali-ar, kali-bi, kali-c, kali-s, kali-sil, lach, mag-c, merc, nat-ar, nat-c, nat-m, nat-p, nat-s, nit-ac, petrola, phos, ran-b, ran-s, rhus-t, rhus-v, sep, sil, sulph, urt-u, verat, vip, zinc.

  - Crusty, moist: alum, anac, anthraci, ars, bar-c, calc, carbn-s, cic, clem, dulc, graph, hell, hep, kali-s, lyc, merc. mez, olnd, petr, phos, plb, ran-b, rhus-t, ruta, sep, sil, staph, sulph.

  - Crusty, yellow: ant-c, aur, aur-m, bar-m, calc, calc-s, carb-v, cic, cupr, dulc, hyper, iod, kali-bi, kali-s, kreos, med, merc, mez, nat-p, petr, ph-ac, spong, staph, sulph, viol-t.

  - Phagedenic: alum, alum-sil, am-c, ars, bar-c, bar-s, borx, calc, calc-sil, carb-v, carbn-s, caust, cham, chel, clem, con, croc, graph, hell, hep, kali-ars, kali-c, kali-sil, lach, lyc, mag-c, mang, merc, mur-ac, nat-c, nat-m, nat-p, nit-ac, nux-v, olnd, par, petr, ph-ac, phos, plb, psor, rhus-t, sars, sep, sil, squil, staph, sulph, tarax, viol-t.

- Pustules: agar, am-c, am-m, anac, ant-c, ant-s-aur, ant-t, arn, ars, ars-br, ars-i, ars-s-f, aur, aur-m, aur-s, bell, brom, bry, bufo, calad, calc, calc-p, calc-s, calc-sil, carb-ac, carb-v, carbn-s, caust, cham, chel, cic, cina, cinnb, clem, coc, con, cop, crot-h, crot-t, cund, cupr-ar, cycl, dulc, euph, fl-ac, gnaph, graph, hep, hippoz, hydrc, hyos, iod, iris. jug-c, jug-r, kali-ar, kali-bi, kali-br, kali-c, kali-chl, kali-i, kali-s, kali-sil, kreos, lach, lyc, mag-m, merc, merc-i-f, merc-i-r, mez, marc-ps, nat-c, nat-m, nit-ac, nux-v, op, petr. ph-ac, phos, podo, psor, puls, ran-b, rhus-t, rhus-v, sars, sec, sep, sil, sol-o, squil, staph, still, sulph-i, sulph, tab, tarent, tarent-c, tell, thuj, vario, viol-t, zinc.
  - Bathing agg.: dulc.
  - Black: ant-t, anthraci, bry, kali-bi, lach, mur-ac, nat-c, rhus-t, thuj.
  - Bleeding: ant-t.
  - Fetid: anthraci, ars, bufo, viol-t.
  - Thin pustules, breaking and discharging ichorous pus corroding the skin and spreading about: ant-t.
  - Vesicular, phagedenic: am-c, ars, borx, calc, caust, cham, clem, graph, hep, kali-c, mag-c, mang, merc, nat-c, nit-ac, petr, sep, sil, sulph.

Location:

- **Head, eruptions.**
  - Impetigo: Ars, arum-t, bar-c, calc, calc-p, caust, con, hep, iris, merc, petr, phos, rhus-t, rhus-v, sil, sulph, viol-t.
  - Margin of the hair: Nat-m.
- **Face, eruptions.**
  - Impetigo: Ant-c, ars, calc, cic, con, crot-t, dulc, graph, hep, kali-bi, kreos, lyc, merc, mez, nit-ac, rhus-t, sep, viol-t.

- **Forehead:** ant-c, kreos, led, merc, rhus-t, sep, sulph, viol-t.
- **Lips; around:** tarent.
  - Eczema, accompanied by, impetigo: bac.
- **Back, eruptions**
  - Impetigo: nat-m, petr.
- **Extremities, eruptions**
  - Impetigo: carbn-s.
- **Foot, back of**
  - Impetigo: carbn-s.

The reader is requested to read the chapter on eczema and refer its therapeutics along with the current chapter.

- **Skin, eruptions**
  - Crusty: agar, alum-p, alumn, am-c, am-m, ambr, anac, ant-c, ant-t, anthraci, apis, ars, ars-i, aur, aur-ar, aur-m, aur-s, bar-c, bar-m, bar-s, bell, bov, bry, calc, calc-i, calc-s, calc-sil, caps, carb-v, carbn-s, caust, cham, chel, chrysar, cic, cist, clem, com, con, dulc, elaps, fl-ac, graph, hell, hep, jug-c, kali-ar, kali-bi, kali-c, kali-chl, kali-i, kali-m, kali-p, kali-s, kreos, lach, lappa, led, lith-c, lyc, mag-c, med, merc, merc-i-r, mez, mur-ac, nat-m, nat-p, nit-ac, nux-v, olnd, paeon, par, petr, ph-ac, phos, phyt, plb, psor, puls, ran-b, rhus-t, rhus-v, sabad, sabin, sang, sars, sep, sil, spong, squil, staph, sul-ac, sulph, tarent, tell, thuj, vac, verat, vinc, viol-t, vip, ziŋc, zinc-p.
  - Bleeding: merc, mez.
  - Body; over whole: ars, dulc, psor.
  - Brown: am-c, ant-c, berb, dulc.
  - Burning: am-c, ant-c, calc, cic, puls, sars.
  - Fetid: graph, lyc, med, merc, plb, psor, staph, sulph.
  - Greenish: ant-c, calc, petr, sulph.
  - Honey coloured: carb-v.

- Inflamed: calc, lyc.
- Moist: alum, anac, anthraci, ars, bar-c, calc, carbn-s, cic, clem, dulc, graph, hell, hep, kali-s, lyc, merc, mez, olnd, petr, phos, plb, ran-b, rhus-t, ruta, sep, sil, staph, sulph.
- Offensive: mez.
- Oozing, greenish, bloody: ant-c.
- Suppurating: ars, plb, sil, sulph.
- Yellow: ant-c, aur, aur-m, bar-m, calc, calc-s, carb-v, cic, cupr, dulc, hyper, iod, kali-bi, kali-s, kreos, med, merc, mez, nat-p, petr, ph-ac, spong, staph, sulph, viol-t.

- **Skin, eruptions**
  - Vesicular:
    - Crusty: bov, chrysar, mez, ran-b.
- **Extremities, eruptions:**
  - Knee, crusty: psor, sil.
    - Hollow of, crusty: bov.
    - Moist: graph, merc, sep.
  - Hand, crusty: anthraci, graph, petr, sanic.
    - Palms: Anthraci.
- **Face, eruptions**
  - Crusty, scabby: aethi-a, anac, ant-c, ars, aur-s, bar-c, bar-m, bar-s, calc, calc-i, carbn-s, caust, chel, cic, cist, clem, con, cory, dulc, elaps, fl-ac, graph, hep, hyper, jug-c, kali-bi, lach, lappa, led, lith-c, lyc, merc, merc-i-r, mez, mur-ac, nit-ac, petr, ph-ac, psor, rhus-t, sars, sul-ac, sul-i, sulph, syph, thuj, vac, viol-t, zinc.
- **Eye, eruptions**
  - Eyebrows about, crusty: anan, fl-ac, nat-m, sep, spong.

- **Skin, eruptions,**
  - Discharging: aethi-a, alum, alum-p, alum-sil, anac, anag, ant-c, ars, ars-i, ars-s-f, bar-c, bell, bov, bry, bufo, cact, cadm-s, calc, calc-s, canth, caps, carb-an, carb-v, carbn-s, caust, cham, cic, cist, clem, con, crot-h, cupr, dulc graph, hell, hep, hydr, iod, jug-c, kali-ar, kali-br, kali-c, kali-p, kali-s, kali-sil, kreos, lacer, lach, led, lyc, manc, merc, mez, mur-ac, narc-ps, nat-ar, nat-c, nat-m, nat-p, nat-s, nit-ac, olnd, petr, ph-ac, phos, phyt, psor, ran-b, rhus-t, rhus-v, ruta, sabin, sars, sec, sel, sep, sil, sol-ni, squil, staph, still, sul-ac, sul-i, sulph, tarax, tell, thuj, vinca, viol-t, zinc, zinc-p.
  - Bloody: ant-c, calc, crot-h, lach, merc, nux-v.
  - Corrosive: ars, ars-s-f, calc, caps, carbn-s, clem, con, graph, kali-bi, merc, merc-i-f, merc-i-r, nat-m, ran-s, rhus-t, sulph, thuj.
  - Glutinous: bufo, calc, carbn-s, graph, mez, nat-m, sulph.
  - Golden crystals dries into: graph.
  - Greenish: ant-c, kali-chlo, rhus-t, sec.
  - Honey like: ant-c, graph, nat-p.
  - Ichorous: ant-t, clem, ran-s, rhus-t.
  - Offensive: kali-p, psor.
  - Pus: clem, dulc, graph, hep, lyc, mez, nat-c, nat-m. nit-ac, psor, sec, sulph.
  - Thick: graph, nat-c, psor.
  - Thin: cupr, dulc, hell, nat-m, petr, psor, rhus-t, rhus-v, sol-ni.
    - Yellow: alum, alum-p, anac, ant-c, ars, ars-s-f, bar-c, bar-s, calc, canth, carbo-an, carb-v, carbn-s, caust, clem, cupr, dulc, graph, hep, iod, kali-c, kali-s, lach, lyc, merc, mez, nat-m, nat-c, nat-p, nat-s, nit-ac, phos, psor, puls, rhus-t, sep, sil, sol-ni, sulph, thuj, viol-t.
- **Head, eruptions**
  - Crusts, scabs

- Moist: anan, bar-c, calc, graph, hep, med, psor, ruta, staph.
- Oozing: med, petr.
- White: alum, calc, mez, nat-m, tell, thuj.
- With thick white pus beneath: mez.
- Yellow: calc, calc-s, cic, dulc, kali-bi, kali-s, med, merc, nat-p, petr, psor, sep, spong. staph, sulph, viol-t.
- Moist: alum, anan, ars, bad, bar-c, bar-m, bar-s, calc, calc-s, carbn-s, cham, cic, clem, graph, hell, hep, hydr, kali-ar, kali-bi, kali-s, kali-sil, kreos, lyc, merc, mez, nat-m, nat-s, nit-ac, olnd, petr, phyt, psor, rhus-t, sars, sel, sep, sil, staph, sulph, tab, thuj, tub, ust, vinc, viol-t.
  - Eats the hair; that: ars, kali-bi, merc, mez, nat-m, psor, rhus-t.
  - Glutinous moisture: graph, kali-s, nat-m, sulph.
  - Yellow: clem, iris, kali-s, nat-m, sulph.
- Scurfy, moist: alum, anan, bar-c, calc, graph, nit-ac.
- **Ear, eruptions,**
  - Moist: ant-c, bov, calc, graph, hep, kali-bi, kreos, lyc, merc, mez, nat-m, nat-p, otit-m-xyz, petr, psor, ptel, puls, rhus-t., rhus-v, sanic, staph.
  - About the ears, moist: kreos.
  - Behind the ears, moist: am-m, ant-c, aur, calc, carb-v, caust, graph, kali-c, lyc, mez, nit-ac, olnd, petr, phos, psor, ptel, rhus-t, rhus-v, sanic, sep, sil, staph, tub.
  - Scabby; exuding a glutinous moisture, sore on touch: thuj.
    - Margins, moist: sil.
- **Face, eruptions**
  - Moist: ant-c, ars, ars-br, ars-i, calc, carb-v, carbn-s, carc, caust, cham, cic, clem, con, dulc, graph, hep, kreos, lyc, merc, mez, nat-ar, nat-c, nat-m, nit-ac, olnd, petr, ph-ac, psor, rhus-t, sars, sep, sil, squil, sulph, thuj, vinca, viol-t.

- Eyebrows: mez.
- Fetid: ars-br, cic, merc.
- Margin of hair: mez
- Nose: aur-m-n, carb-v, graph, nat-c, thuj.
- Scratching after: kali-c, sars, sulph.
- Septum: vinc.
- Wings: thuj.
- Yellow: lyc, rhus-t, viol-t.
- **External throat, eruptions**
  - Moist: caust, merc.
- **Abdomen, eruptions**
  - Moist: merc.
  - Groin, before menses; right: sars.
- **Back, eruptions**
  - Moist: clem, nat-m, psor.
    - Coccyx; on: arum-t, graph, led, nit-ac.
    - Sacrum; on: graph, led.
    - Cervical region, moist: caust, clem.
- **Extremities, eruptions**
  - Moist: bry, merc, nat-m.
    - Upper limbs: alum, bov, con, kreos, rhus-t.
    - Purulent discharge: lyc, rhus-t.
    - Upper limbs, scabs: alum, staph.
    - Forearm: alum, merc, mez, rhus-t.
    - Hand: cist, clem, kali-c, kali-s, mang, merc, mez, petr, ran-s, rhus-t.
    - Hand, back of: bov, kreos, mez.
    - Between the fingers: graph.
    - Lower limbs: bov, bry, chel, kreos, merc, nat-m.
    - Thigh: crot-t, graph, merc, nat-m.
    - Leg: apis, bry, calc, graph, kali-br, merc, petr, rhus-t, tarent-c.
    - Ankle: chel.

INFLAMMATORY DISEASES
OF THE HAIR FOLLICLE

The various diseases under this heading are folliculitis, furuncle, carbuncle, sycosis, etc.

FOLLICULITIS

It is the inflammation of the hair follicles and is generally used to denote follicular infection with pyogenic organisms.

The commonest causative organism is staphylococcus.

Pathogenesis

The use of infected blades for hair removal is a common initiating event.

Distribution

The commonest sites for affection are the beard and the moustash areas in males and the anterior portion of the legs. Axillae, pubic region, scalp or other body sites with terminal (thick) hair may also be affected.

Clinical Features

There are two varieties known:

1. *Superficial folliculitis:* It is an extremely common condition in which the inflammatory changes are confined to the ostium or extend only slightly below it, and which heals without scar formation.

    Superficial folliculitis is not always primarily or exclusively infective in origin. Physical or chemical injury to the skin may be associated with a folliculitis, the pustules of which may be sterile or may contain coagulase-negative staphylococci. Occupational contact with mineral oils or therapeutic or occupational exposure to tar products very typically produces such lesions, which in the case of oil folliculitis are associated with conspicuous oil plugging of many follicles. Other chemical irritants can cause folliculitis, which may be the only visible change, or may accompany an eczematous reaction. Beneath adhesive plasters or adhesive dressings, a sterile folliculitis is common. Following epilation, a traumatic folliculitis may develop.

It involves the upper part of the follicle (infundibulum) with acute (neutrophilic) inflammation and pustule formation and heals without follicular scaring (permanent loss of involved hair). Clinically, tiny follicular pustules grouped together with a narrow rim of erythema are seen.

2. *Deep folliculitis:* It involves the whole length of the follicle upto the level of deep dermis and heals with follicular scarring. Erythematous follicular papules, 2-3mm in diameter, topped by tiny pustules characterizes this condition. Hair shaft of the involved follicle can be pulled out with a light tug.

Differential Diagnosis

Follicular pustules are readily confused by the inexperienced with the non-follicular lesions of pustular miliaria, which should be considered when a widespread papulopustular eruption develops in hot and humid conditions, on previously normal skin, or studding an existing inflammatory dermatitis. Follicular pustules are also a feature of subcorneal pustular dermatosis, in which they are grouped around the margins of plaques of erythema and scaling. Follicular pustules may occur in ringworm. The more-or-less simultaneous development of pustules on a circumscribed, red and oedematous or scaling plaque should arouse suspicion.

FURUNCULOSIS

Synonym

Boil.

Definition

A furuncle is an acute, usually necrotic, infection of a hair follicle with S. aureus. Multiple boils are given the name of furunculoses.

Etiology

The causative organism in these conditions is staphylococcus aureus, less frequently other staphylococci.

It is relatively uncommon in early childhood, but increase rapidly in frequency with the approach of puberty, and in adolescence and early adult life. Furunculosis is a common skin problem, very prevalent in the tropics. It is more common in summer, especially in the monsoon season. Mechanical damage to the skin, even the friction of collars and belts, may determine the distribution of the lesions. Malnutrition is an important predisposing factor in some countries. Diabetes is widely believed to predispose to furunculosis. Furunculosis is common in-patients infected with HIV.

Maceration of skin, dusty and dirty environments and the ingestion of too many carbohydrates, predispose to furunculosis. The eating of too many mangoes has a similar effect (mango boils). A stye is a boil around an eyelash. When one deals with chronic furunculosis, the following predisposing causes must always be kept in mind.

Constitutional

- Diabetes mellitus.
- Chronic nephritis.
- Poor general health: malnutrition, worries, anxieties, etc.
- Seborrheic dermatitis.
- Ichthyosis.

Environmental

- Oily occupations or dusty jobs.
- Friction or changing at work or by rough garments.
- Scabies, pediculoses, etc.

Pathology

A furuncle is an abscess of a hair follicle, usually of vellus type. The perifollicular abscess is followed by necrosis with destruction of the follicle.

Clinical Features

A furuncle first presents as a small, follicular, inflammatory nodule, soon becoming pustular and then necrotic and healing after discharge of a necrotic core to leave a violaceous macule and, ultimately, a permanent scar. The rate of development varies greatly, and necrosis may occur within 2 days or only after 2 or 3 weeks. Tenderness is invariable, and in the more acute and larger lesions there may be throbbing pain. Lesions in the nose or external ear canal can cause very severe pain. The lesions may be single or multiple, and tend to appear in crops. Occasionally, there may be fever and mild constitutional symptoms. Pyaemia and septicaemia are favoured by malnutrition. On the upper lip and cheek, cavernous sinus thrombosis is a rare and dangerous complication.

The sites commonly involved are the face and neck, the arms, wrists and fingers, the buttocks and the anogenital region. Attacks may consist of a single crop, or of multiple crops, at irregular intervals with or without periods of freedom. The prognosis cannot be reliably determined during a first attack. In some individuals, crops continue to develop for many months, or even years.

In HIV disease, furuncles may coalesce into violaceous plaques.

Differential Diagnosis

Other pustular lesions must be differentiated. Furuncles are deep-seated nodules, in contrast to the lesions of superficial staphylococcal folliculitis. The vesicopustules of disseminated herpes simplex are umbilicated and appear simultaneously in large numbers on sites of active or healed eczema. The pustules of acne are but one type of lesion in a polymorphic syndrome. They are associated with papules and comedones, and are usually confined to the face and trunk. Pustules can also occur in halogen eruptions, usually symmetrical and of rapid onset. Nodules and abscesses occur mainly in the axillae and perineum in hidradenitis. Single or few, large, suppurating nodules on exposed skin raise the possibility of myiasis.

Prognosis

The course of the untreated disease is infinitely variable and the prognosis cannot be reliably determined during a first episode. Some patients suffer only one attack while others continue to develop recurrences over months or years, with or without periods of freedom.

HOMEOPATHIC APPROACH TO FURUNCULOSIS

Furuncles or boils are one of the commonest conditions that every homeopath has an opportunity to treat. Patients present to us either during acute stage or with recurrent tendency to develop furuncles.

*   When one is dealing with chronic tendency to boils, one must improve the general state of health by making necessary dietetic changes and encouraging the patients to eat fresh fruits and plenty of green leafy vegetables.

*   Worries and anxieties are known culprits that predispose an individual to develop recurrent boils.

*   Investigations to rule out diabetes mellitus and chronic nephritis should be advised.

*   Seborrheic diathesis if present should be tackled accordingly.

*   Overall hygiene and cleanliness should be maintained.

*   Eating excessive amount of carbohydrates and fatty foods, e.g. chocolates, mangoes should be strictly avoided as they predispose individuals to develop boils.

- Local applications of magnesium sulphate paste should never be encouraged.

For selecting the right remedy, the following points should be considered.

- Note whether boils are matured or not.

- Whether there is more inflammation than suppuration or vice versa.

- Overall look of the boil that is red, pale yellow, dark red, blackish, etc.

- The type of pain with its modalities should be inquired.

- In chronic conditions, itching becomes an important symptom and hence it has to be thoroughly analyzed.

- The lower potencies are to be selected to enhance the suppuration. Higher potencies are selected to abort the suppuration.

Staphylococcus aureus is the causative organism most commonly cultured from the discharge of the fununcle. Hence, the use of Staphylococcinum in recurrent and chronic cases should be employed.

Finally in obstinate cases, I have found encouraging results when patients are exposed to:

1. Sea bathing

2. Bathing in natural Sulphur spring baths.

Being strongly tubercular miasm remedies like Tuberculinum, Bacillinum, and Koch's Lymph Node are of immense value as intercurrent remedies.

Some Important Homeopathic Remedies for Furunculosis

Abrotanum: Tendency to boils in marasmic children. The skin develops purplish discoloration after the boil heals. The emaciation progresses with good appetite.

Aethusa cynapium: Boils associated with enlargement of lymphatic glands. The skin is cold and covered with cool clammy sweat. It is especially useful in children during dentition who have tendency to develop summer boils.

Anantherum muriaticum: One of the remedies that is full of suppuration. Patient has tendency to develop boils, abscesses and ulcers. The important concomitant is offensive foot sweat and diseased deformed nails.

Anthracinum: Purulent focus with tendency to develop succession of boils. The boils have an angry look, may be discolored, black or blue at the later stage. There is terrible burning sensation with great prostration.

Antimonium crudum: Individuals with a tendency to grow fat and have gastric derangement with boils. Itching and burning sensation, which is < at night. Skin is extremely sensitive to cold bathing.

Arnica montana: Small painful boils one after the other, which are extremely sore. Small boils in crops. Pain is more than the swelling (opposite of Rhus tox.).

Arsenicum album: Furunculosis with burning, as if coals of fire were put on the affected part. Cutting and burning pains < after midnight > warm fomentation. Indicated when Anthracinum fails.

Belladonna: Boils are red during stage of inflammation with throbbing pain without pus. Blood-boils.

Bellis perennis: Boils all over the body, which are sensitive to touch. Boil begins as a small pimple with burning pain and then gradually turns into dark fiery purple-colored furuncle. When boils rupture it liberates acrid pus, which destroys the surrounding hair. Pain within boil is < application of heat > cold application.

Calcarea carbonica: Skin is cold, unhealthy, and flaccid. Blood boils, which are recurrent in nature. Skin is extremely unhealthy and every injury tends to suppurate. Boils appear big but when rupture, liberate too little pus. Boils in emaciated children with big head, big belly who sweat easily and are extremely sensitive to cold.

Calcarea hypophosphorosa: Suited to persons who become pale, weak with violent drenching sweat, rapid emaciation with extreme debility due to suffering from continued abscesses having reduced the vitality.

Calcarea picrica: Prime remedy in recurring or chronic boils, particularly when located on parts thinly covered with muscle tissue, as on skin, bones, coccyx, and auditory canal. The boils appear to be small but compared to its size they are excessively painful.

Calcarea sulphurica: Abscesses slow to heal after rupture, with a continuous discharge of yellow pus. Patient desires open air but sensitive to drafts. Purulent exudations in or upon the skin. Discharge on drying up form scabs of various colors like green, brown or yellow. Tendency to furunculosis.

Carbo vegetabilis: Tendency to furunculosis. The skin is blue in colour, moist with hot perspiration. Sensation of burning within the furuncles. Discharges are offensive; pus smells like asafoetida. Tendency to develop furuncles with systemic illnesses likes typhoid, cholera, septicaemia, etc.

Carbolicum acidum: Furuncles on lumbar region with diabetes. Pus with a very foul odor from several openings, severe prostration. Intensely foul breath.

Echinacea angustfolia: Recurring furunculosis. This remedy helps in correction of blood dyscrasias and hence it is useful in septic conditions like furunculosis. Discharge from furuncle is extremely offensive. Due to septic condition, there is pyrexia with chills and sweat. The important concomitants are nausea with chilliness and weakness with aching in muscles.

Ferrum iodatum: Crops of boils in anemic emaciated individuals with tendency to develop goiter. Debility following draining upon vital forces.

Gunpowder: Blood poisoning and septic states. Introduced by Dr. Clarke. Acts as a protective against wound infection. Gunpowder consists of a combination of Nitre with Sulphur and charcoal; therefore one may get symptoms suggestive of Sulphur, Carboveg. and Kalium nitricum.

Hepar sulphur: In early stage of pus formation. Excessive sensitiveness of part with sharp, sticking pains. It helps to stop formation of pus or aid in its absorption. If there is oozing of pus, then it is indicated when the pus is thick, yellow and the patient is sensitive to touch. Patient is chilly yet feels better in wet weather. The skin is unhealthy; every little injury suppurates.

Hippozaeninum: Nosode introduced by Dr. Garth Wilkinson. It promises useful service in the treatment of pyaemic states with lymphatic involvements. The boils fail to heal and gradually progress to ulceration.

Ichthyolum: Its action on the skin is prompt and useful. Crops of boils associated with itching. Tendency to develop boils in individuals with uric acid and tubercular diathesis.

Lachesis mutus: Boils or furuncles surrounded by bluish areola. Usually surrounded by small pimples and are extremely sensitive to touch. Discharge from the lesion is bloody, foul, pus containing dark particles like charred straw. There is burning, throbbing, constricting pain in furuncle < at night, during sleep, heat of summer, slightest touch, < pressure > open air, local application of heat. However, the striking modality is that patient feels better when the boil ruptures and free flow of discharge sets in.

Ledum palustre: Development of boil or furuncle after injury with a sharp needle. There is accumulation of foul pus within the boil. Patient feels locally > cold fomentation.

Lycopodium clavatum: Boils that do not mature but remain blue. Tendency to develop blood boils. Sites of old boils indurate and form nodules that remain long. The discharge from the boil is thick yellowish offensive. Boils are associated with urinary, gastric and hepatic disorders.

Myristica sebifera: Great antiseptic power. It hastens suppuration and shortens its duration. Furuncles that develop on end of fingers and phalanges.

Morbillinum: Recurrent boils in the external auditory meatus with terrible pain, having past history of measles.

Oleum myristicae: A remedy for boils and furuncles to be used in obstinate cases.

Operculina turpenthum: Furuncles that are associated with GIT upset. The lymphatic glands are enlarged and indurated. It is an excellent remedy when boils and furuncles suppurate very slowly.

Phosphoricum acidum: Boils and furuncles after fever. The discharge is horribly offensive. Furuncles that develop on buttocks. Furuncles that proliferate deep into soft tissues and affect the bony structure producing osteitis and periosteitis.

Phytolacca decandra: Inherent disposition to develop boils and furuncles associated with swelling and induration of glands. The pus is watery, fetid and ichorous. Furuncles and boils, which penetrate deep into the soft tissues thereby affecting, bone and joints. Presence of furuncles and boils in an individual with syphilitic dyscrasia.

Picricum acidum: Tendency to develop abscesses and boils during summer. Furuncles that chiefly affect nape of the neck. It is chiefly indicated in grave and serious conditions, e.g. toxemia, uremia, pernicious anemia, after burns. There is presence of tired, heavy feeling all over the body, especially in the limbs < on slightest exertion.

Secale cornutum: Furuncles in thin, scrawny feeble individual of cachectic appearance. There is a burning sensation in furuncles > local application of heat. The discharge is very offensive bloody and greenish. The abscess matures very slowly.

Silicea terra: Boils and pustules practically on each and every part of the body, which are painfully sensitive. The discharge is highly offensive, purulent, bloody. Patient gets improvement by applying local heat. The furuncles have tendency to corrode soft tissue and spread deep in the bones.

Stramonium: Chronic abscesses with severe pain characterized by shiny red flush. Hip joint is chiefly affected.

Sulphur: Unhealthy skin that develops furuncles everywhere which refuses to heal. The skin is dry, rough and wrinkled. Presence of voluptuous itching < at night and in bed. The suppuration is characterized by presence of air bubbles in it. There is severe burning sensation in the furuncle, which is < by local application of heat.

Tarentula cubensis: A useful remedy in toxic and septic condition where the progress of symptoms is rapid with alarming prostration with atrocious burning and sharp stinging pain. Furuncles are extremely painful with bluish, black, purplish discoloration. Symptoms < at night.

REPERTORY

Abrot, aeth, agar, aloe, alum, alumn, am-c, am-m, anac, anan, anth, ant-c, ant-t, apis, arn, ars, ars-i, aur, bar-c, bell, bell-p, bov, brom, bry, bufo, calc, calc-hp, calc-picr, calc-p, calc-s, carb-an, carb-s, carb-v, chin, chin-a, cist, cocc, coc-c, colch, colo, con, crot-h, dulc, echi, elaps, euph, ferr-i, gels, graph, grat, ham, hep, hippoz, hydras, hyos, ichth, ign, ind, iod, iris, jug-r, kali-ars, kali-i, kali-m, kali-n, kreos, lach, laur, led, lyc, mag-c, mag-m, med, merc, merc-i-r, mez, mur-ac, nat-a, nat-m, nat-p, nit-ac, nux-m, nux-v, ol-myr, oper, op, petr, ph-ac, phos, phyt, pic-ac, plb, psor, ptel, puls, rhus-r, rhus-t, sars, sec, sep, sil, spong, stann, staph, stram, sulph, sulph-i, sul-ac, tarent, thuj, tub, zinc, zinc-ox.

- **Aborting, leaving induration:** cinch, lach, sil.
- **Blind:** fago, lyc.

- **Blood boils:** alum, arn, aur-m, bar-c, bell, bry, calc, cypr, euph, hep, hyos, iod, iris, kali-bi, lach, led, lyc, mag-c, mag-m, mur-ac, nat-m, nit-ac, phos, ph-ac, sec, sep, sil, sulph, sul-ac, syph, thuj.
- **Blood boils instead of asthma:** calc.
- **Blood boils, large:** hyos.
- **Blood boils during new moon:** calc.
- **Blood boils pricking when touched:** mur-ac.
- **Blood boils after abuse of sulphur:** bell.
- **Blood boils after abuse of sulphur:** bell.
- **Burning with:** anthr, ars, carb-v, tarent.
- **Blue:** anthr, bufo, crot-h, lach.
- **Body all over:** viol-t.
- **Crops of:** echi, sil, sul, syph.
- **Dark bluish red:** lach, sec.
- **Debilitating:** ars, sec.
- **Greenish pus:** sec.
- **Impotency with:** pic-ac.
- **Injured places:** dulc.
- **Inflamed:** bell, merc.
- **Inflammation and pain predominates:** tarent.
- **Large:** Ant-t, apis, bufo, crot-h, hep, hyos, lach, lyc, merc, nat-c, nit-ac, nux-v, petr, phos, sil, viol-t.
- **Large red borders, near small of back:** thuj.
- **Boils:** abrot, agar, alum, alum-p, alum-sil, alumn, an-c, am-m, ambro, anac, anan, ant-c, ant-t, anth, anthr, apis, arn, ars, ars-i, ars-s-f, aur, aur-ar, aur-s, bar-c, bell, bell-p, brom, bry, bufo, cadm-s, calc, calc-chln, calc-i, calc-m, calc-p, calc-pic, calc-s, calc-sil, carb-an, carb-v, carbn-s, chin, chinin-ar, cist, coc-c, cocc, coccal, con, crot-h, dulc, elaps, elat, euph, graph, hep, hippoz, hyos, ign, iod, jug-r, kali-bi, kali-i, kali-n, kreos, lach,

laur, led, lyc, mag-c, mag-m, maland, mang-coll, merc, mez, mur-ac, nat-ar, nat-c, nat-m, nat-p, nat-sal, nit-ac, nux-m, nux-v, petr, ph-ac, phos, phyt, pic-ac, psor, puls, rhus-t, rhus-v, sabin, sapin, sars, sec, sep, sil, sol-a, spong, stann, staph, stram, strych-g, sul-ac, sul-i, sulph tarent, thuj, urin, zinc, zinc-p.

- **Furuncles:** abrot, alum, anac, apis, ars, calad, calc-s, cina, merc, sil, sulph.

- **Boils and Furuncles.**

  - Aborting, leaving induration: chin, lach, sil.

  - Blind: fago, lyc.

  - Another, as soon as the first boil is heated; succeeded by: sulph.

  - Blood boils: alum, alum-p, arn, bell, bry, calc, euph, hyos, iod, iris, kali-bi, led, lyc, mag-c, mag-m, mur-ac, nat-m, nit-ac, ph-ac, phos, sec, sep, sil, sul-ac, sul-i, sulph, thuj, zinc.

    - Instead of asthma: calc.

    - Large: hyos.

    - During new moon: calc.

    - Pricking when touched: mur-ac.

    - After abuse of Sulphur: bell.

  - Blue: anthr, bufo, crot-h, lach.

  - Burning with: anthr, ars, carb-v, tarent.

  - Body all over: biol-t.

  - Chronic body parts over: calc-pic.

  - Chronic, could not sit or lie: apis.

  - Carbuncular, small, discharge slowly and show dark red streaks, pains intolerable, could not sleep for 3 night: med.

  - Commence with small blisters: cist.

  - Crops, of: echi, sil, sulph, syph.

- Crops, in, on various parts of body, painful with inflamed base, terminating in suppuration, discharging unhealthy pus, sometimes bloody, healing up soon, followed by another crop: sulph.
- Dark bluish red: lach, sec.
- Debilitating: ars, sec.
- Diabetes, in: ph-ac, sec, tarent.
- Epidemic of various sizes from a small pustule to a large boil, the latter becoming carbuncular and surrounded by little pustules: kali-i.
  - As if it would form: ars-m.
- Fever low, parts bluish, discharge scanty, tardy or dark fluid, unhealthy: crot-h.
- Frequent: fl-ac.
- Greenish pus: sec.
- Impotency with: pic-ac.
- Indigestion, from: mag-c.
- Inflamed: mell, merc.
- Injured places on: dulc.
- Long inflamed, suppuration commencing with blisters: hep.
- Itch, sequelae of: calc, sulph.
- Inflammation and pain predominates: tarent.
- Large: ant-t, apis, bufo, crot-h, hep, hyos, lach, lyc, merc, nat-c, nit-ac, nux-v, petr, phos, sil, viol-t.
  - Painful: cob.
  - Burning, stinging: apis.
  - Large red borders near small of back: thuj.
  - Mature do not mature, but remain blue: lyc.
    - And heal slowly: sec.
    - Do not: sanic.

- Slowly: hep, sil, sulph.
- Menses at: merc.
  - During: med.
- Multiple: arn, ars, nux-v, sulph.
- Many openings with: hep, lyc, nit-ac.
- Liver, with functional derangement of: sep.
- Malignant, painful turn blue and spread: lach.
- Painful: ars, hep, sec.
  - Small: kali-bi.
  - Small indolent: sep.
  - To touch: spong.
- Painless: nat-c.
- Periodical: anthr, ars, hyos, iod, lyc, merc, nit-ac, phos, phyt, sil, staph, sulph.
  - 2 or 3 inches apart, some popular with inflamed ar eas, other pustular: hydr.
- Phagedenic: borx.
- Predisposition, eradicate: calc.
- Pus has formed, after: merc.
- Recurring frequently: arn, ars, ant-c, aster, berb, calc, calc-mur, calc-p, calc-pic, echi, iod, hep, merc, nux-v, sulph, tub.
- Small: arn, bar-c, bell, dulc, fl-ac, grat, hydr, iod, kali-i, lyc, mag-c, mag-m, nat-m, nux-v, sulph, tarent, ust, viol-t, zinc.
- Scarlet red: apis, bell.
- Spring, in the: bell, crot-h, lach.
- Sore: arn, hep, lappa, pic-ac, sec, tub.
- Stinging, burning: apis.
  - Stinging on touch: mur-ac, sars, sil.

- Several small ones unite: nux-v.
- Successions of: anthr, arn, sulph.
- Sudden appearance: hep.
  - Sudden appearance with day blindness: sil.
- Suppurating, often leaving scars: kali-i.
- Suppuration to hasten: berb, merc, hep.
- Ulcers, boils, from: calc-p.
- Vaccination, after: ant-t.

Locations

- **Head:** anac, ant-t, arn, ars, bar-c, bell, calc, hep, kali-bi, kali-c, kali-i, led, mag-m, mez, mur-ac, nit-ac, psor, rhus-t, sulph.
  - Forehead: am-c, bar-c, carb-an, led, mag-c, phos, ptel, rhus-v, sep.
  - Eyes above the: calc-s, nat-m, sil.
  - Occiput: kali-bi, lyc, nat-c.
  - Temple, right: mur-ac.
- **Eyes**
  - Eyelids, on: ant-c, arg-met, carbn-s, hydrog, lyc, merc, puls, sep, sil, sulph, tell.
  - Right lid under: pall.
  - Canthi: bell, bry, calc, kali-c, lach, lyc, nat-c, petr, puls, sil.
  - Left, inner: stann.
  - Margins: arg-met, hydrog, puls, sep.
- **Ear:** carc, kali-c, pic-ac, sil, spong, sulph, syph.
  - Behind the ears: Ang, bry, calc, carc, con, nat-c, phyt, sulph, thuj.
  - Below the ears: calc.
  - External ear: nat-m, spong.
  - Front of ears: bry, carb-v, laur, sulph.
  - Lobes on: nat-m.

- Meatus: bell, bov, calc-pic, crot-h, ferr-pic, merc, pic-ac, puls, rhus-t, sil, sulph.
- **Face:** alum, am-c, anan, ant-c, arn, bar-c, bar-i, bar-s, bell, bry, calc, calc-p, calc-s, calc-sil, carb-v, chin, cina, coloc, hep, hyos, iod, iris, kali-ar, kali-br, kali-i, lappa, led, mez, mur-ac, nat-m, nit-ac, rhus-v, sars, sil, sul-i, sulph.
  - Blood boils, small: alum, iris, sil.
  - Menses during: med.
  - Painful: hep.
  - Repeating: alum.
  - Chin: am-c, cob, hep, lyc, nat-c, nit-ac, sil.
    - Right side of: cob, nat-c.
    - Under: carb-v.
  - Lips: hep, lach, nat-c, petr.
  - Mouth, corner of: am-c, ant-c.
- **Nose:** acon, alum, am-c, anan, cadm-s, carb-an, con, hep, mag-m, phos, sars, sil.
  - Inside: alum, am-c, carb-an, sep, sil, tub.
  - Tip: acon, am-c, anan, apis, borx, carb-an, tub.
- **Jaw, large furuncle in the region of the left lower jaw:** cob.
- **Gums:** Agn, anan, arn, aur, carb-an, carb-v, caust, chel, euph, jug-r, kali-chl, kali-i, lac-c, lyc, merc, mill, nat-m, nat-p, nat-s, nux-v, petr, ph-ac, phos, plan, plb, sanic, sil, staph, sulph.
  - Small, near left upper canine, painful to touch: agn.
- **External throat, sides of neck:** arg, caust, coloc, graph, kali-i, mag-c, nat-m, nit-ac, phyt, rhus-v, sec, sep.
  - Blood boils: arn, caust, sep, sil.
- **Abdomen:** am-m, phos, rhus-t, sec, zinc.
  - Inguinal region: ars, merc, nit-ac, phos, rhus-t, stram.
- **Anus:** ant-c, calc-p, carb-an, caust, nit-ac, petr.
  - Near anus, with fistula: berb.

- **Perineum:** alum, ant-c.

- **Genitalia, pubes:** apis, rhus-t.

- **Chest:** am-c, chin, hep, lach, kali-i, mag-c, mag-m, phos, psor, sulph.

- **Back:** caust, coloc, crot-h, graph, kali-bi, kali-i, lach, mur-ac, ph-ac, phyt, sanic, sul-ac, sulph, tarent, tarent-c, thuj, zinc.

  - Blood boils: carb-an, caust, graph, hep, iris, kali-bi, mur-ac, nat-m, sul-ac, thuj, zinc.

    - Stinging on touch: mur-ac.

    - Groups in: berb.

  - Cervical region: androc, calc, carb-an, coloc, crot-h, cupr, dig, graph, hep, indg, kali-i, lach, nat-m, nit-ac, petr, phos, psor, rhus-v, sec, sil, sulph, thuj, ust.

  - Dorsal region, scapulae: am-c, bell, led, lyc, nit-ac, zinc.

    - Shoulders, between: iod, tarent-c, zinc.

- **Lumbar region:** hep, psor, rhus-t, thuj.

- **Sacrum:** aeth, thuj.

- **Extremities:** all-c, alum-sil, am-c, apoc, ars, ars-s-f, aur-m, bell, brom, calc, carbn-s, clem, cob, elaps, graph, guare, hep, hyos, iris, kali-bi, kali-n, lyc, merc, mez, nat-m, nit-ac, nux-v, petr, ph-ac, psor, rat, rhus-t, rhus-v, sec, sep, stram, sulph, thuj.

  - Upper limbs: aloe, am-c, ars, bar-c, bell, brom, calc, calc-sil, carb-an, carb-v, cob, coloc, elaps, graph, guare, iod, iris, kali-n, lyc, mag-m, mez, petr, ph-ac, rhus-t, sil, sulph, syph, zinc.

  - Shoulder: am-c, am-m, bell, hydr, kali-n, nit-ac, ph-ac, sulph.

    - Blood boils, large: calc, jug-r, lyc, zinc.

  - Upper arm: aloe, bar-c, carb-v, coloc, crot-h, iod, jug-r, mez, sil, zinc.

  - Forearm: calc, carb-v, cob, iod, lach, lyc, mag-m, nat-s, petr, sil.

- Wrist: iod, sanic.
- Hands: calc, coloc, crib, lach, led, lyc, psor.
  - Small boils: iris.
  - Back of hand: calc.
  - Fingers: calc, lach, sil.
  - Joints: calc.
  - Thumb: hep, kali-n.
- Lower limbs: all-c, am-c, apoc, ars, aur-m, bell, carbn-s, clem, hep, hyos, kali-bi, nat-m, nit-ac, nux-v, petr, ph-ac, phos, rhus-t, rhus-v, sec, sep, sil, stram, sulph, thuj.
- Nates: acon, agar, alum, alum-p, am-c, aur-m, bar-c, bart, borx, cadm-s, calad, graph, hep, indg, lyc, nit-ac, ph-ac, phos, plb, psor, rat, sabin, sars, sec, sep, sil, sulph, thuj.
  - Blood boils: aur-m, hep, lyc.
- Thigh: acon, agar, all-s, alum, alum-p, am-c, androc, apoc, aur-m, bell, calc, calc-sil, carbn-s, clem, cocc, hep, hyos, ign, kali-bi, lach, lyc, mag-c, nit-ac, nux-v, petr, ph-ac, phos, plb, puls, rhus-v, sep, sil, thuj.
  - Right: calc, hell, kali-bi, kali-c, rhus-v.
- Knee: am-c, calc, nat-m, nux-v.
- Legs: anan, anthr, ars, calc, castor-eq, mag-c, nit-ac, nux-v, petr, rhus-t, sil.
  - Blood boils: mag-c.
  - Calf: bell, sil.
- Ankle: merc.
- Foot: anan, calc, led, lyc, sars, sil, stram.
  - Sole of foot: rat.
  - Heel: calc, lach.
- Toes: cocc.
- Lower limb, itching at the site of a previous boil: graph.

CARBUNCLE

In French, Spanish and some other Latin languages, 'anthrax' is the term commonly applied to a carbuncle, whilst 'charbon' (French), or a similar related word, describes infection with Bacillus anthracis.

Etiology

A carbuncle is a deep infection of a group of contiguous follicles with S. aureus, accompanied by intense inflammatory changes in the surrounding and underlying connective tissues, including the subcutaneous fat. Carbuncles occur predominantly in men, and usually in middle or old age. They may be seen in the apparently healthy but are more common in the presence of diabetes, malnutrition, cardiac failure, drug addiction or severe generalized dermatoses, such as exfoliative dermatitis or pemphigus, and during prolonged steroid therapy.

Clinical Features

The term carbuncle is derived from the Latin word for a small, fiery coal, and describes the painful, hard, red lump that is the initial stage of the infection. It is at first smooth, dome-shaped and acutely tender. It increases in size for a few days, to reach a diameter of 3-10 cm or occasionally more. Suppuration begins after some 5-7 days, and pus is discharged from the multiple follicular orifices. Necrosis of the intervening skin leaves a yellow slough surmounting a crateriform nodule. In some cases, the necrosis develops more acutely without a preliminary follicular discharge, and the entire central core of the lesion is shed, to leave a deep ulcer with a purulent floor. Most lesions are on the back of the neck, the shoulders or the hips and thighs, and although usually solitary may be multiple or associated with one or more furuncles.

Constitutional symptoms may accompany, or even precede by some hours, the development of the carbuncle. Fever may be high, and malaise and prostration may be extreme if the carbuncle is large or the patient's general condition poor.

In favourable cases, healing slowly takes place to leave a scar. In the frail and ill, death may occur from toxemia or from metastatic infection.

DIAGNOSIS

Anthrax presents the only important problem. In the typical case, the hemorrhagic crust and the vesicular margin are quite unlike a carbuncle, but sometimes certain clinical differentiation is difficult. A swab must be taken, but treatment should not be postponed until bacteriological confirmation is available.

HOMEOPATHIC APPROACH TO CARBUNCLES

Carbuncle is a disease peculiar to people of a debilitated, broken-down constitution, and attacks them usually about or past the middle period of life. It is but seldom seen on the extremities, or what is more singular, on the anterior surface of the body. The back of the neck is the usual seat. When it is situated on or near the head, or when it is of large size, the patient may die, passing into a septicemic condition. Carbuncle begins with inflammation, swelling, and some pain; the swelling is flat, circular, and of a dusky red hue; usually it is but very slightly elevated above the surrounding skin. When sloughing is about to occur, the skin covering it becomes darker, undermined, and finally breaks down around the edges, leaving fissures through which exudes a thin, badly-colored, unhealthy pus.

The points of distinction between boils and carbuncles are sufficiently well marked to prevent the possibility of confusion. Boils have a small slough, and copious discharge of pus; carbuncles have an immense slough, while the suppurative action is mild or deficient. Again, boils are elevated above the surrounding integument considerably, and are of a conical shape; carbuncles are nearly always on a level with, or but slightly raised above the skin, and are flat. These formations vary in size from one or two inches in diameter, to six, or even more. They seldom attack young people, or those of a robust habit. Carbuncle is a combination of

F-23

several furuncles and accompanied with gangrenous changes. It usually occurs in integuments along the dorsal spine, nape of neck, inguinal and sternal. Carbuncles can occur in both cachetic and robust people. They begin and run their course with great pains.

For selecting the right remedy, the following points should be considered.

- Note the location of the carbuncle.
- Overall look of the carbuncle, whether it is red, pale yellow, dark red, blackish, purplish, etc.
- The description of the carbuncle and the condition of the surrounding parts.
- The type of pain with its modalities should be inquired.
- Any associated features or pathological condition should also be considered.
- The lower potencies are to be selected to enhance the suppuration. Higher potencies are selected to abort the suppuration.

Some Important Homeopathic Remedies for Carbuncles

Abroma augusta: Diabetic carbuncle associated with albuminuria, dry skin, itching and burning after scratching, worse night. Boils in summer. Excessive debility.

Achyaranthes aspera: Carbuncles, ulcers. Burning pain all over body.

Agaricus muscaris: Carbuncle on front side of the left thigh.

Anthracinum: Ulceration, sloughing and intolerable burning. Arsenic like symptoms but when Arsenic fails to relieve the burning pains. Discharges are ichorous, offensive, pus like. Carbuncles in the head, near temples and ears, omentum, intestinal tract, forearm and back. Marked chilliness associated with great debility. General loss of appetite. Erysipelatous inflammation around carbuncles. Dark red, indurated and ulcerated. Dusky red appearance.

Apis mellifica: Burning and stinging pains in the carbuncles. Edema, waxy pale face and look of skin. Skin white almost transparent.

Arnica montana: Carbuncles on thigh. Sore, bruised feeling of the affected part. Dusky, mottled appearance of the affected part.

Arsenicum album: Skin looks white. Burning, itching; painful after scratching. Burning as if coals of fire on affected parts. Pains are worse after midnight and better by heat. Sensation of swelling as though boiling water were running through. Great irritability of mind and body worse midnight.

Asimina triloba: Carbuncle on thigh.

Boricum acidum: Used for a wet dressing over the carbuncle.

Bufo rana: Carbuncle on the neck and back. Useful at the commencement of the carbuncle. Blueness extending far around the carbuncle; red and purplish skin.

Calcarea sulphurica: Carbuncle on the back discharging pus.

Calendula officinalis: A most remarkable healing agent, applied locally. Useful for open wounds, parts that will not heal, ulcers, etc. Promotes healthy granulations and rapid healing by first intention. Pain is excessive and out of all proportion to injury. Has remarkable power to produce local exudation and helps to make acrid discharge healthy and free. In carbuncle, promotes favorable cicatrization, with least amount of suppuration. Carbuncles with slough, proud flesh, and raised edges.

Carbo vegetabilis: Induration of lymphatics around carbuncles. Affected parts are bluish or livid. Discharges are offensive, ichorous, fetid and associated with burning pains like Arsenic, but without the extreme restlessness of the latter. Carbuncle becomes gangrenous. Also charcoal poultice can be applied locally over the carbuncle.

Crotalus horridus: Tendency to carbuncle. Carbuncles begin on back and neck with pustular eruptions. Suppuration and gangrenous condition. Bluish appearance of the carbuncles. Skin appears purplish and mottled with edema around the carbuncles which pits on pressure. Profuse hemorrhages on touch. Debilitated, broken down constitution; marked prostration. Diabetic carbuncle.

Cynodon dactylon: Carbuncles with bleeding from nose.

Echinacea angustifolia: Carbuncles with bluish discoloration, intense pain and profuse foul smelling discharges. Septic state with marked prostration, debility and progressive emaciation. Intense itching and burning of skin on neck. White coating of tongue with red edges. Can be applied externally .

Euphorbium officinarum: Terrible burning pains of the affected parts worse at night, rest. Pains are accompanied with restlessness, weakness and chilliness (Ars.). Indolent ulcers with biting and burning pains. When Anthracinum though indicated but fails to relieve.

Gunpowder: The remedy was introduced by Dr. Clarke and is extremely useful for blood poisoning and septic states. Acts as a protective against wound infection. Carbuncles with excessive suppuration and very offensive discharge and there are no indications of healing. Gunpowder consists of a combination of Nitre with Sulphur and charcoal; therefore one may get symptoms suggestive of Sulphur, Carbo vegetabilis. and Kalium nitricum.

Gymnema sylvestra: Diabetic carbuncle

Hepar Sulphur: Intense pain with sleeplessness. Carbuncles with corroding edges.

Hippozaeninum: This powerful nosode introduced by Dr. J. J. Garth Wilkinson. It promises useful service in the treatment of pyaemic states with lymphatic involvements. The boils fail to heal and gradually progress to ulceration. Carbuncles in patients suffering from tuberculosis and malignancy. All glands swollen; painful; form abscesses. Lymphatic swellings. Nodules of muscles of arms. Pustules and abscesses.

Lachesis mutus: It is a very useful remedy when the surface is swollen and pus forms very slowly. Thin, sanious and offensive pus. Dark bluish, purplish appearance of the affected parts. Dark red streaks running along the lymphatics. There is great burning, relieved by washing in cold water. Small boils surrounding the main sore. Carbuncles which slough and are very offensive. Inability to bear any bandage. Diabetic carbuncle. Prostration.

Medorrhinum: Intolerable pain in carbuncles.

Muriaticum acidum: Carbuncles accompanied by septic condition with high fever and great prostration. Carbuncles; foul-smelling ulcers on lower extremities. Patient becomes so weak she slides down the bed. Decomposition of fluids. Loud moaning with great restlessness. Tongue, pale, swollen, dry, leathery, paralyzed. Deep ulcers on tongue. Fetid breath. Sordes on teeth. Pulse rapid, feeble, and small. Intermits every third beat. Frequent desire to urinate, but cannot urinate without having the bowels move at the same time.

Mysristica sebifera: A remedy of great antiseptic powers. Carbuncles often extending deep up to periosteum. Coppery taste in the mouth and burning in throat. Tongue white and cracked. Phlegmonous inflammations. Hastens suppuration and shortens its duration. Acts more powerfully often than Hepar sulph. or Silicea.

Nitricum acidum: Carbuncles with many openings and intolerable stinging pains as if from a splinter. Carbuncles about the anus. Tendency to hemorrhages. Excessive debility with night sweat.

Phytolacca decandra: The patient has inherent disposition to develop boils, furuncles and carbuncles associated with swelling and induration of glands. The pus is watery, fetid and ichorous. Carbuncles which penetrate deep into the soft tissues thereby affecting bones. The skin becomes dry, shrunken, pale. Papular and pustular lesions. There is itching, but too sore to allow any scratching, or made worse by scratching. The skin is hot and dry. Erythematous blotches. Irregular, slightly raised, pale red ending in dark red or purple spots. Worse in damp, cold weather, night. Better in warmth, dry weather. Aching, soreness, restlessness, prostration are marked associated symptoms with glandular affections.

Rhus toxicodendron: Indicated during the first stage of development of carbuncle. Confluent blisters, containing a milky or watery fluid with peeling of skin. The skin appears red and swollen. The bullous eruption suppurates very easily. There is sensation of burning and itching which is worse by scratching and better by local application of heat. Slow local development, frequent remission; dark-red erysipelatous, with little blisters or oedema. Overall, the patient is worse in the night and wet weather and better in dry weather. External coldness of skin, but doesn't mind cold air. Chilly with coldness of single parts or of one side only; better hot things. The patient has an irresistible desire to move, or change position, with great relief for a short time.

Secale cornutum: Carbuncles with ecchymosis. Cannot bear any external warmth. Livid spots, purplish, blackish discoloration. Burning, lightening like pains. Greenish pus. Carbuncles turning gangrenous. Skin unhealthy, withered, wrinkled and shriveled. Unhealthy skin. Carbuncles in diabetics and patients suffering from neurological diseases. Tendency to hemorrhages with dark, black, clotted blood.

Silicea terra: Soggy and wilted skin. Carbuncles appear in crops on back, between the shoulders and nape of neck. Carbuncles with offensive odor and proud flesh associated with great induration. Stinging pains worse on touch, better by hot application. Patient has a great thirst, is very restlessness and has a red tip of tongue. Glandular enlargement associated with carbuncles. Lack of vital heat.

Staphylococcinum: Diabetes accompanied by carbuncles. Flushes of heat. Desire spicy and sweets. Concomitant – early morning diarrhea, cramping and griping in abdomen before stools. Face is chapped. Styes in eyes. Otorrhea.

Tarentula cubensis: Sloughing carbuncle with extreme prostration. Redness around carbuncle. Carbuncle associated with diarrhea and intermittent fever of evening exacerbation, sweat, and anxiety. Excessive atrocious pain in carbuncles. An indication is an early marked black core center.

Vipera berus: Carbuncles with bursting sensation better by elevating the affected part.

REPERTORY

Acon, agar, ant-t, antho, anthrac, apis, arn, ars, ars-s-f, asim, bell, both, bov, bry, bufo, calc-chln, calc-s, calen, caps, carb-ac, carb-an, carb-v, chin, coloc.,crot-c, crot-h, cupr-ar, echi, euph, hep, hippoz, hyos, ins, iod, jug-r, kali-p, kreos, lach, lappa, led, lyc, merc, mur-ac, mygal, myris, nit-ac, op, ph-ac, phyt, pic-ac, pyrog, rhus-t, sang, scol, sec, ser-febr-s, sil, staphycoc, stram, strych-g, sul-ac, sulph, tarent, tarent-c$_1$

- **Accompanied by** — Diabetes.
    - Diabetes: abrom-a, ars, cephd-i, crot-h, graph, gymne, ins, kreos, lach, led, ph-ac.
    - Pain, bursting: Vip.
- **Burning:** anthraci, apis, ars, coloc, crot-c, crot-h, hep, tarent-c.
- **Chronic:** stram.
- **First stage:** echi, rhus-t.
- **Foul smelling:** anthraci, lach.
- **Openings; with many:** hep, lyc, nit-ac.
- **Purple - vesicles around; with small:** crot-c, lach.
- **Red**
    - Bluish red: lach.
    - Scarlet red: apis, bell.
- **Stinging:** apis, carb-an, nit-ac.

Locations

- **Head:** anthracin, ars, crot-h, hep, lach, sil, sulph.

- **Face**
  - Chin, on: lyc.
- **Rectum**
  - Anus, about: nit-ac.
- **Urethra:** acon, ars, borx, clac, carb-v, dulc, graph, hep, lach, merc, nit-ac, nux-v, puls, sulph.
- **Back:** anthracin, ars, crot-h, lach, sil, tarent.
- **Extremities:** anthracin, arn, ars, hep, lach, sil, sulph, tarent-c.
- **Forearms:** hep.
- **Nates:** agar, thuj.
- **Thighs:** agar, arn, asim, hep.

SYCOSIS

Sycosis is a subacute or chronic pyogenic infection involving the whole depth of the follicle. If the follicles are destroyed with clinically evident scarring, the term lupoid sycosis, or its cumbersome synonym ulerythema sycosiforme, is applied. Folliculitis decalvans is essentially the same process involving the scalp. Many sites may be involved in the same individual.

Etiology

In order of frequency, the beard region, neck, scalp, legs, arms, pubic regions are most often involved. Sycosis occurs only in males after puberty, and commonly involves the follicles of the beard. Many patients are seborrheic, with a greasy complexion and chronic blepharitis. The most common causative organism is Staphylococcus aureus; less commonly, other staphylococci. Discharges from nose, throat and teeth are the source of these organisms. They may enter the skin through slight injuries or abrasions caused by shaving. Use of unhygienic shaving kit, blunt razors, fine shaving by stretching the skin and shaving against the grain of hair tend to cause sycosis. Workers handling or coming in contact with oil tend to develop oil acne, which must be distinguished from primary sycosis. Predisposing causes are many. Clerical and other indoor workers are affected more often than those who work in the open air. Seborrheic diathesis is a common feature. Sedentary habits, under-nutrition or obesity diabetes, unhygienic living, neurotic temperament and emotional strain are the common predisposing factors.

Pathology

The affected follicle is packed with polymorphonuclear leukocytes, which infiltrate its wall. Around the follicle there is a chronic granulomatous infiltrate in which lymphocytes, plasma cells, histiocytes and foreign-body giant cells are conspicuous. The sebaceous gland, or the whole follicle, may be destroyed and replaced by scar tissue.

Clinical Features

The essential lesion is an edematous, red, follicular papule or pustule centred on a hair. The individual papules remain discrete, but if neighbouring follicles are involved the perifollicular edema may coalesce, to produce the raised plaques studded with pustules which suggested the appearance of a ripe fig to the ancient author who coined the term sycosis. Some rupture to discharge beads of pus, the rest dry up to form crusts. Folliculitis develops rapidly, involving more and more follicles. Soon the infection becomes chronic, the skin looks congested, swollen and infiltrated. In more chronic forms, the lesions are typically clustered into plaques, especially on the upper lip and chin, and may persist for very long periods. There is often some crusting and scaling, but the hair are retained and there is no evident scarring. Usually, no pain is present; itching and burning are the only symptoms. There is no oozing and weeping at any stage; this feature helps in differentiating the disease from follicular infective eczema in which the whole of the beard region is rapidly involved and oozing is a dominant feature.

HOMEOPATHIC APPROACH OF SYCOSIS BARBAE

Cases of chronic folliculitis come in plenty to a homeopath, as the course is chronic and frequently the disease recurs with conventional treatment. I would like to stress the following points for the same:

1. Removing the causes viz. eliminating the septic focus from the nose, throat, teeth, etc; change from dusty environments; improving the general health with tonics and exercises.

2. Avoiding trauma to the affected parts viz. by shaving in one direction; by keeping away from use of strong soaps and irritating oil like mustard oil (sarson ka tel); by using sharp razor blades to prevent repeated shavings; by keeping the hair short and by refraining from fine shaving which would necessitate stretching of skin. In resistant cases, shaving should be avoided.

3. Under no circumstances X-ray therapy or staphylococcin vaccine should be permitted as it suppresses the expression of disease thereby making the disease more chronic.

4. For annoying itching and burning sensation locally a mixture consisting of Calendula external with water in 1:1 ratio.

5. Folliculitis is a disease which is characterized by remissions and relapses and hence all due care should be taken whilst revaluating the condition.

    In the repertory you will find the condition under the rubric

    Face- eruption- beard – folliculitis.

    Cicuta vir. and Natrium sulph. have been successfully used by in my practice for this condition.

Some Important Homeopathic Remedies

Antimonium tartaricum: Eruption around the mouth. Thick pustular eruption like pocks which leave bluish red marks on healing, leaving ugly blue, red scars. The most characteristic symptom is that the individual pustule is as large as a pea and distended with pus. Profuse salivation with thick, white, pasty tongue.

Calcarea carbonica: The skin of the face is rough and dry covered by humid, scabby eruptions in the form of clusters with burning pain. There is scanty discharge of thin pus. The face appears pale, puffy and pasty with swelling of lower lip. Lips are full of cracks and they bleed easily. The submaxillary glands are swollen.

Cicuta virosa: Eruptions are present on the face, are confluent, purulent and of a deep red colour. There is formation of burning scab with yellowish serum on the upper lip, cheeks and chin. Also thick honey scurf is present on chin, upper lip and lower portion of cheek. The eruption is accompanied with swelling of submaxillary gland and insatiable appetite.

Graphites: Eruptions that affect the skin around the nose, mouth and lips. They are full of cracks, which ooze glutinous discharge, which forms into thick crust. There is presence of itching and burning sensation along with stinging pains. The itching is worse at night and by warmth of bed. The other concomitants are constipation, tendency to obesity and disposition to catch cold.

Kalium bichromicum: The eruptions of Kali-bi. resemble those of small pox. Presence of vesiculopustulous eruptions with burning pains and tendency for ulceration. The discharges from the eruption are yellow, sticky, acrid and offensive. Presence of itching < from heat, hot weather, on undressing. It is specially indicated for persons who are fleshy, fat, light complexioned, who are subjected to catarrh and to syphilitic history.

Lithium carbonicum: Excessive dryness of skin with presence of scabby, tettery eruption on hands, head and cheeks which are preceded by red raw skin. There is presence of dull, stitching pain in the eruption, which ultimately ends in itching. Barber's itch is more prominent on the right side of the face. Uric acid diathesis and rheumatic complaints are associated concomitants.

Lycopodium clavatum: Eruptions that affect the face, behind the ears, corners of the mouth in patches, characterized by loss of hair with oozing of watery or yellowish fluid. Tendency to form cracks and ulcerations in the eruption, which tend to later on heal. Offensive perspiration, right-sided affection and 4-8 p.m. aggravation are important concomitants.

Mercurius iodatus ruber: Presence of vesicular papular eruptions on the face especially on the cheek. The eruptions are full of small fissures and cracks. Presence of sycosis barbae in patients with a syphilitic background.

Rhus toxicodendron: Corners of the mouth, lips are surrounded by erythematous vesicular eruptions with oozing of watery, yellowish fluid. There is formation of painful yellow crust. Itching < by scratching, by warmth (Rhus-v. is better by hot application).

Staphysagria: Thick scabs that itch violently. Biting and itching sensation as of vermin, which changes place on scratching. The skin symptoms alternate with joint pain.

Sulphur iodatum: Obstinate cases of barber's itch where papular eruption on the face is prone to suppuration. Itching < warm room, < warm application. Discharges are acrid and produce burning sensation wherever it comes in contact with the skin. Lymph nodes surrounding the eruptions are enlarged and swollen.

Thuja occidentalis: Beard and whiskers. Foul pustules with sunken apices. Eruptions itch or burn violently whenever the patient applies cold water. Greasy skin, presence of warts, sweetish odor of perspiration.

SYCOSIS NUCHAE

On the back of the neck, sycosis has a tendency to produce small, keloidal papules and nodules (Acne keloides nuchae) that are chronic and relapsing. It starts as discrete, follicular papules, some of which turn into pustules, others develop into firm nodules or plaques of thick scar like tissue by coalescence. The hair appears twisted and tangled. Marked itching and occasionally pain accompany it.

SYCOSIS LUPOIDES

In lupoid sycosis, the follicles are destroyed by scarring, and active papules and pustules fringe the advancing margin around a pink atrophic scar. Granulomatous inflammatory changes may give the papules a lupoid appearance. The process usually begins in front of one ear or under the chin and extends irregularly in any direction. The scalp may be extensively involved. Rarely, a similar process affects axillary and pubic hair, or the lower legs, thighs and arms. Lupoid sycosis tends to persist indefinitely, although the rate of extension may vary from time to time.

FOLLICULITIS DECALVANS

It is comparatively an acute and severe skin disease involving the scalp. Furunculoses, abscesses and cicatrical alopecia are the important clinical features.

Differential Diagnosis

The most frequent misdiagnosis is certainly the *pseudofolliculitis* caused by ingrowing hairs. The papules and pustules are irregularly scattered over the sides of the neck and the angles of the jaw and are not grouped but may lie in skinfolds.

Tinea barbae can be distinguished from this condition by the presence of deep seated, indurated, boggy swellings and microscopic examination for fungus.

Secondary eczematization and follicular infective eczema, on the other hand, can be distinguished by the features described above.

Impetigo has special features like interfollicular epidermal involvement, tense bullae and stuck-on honey-coloured crusts, etc. In etiological diagnosis, *seborrheic diathesis* and/or *acute seborrheic dermatitis* must be seriously considered.

Mycotic sycosis, a kerion of the beard, usually occurs on the chin or cheeks. The oedematous plaque of grouped pustules of acute onset is easily recognized. The diagnosis is suggested by the patient's contact with cattle, and confirmed by mycological examination.

Lupoid sycosis rarely simulates *lupus vulgaris*. The presence of pustules establishes the diagnosis. Biopsy can be undertaken if doubt remains. The scarring of lupoid sycosis may have medicolegal implications if the patient falsely attributes it to the use of radiotherapy during its early stages.

Prognosis

The course of sycosis is chronic; exacerbation and remissions mark it. The disease can continue for years. The prognosis is good if proper treatment is given and the patient co-operates. Only a very small % of cases is intractable.

ANGULAR STOMATITIS

Synonym

Perleche.

Clinical Features

It is characterized by linear cracks at the angles of the mouth.

Malnutrition particularly deficiency of riboflavin, monilial infection, low grade pyogenic infection, as a feature of seborrheic dermatitis, or a complication brought on by an ill fitting or a sensitizing denture or by pipe smoking are several known exciting factors.

Clinically, it is seen as erythema and as a crack covered by yellowish crust. It is usually a chronic condition and the prognosis depends upon the cause. Thus it is important that the physician examines the patient throughly rather then merely relying on the use of vitamins for treating the same.

A HOMEOPATHIC APPROACH TO ANGULAR STOMATITIS

First of all the homeopathic physician has to decide whether the person is well nourished or not. If a person is ill nourished then dietetic advice and vitamin supplement has to be given. If the patient is well nourished, then one must try and find out the exact cause like monilial infection, seborrhoeic dermatitis etc. Since the lesions are characterized by deep cracks, it indicates a dominant syphilitic miasm. The crusts formed in the lesion should be gradually removed with the help of a solution prepared by mixing Calendula and water in ratio 1:2. And on the raw surface, Calendula ointment should be applied. The above application is only meant for the protection of the raw surface from the environment. The rest of the approach remains same as that of impetigo.

The following rare remedies should be remembered for this condition:

Alloxanum, Abroma augusta, Morgan pure, Natrium arsenicosum, Syphilinum, Capsella bursa pestoris, Vaccininum.

Kent's Repertory should be referred for the therapeutic utility as

Face – Cracked – Corners of the mouth.

Some Important Homeopathic Remedies

Antimonium crudum: Cracks at the corners of mouth. They are small, sore with presence of thick, yellow crusts on top. The tongue is coated thick white and the patient is extremely thirstless. The cracks are associated with gastrointestinal disturbances.

Cundurango: Cracks are extremely painful to slightest touch. They are associated with digestive disturbances. Presence of angular stomatitis in cancerous diathesis; stricture of esophagus.

Graphites: Presence of rawness in the cracks. They bleed easily and ooze out gluey moisture, which turns into a crust. The cracks are usually associated with eczema. There is a sour foul odor from mouth and there is a sensation as if a cobweb is present on the face. The cracks are associated with gastric and menstrual disturbances. Burning blisters on tongue, salivation.

Nitricum acidum: Angles of lips are raw, cracked and scabby. The cracks are very painful, pricking pain like a splinter is a characteristic symptom which is worse when touched and at night. The cracks turn into ulcers which oozes acrid, thin bloody, offensive, dirty brown discharge. The tongue is also fissured or mapped. Presence of aphthous stomatitis in individuals who have history of abuse of mercury.

Silicea terra: Cracks are indurated, situated at the corners of lips. Cracks are also present in the lips. The cracks suddenly become painful and they suppurate easily. There is presence of itching sensation in cracks. Cracks are present in individuals with scrofulous diathesis. Mouth is sensitive to cold water. Sensation of hair on tongue.

■

Chapter-18

Fungal Infection of the Skin

Introduction

Fungal infections are caused by non-photosynthetic vegetable parasites called fungi, which can be broadly divided into two basic forms, moulds and yeasts. Fungi are capable of colonizing almost any environment, and generally play an invaluable role in the decomposition and recycling of organic matter. They tend to produce harmful effects by producing mycotoxins, by evoking allergic reactions or by direct tissue invasion. They reproduce both sexually and asexually, sometimes simultaneously.

Fungal infections can be broadly classified into superficial, subcutaneous and deep infections on the basis of degree of tissue invasion in reference to skin and mucous membranes.

Classification

1. Superficial & Cutaneous Mycoses

This category consists of infections affecting the hair, skin and nails alone, and here too there is a division into:

- 'Superficial mycoses', where there is no significant histopathological inflammatory response in the host. E.g.

Malassezia infections (pityriasis versicolor, seborrheic dermatitis, malassezia folliculitis, tinea nigra, and black and white piedra); and,

- *'Cutaneous mycoses'*, where there are pathological changes occurring in the host tissue inspite of the fungus being confined to the stratum corneum. E.g. Dermatophytosis (tinea corporis, tinea pedis, tinea capitis), Candidosis (cutaneous, oropharyngeal, vaginal), and a range of non-dermatophyte infections of the skin and nails, such as dermatomycoses caused by scytalidium species and onychomycosis caused by other non-dermatophyte moulds).

Laboratory diagnosis of superficial and cutaneous mycoses relies on the direct microscopical observation of the pathogen in samples from the affected area. Also, a culture can then be done with the specific identification of the fungus.

2. Subcutaneous Mycoses

- Mycetoma.
- Sporotrichosis.
- Chromoblastomycosis.
- Phaeohyphomycosis.
- Rhinisporidiosis.
- Lobomycosis.
- Phycomycosis.

3. Systemic Mycoses

- *Pathogenic:* Histoplasmosis, Blastomycosis, Paracoccidio-idomycosis, and Coccidioidomycosis.

- *Opportunistic:* Cryptococcosis, Aspergillosis, Mucormyco-sis, and Candidiasis.

SUPERFICIAL & CUTANEOUS MYCOSES

PITYRIASIS VERSICOLOR

Synonym

Tinea versicolor; Dermatomycosis furfuracea; Tinea flavea; Liver spots; Chromophytosis.

Definition

It is a commonly seen, asymptomatic and benign, superficial fungal infection of the skin caused by Malassezia yeasts, and characterized by discrete or concrescent, scaly, hypopigmented or hyperpigmented macules and patches, mainly on the upper trunk. In predisposed patients, the condition may recur chronically.

Etiology & Incidence

Malassezia furfur is the complex species of thick-walled, spherical yeast known to cause this condition. They are especially dense in the scalp, the upper trunk and the flexures. Pityrosporon orbiculare, P. ovale and M. ovalis are synonyms for M. furfur.

In quite a few cases a strongly positive family history is seen, which could be related to either a genetically determined host-susceptibility factor, or the greater opportunity for heavy colonization by the yeast. Transmission from one person to another can also take place.

This condition is especially common in the tropical, humid and warm countries, where the individual tends to perspire easily. Its peak incidence is in the late teens (especially the early 20's), and is rarely seen in young children and in the aged.

Pityriasis versicolor is also seen to occur more commonly in the following conditions – Cushing's syndrome, malnutrition, pregnancy and oral contraceptives, and in those who tend to apply a lot of oil to the skin

Histopathogenesis

Hyperkeratosis, parakeratosis and slight acanthosis, with a mild inflammatory infiltrate in the upper dermis are the characteristic features. A marked accumulation of Langerhans' cells in the epidermis, reduced expression of cellular activation markers, and the presence of macrophages and T cells are also seen.

M. furfur is seen in the upper layers of the stratum corneum, invading even the keratinized cells. M. furfur is a member of normal human cutaneous flora and can be found on normal skin as well as in skin regions demonstrating cutaneous disease. In this condition though, the organism is found in both the yeast (spore) stage and the filamentous (hyphal) form.

The hypopigmentation of the skin could be the result of dicarboxylic acids produced by the fungus, resulting in inhibition of a necessary enzyme of melanocyte pigment formation. The hyperpigmented lesions seen in fair-skinned individuals can be due to the abnormally large melanosomes and a thicker keratin layer.

Clinical Features

This condition is termed 'versicolor' (*versi* - several) since the patient often presents with lesions that tend to assume variable colors like yellow, white, reddish brown, dark brown, or at times even black. They occur in irregular and many a times confluent patches, with a mild irritation of the skin. Patients often complain that the involved skin lesions fail to tan in the summer.

The primary lesion is a sharply demarcated, at times red, macule, covered by fine dust-like scales. This lesion then spreads to involve large, confluent areas, with scattered oval patches and outlying macules. The scales may at times not be easily visible, but can be made more obvious by abrading the lesion with a blade, pin or a not-so-sharp knife (Scratch sign).

The lesions occur at any site on the body, especially the upper trunk and the parts that tend to perspire a lot. The lesions can spread to the upper arms, axilla, neck, abdomen, groins, and inframammary folds (in females).

Diagnosis

- With the Wood's lamp, the scaly lesions may show pale-yellow, golden yellow, or coppery-orange fluorescence. However, in some cases, the lesions will appear darker than unaffected skin under Wood's light, but will not fluoresce.

- Scraping the lesions and mounting them in 10% KOH solution confirms diagnosis by showing clusters of spherical, thick-walled yeasts and coarse mycelium with short broad filaments (hyphae), resembling 'spaghetti and meat balls'.

Differential Diagnosis

- The Pityriasis versicolor patches can resemble vitiligo and chloasma, but the absence of scaling is the latter two help differentiation.

- Seborrhoeic dermatitis, pityriasis rosea, psoriasis, secondary syphilis, pinta and tinea corporis, show more inflammatory change than pityriasis versicolor, and none of these ever has the even branny scale of the latter condition.

- Erythrasma can mimic or coexist with pityriasis versicolor, having similar pigmentary change and scaling, but satellite lesions are less commonly seen in it, and there is a pink fluorescence under the Wood's lamp.

Treatment

- Patients should be told that tinea versicolor is caused by a fungus that is normally present on the skin surface and is thus not a contagious illness.

- The condition does not leave any permanent scar or pigmentary changes, and any skin color alterations resolve within 1-2 months after treatment has been initiated.

- Recurrence is common, and prophylactic therapy may help reduce the high rate of recurrence.

SEBORRHEIC DERMATITIS

It is a chronic and commonly seen, scaly condition, affecting the face, nasolabial folds, upper trunk, and the scalp (dandruff). It has red, sharply marginated papulosquamous lesions covered with greasy scales.

This condition is explained in detail in the chapter 'Eczema and Dermatitis'.

MALASSEZIA FOLLICULITIS

This condition, which is also associated with Malassezia yeasts, is characterized by itchy, diffusely scattered, follicular eruptions (papules and pustules) on the back, upper trunk and shoulders.

It is most often seen in teenagers or young adult males, especially after exposure to too much sun.

Diagnosis

Biopsies taken from typical cases show clusters of yeasts within follicles surrounded by inflammatory cells, which are distinguishable from the colonization of follicular openings that can be seen in normal individuals.

Differential Diagnosis

The lesions may resemble acne, but the itching and the characteristic distribution tend to distinguish them from it.

TINEA NIGRA

Synonym

Tinea nigra palmaris; Keratomycosis nigricans palmaris; Pityriasis nigra.

Definition

It is an asymptomatic superficial fungal infection generally affecting the skin of the palms and characterized by deeply pigmented, macular, non-scaly patches.

Etiology

It is caused by Phaeo-annellomyces werneckii (also called as Exophiala werneckii or Hortaea werneckii).

Histopathology

Thickening of the stratum corneum is seen along with the presence of filaments (hyphae). There is hardly any inflammatory reaction in the dermis.

Clinical Features

The lesions are benign, macular, non-scaly, and sharply defined patches, of a characteristic brown or black colour resembling a silver nitrate stain.

The site of affection is usually always the palms, though the soles, neck and trunk may also be affected.

Differential Diagnosis

The black colour and the absence of scaling differentiate the condition from pityriasis versicolor.

• The pigmented lesions of Addison's disease, syphilis, pinta and junctional naevi of the palm may have to be differentiated, and mycological examination of scales is usually required.

Diagnosis

• Microscopy of infected epidermal scales in KOH mounts reveals brown, branched, closely septate hyphae, and elongated budding cells.

• Cultures of the causative organism can also be grown.

BLACK PIEDRA

Synonym

Tinea nodosa; Trichomycosis nodularis.

Definition

It is a fungal infection confined to hair shafts, where there is the formation of hard, dark, and superficial nodules.

Etiology & Incidence

It is caused by the fungus Piedraia hortae, occuring especially in the humid, wet, and tropical regions.

Clinical Features

There is the formation of multiple, very tiny (about 1mm or more in diameter), black, firmly adherent, rough and hard nodules on the hairs of the scalp, and occasionally on the hair of the beard, moustache or pubic area. These nodules with the fungi in it can rupture and grow on the outside of the hair cuticle, at times involving the complete hair shaft, causing the hair to break easily.

Histopathology

The nodules consist of closely packed, brown hyphae held together by a cement-like substance. In the thicker areas of the nodule, club-shaped asci containing eight elongated ascospores may be formed, with a polar filament at each end. Piedraia hortae is characteristically the only fungus that produces sexual spores in its parasitic phase.

Treatment

Shaving or cutting off the hair is an effective cure.

WHITE PIEDRA

Synonym

Trichosporosis nodosa.

Definition

A fungal infection that is confined to hair shafts with the formation of soft, white, grey or brownish, superficial nodules.

Etiology

Trichosporon ovoides is the causative organism.

Clinical Features

In this condition there is the formation of tiny, soft, white or light-brownish nodules on the hairs of the beard, moustache and genital areas. The scalp is less often involved. These nodules are transparent and can be easily detached from the hair. The fungus tends to grow both within and on the outside of the hair shaft causing it to break easily.

Histopathology

The nodules of white piedra are in the form of a sheath extending around and also growing within the hair shaft. The hyphae with arthroconidia and budding blastoconidia may also be seen

Treatment

Shaving or cutting the hair can cure this condition.

DERMATOPHYTOSIS

Synonym

Ringworm, Tinea.

Definition

Dermatophytosis is a superficial fungal infection caused by

the dermatophytes, which invade the dead keratinized tissue of the skin, hair and nails.

Etiology

Several species of dermatophytes tend to infect the human race, and they belong to three genera Trichophyton (T. rubrum, T. tonsurans, T. interdigitale), Epidermophyton (E. floccosum), and Microsporum (M. canis).

The infection may spread from person to person (anthropophilic), animal to person (zoophilic) or soil to person (geophilic). Characteristically, the zoophilic species tend to produce highly inflammatory reactions in humans, followed by a spontaneous cure, whereas anthropophilic species tend to produce mild but chronic lesions.

Predisposing factors to this condition are – warm, humid climate, poor nutrition and hygiene, obesity, diabetes mellitus and debilitating illness.

Pathogenesis of Infection

Invasion of the epidermis by dermatophytes follows a common pattern starting with adherence of the infectious arthroconidia to the keratinocytes, followed by penetration through and between the cells, and the development of a host response.

Histopathology

The histological finding varies according to the keratin destruction and the inflammatory host response. There can be a simple hyperkeratosis with hyper- or hypogranulosis, spongiosis, mononuclear invasion, and mild or moderate acanthosis seen in a few cases; or there can be pustular, highly inflammatory keratin seen (especially in the zoophilic infections). In a few cases, an erythema multiforme-like process with subepidermal bullae and leucocytic infiltration can be seen. In the classical annular ringworm, the border of the lesion is marked by clear inflammatory changes including a perivascular infiltrate of lymphocytes. By contrast, in the center of the lesion there is hardly any inflammation.

Classification

Clinically, tineas are classified according to the site of body infected.

- Tinea corporis is infection of the trunk and extremities.
- Tinea capitis is the infection of the scalp and its hair.
- Tinea manuum and tinea pedis is infection of palms, soles and interdigital webs.
- Tinea cruris is infection of the groin.
- Tinea barbae is infection of the beard area and neck.
- Tinea facia is infection of the face.
- Tinea unguium (onychomycosis) is infection of the nail.

The presence of humid or moist skin is very favorable for the establishment of the fungal infection.

TINEA CORPORIS

Synonym

Ringworm of the body; Tinea circinata.

Definition

Ringworm infection here occurs on the skin areas with less hair, like the trunk and limbs.

Etiology

It is caused most often by trichophyton species, especially T. rubrum.

Clinical Features

The lesion starts as a papule, which spreads in a ring-like form peripherally, with a central clearing. The lesions are characteristically circular with a sharply defined, active and raised edge, consisting of vesicles and scaling. Single lesions occur, or there may be multiple plaques, that may coalesce into large lesions. The sites most often involved are the waist, axillae, buttocks and extrimities but not the groins, palms and soles.

The central skin of the lesions may show postinflammatory pigmentation, a change of texture or residual erythematous dermal nodules.

Differential Diagnosis

- Seborrheic dermatitis can be confused with it, but it is usually symmetrical and there is often associated infection of the scalp and intertrigo at the skin folds.

- Intertrigo with scabies where the lesions occur at the flexural and moist sites, which are also sites of predilection for tinea corporis.

- Tinea versicolor and pityriasis rosea also have symmetrical lesions, especially confined to the trunk and proximal parts of the limbs, but the herald patch, if seen, is almost impossible to differentiate from ringworm without microscopic examination of the scales.

- Impetigo circinata especially in children.

- Psoriasis can appear similar to corporeal infection in a few cases where the distribution is not quite typical. The lesions in psoriasis occur especially on the knees, elbows and scalp, with associated lesions and pitting of the nails.

- Nummular eczema is a commonly confused with tinea corporis.

- Tuberculoid leprosy where minimal infiltration in the periphery mimics the active border of tinea corporis.

- Lichenification of a patch of tinea, of the leg for example, can mimic lichen simplex very closely.

Complications

- Due to constant scratching, the skin can get red and inflamed with eczematous oozing and crust formation.

- There can be secondary pyogenic infection of the ringworm lesions.
- There can be dissemination in immunocompromised individuals.

TINEA CAPITIS

Here there is fungal infection of the scalp, and is already discussed in detail in the chapter 'Diseases of the hair'.

TINEA BARBAE

Synonym

Ringworm of the beard area.

Definition

This is a condition seen in adult males, where there is ringworm infection of the coarse hair and beard and moustache areas of the face.

Etiology

T. verrucosum and T. mentagrophytes var. mentagrophytes are common causes. In a few cases M. canis, T. violaceum, T. schoenleinii, T. megninii and T. rubrum can also cause this condition.

It is especially acquired from a barber's instruments or from animals.

Pathogenesis

Large-spored ectothrix invasion with the spores in chains is seen usually.

Clinical Features

There is a highly inflammatory, pustular folliculitis seen, where the hair of the beard or moustache regions are surrounded by red, inflammatory papules or pustules or scales, usually with seropurulent exudation or crusting. There is a little irritation, itching, and slight pain in the affected areas. Also, the hair in the affected areas are weak and loose and can be painlessly and easily plucked.

There are two types of this condition seen:

- The non-inflammatory type, where the lesions spread peripherally and clear at the center.

- The inflammatory type, where the lesions are of a deeper type with pustules and scale formation.

The lesions may persist for months and tend to resolve spontaneously. The inflammatory type causes cicatricial alopecia on healing.

Differential Diagnosis

- Boils on the face tend to be much more painful than the tineal lesions. Also, though there are loosened hairs seen in boils, they are not so profound as seen in tinea barbae.

- Milder cases of tinea need to be distinguished from bacterial folliculitis, acne, rosacea and pseudofolliculitis.

TINEA FACIEI

Synonym

Ringworm of the face, Tinea faciale.

Definition

This is seen especially in females and young children, where the glabrous skin of the face is infected with a dermatophyte fungus.

Etiology

T. mentagrophytes var. mentagrophytes and T. rubrum are especially known to cause this condition, though M. audouinii and M. canis are also common causative agents.

Pathogenesis

The fungal spread can occur either by direct contact with a pet or can be a secondary spread from pre-existing tinea of another body site.

Clinical Features

The most commonly seen complaints are that of itching, erythema, burning and exacerbation after sun exposure. History of exposure to animals can be obtained in most of the cases. Annular or circinate lesions are seen in quite a few cases, with an indurated and raised margin, and slight scaling. In other cases, simple papular lesions or completely flat erythematous patches are seen.

Differential Diagnosis

- Due to the sensitivity of the lesions to sunlight, very little scaling and different types of lesions seen in this condition, it is frequently confused with discoid lupus erythematosus (DLE) and polymorphic light eruption. Diagnosis can be established by careful examination of the scrapings taken from the skin surface.

- Bowenoid solar keratoses, psoriasis, impetigo, rosacea, seborrheic dermatitis and benign lymphocytic infiltrates are other conditions that need to be differentiated.

TINEA PEDIS

Synonym

Foot ringworm.

Definition

This condition is defined as ringworm infection of the feet or the toes.

Etiology

T. rubrum, T. mentagrophytes var. interdigitale and E.

floccosum are the three main fungi responsible for foot ringworm. Mixed infections are common. Also, a few zoophilic fungi are known to cause tinea pedis.

Pathogenesis

It is a commonly seen condition resulting from wearing of socks and closed shoes, which causes maceration of the toe-cleft skin. It is especially seen in adult males and not so much in children and females. The infection tends to spread from use of a common family bathroom or pool.

In chronic tinea pedis, resident bacteria like large-colony coryneforms can act as important copathogens.

Clinical Features

In the intertriginous dermatitis form of tinea pedis, there is scaling, maceration and fissuring of skin of the interdigital areas, occasionally spreading to involve the posterior surface of the toes and the soles. The condition tends to be very chronic and persistent, often affecting only one foot, with the itching getting worse in the summer. In the infections resulting from T. rubrum, chronic squamous hyperkeratotic lesions are seen, affecting especially the soles, heels and sides of the feet. The affected area becomes pink and is covered with fine silvery white scales. The dorsal surfaces of the toes and feet are not often affected, but the nails tend to be commonly affected. In cases where the person has a tendency to excessive perspiration, the symptoms tend to get more severe. The excessive perspiration can also be a result of the tineal infection, along with an offensive odor of the part and secondary bacterial infection, with fissures in the toe clefts.

In cases of tinea resulting from T. mentagrophytes var. inter-digitale, the clinical symptoms may vary from mild insignificant scaling or fissuring of the toe clefts, to severe acute inflammatory reactions affecting all parts of the feet. A vesiculobullous reaction, extending over the whole sole, is more commonly seen in tinea pedis resulting from this fungal type. The vesicles become pustules, which then rupture and leave collarettes of scaling with normal intervening skin, or there can be various degrees of scaling and inflammation. Spontaneous cure tends to occur, but there can be recurrence in warm and humid weather.

E. floccosum produces a similar chronic vesicular infection of the sole as seen in the above type, or there is a chronic dry hyperkeratotic condition seen like that caused by T. rubrum. Here in this type there is a significantly lesser toenail involvement than in the other two types.

Differential Diagnosis

- Erythrasma, where too the lesions are restricted to the toe cleft, can be differentiated from tinea pedis due to it rarely causing any fissures. Also in the Wood's lamp, a pink fluorescence can be seen for erythrasma.

- Candidosis is differentiated from tinea pedis due to a build-up of rather more white macerated skin.

- Bacterial infections of the sole can also cause inflammation and foul odor. These may or may not coexist with tinea pedis. Swabs and scrapings for bacterial and ringworm organisms can be done. Also the Wood's lamp may show a greenish blue for Pseudomonas infections

- Soft corns or callosities sometimes with sinus formation are common in the lateral toe clefts, especially in women.

- In younger children, juvenile plantar dermatosis needs to be ruled out.

- In cases where the soles of the feet, especially the heels, are involved more than the toe cleft, pustular psoriasis must be ruled out.

- Psoriasis, pityriasis rubra pilaris, Reiter's syndrome, and contact dermatitis from nylon dyes or shoe materials need to be differentiated, by checking the skin scrapings for tinea pedis.

Treatment

- Infected individuals should avoid exposing others to their infection by not walking barefoot on the floors of communal changing rooms, and by avoiding swimming.
- Frequent washing of the floors of shower rooms, bathtubs, and the sides of swimming pool reduces the prevalence of this condition in the society.

TINEA MANNUM

Synonym

Ringworm of the hand.

Definition

Here there is fungal infection of the palm and interdigital areas of the hand, and it usually occurs in association with tinea pedis.

Etiology

T. rubrum is the commonest cause for this condition, with E. floccosum, T. mentagrophytes var. interdigitale, T. violaceum and T. mentagrophytes var. erinacei involved in a few cases.

Pathogenesis

The spread can occur via animals or from a pre-existing foot infection with or without toenail involvement. T. mentagrophytes var. interdigitale ringworm infections can occur under worn metal rings or wristwatches, anatomical deformities, or frequent occupational usage predispose to maceration between the fingers. Poor peripheral circulation and tylosis are other possible predisposing factors to it.

Clinical Features

Unilateral involvement of a palm is seen, which becomes dry and hyperkeratotic, with mild scaling, especially around the palmar creases. Crescentic, exfoliating scales; circumscribed, vesicular patches; discrete, red papular and follicular scaly patches; and erythematous, scaly sheets on the dorsal surface of the hand are other clinical variants seen.

Differential Diagnosis

- Contact dermatitis, psoriasis, pityriasis rubra pilaris, constitutional eczemas, tylosis, syphilis and post-streptococcal peeling need to be differentiated by examining the skin scrapings histologically.

- Candidosis and bacterial intertrigo should also be ruled out in ring and web-space infections.

Treatment

Prompt treatment of tinea pedis (since tinea manuum is directly related to the level of tinea pedis in the society) and the use of separate towels is necessary to control the spread of this condition.

TINEA CRURIS

Synonym

Ringworm of the groin; Dhobi itch; Eczema marginatum.

Definition

This is an infection of the groins by a type of dermatophyte.

Etiology

T. rubrum is the most frequently seen cause, and T. mentagrophytes var. interdigitale and E. floccosum are other causes.

Pathogenesis

Ringworm of the groins is a commonly seen condition, especially in the tropical countries, where there is a warm and humid weather. It is especially common in males rather than females. Obesity, moisture, warmth and friction are the important factors for its existence.

In most of the cases autoinfection from the foot to the groin is common, but also sharing of towels and other clothing is also important.

Clinical Features

Itching of the groins is the most predominant symptom. Initial lesions consist of erythematous plaques, curved with sharp margins extending from the groin down the thighs. There can be marked scaling with dermal nodules forming a bead-like structure along the margins of the lesion, with slight central clearing. There are occasional pustules seen, but rarely any vesiculation. Lesions may spread to the scrotum, penis, buttocks, lower back and the abdomen.

Differential Diagnosis

- Candidosis is usually seen more often in females, and it doesn't seem to have the characteristic raised beaded margin. Instead it has white pustules with numerous and small satellite lesions, with a frayed peeling edge that occurs as the tiny pustules rupture.

- Pityriasis versicolor and erythrasma are usually non-inflammatory and asymptomatic, and rarely has any central clearing.

- Intertrigo with heavy bacterial colonization is especially seen in the obese people, where there may be a sharp margin, but it is usually a simple curve where the opposed skin surfaces meet.

- Psoriasis and mycosis fungoides may occasionally mimic tinea cruris, but characteristic lesions in other sites can usually be found.

- In atopic eczema there may be lichenification, but these changes usually extend up towards the hip.

Treatment

By avoiding the sharing of towels and by wearing the right kind of clothing, one can control the spread of tinea cruris.

TINEA UNGUIUM

Synonym

Ringworm of the nails; Onchomycosis due to dermatophytes.

Definition

Here there is invasion of the nail plates by the dermatophytes.

Etiology

T. rubrum, T. mentagrophytes var. interdigitale and E. floccosum are the common dermatophytes known to cause this condition with associated foot and hand infections.

T. tonsurans, T. violaceum and T. schoenleinii are the common dermatophytes known to cause this condition with associated scalp infections.

In the great majority of cases they are associated with tinea pedis or tinea manuum. T. rubrum predominates in fingernail and toenail infections. T. mentagrophytes var. interdigitale tends to affect especially the great toenail. E. floccosum, however, seems to be less capable of invading the hard keratin of the nail.

Invasion of the nail plate usually occurs either from the lateral nailfold or from the free edge, and an elaborate network of channels and lacunae is formed, leading to opacity and eventually destruction and crumbling of the nail-plate. Subungual hyperkeratosis can also occur. Tinea unguium is largely a disease of the adults, but children, especially those in institutions and in households where the adults are infected with T. rubrum, may be infected from time to time. A poor peripheral circulation and poor susceptibility can make this condition chronic. Traumatized nails and nails of elderly people are more susceptible to infection.

Clinical Features

Three distinct clinical patterns are seen.

- *Distal and Lateral Subungual Onychomycosis (DLSO)* is the most common form of infection, which usually presents itself as a white or yellow streak or patch at the free edge of the nail plate, often near the lateral nailfold. This spreads towards the base of the nail and may occasionally become darker, brown or black. The nailplate becomes thick, and may crack as it is pushed up by the accumulation of soft, subungual hyperkeratosis. In chronic cases, there is massive destruction of the nailplate (Total Dystrophic Onychomycosis, TDO). Although commonly starting with a single affected nail, other digits later become invaded.

- *Superficial White Onychomycosis (SWO)* is where the dorsal surface of the nail plate is eroded in well-circumscribed, powdery white patches, often away from the free edge. It is distinguishable from other causes of leukonychia by the powdery nature of the white material, which can easily be scraped away. The whole surface of the nail plate may be affected in such a way. Toenails are usually affected, but in AIDS patients SWO of both toe and fingernails has been reported.

- *Proximal subungual onychomycosis* is a form seen especially in AIDS patients. Here there is rapid invasion of the nail plate from the posterior nail fold, producing a white nail with only marginal increase in thickness.

Differential Diagnosis

- Psoriatic lesions of the nails can resemble ringworm of the nails, where there are destructive changes of the nail plate and nail bed. The distinguishing feature is the fine pitting of the dorsal nail plate, which is never seen in fungal infections.

- In cases of eczema, there is an irregular buckling of the nail.

- Lichen planus causes a ridge or dysplastic changes of the nail.

- Paronychia, due either to bacteria or to Candida, usually affects the nail plate proximally, and laterally, while the free edge is often spared, at least initially. Also there is no swelling of the nail fold seen in dermatophyte infections, with a purulent discharge, which is never seen tinea unguium.

- Nail dystrophies can be distinguished from this condition by checking out the scrapings and also since they are usually symmetrical affections, whereas fungal infections are usually asymmetrical.

STEROID-MODIFIED TINEA

Synonym

Tinea incognito.

Definition

These are ringworm infections modified by systemic or topical corticosteroids prescribed for some pre-existing pathology or given mistakenly for the treatment of misdiagnosed tinea.

Pathogenesis & Clinical Features

In this type there is hardly any inflammatory response seen, which is almost totally suppressed by the corticosteroids. The resistance to infection mediated by the immune response, especially the cell-mediated response, could be diminished by the corticosteroids. Thus the infection is less likely to be diagnosed, plus the patient has been rendered more susceptible to that infection.

There is hardly any scaling or the typical raised margin with central clearing. The inflammation is reduced to a few nondescript nodules, with a bruise-like, brownish discoloration, especially in the groins. In other areas, like the face, there can be superimposed perioral dermatitis with papules and tiny pustules. In cases of chronic overuse of steroids, there is atrophy, telangiectasia and striae likely to be seen, which represent the whorls of fungal growth.

Diagnosis

- Candidosis needs to be differentiated after the stopping of therapy and performing mycological investigations like skin scrapings.

Laboratory diagnosis of dermatophytosis

The diagnosis of ringworm infection is done through histological examination of the skin, hair and nail samples, and through growth of the primary culture or by using a media. The dermatophytic fungi are seen as highly refractile, long, undulating, branched and septate hyphae, along with the spores in skin scales. Also, the lesions of certain types of *Tinea capitis* fluoresce when examined under Wood's lamp, emitting ultraviolet rays.

Complications

- Cellulitis of the lower extremities can occur in a few cases, resulting from interdigital fungal infection due to a breach in the skin followed by inoculation of the opportunistic bacteria.
- Also, in patients with impaired cell-mediated immune function and AIDS, atypical and locally aggressive presentations of dermatophyte infection may occur, resulting in extensive skin involvement, superadded cutaneous infections, subcutaneous abscesses and dissemination.

Treatment

- Patients who tend to sweat a lot should change their clothes frequently, wear cotton undergarments and socks and avoid the use of any synthetic material.
- Clothes, especially the underwear, and towels should be boiled in hot water in those who have already been infected.
- Bathrooms and bathtubs should be regularly cleaned and scrubbed with soap and warm water.
- Footwear should be of the open and comfortable type permitting sufficient aeration.
- Intertriginous areas like the groins, armpits, etc. should be kept clean and dry.
- One should shampoo the hair immediately after visit to the barber's shop.

CANDIDOSIS

Synonym

Candidiasis, moniliasis, thrush.

Definition

Candidosis is an infection caused by any of the species of the yeast Candida, especially Candida albicans, resulting in superficial infections of the mucous membranes and skin, and in a few rare cases internal organs may also be severely involved resulting in septicaemia, endocarditis and meningitis.

Etiology

Candida albicans is an oval yeast, producing budding cells, pseudohyphae and true hyphae. They have the ability to simultaneously display several morphological forms and are thus termed as polymorphic. This organism is a common commensal in the mouth, vagina and GI tract in healthy individuals. Apart from C. albicans, the genus Candida includes over 100 species, most of which do not infest the humans, except in a few immunosuppressed cases like in AIDS patients and in those being nursed in intensive care units.

Predisposing Factors

The very old, the very young and the very ill are susceptible to candidosis. Also, in cases of oral thrush, the predisposing factors include the carbohydrate level in the mouth, presence of any food debris, inadequate oral hygiene, wearing of dentures, less flow of saliva, etc. Also patients with diabetes, Sjögren's syndrome, AIDS, leukemia, or obesity are also known to be prone to candidosis. Also, persons with hyperhidrosis, or who are on systemic antibiotics, immunosuppressive drugs, systemic or prolonged steroids, and oral contraceptives are known to develop candidiosis.

Histopathology

There is the presence of the yeast in the stratum corneum, along

with inflammatory changes and the formation of a pseudomembrane
of epithelial and inflammatory cells. In the oral epithelium and in
the cutaneous epidermis, the inflammatory infiltrate consists
predominantly of polymorphs, which may form microabscesses or
subcorneal pustules. There is then a resultant splitting of the
epidermis. In the dermis there is a mixture of lymphocytes, plasma
cells and histiocytes. In chronic cases, hyperplasia with
parakeratosis and acanthosis of the epithelium is associated with a
mixed inflammatory infiltrate.

Clinical Syndromes of Candidosis

A. Oral candidosis

1. **Pseudomembranous Candidosis/Candidiasis/Oral Thrush:**
    Here the characteristic feature is the sharply defined patch or
    patches of creamy, crumbly, curd-like, white pseudomembrane,
    which, when removed, leaves an underlying erythematous base.
    This pseudomembrane consists of desquamated epithelial cells,
    fibrin, leukocytes and fungal mycelium that tend to attach to
    the inflamed epithelium. The sites affected are the buccal
    mucosa of the cheek, the gums and the palate. In old patients
    or in the immunocompromised, the tongue, pharynx and
    esophagus may be affected, with ulceration and erosion of the
    mucous membrane. This condition is also especially common
    in infants in the first few weeks of life, and is also seen in
    those with AIDS. There is inadequate food intake due to the
    pain and soreness of lesions. Secondary bacterial infections
    are common.

2. **Erythematous candidosis (atrophic oral candidiasis;
    denture-sore mouth; denture stomatitis):** Here there is a
    marked soreness with erosion, dusky-colored erythema and
    atrophic, shiny erythematous mucous membranes, with edema,
    especially on the dorsum of the tongue and in the denture-
    bearing area. It usually occurs as a complication of pseudo-
    membranous candidosis, and in those wearing dentures or
    orthodontic appliances. In chronic cases there is secondary
    papillomatosis and angular cheilitis that develops.

3. **Chronic plaque-like Candidosis (chronic hyperplastic candidiasis; candida leukoplakia):** This condition has persistent, firm, irregular, white oral plaques, with slight soreness and roughness, especially on the cheek and tongue. These plaques cannot be removed and are surrounded by a margin of erythema. Adult males are especially affected. Smokers are prone to develop this type of oral candidosis. These need to be differentiated from leukoplakia.

4. **Chronic Nodular Candidosis:** This rare form of candidosis, often seen in certain patients with chronic mucocutaneous candidosis, produces a cobbled appearance of the tongue.

5. **Angular Cheilitis (angular stomatitis; perleche):** Here there is fissuring, maceration and soreness of the angles of the mucosa of the mouth, extending outwards to the folds of the facial skin. This can be a result of interplay of a lot many organisms, though Candida is the most common. It is especially seen due to excessive moisture resulting from persistent salivation or constant licking of the lips. It is also seen in patients wearing chronic dentures.

6. **Median rhomboid glossitis:** This is a condition where there is a diamond-shaped lesion on the dorsum of the tongue, with loss of papillae.

7. **Candidosis and local steroids:** Local applications of steroids, in the form of creams, mouthwashes, lozenges, and aerosols (used for treatment of chronic aphthosis, lichen planus, or asthma) can result in diminished local immunity in this area, leading to development of candidosis.

8. **Other Conditions Associated with Candida in the mouth:** Candidosis can be a result of super-infection over other oral conditions like lichen planus, leukokeratosis and white-sponge naevus.

B. Candidosis of the skin and genital mucous membranes

Most of the candidal infections of the skin occur at skin folds or over parts that are kept moist or poorly ventilated. Also mucous membranes and orifices of the body are frequently affected areas of the body.

1. **Candida Intertrigo (Flexural candidosis):** This is especially seen in obese individuals, where there is erythema of the skin folds with a slight moist exudation. It can spread and form an irregular edge with formation of tiny pustules that rupture to form tiny erosions, with peeling of the superficial layer of the skin. Soreness and itching of lesions is marked. There are satellite lesions typically occuring in the form of pustules or papules. In cases where there is involvement of the web spaces of the toes or fingers, marked maceration with a thick, white, horny layer is usually seen. There is also candidal infestation with maceration of the skin occuring in areas around metal rings or dressings.

2. **Candida affecting the nails:** There is onychia and paronychia, with inflammation of the posterior nail fold and erosion of the edges of the nails, which are discolored, as a result of candida infestation.

3. **Vulvovaginitis (vulvovaginal thrush):** This is a commonly seen condition where the woman complains of itching and soreness of the genitalia, with dyspareunia and a thick, creamish white discharge. It is commonly seen in pregnant woman, and in those who are sexually active. On examination there is a dusky-red erythema of the vaginal mucous membrane and the vulval skin, with white and curdled particles of discharge.

   The rash can extend to the perineal and groin region. In a few' severe cases there is formation of pustules with fringed and irregular margins. In chronic cases, the vaginal mucosa may become glazed and atrophic.

4. **Candida Balanitis:** This condition is especially seen in the uncircumcised and the diabetics, where there is development of tiny papules on the glans penis a few hours after intercourse. These then form white pustules or vesicles and rupture, leaving a peeling erosive edge covered with a soft white material, with minimal soreness and irritation. Involvement of the groins can

occur along with the glans and prepuce, especially during the hot summer days.

The skin of the glans penis, especially in the uncircumcised, may sometimes be colonized by Candida asymptomatically. When Candida balanitis develops, it is usual to find either abundant vaginal candida carriage or frank vulvovaginitis in the sexual partner.

5. **Perianal and scrotal candidosis:** It begins as an erythema with soreness and irritation around the anal margin, which spreads to the nates and the scrotum. There is formation of erosions with white discharge and marginal pustules over the perianal skin.

6. **Napkin Candidosis:** Candida albicans is normally also present in the genital area of infants, but it tends to get worse in cases of napkin rash. There is formation of sub-corneal pustules, with a fringed and irregular border in typical cases.

7. **Nodular or granulomatous candidosis of the napkin area (granuloma gluteale infantum):** Here there is formation of bluish or brownish nodular eruptions over the buttocks, genitalia, upper thighs and pubis

Diagnosis

- Histological examination reveals the oval, budding candida yeasts with hyphal elements.

- The Germ tube test and Slide agglutination tests are diagnostic for candidosis.

Differential Diagnosis

- Tinea, seborrhoeic dermatitis, bacterial intertrigo, flexural psoriasis, and flexural Darier's disease need to be differentiated from candida, usually by histological examination of the swab or scraping collected during the acute phase of the illness.

- Trichomonas infection and bacterial vulvovaginitis should also be considered for differential diagnosis.

INFECTIONS CAUSED BY SCYTALIDIUM SPECIES

Etiology

This condition is caused by Scytalidium dimidiatum, which is a weak secondary pathogen of higher plants, found mainly in tropical areas. This grey to black mould is now recognized as the cause of ringworm-like infections of the palms, soles, toe webs and nails. S. hyalinum is a similar but non-pigmented organism, which can also mimic tinea pedis and manuum and invade the nail plate.

Clinical Features

There are hardly any symptoms produced except for a few changes in the nails at their lateral and distal edges, making it weak and break off or fissure transversely. There is paronychia and increased pigmentation in the nail plate or longitudinal pigmented streaking. There is also the involvement of thickly keratinized skin like the palms and soles.

Laboratory Diagnosis

Direct microscopy reveals the S. dimidiatum, though in a few cases brown or hyaline hyphae can also be seen.

Onychomycosis from non-dermatophyte moulds

Onchomycosis is a term used for any fungal infection of the nail plate. The most common organisms responsible for it are the dermatophytes, candida, and scytalidium, which are already covered. In this section we will deal with other non-dermatophyte moulds, affecting especially the toenails

SCOPULARIOPSIS INFECTIONS

Scopulariopsis brevicaulis is a common saprophytic mould that causes nail dystrophy, which is indistinguishable from that caused by a ringworm infection. The only distinguishing feature is that in chronic and severe infestations there is presence of brown spores that tend to give a cinnamon colour to the nail, especially at the area of subungual hyperkeratosis. The great toenails are most often affected, but it can occur in the other toenails or fingernails. Also, it can occur in association with dermatophyte infections of the skin, though scopulariopsis by itself doesn't affect the skin.

Laboratory Diagnosis

On examination, the fungi are seen as spherical or lemon-shaped ones with a single flat basal facet.

Superficial white Onchomycosis

This appears similar to onychomycosis caused by Trichophyton mentagrophytes var. interdigitale, but here the distinguishing feature is the lack of accompanying skin lesions. Acremonium strictum, Aspergillus terreus and Fusarium species are the ones seen most often to cause it.

Laboratory Diagnosis

There are bizarre atypical hyphal forms of the fungi seen with extensive leaf-like hyphae.

Onchomycosis caused by onchocola canadensis

There is a yellowish or greyish discoloration of the nails with hyperkeratosis and build-up of subungual debris. Microscopical examination reveals irregular hyaline, or brownish hyphae with barrel-shaped or round arthroconidia.

Miscellaneous Mould Infections

Pseudeurotium ovalis, Pyrenochaeta unguius hominis, Lasiodiploidea theobromae, Curvularia lunata and other moulds can also be responsible for onychomycosis. Toenails are especially affected.

SUBCUTANEOUS MYCOSES

These are tropical infections that occur sporadically following accidental inoculation with environmental fungi, into the dermis or subcutaneous tissue through a penetrating injury. Sporotrichosis, mycetoma and chromoblastomycosis are the most common types of subcutaneous mycoses seen; the less common ones include phaeohyphomycosis, lobomycosis, rhinosporidiosis and subcutaneous zygomycosis.

Laboratory Methods

- Direct microscopic or histological examination of the material will reveal the causative organism.

- In a few cases culture may need to be done.

MYCETOMA

Synonym

Maduromycosis; Madura foot.

Definition

Mycetoma is a chronic destructive subcutaenous infection caused either by fungi (eumycetomas) or actinomycetes or filamentous bacteria (actinomycetomas), with a tendency to form large colonies of the causative organisms within abscesses in tissues. These are discharged as granular matter (grains) through sinuses to the surface of the skin.

Etiology

It is caused by the various species of fungi (eumycetoma) and aerobic actinomycetes (actinomycetoma), occuring as saprophytes in the soil or on plants in the tropical countries, which get implanted subcutaneously into the skin due to a penetrating injury.

Histopathology

There is a chronic inflammatory reaction resulting in neutrophilic abscess formation, with scattered giant cells and fibrosis. The colorful grains (red, white, yellow, or black granules) that are characteristic of this condition are the collection of microcolonies of the organism, which are present at the center of the inflammatory response, and are slowly discharged with the pus through the multiple sinuses onto the skin surface. There is a slow destruction of the underlying tissues, muscles and bones.

A haematoxylin and eosin preparation is sufficient to distinguish between eumycetoma and actinomycetoma.

Clinical Features

Most of the lesions occur on the feet or the lower half of the leg, since they result from penetrating injury. Hands, shoulders or buttocks can be rarely affected. The lesions are not contagious.

The lesions start insidiously, with a firm, painless nodule palpable initially, which then forms a papule or pustule that then breaks down to form multiple draining sinuses onto the skin surface. The discharge may be purulent or seropurulent. There is hardly any pain inspite of the marked swelling and induration of the part. The disease then progresses into the underlying bones and joints gives rise to periostitis, osteomyelitis and arthritis.

In a few severe cases gross destruction of the bone may result in deformity of the part. The sinuses remain open for months or tend to close and reopen again, or may be replaced by new sinuses.

Diagnosis

The pus should be examined under the microscope for the presence of grains. If there are no discharging sinuses, biopsy may be required. The grains are examined by direct microscopy, histopathology and culture.

Black grains are always due to fungi (eumycetomas) and red grains to an actinomycete. Also, if the infection is eumycotic, the grains will consist of masses of fungal mycelium with thicker hyphae (2-6 mm in diameter). Actinomycotic grains will be seen to consist of masses of much narrower hyphae (0.5-1.0 mm in diameter).

Differential Diagnosis

• This condition needs to be differentiated from chronic osteomyelitis, especially in the initial stages.

SPOROTRICHOSIS

Definition

Sporotrichosis is an acute or chronic fungal infection of the subcutaneous and rarely the systemic tissues, due to Sporothrix schenckii.

Etiology

This condition occurs due to the fungus S. schenckii, which tends to usually grow on decaying vegetable matter. The fungus tends to enter the human skin through trauma or a minor puncture wound (due to a thorn or splinter or insect bite). In a few cases, there is systemic affection due to inhalation of this fungus, where the portal of entry is through the lung.

Histology

The fungus S. schenckii either remains localized in the subcutaneous tissue, or can spread locally through the lymphatics or can rarely, after pulmonary infection, be widely disseminated in the bloodstream. There is a mixed granulomatous reaction with neutrophil foci. The fungus is seen as small (3-5μm), cigar-shaped or oval yeasts, surrounded by a thick, eosiniphilic substance that looks like it is radiating away from the yeast, forming the distinctive asteroid bodies.

Clinical Features

Cutaneous sporotrichosis is divided into two main types, the lymphangitic and the fixed forms, of which the lymphangitic is the most common, resulting from implantation of the spores in a wound. Occasionally atypical varieties such as mycetoma-like or cellulitic forms can occur.

In the lymphangitic type the lesions are especially on exposed surfaces like the extremities, where a nodule or pustule forms initially, which breaks down to form a small ulcer. There is then an insiduous involvement of lymphatics from the draining area and a chain of lymphatic nodules develops, which soften and ulcerate and are connected by tender lymphatic cords. There is a thin purulent discharge oozing from the primary lesion and a few early lymphatic nodules, and as the disease becomes chronic, the regional lymph nodes become swollen and may break down. The primary lesion may heal spontaneously leaving the lymphatic nodes enlarged.

In the fixed variety, the pathogen remains more or less localized at the point of inoculation. The lesions may be acneiform, nodular, ulcerated or verrucous, or in a few cases there can be infiltrated plaques or red, scaly patches.

In systemic affection, which is especially seen in persons with low immunity, the inhaled fungus produces local pulmonary disease or focal or widely disseminated lesions in the joints, meninges and skin.

Diagnosis

The fungus is rarely detected in the infected tissues, but fluorescent antibody techniques can help in the diagnosis of this condition. Culture of the fungus will also confirm diagnosis.

Differential Diagnosis

• It simulates granulomatous lesions of almost any other origin, and a history of injury has to be looked into.

• Mycobacterial infections and leishmaniasis may also simulate this condition.

CHROMOBLASTOMYCOSIS

Synonym

Chromomycosis; Verrucous dermatitis.

Definition

Chromomycosis is a chronic fungal infection of the skin and subcutaneous tissues, usually affecting one leg or foot, and is caused by pigmented fungi, which produce thick-walled clusters (sclerotic or muriform bodies) in the tissues, characterized by the production of slow-growing exophytic lesions.

Etiology

Five dematiaceous fungi are the main causative agents - Cladosporium carrionii, Phialophora verrucosa, Fonsecaea pedrosoi, F. compacta and Rhinocladiella aquaspersa.

Trauma or puncture wounds from wood products and soil exposure results in implantation of the organism. Thus is especially seen in rural communities. It occurs more often in men than in women, especially in the 20-50 year group.

Histopathology

There is a granulomatous reaction with formation of pseudotubercles containing giant cells with isolated areas of microabscess formation. There is also a focal round cell infiltration in the superficial layers of the dermis. The fungus occurs in the form of golden brown, spherical cells with thick, dark cell walls and coarsely granular, pigmented protoplasm. The cells are characteristically divided in several planes of division by thick septa and are termed muriform or sclerotic cells. The fungi appear in clusters of spherical cells. The tissue between the granulomatous nodules shows chronic fibrosis. When ulceration has occurred there is usually secondary bacterial infection.

Clinical Features

It usually affects the exposed foot, leg, arm or face. The initial lesion is a small, pink, scaly papule or wart-like growth, which slowly expands into a hypertrophic plaque. The lesion is usually painless unless the presence of secondary infection causes itching and pain. Satellite lesions are produced by scratching, and there may be lymphatic spread to adjacent areas. The limb is swollen up and at the distal end is covered by various nodular, tumorous, verrucous lesions, which when extensive looks like a cauliflower. Cicatricial nodular lesions can also form, which spread peripherally and heal at the center by sclerosis. There can be associated keloid formation. Squamous carcinomas may develop in chronic lesions. The whole disease progress is a slow one and can take years to develop completely. In a few rare cases metastases through the blood circulation can occur.

Diagnosis

- Biopsy will reveal deeply pigmented, thick-walled, muriform or sclerotic cells, though in a few cases only pigmented hyphae may be seen.

- Culture of material for the associated fungi will also help establish the diagnosis.

Differential Diagnosis

- Blastomycosis needs to be ruled out, by checking for the absence of a sharp border containing minute abscesses.

- Also rule out cutaneous tuberculosis, leishmaniasis, syphilis and yaws.

PHAEOHYPHOMYCOSIS

Synonym

Phaeomycotic subcutaneous cyst.

Definition

This is a heterogeneous group of mycotic infections caused by a range of brown-pigmented (dematiaceous) fungi, which form pigmented hyphae in tissue, resulting in the formation of localized, subcutaneous or intramuscular cyst or abscess formation. Systemic phaeohyphomycosis is seen in immunocompromised patients.

Etiology

The most commonly seen fungi known to cause it are Exophiala jeanselmei, Exophiala dermatitidis, Bipolaris species, and Alternaria alternata.

Implantation from an exogenous source like plant tissue fragments can be responsible.

Clinical Features

The initial lesions consists of a firm, sometimes tender nodule, which may develop into a large cyst up to several centimetres in diameter. The overlying epidermis is not conspicuously thickened. Lesions similar to dermatophytosis and tinea nigra can also be seen. There is no tendency towards lymphatic spread, and dissemination is exceedingly uncommon.

LOBOMYCOSIS

Synonym

Keloidal blastomycosis; Lobo's disease.

Definition

This condition is characterized by keloidal skin lesions occuring on any part of the body, which remains fairly well localized and apparently do not affect the general health of the patient. In long-standing cases, there is involvement of regional lymph nodes.

Etiology

Loboa loboi is the causative fungus and is said to be present in water, soil or forest vegetation.

Histopathology

Granulomatous changes are seen with abundance of giant cells and round or lemon-shaped fungi in the lesions. Epidermis is atrophic.

Clinical Features

The lesions, which are keloidal, with or without fistulas, can occur on any part of the body, but are usually on exposed parts, legs, arms and face. There is no marked lymphangitis and no visceral dissemination, except in long-standing cases. Old chronic lesions present as elevated crusted fungoid plaques, especially around the ears. Squamous carcinomas may occasionally develop in chronic lesions.

Differential Diagnosis

Clinically, the disease most closely resembles chromoblastomycosis. Microscopic examination of biopsy material will establish the diagnosis.

RHINISPORIDIOSIS

Definition & Etiology

It is a chronic granulomatous mycosis caused by Rhinosporidium seeberi, where there is development of polyps of the mucous membrane.

Histopathology

It resembles a nasal polyp, but has conspicuous sharply defined globular cysts up to 0.5mm in diameter, with occasional microabscesses.

Clinical Features

There is development of pedunculated vascular polyps on the mucous membrane of the nose, nasopharynx, soft palate, and in a few cases the conjunctiva, lacrimal sac, genitals or skin may be involved.

These polyps become hyperplastic, reaching an enormous size, with a pink, red or purple surface, and a lobulated, cauliflower-like appearance. Close examination of the surface reveals small, white spots, which represent mature sporangia of the fungus. The disease may last for many years, and is not contagious.

Noseblock and difficulty in breathing is usually the main complaint, when the polyps are in the nose. If the genitalia are involved, the lesions look like condylomas. In cases of involvement of the eye, there is conjunctivitis and photophobia, and in a few cases eversion of the lid due to the weight of the polyp.

Diagnosis

The diagnosis depends on the detection of sporangia on the surface of the polyp or in its sections. They can be seen as firm, white cysts on or just below the surface. Microscopically, these are single, thick-walled and spherical, and when fully differentiated are packed with numerous rounded endospores.

Differential Diagnosis

In cases of atypical lesions, differentiation from warts, condylomas and hemorrhoids is necessary.

PHYCOMYCOSIS

Synonym

Basidiobolomycosis; Subcutaneous zygomycosis; Conidiobolomycosis; Rhinoentomophthoromycosis.

Definition

It is a localized subcutaneous and predominantly tropical mycosis characterized by chronic hard swelling of subcutaneous tissue.

Etiology

Phycomycosis is caused by Basidiobolus ranarum or Conidiobolus coronatus (rhinoentomophthoromycosis).

Histopathology

The lesion is an eosinophilic granuloma lying deep in the subcutaneous tissue and largely replacing fat. Wide, sparsely septate hyphae, branching at right angles, are scattered throughout the granuloma and there is often dense fibrosis.

Clinical Features

The lesion is a slowly growing, painless, subcutaneous, smooth but hard, disc-shaped swelling originating from the limbs, nasal mucosae or sinuses. It may be single, or multiple.

The lesion is usually lobulated, and can be raised up by inserting the fingers underneath it. The overlying skin may be tense, oedematous, desquamating, hyperpigmented or normal.

Diagnosis

The diagnosis is usually established histologically by biopsy, but culture is not difficult.

SYSTEMIC MYCOSES

HISTOPLASMOSIS

A highly infectious mycosis caused by Histoplasma capsulatum and affecting primarily the lungs, where it is generally asymptomatic. The fungus is intra-cellular, parasitizing the reticuloendothelial system and involving the spleen, liver, kidney, central nervous system and other organs. Rarely, the disease may become chronic, progressive and fatal.

BLASTOMYCOSIS

It is a chronic granulomatous and suppurative mycosis caused by Blastomyces dermatitidis, affecting primarily the lungs but with disseminating forms affecting skin, bones, central nervous system and other sites.

PARACOCCIDIOIDOMYCOSIS

It is a chronic granulomatous fungal infection caused by Paracoccidioides brasiliensis, affecting the skin, mucous membranes, lymph nodes and internal organs.

COCCIDIOIDOMYCOSIS

It is a (primary) respiratory fungal infection caused by Coccidioides immitis, which may become progressive and disseminated, with severe or fatal forms.

CRYPTOCOCCOSIS

It is an acute, subacute or chronic infection caused by the encapsulated yeast Cryptococcus neoformans. There is a marked predilection for the brain and meninges, although the lungs and occasionally the skin and other parts of the body may be involved.

CANDIDIASIS

In most cases of systemic candidosis, the causal organism originates in the patient's own gastrointestinal tract. Invasion by Candida along intravenous infusion lines is also important, and maceration or signs suggestive of cutaneous candidosis on adjacent skin should not be ignored. Drug addicts are particularly at risk.

Typical lesions start as macules, become papular or nodular, and may show a pale centre. Some are likely to be hemorrhagic and may break down to form ecthyma gangrenosum-like lesions. Fever, diffuse muscle tenderness and an erythematous macular rash are regarded as an indication for prompt skin biopsy in any compromised patient.

HOMEOPATHIC APPROACH TO FUNGAL INFECTIONS

It will be one of the most common complaints in the homeopathic practice. The patient may visit the homeopath with various presentations as:

1. Circular discoloured patches.
2. Itching.
3. Disfigured nails.

Sometimes the patient may be asymptomatic as in the case when nails are affected. In such asymptomatic cases the constitutional remedy should be considered.

Much depends on the personal hygiene and care of skin of the patient. The following advice will be beneficial if it is passed to the patient while starting the homeopathic treatment.

1. To keep the linen and garments clean and to discourage wearing each other's garments. This is especially true among children who frequently wear each other's cap while playing games.

2. The affected part should be washed daily and twice during summer season with soap, preferably Calendula and hot water.

3. To soothe the irritated skin, locally, an ointment prepared by mixing olive oil and calendula external in 1:1 proportion should be applied.

4. It is essential while treating the patient's infection, especially tinea corporis, to remove the source of infection, either from infected human beings or animals.

5. In cases of tinea cruris, the under clothing must be sterilized properly amd avoid the use of public lavatories.

6. In cases of tinea on the feet, the patient is adviced to wear open type shoes and sandals and dry the feet properly after bathing; after removing the shoes they should be exposed to mild sun and fresh air.

Avoid antifungal agents as these only suppress the lesion and permit the disease to enter deep into the system affecting the vital organs. Also, prolonged use of antifungal agents brings resistance as a result the infection spreads throughout the body.

Some Important Therapeutic Hints

PITYRIASIS VERSICOLOR

Here one has to start treatment in a classical way by giving the constitutional remedy. Pityriasis versicolor can be found in the repertory under 'Skin-Eruptions-Scaly'. You'll find many remedies – around 90 remedies – in it. This rubric should not be used directly in such patients; however, one can have a general knowledge of remedies for this particular disease, using it. The approach has always got to be very constitutional.

Sometimes it so happens in this particular disease that due to excessive tropical climate and due to excessive humidity, a person is highly prone to such kind of condition, and as a preventive for such particular illness, I tell my patients to regularly massage their body, as a preventive, with *Phytolacca* mother tincture. This is one such remedy, which when applied to the skin, prevents pityriasis, and even if there are some good symptoms of Phytolacca in the lesion, its one of the good remedies.

The most important description of Phytolacca will be, the itching is always worse by scratching. So the more he scratches, the more it becomes worse. The eruptions are extremely itchy. The rest of the surrounding skin around the lesion is extremely dry. This is also a very important aspect of this remedy. Although Phytolacca may not have many modalities or many sensations as far as this condition is concerned, its general symptoms are extremely important. Aggravation from cold wet weather is one important symptom of this remedy, and since pityriasis is a common condition in wet weather, it becomes an important remedy for this condition.

Another very important remedy useful to me as an intercurrent in pityriasis is *Tuberculinum Koch's*.

TINEA CORPORIS

This ringworm infection is another very commonly seen condition, which we also need to note to treat constitutionally. The intercurrent remedy very useful for such condition is *Bacillinum*, but there are many other good small remedies that have been very useful to me like:

- *Chrysophanicum acid*, a remedy that Clarke has very beautifully described.

- The *Juglans group* of remedies (*Juglans Cinerea* and *Juglans Regia*) is also very important for this condition.

- The remedy *Lappa Articum* is another useful remedy, which I use as a preventive medicine for those who are prone to develop ringworm, in people who stay in a dirty atmosphere, unhygienic surrounding. I request patients to apply the mother tincture of this remedy as a preventive measure on certain areas of the skin that are highly prone to be infested with ringworm.

- *Tela Aranea* is one such remedy that is the most specific remedies for this condition.

- *Oleum Jecoris Aselli* is one another remedy, the mother tincture of which can be massaged on a child infested with or prone to develop ringworm.

- The major approach is to use a constitutional remedy.

TINEA PEDIS

For ringworm infection between the toes, in addition to asking the patient to take a good hygienic care, I ask them to massage their toes with *Petroleum* mother tincture. This remedy is especially useful in cases of athletic people who are highly prone to wearing socks that are wet from perspiration. Otherwise the constitutional approach is very important for a very deep-seated chronic tinea pedis.

TINEA UNGUM

Intercurrent remedies like *Psorinum* has been useful to me when there has been ringworm of the nails, especially tinea ungum. Here what I have seen is that recovery takes place very slow, and one has to take many years of homeopathic treatment. One remedy, called *X-ray* in the potentized form has been very useful to me, and intercurrent remedies like *Tuberculinum* and *Syphilinum*, have been useful to me in the above condition.

CANDIDIASIS

For this condition, the nosode *Monilia Albicans*, is not only a good remedy for this condition, but has a detailed proving in Julians materia medica, and is used in many other conditions besides candidiasis, one of which is chronic leucorrhea. *Medorrhinum* is another very good intercurrent remedy useful in this condition. Candidiasis, like any other condition, also requires a constitutional approach.

An important thing is to have an anti-candidial diet, and avoid fermented food or food that contains yeast in it, like bread, wine, etc.

Some Important Homeopathic Remedies

Bacillinum is often used as *an intercurrent remedy.*

Rare remedies like Sulphurosum acidicum and *Mica should be considered.*

Agar, anac, anag, ant-c, ant-t, ars, ars-i, bac, bar-c, bar-s, calc, calc-i, chrysar, clem, dulc, eup-per, graph, hell, hep, iod, jug-c, jug-r, kali-c, kali-s, lith-c, lyc, mag-c, med, mez, lappa, nat-ar, nat-c, nat-m, olean, phos, phyt, psor, rhus-t, semp, sep, spong, sulph, sul-ac, tell, tub, ust, vinca, viol-tr.

Tinea capitis

Ars, bac, bar-m, calc, chrysar, dulc, graph, kali-s, mez, petr, psor, sep, sil, sulph, tell, tub, viol-tr.

Tinea versicolor

Bac, chrysar, mez, nat-ar, sep, sulph, tell, tor.

For further therapeutics kindly refer to the chapter on therapeutics of eczema and herpes.

REPERTORY

- **Head, eruptions**
    - Ringworm: Bapt, bar-m, caust, dulc, iris, mez, nat-c, phys, psor, querc-r-g-s, tub, vinc.
    - Herpes, circinatus: Ars, bac, bar-m, calc, chrysar, dulc, graph, kali-s, med, mez, petr, phyt, por, sep, sil, sulph, tell, tub, viol-t.

- **Face, eruptions**
    - Herpes, circinatus: Anag, bar-c, calc, cinnb, clem, dulc, graph, hell, kali-chl, lith-c, lyc, med, nat-c, nat-m, phos, sep, sulph, tarent, tell, tub.
- **Skin, eruptions**
    - Pityriasis versicolor: Bac, carb-ac, caul, chrys-ac, dulc, lyc, mez, nat-ar, sep, sul-ac, tell
    - Herpetic, circinate: Anac, anag, ars-s-f, bac, bar-c, bar-s, calc, calc-ar, chrysar, clem, dulc, dys, equis-h, eup-per, graph, hell, hep, iod, lach, lith-c, mag-c, med, morg, morg-p, nat-c, nat-m, par, phos, phyt, psor, rad-br, sanic, semp, sep, spong, sulph, syc, tell, thuj, tub.

■

Chapter-19

Lichen Planus and Lichenoid Disorders

Introduction

The term 'lichen' is described in dictionaries as being probably derived from the Greek verb 'to lick'. However, no explanation is forthcoming as to how such a word of this original meaning could be adapted to a noun both in Greek and Latin for those symbiotic forms of plant life that are now called lichens, and also dermatoses that only vaguely resemble the botanical formations because they present to the eye a surface pattern of more or less closely agminated papules.

Definition

Lichenoid tissue reactions are those exhibiting epidermal basal cell damage as the primary event, which then initiates the cascade of changes, which are seen and recognized in the fully developed histopathology of LP.

In other words, where one sees histological damage to the lower epidermis, and a grouped chronic inflammatory infiltrate in the papillary dermis that disturbs the interface between the epidermis and dermis, then that dermatosis can be classified as a lichenoid dermatitis no matter what the overall clinical appearances. The prototype of all lichenoid eruptions is LP itself but a number of other diseases may develop a lichenoid tissue reaction.

Etiopathogenesis

Considerable evidence now exists that the underlying processes involved in the pathogenesis of LP are immunologically mediated. The observation that Langerhans' cells are increased in the earliest lesions has been taken to indicate that the Langerhans' cells may be processing antigens prior to their presentation to lymphocytes. The dermal infiltrate largely consists of T cells.

In addition to Langerhans' cells, dermal dendritic cells, expressing factor XIIIa and lysozyme-positive histiocytes, are present and appear to play an important role in LP. A constant feature of dermal lymphocytic infiltrates in lichenoid tissue reactions is their affinity for the epidermis (epidermotropism).

Whatever the immunological stimulus, it is known that LP can occur in families, and in these affected individuals an increased frequency of HLA-B7 has been noted.

In tropical countries, a lichen planus like eruption is brought about by chloroquine, non-steroidal anti-inflammatory drug like brufen.

Histology

In a fully developed LP papule, on biopsy, the centre of the papule corresponds to an area of irregular acanthosis of the epidermis with hypergranulosis and compact hyperkeratosis. A focal increase in thickness of the granular layer and infiltrate corresponds to the presence of Wickham's striae. In the centre of the papule the rete ridges appear flattened or effaced ('saw-tooth' appearance). The damage to the lower epidermis results in a number of histological changes as follows:

1. Colloid bodies.
2. Melanin pigmentary incontinence.
3. Epidermal changes.
4. 'Band-like' inflammatory infiltrate.

Clinical Features

LICHEN PLANUS

It usually affects young and middle aged people. The disease is non-infectious.

Flat topped, polygonal, violaceous, erythematous, 2-10 mm papules covered with scanty scales are characteristic. Application of oil on the surface of the papules demonstrates cris-scross white lines termed as Wickham's striae. Initial lesions are tiny 1-2 mm skin colored papules whereas later, coalescence of the lesions may lead to the formation of larger (25cm) plaques. Occurrence of lesions within scratch marks is an indication of Koebner phenomenon (as seen in psoriasis).

The overall colour is also often characteristic, and is described as violaceous. This is most obvious in older lesions, especially when they become hypertrophic.

The rash is bilateral and asymmetrical. Flexor aspects of wrists and forearms, shins, ankles, dorsa of the feet, anterior thighs and flanks are sites of predilection. In about half the number of cases affected, lesions also occur in the mouth, buccal mucosa, less commonly, on the lips, tongue and genitalia, as dead white spots, streaks and plaques, or like lacy network. The disease is seldom seen on the scalp, the palms and soles. The mucus membrane lesions are usually asymptomatic, but sometimes cause a little burning and irritation.

Nails are affected only in some cases. The first change is seen near the cuticle and gradually it extends forward with the growth of the nail. This results in a nail with rough surface and marked longitudinal striations. If the thinning is severe, the cuticle may grow forward as a pannus. Rarely there may be permanent shedding of the nail.

Although a few cases evolve rapidly and clear within a few weeks, the onset in most cases is insidious and it is some weeks or months before the patient seeks advice. The skin lesions subside within 9 months in about 50% of cases, and in 85% have cleared within 18 months. Chronicity is usually attributable to the development of local hypertrophic lesions or to mucous membrane involvement. Mucosal LP tends to be a particularly long-lasting disease in some cases.

Itching is a fairly consistent feature in LP, but is occasionally completely absent. When present, it ranges from occasional mild irritation to more or less continuous, severe itching, which interferes with sleep and makes life almost intolerable. Hypertrophic lesions usually itch severely. Paradoxically, even when itching is severe, one seldom finds evidence of scratching, as the patient rubs, rather than scratches, to gain relief. Itching at sites without visible skin lesions can occur. Burning and stinging are less common complaints. In the mouth, the patient may complain of discomfort, stinging or pain; ulcerated lesions are especially painful. Great discomfort may be caused by hot foods and drinks.

Morphological Variations of Lichen Planus

- **Annular:** Ring like lesions with central clearing and raised from periphery. Lichenoid eruption following an insect bite commonly produces this type of lesion on the exposed parts of the body, particularly the face.

- **Vesicular and bullous:** Rare.

- **Linear:** Due to Koebner phenomenon.

- **Hypotrophic:** Large thick plaque on the skin, ankle and foot. The development of hypertrophic lesions greatly lengthens the course of the disease, as they may persist for many years. When such lesions eventually clear, an area of pigmentation and scarring may remain and there is often some degree of atrophy.

- **Atrophic:** Macular (flat) lesions.

- **Follicular:** Lichen plano-pilaris Conical papules with center keratin plug. A common consequence is scarring alopecia of the scalp (Graham-Little Syndrome). Follicular LP must be distinguished by biopsy from keratosis pilaris, Darier's disease, follicular mucinosis, lichen scrofulorosum and, in the scalp, from lupus erythematosus.

- **Actinic LP** (lichen planus subtropicus): The lesions occur on the exposed skin (usually the face) and are characterized by well-defined nummular patches, which have a deeply hyperpigmented centre surrounded by a striking hypopigmented zone.

- **LP Pigmentosus:** The macular hyperpigmentation involves chiefly the face and upper limbs, although it can be more widespread. The mucous membranes, palms and soles are usually not involved, but involvement of mucous membranes has been observed.

- **Guttate LP:** This term may be reserved for two clinical types in which lesions are widely scattered and remain discrete. The lesions may all be small, 1-2 mm across, or larger, up to 1cm. These forms have a relatively good prognosis, and individual lesions seldom become chronic. Early in an attack, guttate psoriasis may be suspected, but the diagnosis becomes obvious quite quickly and can easily be resolved by the histopathological findings.

- **Lichen plannus verrucosus:** It occurs as hyperkeratotic, verrucous, violaceous nodules and patches on the legs. Itching is severe.

Variation Based on Distribution

- *Acute generalized lichen planus:* The onset is sudden. The course short and the rash generalized. In the early stages, the eruption may not be typical, but characteristic lesions soon become visible. It may merge into chronic lichen planus.

- *Chronic localised:* Common around ankles and wrists.

- *Segmental:* Involves one nerve segment.

- *Oral*: Papules arranged in an annular or lace-like pattern.

- *Nail:* Thin striated nails with pterygium (extension of proximal nail fold on the nail plate) formation.

Diagnosis

- Demonstration of typical lesion – polyhedral, firm, violaceous (may be difficult to detect in dark skinned people), flat topped papules with Wickham's striae and very thin adherent scales.

- Distribution on flexors, genitalia and mouth.

- Pruritus.

- A chronic course.

- A typical histology.

Differential Diagnosis

The only differential diagnosis to be considered in a typical case is that of lichenoid eruptions induced by drugs or colour developer, and this must be based on the history. Less typical cases of LP may be mistaken for plane warts, eczematous eruptions with lichenification from scratching, pityriasis rosea, lichen simplex chronicus and other lichenoid eruptions such as lichen amyloidosus (papular). The occasional cases of LP without itching must be distinguished from secondary syphilis. The differential diagnosis of the special variants has already been mentioned. In any case of doubt, a biopsy should establish the diagnosis. The mucous lesions of lichen planus must be differentiated from the lesions of leukoplakia, the mucous patches of syphilis and aphthous stomatitis. On the scalp it must be distinguished from discoid lupus erythematosus, pseudo-pelade, favus, etc.

Other Lichenoid Eruptions

LICHEN SCROFULOROSUM

It is an uncommon questionable tuberculide. It affects children with or without systemic tuberculosis. The shoulders and trunk are the sites involved. Clinically, the lesions consist of patches of grouped, firm, follicular, bluish-red indolent papules with central spines. It itches slightly. Histopathology is tuberculoid. Tuberculin test is negative.

LICHEN SPINULOSUS

It is characterized by pinhead sized, follicular, flesh coloured papules with horny spines. The papules are grouped in patches. Children are commonly affected. Sites of affection are the abdomen, buttocks and legs. The condition is asymptomatic, and clears up with a good nourishing diet containing plenty of animal fats, extra vitamins, tonics and the local application of animal fats or cod liver oil.

LICHEN SYPHILITICUS

Follicular papules with induration; slight itching; lymphadenopathy mucous patches and a history of exposure. The VDRL is positive.

LICHEN SIMPLEX CHRONICUS

Lichenification or neurodermatitis is another term. Affecting more commonly neurotic people who are prone to chronic scratching and rubbing of skin under stress and anxiety. It is common amongst young people and menopausal women. The integument becomes thickened, infiltrated and pigmented; the criss-cross markings become more prominent. Margins are irregular but usually well defined. There may be one or several localized patches. Occasionally an extensive disseminated variety is seen.

Sites: Nape of neck, arms, ano-genital area, scrotum, back of knees, legs and ankles.

Chronic eczemas may become lichenified through constant scratching. Lichenification is a prominent feature of atopic eczema. In the dark Indian skin, lichenification occurs early. Differential diagnosis is from lichenified eczemas, atopic dermatitis, lichen planus hypertrophicus.

LICHENOID DRUG ERUPTIONS

These occur commonly in the tropics and in dark skinned people. An idiosyncrasy to certain drugs, e.g. brufen (NSAID) arsphenamine, gold, chloroquine, onepacrine, hydroxychloroquine, quinine and certain phenothiazine derivatives, para-amino-salicylic acid, thiazide diuretics and aminophenazole (Daptazole) may result in lichenoid eruption which may simulate lichen planus. Contact with chemicals used in the processing of coloured photographic films may, in sensitized individuals, produce similar eruptions.

LICHEN NITIDUS

It consists of discrete, pink or flesh coloured, asymptomatic papules grouped in patches. The typical sites are the genitalia, inner sides of thighs, lower abdomen and at times wrists. It is a benign disease.

LICHEN STRIATUS

An uncommon form occurring in children. It usually affects upper limbs and occasionally the legs. Lesions consist of flesh colored or darker lichenoid papules arranged in a linear fashion, usually unilateral and along the long axis of a limb. Streak may be only a few centimeters in length or extend along the long axis suggesting a linear naevus. Histopathology is non-specific. No active treatment is necessary as the eruption has a tendency to disappear spontaneously.

LICHEN URTICATUS

Synonym: Papular urticaria. Refer to chapter of Urticaria.

LICHEN AMYLOIDOSES

Localized variety of primary cutaneous amyloidosis. Itching papules, nodules or plaques, yellowish brown in color, combined with pigmentation. A biopsy and Congo Red test help in diagnosis.

LICHEN SCLEROSUS ET ATROPHICUS

It is essentially confined to the cutaneous portion of he vulva, anogenital region, trunk and shoulders. Irregular, whitish papules and plaques with keratotic plugs or central delling characterizes it; later white tissue paper like wrinkled patches develop. Minimal pruritus.

Histology

Hyperkeratosis, follicular plugging, epidermal atrophy, band of hyalinized collagen below the epidermis, dilated capillaries and a band of round cell infiltration. It is a chronic disease, allopathic treatment being unsatisfactory.

LICHEN MYXEDEMATOSES

A very rare but definite entity, practically independent of thyroid pathology. Lesions consist of discrete, localized papular, annular or discoid, lichenoid plaques. This is associated with infiltration and at times lymphedema. Itching is only minimal. General health is not affected. Basal metabolic rate, erythrocyte sedimentation rate and other tests for metabolic defect are nominal except the blood lipids may show slight change. Thyroid extract may benefit an occasional patient.

Prognosis

Occasional cases clear in a few weeks, but most acute and subacute attacks will last 6-9 months unless treated with systemic corticosteroids or the potent topical steroids. The first feature to disappear is itching. The papule then flattens, but is often replaced by a corresponding area of pigmentation. If hypertrophic patches develop, they are likely to persist for many more months, and occasionally for 20 years or more. The development of large, annular lesions is also a poor prognostic sign in terms of longevity of the disease. When hair fall occurs, it is usually permanent. Mucous membrane lesions clear more slowly than those on the skin and may remain visible for years after all evidence of the skin lesions has cleared.

HOMEOPATHIC APPROACH TO LICHEN PLANUS

Lichen planus should be considered as a constitutional disorder and not merely a local disease. Relapses and remissions characterize the disease and the course of the illness is chronic. Hence, case should be taken to treat the disease at its earliest, so that we can give relief to the patient from the pruritus, which is one of the most annoying symptoms of the disease.

Psychogenic stress is known to induce the relapse in many individuals; hence, while taking the history of the patient, it is important to discuss the mental state in great detail. At no cost corticosteroid should be advised to the patient. If he is already on corticosteroid, then it should be tapered off at the earliest. Soothing lotion preferably calendula mother tincture 1:10 dilution should be advised. The following points should be considered while taking the history:

1. Psychosomatic aspects of the patient.

2. Pruritus should be enquired into in detail with its modalities and concomitant.

3. Lichen planus is known to have many variants hence sound knowledge of its manifestations should be known to the treating physician. Psychotherapy in obstinate cases can be given along with homeopathic drugs.

Certain variants of lichen planus and lichen striatus are known to disappear spontaneously. Hence, one should be aware of the natural course of the disease.

Drugs given below are found useful in cases of lichen planus. The reader is advised to refer the therapeutics of Eczema and Psoriasis for its characteristic symptoms.

Some Important Homeopathic Remedies

agar, alum, am-m, anac, ant-c, anan, apis, ars, ars-i, bell, bov, bry, calad, castn-v, chinin-ar, dulc, iod, jug-c, kali-ars, kali-bi, kali-i, kreos, led, lyc, merc, merc-s, nabal, nat-c, plan, phyt, rumx, sep, sars, staph, sulph, sul-i, til.

REPERTORY

- **Skin, eruptions**

    -   Lichen: Agar, anthraco, apis, ars, ars-i, aur, dulc, jug-c, mang, phyt, rhus-t, rumx, sulph, til.

- Lichen planus: Sul-i, sulph, syph.
- Papular: Allox, aur, calc, caust, cham, cycl, gels, grin, hippoz, hydrc, iod, kali-bi, kali-c, kali-i, kali-s, lyc, merc, narc-ps, petr, phos, pic-ac, psor, sep, sil, sulph, syph, thiop, zinc.
- Itching: Allox, beryl.
- Flat: Am-c, ang, ant-c, ant-t, ars, asaf, bell, carb-an, euph, lach, lyc, merc, nat-c, nit-ac, petr, ph-ac, phos, puls, ran-b, sel, sep, sil, staph, sulph, thuj.

■

Chapter-20

Psoriasis

Definition

A common, genetically determined, inflammatory and proliferative disease of the skin, the most characteristic lesions consisting of chronic, sharply demarcated, dull-red, scaly plaques, particularly on the extensor prominences and in the scalp.

The disease is enormously variable in duration and extent and morphological variants are common.

Incidence

Contrary to earlier belief, it is fairly common in the tropics; though undoubtedly, it is more prevalent in the temperate climate.

Females tend to develop psoriasis earlier than males. A German study, evaluation of the age of onset revealed two peaks—an early one at 16-22 years, and a later one at 57-60 years.

Patients with a family history of psoriasis tend to have an earlier age of onset. Siblings of patients with onset before 15 years were also more than three times as likely to have psoriasis as siblings of patients with age of onset after 30 years.

The earlier age of onset in females suggests a greater incidence in young females than young males. However, the incidence of psoriasis in adult men and women is usually reported to be about equal.

Psoriasis is a chronic disease; its course is punctuated by intermissions and remissions. Attacks are more common in winter than summer; the eruption has a natural tendency to clear up with the warm weather. In the tropics a fair number of attacks develop in the monsoon (rainy season).

Etiology

The exact etiology is still unknown.

Genetic predisposition

The evidence that psoriasis may be inherited is beyond doubt, and rests on population surveys, twin and other family analyses and HLA studies. There has, however, been controversy over the mode of inheritance.

Provocation and exacerbation

According to most workers, it is a heredio-familial disease brought on by:

Trauma

- Psoriasis at the site of an injury is well known (see Köbner phenomenon, below). A wide range of injurious local stimuli, including physical, chemical, electrical, surgical, infective and inflammatory insults has been recognized to elicit psoriatic lesions.

Infection

- The role of streptococcal infection, especially in the throat, in provoking acute guttate psoriasis has long been recognized.

Endocrine factors

- The early report that there are peaks of incidence at puberty and at the menopause has been supported by more recent findings. Generalized pustular psoriasis may be provoked by pregnancy and may exacerbate premenstrually, and may also be provoked by high-dose oestrogen therapy.

Sunlight

- Although sunlight is generally beneficial, a small minority of psoriatics is provoked by strong sunlight and suffers summer exacerbation in exposed skin. Photosensitivity in psoriasis was significantly associated with skin type I, advanced age and female sex.

Metabolic factors

- Hypocalcemia (e.g. following accidental parathyroidectomy) and dialysis have precipitated psoriasis.

Drugs

- The most frequent associations include the administration of lithium, adrenergic blocking agents and antimalarials, and the withdrawal of systemically administered corticosteroids. Withdrawal of the latter, as well as of the potent topical steroid clobetasol propionate, is particularly associated with outbreaks of generalized pustular psoriasis.

Psychogenic factors

- Various studies have shown a positive correlation between stress and the severity of the disease. It is possible that psychological stress may be associated with a diminished capacity to cope with regular treatment, and that this may lead to deterioration, especially in severe cases.

Alcohol and smoking

- A Finnish study confirmed that alcohol is a risk factor for psoriasis in young and middle-aged men, and suggested that psoriasis may sustain drinking. It seems unlikely that alcohol directly exacerbates psoriasis, in view of the marked differences in its consumption between the sexes. It is possible that excessive alcohol consumption may lead to reduced therapeutic compliance, and also that it is a symptom of stress caused by severe skin disease. The association between smoking and psoriasis has been reviewed; reports suggest an increased risk for both palmoplantar pustulosis and chronic plaque psoriasis.

Acquired immunodeficiency syndrome

- The association between severe psoriasis, psoriatic arthropathy and human immunodeficiency virus (HIV) infection is well recognized. The mechanism of worsening of psoriasis in these circumstances is unclear. Furthermore, the knowledge that psoriasis may be aggravated by AIDS, a disease in which the helper T cell is the major target, and the evidence that psoriasis may be greatly improved by cyclosporin, which inhibits helper T cell function, create a paradox that remains to be fully explained.

Pathogenesis

Psoriasis is characterised by three main pathogenic features:

- Abnormal differentiation.
- Keratinocyte hyperproliferation.
- Inflammation.

Accelerated epidermopeisis (3 to 4 days instead of 28 days in normal skin) has been considered as the prime pathological event. The abnormality in psoriatic epidermis appears to be the result of an increased recruitment of cycling cells from the resting fraction, thus producing an increased growth fraction. The heightened rate of epidermopoesis or the heightened proportion of epidermal cells participating in the proliferative process, which ever be the cause, result in increased production of keratin.

Histochemical studies have revealed an increase in both oxidative and anaerobic metabolism with increased pentose, glycogen, purines, sulphydral groups and soluble proteins and decrease in activity of dipeptidases.

It has been discovered that apparently normal skin of both the psoriatics and their relations show these changes in miniature – 'latent psoriasis'.

Histology

(i) Parakeratosis,

(ii) Thinning of supra-papillary portion of the stratum malpighii,

(iii) Elongation of ridges,

(iv) Oedema and clubbing of papillae,

(v) Micro-abscesses of Munro,

(vi) Dilated and tortuous capillaries in upper demis,

(vii) Oedema and round-cell infiltration in the papillae and upper demis.

Clinical Features

Modes of onset

- The first manifestation of psoriasis may occur at any age. Males are a little more affected than females. Its duration may vary from a few weeks to a whole lifetime. The course is unpredictable and the variations numerous. Certain patterns are, however, more common than others.

Distribution

- Typical distribution is extensor. The areas commonly affected are the scalp, back of elbows, front of knees and legs and the lower part of the back of the trunk. The nails, the palms and the soles may also be affected in the average case; but the mucous membranes may be rarely involved. The eruption is usually symmetrical.

Morphology of Common Chronic Stable Plaque Psoriasis (Psoriasis Vulgaris)

- The early lesions are guttate erythematous macules, which from the beginning are covered with dry, silvery scales, which typically do not extend all the way to the edge of the erythematous area. The patches increase in size by peripheral extension and coalescence and become thicker in size through the accumulation of scales. The scales are micaceous and are looser toward the periphery of the patch, althogh adherent in the center. When a psoriatic lesion is scratched with the point of a dissecting forceps, a candle-grease like scale can be repeatedly produced even from the non-scaling lesions. This is called the candle-grease sign (Tache de bouge). The complete removal of a scale produces pinpoint bleeding (Auspitz sign).

• Psoriasis is normally characterized by the absence of itching, but in tropical countries, patients complain of slight or moderate pruritis, which, if accompanied by secondary psychogenic stress and lichenification, is more, marked. Psoriatic lesions may develop along the scratch lines in the active phase; this is called Koebner's phenomenon (other common diseases in which Koebner's phenomenon occurs are warts and lichen planus).

Morphological Variations

Psoriasis figurata / annulata / gyrata

When the patches reach a diameter of about 5cm, they may cease spreading and undergo involution in the center, so that annular, lobulated and gyrate figures are produced.

Psoriasis follicularis

Tiny, scaly lesions are located at the orifice of the pilosebaceous follicles.

Psoriasis ostracea

Old patches may be thickened and tough, and covered with lamellar scales like the outside of an oyster shell.

Psoriasis guttate

Lesions are of the size of water drops.

Psoriasis discoidea

Solid patches persists in the patches in which central involution does not occur.

Psoriasis rupoides

Crustaceous lesions resembling syphilitic rupia.

Variations According to the Sites

Scalp

Often, very thick plaques develop, especially at the occiput. The whole scalp may be diffusely involved, or multiple discrete plaques of varying size may be seen. A morphological entity consisting of plaques of asbestos-like scaling, firmly adherent to the scalp and associated hair, has been termed pityriasis (tinea) amiantacea. Hair loss, sometimes cicatricial, is seen in pityriasis amiantacea. Otherwise, common scalp psoriasis is not a frequent cause of alopecia, although it may occur. Psoriatic erythroderma is associated with severe hair loss, as is vigorous local treatment. Hair-shaft abnormalities have been described on electron microscopy, but the rate of hair growth is normal.

Penis

A solitary patch on the glans of the uncircumcised male lacks scales, but its colour and well-defined edge are usually distinctive. Where confirmatory signs elsewhere are absent, a diagnostic biopsy may be necessary, as it may resemble erythroplasia or Zoon's plasma cell balanitis.

Flexural (inverse) Psoriasis

It is also called as volar psoriasis. It is so called as it selectively involves folds, recesses, and flexor surfaces ears, axillae, groins, inframammary folds, navel, intergluteal crease, glans penis, lips and above all, the palms, soles and nails.

Palmoplantar Psoriasis

On the palms and soles psoriasis may present as typical scaly patches on which a fine, silvery scale can be evoked by scratching; as less well-defined plaques resembling lichen simplex or hyperkeratotic eczema; or as a pustulosis. Mixed forms occasionally occur. It may often be difficult to distinguish the psoriasis from eczema, with which it may sometimes alternate.

Nail involvement

Nails show three types of lesions (a) pitting, (b) separation of the distal portion of the nail from the nail bed and walls, and (c) thickening of the nail, accompanied by the collection of hyperkeratotic debris under the nail.

Clinical Variants

GUTTATE PSORIASIS

As described under morphological variations, this type of psoriasis is characterised by lesions that are of the size of water drops. Though the normal course of psoriasis is chronic, there occurs occasionally an acute attack in the form of guttate psoriasis. It is seen particularly in children and young adults, and often precipitated after acute streptococcal infections, either by an acute illness like tonsillitis or a sharp mental stress or physical injury. They are scattered more or less evenly over the body, particularly on the trunk and proximal part of the limbs, rarely on the soles but not infrequently on the face, ears and scalp. The lesions on the face are often sparse, difficult to see and disappear quickly. The diagnosis is made chiefly on the nature of the scaling, the general distribution and evidence for preceding infection.

RUPIOID, ELEPHANTINE AND OSTRACEOUS PSORIASIS

These terms describe plaques associated with gross hyperkeratosis. Rupioid psoriasis refers to limpet-like, cone-shaped lesions. The term elephantine psoriasis might be used to describe unusual but very persistent, thickly scaling, large plaques that sometimes occur on the back, limbs, hips or elsewhere. Ostraceous psoriasis, an infrequently used term, refers to a ring-like, hyperkeratotic lesion with a concave surface, resembling an oyster shell.

UNSTABLE PSORIASIS

This term, which has no aetiological connotation, may be usefully employed to describe phases of the disease in which activity is marked and the course and immediate outcome unpredictable, for example in stages when a previously stable and chronic form is exacerbated by inappropriate management and threatens to become erythrodermic or pustular; or when localized pustular or ill-defined erythematous lesions appear spontaneously for the first time. Patients may develop such unstable phases repeatedly, settling back again into the classical forms of the disease. Withdrawal of intensive systemic or topical corticosteroid therapy, hypocalcemia, acute infection, overtreatment with tar, dithranol or UV irradiation, and perhaps severe emotional upset, may precipitate this condition.

PUSTULAR PSORIASIS

Rarely psoriasis patients develop generalized pustule formation, which may be complicated by arthritis, exfoliation and constitutional symptoms. Lesions may be de novo or on old patches. Pustules may coalesce to form lakes of pus. Steroids, iodides, salicylates, etc. precipitate condition. Localized psoriasis is confirmed to palms and soles as pinhead pustules on red exfoliating macules. Differentiation is from tinea, acrodermatitis persistant with bacteroid.

ERYTHRODERMIC PSORIASIS

Two forms exist. Chronic lesions may evolve gradually into an exfoliative phase, and can be regarded as extensive plaque psoriasis involving all, or almost all, the cutaneous surface. There are usually some areas of uninvolved skin. The psoriatic characteristics are retained, mild treatment is well tolerated, and the prognosis is good. The second form is part of the spectrum of 'unstable' psoriasis. It may occur at any time, either presenting suddenly and unexpectedly, or ushered in by a period of increasing intolerance to local applications, UV therapy, etc., and of loss of control over the disease. It is more frequent in arthropathic psoriasis. Generalized pustular psoriasis may revert to an erythrodermic state.

It can be precipitated by infections, hypocalcemia, antimalarials, tar and withdrawal of corticosteroids. The characteristics of the disease are often lost, the whole skin is involved, the patient may be febrile and ill, the course is often tumultuous or prolonged, relapses are frequent, and there is an appreciable mortality. In contrast to the stable form, itching is often severe. One has to be very alert with regards to the various metabolic complications of erythroderma. Persistent universal inflammation of the skin may have important consequences for thermoregulation, haemodynamics, intestinal absorption, protein, water and other metabolism.

Atypical Forms of Psoriasis

Linear and zonal lesions

Linear psoriasis may occur in the presence of other typical lesions, as part of the Köebner's phenomenon. Zonal lesions may represent a Köebner's reaction at a site of herpes zoster. True linear psoriasis in the absence of lesions elsewhere is extremely unusual. It may be confused with inflammatory linear verrucous epidermal naevus or may occur as a Köbner response on verrucous epidermal naevi of the non-inflammatory type. True psoriasis arranged in linear bands unilaterally has also been described.

Seborrhoeic psoriasis

There is no reason why a genetically constituted psoriatic should not develop seborrhoeic dermatitis. Lesions involving the scalp, eyebrows and the region of the ears are often of this type, having features of both diseases or changing during the course of observation. Difficulties also occur in the flexures as in the 'napkin psoriasis' of infants and in obese, middle-aged or elderly patients.

Mucosal lesions

True mucosal involvement by psoriasis appears to be rare, but has been associated with cutaneous involvement by pustular, erythrodermic and plaque forms. Various lesions have been described, including grey, yellowish, white or translucent plaques or annular forms, diffuse areas of erythema and the geographic tongue (benign migratory glossitis) with HLA-Cw6 provides further evidence that the two disorders are related.

Ocular lesions

Blepharitis, conjunctivitis, keratitis, xerosis, synblepharon and trichiasis have been recorded. Chronic uveitis has been found particularly in patients with psoriatic arthritis. Uveitis was also reported in patients with generalized pustular psoriasis or psoriatic arthritis, who were receiving treatment with methotrexate. It was unclear whether methotrexate contributed to the ocular lesions.

PSORIASIS AND ITS ASSOCIATIONS TO VARIOUS OTHER CONDITIONS

Other Skin Diseases

Bullous pemphigoid pemphigus, neurofibromatosis, actinic reticuloid, Peutz-Jeghers syndrome, vitiligo, lupus erythematosus and viral warts have been seen to be associated with psoriasis.

Arthritis / Gout

Psoriasis is only one of some 25 diseases for which an association has been suggested.

Hypocalcemia

This is most often seen in pustular psoriasis.

Intestinal Disease and Malabsorption

The psoriasiform character of dermatoses associated with malabsorption states lends support to a possible association. Both Crohn's disease and ulcerative colitis are positively associated with psoriasis.

Cardiovascular Disease

An increased incidence of occlusive vascular disease has been reported in psoriatic patients in retrospective studies.

Relapsing Polychondritis

About 25% of patients with this rare disorder have an associated rheumatic or autoimmune disease. Association with psoriasis has also been reported.

Chronic Recurrent Multifocal Osteomyelitis

This is an unusual, idiopathic entity that manifests with pain and swelling in affected bones, due to non-infective inflammatory lesions, which suggest osteomyelitis on radiological investigation. The syndrome has been reported in children and young adults in association with palmo-plantar pustulosis and with psoriasis in the absence of pustules.

DIAGNOSIS

It is based upon:

1. F/H of psoriasis.
2. Typical distribution of the lesions on scalp, knees, elbows, the front of the legs, back and nails.
3. Well- defined non-indurated, dry, erythematous areas with silvery layer- upon- layer scaling.
4. The candle-grease sign, Koebner's phenomenon and pin-point bleeding upon removal of the scale (Auspitz's sign).
5. Little or no itching.
6. H/O previous attacks and seasonal variations of the disease.
7. Typical histopathology.

Differential Diagnosis

In the majority of cases, the diagnosis of psoriasis is usually easy if the above-mentioned features are borne in mind. Atypical cases may create diagnostic problems.

The following conditions must be particularly considered in differential diagnosis

- *Seborrheic psoriasis:* The scalp patches are diffuse, ill defined and moist; the hair is matted and tangled in the crust; the crusts are greasy. Body lesions affect the flexures, the sternal and inter-scapular regions. Sebo-psoriasis is a condition in which features of both psoriasis and seborrheic dermatitis are seen as indistinguishable.

- *Pityriasis rosea:* A short history, centripetal distribution with herald patches and typical oval lesions with cigaratte paper like centrifugal scaling.

- The flexural lesions must be distinguished from those in tinea cruris, intertrigo, seborrheic dermatitis; the nail lesions, from the lesions in tinea unguium, eczema, paronychia and syphilis; the palmar lesions from the other causes of hyperkeratoses; the guttate variety, from lichen palanus and the erythrodermia type from the other causes of erythroderma.

Course and Prognosis

This remains as unpredictable as it was 150 years ago. 'Psoriasis is at all times and under all forms a very troublesome and, often, an intractable disease, but it is rarely dangerous to life'. 'It is impossible to say, in any particular case, how long the disease will last, whether a relapse will occur, or for what period of time the patient will remain free from psoriasis'.

The disease is non-infectious. General health and longevity are unaffected though the majority of patients suffer from the disease on and off throughout their lives. The course is chronic with varying periods of intermission (from weeks to years). The disease does not leave scars. There is only faint staining which disappears slowly. The nails gradually assume their normal appearance in months after the attack has aborted.

Guttate attacks carry a better prognosis than those of a slower and more diffuse onset, and have longer remissions after treatment. At the other extreme, erythrodermic and pustular forms carry an appreciable mortality and arthropathic forms a considerable morbidity. An early onset and a family history of the disease appear to worsen the prognosis.

Flexural, erythrodermic and pustular psoriasis take longer to heal then the typical variety. The palmer and nail lesions are rather resistant to treatment.

Complications

Infection

- Secondary infection of psoriatic lesions is rarely a problem except during topical steroid therapy under occlusive dressings, when folliculitis and furunculosis are a hazard. However, staphylococci are carried by 50% of psoriatics, especially on the lesions.

Itching

- This is very variable in psoriasis, ranging from complete absence to severe pruritus in a minority of patients. It is more common in unstable forms. Pustular and erythrodermic patterns are more usually accompanied by sensations of burning or tightness. Often, the degree of itching reflects the emotional state of the patient and, if severe, may be a symptom of anxiety or depression.

Arthritis

- *PsoriasisArthropatic.* It is the association of psoriasis of the skin and/or nails with a peripheral and/or spinal arthropathy, and usually a negative serological test for rheumatoid factor. The joints of the fingers, feet, ankles, knees and sacro-iliac are selectively affected; these joints are swollen and painful. The psoriatic eruption and the involvement of the joints may increase or decrease simultaneously. Nail changes are usually present. Radiological changes are characteristic and consist of osteoporosis followed by increased density, diminished joint space, erosion of joint surfaces followed by eventual destruction of the ends of bones. Ultimately, the joints become deformed.

Nephritis and renal failure

- Renal failure due to acute tubular necrosis may rarely result from the oligaemia after loss of albumin into and from the skin in acute pustular psoriasis.

Hepatic failure

- Severe abnormalities of liver function may occur in erythrodermic or pustular psoriasis, and are likely to be related to drugs, alcohol intake and oligaemia.

Amyloidosis

- Amyloidosis of the secondary type is a rare sequel of arthropathic, generalized pustular and severe non-pustular psoriasis. It is an additional cause of renal failure in association with psoriasis, and may follow an aggressive, fatal course.

Treatment

General and non-specific measures

- Attention to the patient's general, physical and psychological health is always worthwhile. Mild anemia, minor but untreated arthritis, an anxiety state or depression, especially in the elderly patient, may all critically lower the patient's tolerance of his or her disability. Rest, mild sedation, removal from a troublesome environment, a holiday or a short stay in hospital may all help to turn the therapeutic tide. Harmless placebos may give comfort and should not be despised.

The treatment should lay stress on

- Impressing upon the patient that the treatment should be continued till the last lesion has disappeared. In this respect, the scalp should not be forgotten. The relapse rate is low, if the attack is completely controlled.
- General health should be maintained. Exciting causes should be eliminated as far as possible.

Homeopathic Approach to Psoriasis

Since modern medicine has a very limited role to play in case of psoriasis, homeopathy comes as a rescue, not only as a palliative, but also as curative in a vast majority of cases. In certain obstinate cases, it is difficult to achieve the cure.

The homeopathic treatment should lay stress on

- Impressing upon the patient that the treatment should be continued till the last lesion has diappeared.

- The general health of the patient should be maintained, and the exciting causes should be studied and eliminated as far as possible.

- The patient's life should be regulated, so that no undue stress affects either body or mind.

- Moderate firm climates, frequent sunbaths, before the onset of winter are very useful in bringing down the relapse rate.

As regards the treatment of individual attacks, the pattern of inquiry and analysis is as follows:

- Adequate information in relation to past and family history should be extracted from the patient, as psoriasis is a herediofamilial disease. Also, past and family history of streptococcal infection, diabetes, gout and injuries (physical and mental) should be inquired because psoriasis is frequently associated with the above conditions.

- Methodical recording of the remission and relapses chronologically is very useful. In every individual there are different exciting factors, aggravating and ameliorating factors, hence they should be recorded after thorough evaluation.

- Individual lesion should be examined in detail for characteristic location, cracks and ulceration, general appearance of the skin, itching with its modalities and any other concomitant symptoms.

- The life situation of the patient including the mental state should be evolved, as it is a known fact that relapses do occur during stressful situation.

Finally a homeopath should always keep in mind that psoriasis is a chronic disease; its course is punctuated by intermissions and remissions. Attacks are more common in winter than in summer. The eruption has natural tendency to clear up in the warm weather.

It is very important in case of children suffering from psoriasis to analyze the life situation in view of the following:

- Ailments from excessive domination.

- Being forced by parents to do things against their wishes.

- Wrongly punished by parents.

- Deceived in friendship.

Some Important Homeopathic Remedies

Arsenicum iodatum, Arsenic album, Calcarea sulph, Calcarea carb, Chrysophanic acid, Clematis, Graphites, Kali ars, Kali sulph, Kali carb, Manganum, Mercurius, Mezereum, Lycopodium, Petroleum, Phytolacca, Phosphorus, Psorinum, Pulsatilla, Rhus tox, Sepia, Silicea, Sarsaparilla, Sulphur, Thyroidinum, Thuja, X-ray.

Uva ursi and Berberis aquefolium are important in the form of local application in cases of psoriasis.

REPERTORY

Alum, am-c, ambr, ars, ars-i, ars-s-f, aur-ar, aur, berb-a, borx, bry, bufo, calc, carb-ac, calc-s, carb-v, canth, chin, cic, clem, cor-r, cupr, dulc, graph, hydrc, iris, iod, kali-ar, kali-br, kali-c, kali-p kali-s, led, lob, lyc, mang, merc, mez, mag-c, merc-c, merc-i-r, nat-m, nit-ac, nuph, petr, ph-ac, phos, phyt, puls, psor, ran-b, rad-br, rhus-t, sars, sep, sil, staph, sulph, sul-i, tell, teucr, thuj, thyr, tub, x-ray.

- **Skin, eruptions, psoriasis:**
  - Diffusa: ars, ars-i, calc, cic, clem, dulc, graph, lyc, mez, merc-i-r, mur-ac, rhus-t, sulph, thuj.
  - Inveterate: calc, carb-ac, clem, kali-ar, mang, merc, petr, puls, rhus-t, sep, sil, sulph.

- Syphilitic: ars-i, ars, aur, cor-r, kali-br, merc, nit-ac, phyt, sars, thuj.

- **Skin, eruptions, desquamating:** acet-ac, agar, am-c, am-m, ars, ars-i, arum-t, aur, ant-t, apis, ars-s-f, bar-c, bell, borx, bov, bufo, calc, calc-s, calc-sil, canth, carb-an, caps, caust, cham, clem, coloc, con, crot-h, cupr, dulc, elaps, euph, frr-p, ferr-iod, graph, hell, kali-s, kali-ar, kali-c, kali-sil, kreos, lach, laur, led, mag-c, manc, medus, merc, mosch, mez, nat-ar, nat-c, nat-m, nat-p, olnd, op, par, petr, plat, plb, ph-ac, phos, ptel, psor, puls, ran-b, ran-s, rhus-t, rhus-v, sep, sec, sil, staph, sulph, sabad, sel, spig, sul-ac, tarax, teucr, thuj, urt-u, verat.
  - Over affected parts: rhus-t.
  - Of hardened pieces: am-c, ant-crud, bor, graph, ran-b, sep, sil, sulph.
  - White scales: ars, calc, como, crot-t, dulc, lyco, merc, sep, sil, thuj.

- **Skin, eruptions, scaly:** am-m, ars, ars-i, aur, bar-m, bell, calad, calc, clem, fl-ac, graph, hydrc, kali-bi, kali-br, kali-s, kreos, led, mag-c, merc, nat-ar, nat-m, nit-ac, olnd, phos, phyt, plb, psor, rhus-t, sars, sep, sil, sulph.

- **Skin, eruptions, crusty:** ant-c, ars, ars-i, calc, calc-s, carbn-s, con, dulc, graph, lyc, merc, mez, nat-m, nit-ac, olnd, petr, ran-b, rhus-t, sil, sulph.
  - Black: ars, bell, chin, vip.
  - Bleeding: merc, mez.
  - Body; over whole: ars, dulc, psor.
  - Brown: am-c, ant-c, berb, dulc.
  - Burning: am-c, ant-c, calc, cic, puls, sars.
  - Dry: ars, ars-i, aur, aur-m, bar-c, calc, chinin-s, graph, lach, led, merc, ran-b, sulph, thuj, viol-t.
  - Elevated: mez.
  - Fetid: graph, lyc, med, merc, plb, psor, staph, sulph.

- Gray: ars, merc, sulph.
- Greenish: ant-c, calc, petr, sulph.
- Hard: ran-b.
- Hay, allergic to: graph.
- Honey colored: carb-v.
- Horny: ant-c, graph, ran-b.
- Inflamed: calc, lyc.
- Mercury, after abuse of: calc, lyc.
- Moist: alum, anac, anthraci, ars, bar-c, calc, carbn-s, cic, clem, dulc, graph, hell, hep, kali-s, lyc, merc, mez, olnd, petr, phos, plb, ran-b, rhus-t, ruta, sep, sil, staph, sulph.
- Offensive: mez.
- Oozing, greenish, bloody: ant-c.
- Crusty, patches: hydr, kali, merc, nit-ac, sabin, sil, thuj, zinc.
- Renewed daily: crot-t.
- Scratching, after: alum, am-c, am-m, ant-c, ars, ars-s-f, bar-c, bell, bov, bry, calc, carb-an, caps, carbn, carb-v, cic, con, dulc, graph hep, kali-ar, kali-c, kali-s, kali-sil, kreos, led, lyc, merc, mez, nat-m, petr, phos, puls, ran-b, rhus-t, sabad, sabin, sars, sep, sil, staph, sulph, thuj, verat, viol-t, zinc, zinc-p.
- Serpiginous: clem, psor, sulph.
- Smarting: puls.
- Suppurating: ars, plb, sil, sulph.
- Thick: aur, merc, mez.
- Warm weather: bov.
- White: alum, calc, mez, nat-m, tell, thuj.
- Yellow: ant-c, aur, aur-m, bar-m, calc, calc-s, carb-v, cic, cupr, dulc, hyper, iod, kali-i, kali-s, kreos, med, merc, mez, nat-p, petr, ph-ac, spong, staph, sulph, viol-t.
- Yellowish-white: mez.

- **Skin, cracks:** aloe, alum-sil, alum, am-c, aesc, ant-c, arn, aur bad, bar-c, bar-s, bry calc, cadm-s, calc-s, corn-a, caust, carban, carbn-s, cham, cycl, graph, hep, hydr, iris, ind, kali-s, kali-c, kali-sil, kreos, lach, lyc, mag-c, mang, merc, nat-c, nat-m, nit-ac, osm, paeon, petr, phos, psor puls, sars, sep, sil, sulph, rhus-t, ruta, teucr, viol-t, zinc, zinc-p.
  - Burning: petr, sars, zinc.
  - Deep, blood: nit-ac, petr, merc, sars, sulph, psor, puls.
  - Fetid: merc.
  - Humid: aloe.
  - Itching: merc, petr.
  - Mercurial: hep, nit-ac, sulph.
  - New skin cracks and burns: sars.
  - Painful: graph, mang, zinc.
  - Summer, agg.: coc-c.
  - Ulcerated: bry, merc.
  - Washing, after: alum, ant-c, bry, calc, calc-s, cham, kali-c, lyc, nit-ac, puls, sars, sep, sulph, rhus-t, zinc.
  - Winter, in: alum, calc, calc-s, carbn-s, graph, petr, psor, sep, sulph.
  - Yellow: merc.

Location

- Eyebrows about: phos.
- Penis, prepuce: graph, sep.
- Scrotum: nit-ac, petr, thuj.
- Back: calc, kali-ar, mez.
- Upper limbs: iris, kali-s, kali-ar, rhus-t, sil.
  - Elbow: iris, kali-ar, kali-s, phos.
  - Forearm: rhus-t.
  - Hand, psoriasis diffusa: ars, calc, clem, carc, graph, kali-bi, lyc, mez, petr, rhus-t, sars, sulph.

- Palm: aur, phos, calc, clem, cor-r, crot-h, graph, hep, kali-s, lyc, med, merc, mez, mur-ac, nat-s, petr, psor, sars, sil, sel, sulph, sul-ac, x-ray.
  - Syphilitic psoriasis: ars, ars-i, aur, merc, phos, sel.
- Back of hand:
  - Chronic psoriasis: ars, aur, bar-c, graph, hep, lyc, maland, petr, phos, phyt, rhus-t, sars, sulph.
  - Syphilitic psoriasis: ars, aur, merc, phos.
- Fingers: graph, lyc, teucr.
  - Nails, about: graph, sep.
  - First finger: anag, teucr.
  - Second finger: anag.
- Knee: iris, psor.
- Leg: kali-ar, phos.
- Foot, sole of: cor-r, phos.
- **Skin, chapping:** aesc, alum, alum-sil, ant-c, arn, aur, bry, calc, calc-sil, carbn-s, cham, cycl, graph, hep, kali-c, kreos, lach, lyc, mang, mag-c, merc, nat-c, nit-ac, petr, puls, rhus-t, sars, sep, sulph, sil, uta, viol-t, zinc.

■

Chapter-21

Erythema

Definition

Erythema is a common primary lesion of the skin where there is redness or hyperemia of the skin, which is either localized or widespread, caused by the dilatation of the superficial cutaneous blood vessels.

Etiology

Localized erythema

- **Trauma:** Injury, pressure, bedsores, intertrigo, napkin rash.
- **Chemical:** Dermatitis and eczema.
- **Mechanical** (Heat, cold, light): Burns, frostbite, sunburn.
- **Infective:** In the early stages of impetigo, insect bite.

Generalized erythema

- Drugs.
- Bacterial toxins.
- Viral infection.
- Erythema Multiforme – resulting from hemolytic streptococcal infection, herpes simplex virus, or drugs (like sulphonamides,

barbiturates, co-trimoxazole, penicillins, phenothiazines, thiazide diuretics, and NSAIDs). In a few cases neoplasia, deep X-ray therapy, collagen diseases and contraceptive pills are also implicated.

- Erythema Induratum – occuring as a result of sensitivity to the tubercle bacilli (or its toxins) and due to sarcoid.

- Erythema Nodosum – resulting from rheumatic fever, infections (streptococcal, tuberculosis, leprosy, histoplasmosis, salmonella, shigella, brucellosis, blastomycosis, coccidiodomycosis, lymphogranuloma inguinale, psittacosis, rickettsial infection, cat scratch fever, tricophytosis), inflammatory bowel disease, drugs (like sulphonamides, oral contraceptives, barbiturates), ulcerative colitis, sarcoidosis, hematologic malignancies, pregnancy, and Bechet's disease.

- Gyrate erythema – resulting from infections, malignancies, or drugs.

- Exanthemata.

- Lupus erythematous.

- Toxic erythemas – due to viral and bacterial infections.

- Syphilis.

Clinical Features

Erythema may take the form of localized or generalized red macules. It may be transient or persistent. Asymmetrical, localized redness is usually due to a local, external cause. It is usually the first symptom seen in inflammatory skin conditions like chemical and thermal burns, insect bites, bacterial infections, dermatitis and eczema. Bilateral and symmetrical widespread erythematous eruptions are usually due to a systemic internal cause.

In every case, an erythematous lesion must be felt for induration or infiltration. Simple erythema has no resistance or infiltration of underlying tissues. Granulomas, however, like tuberculosis and leprosy, have erythema plus infiltration. Generalized erythema and infiltration of the whole integument is called erythroderma.

The distinguishing feature of an erythematous lesion is that the skin over it blanches temporarily under pressure.

A few important erythematous conditions are described below

ERYTHEMA MULTIFORME

It is a self-limiting, recurrent disease, seen to affect young adults in countries with a temperate climate, occuring seasonally during the spring and autumn months. The onset is acute with mild prodromal symptoms like mild fever, malaise and other constitutional symptoms, for about 1-4 weeks.

Then multiple lesions occur, which are sharply marginated, circular, erythematous macules, which become into raised, flattened, edematous papules within 2 days time. The lesion typically has 3 zones – the central dusky purpura, an elevated edematous pale ring, and surrounding macular erythema. The colour of the macular and papular cutaneous lesions can change from crimson red to a purplish or even a bluish colour. Nodules, vesicles and bullae are also common.

The lesions occur symmetrically especially on the palms and soles, dorsal surfaces of hands and feet, extensor limbs, elbows, knees, face, neck and in a few cases the trunk. Mucous membranes are usually spared, but a few lesions may be found in the mouth. These cutaneous lesions are asymptomatic except for mild burning and smarting.

In a few cases though, there is severe erythema multiforme with predominantly extensive bullous eruption of the skin and mucous membranes, sudden onset of high fever, malaise, myalgia and arthralgia. This is termed as *Stevens-Johnson syndrome.* In this syndrome, along with erythema multiforme, there is involvement of the eyes (conjunctivitis, bulla formation, corneal ulceration, uveitis and panophthalmitis, ultimately causing corneal opacities and blindness), urethra and respiratory tract, with blistering and erosion of oral and genital mucosa. *Bullous pemphigoid* is a chronic variant of bullous erythema multiforme in elderly persons.

Pathogenesis

Erythema multiforme represents an immune reaction. Cell-mediated immune mechanisms most likely play the main pathogenic role, with keratinocyte as the primary target.

Histopathology

The most important changes are in the upper dermis and lower epidermis. Some cases have prominent dermal inflammatory changes, with a lymphohistiocytic infiltrate around blood vessels and some oedema and vasodilatation, but little epidermal change. There may also be some vacuolar degeneration of the lower epidermis or individually necrotic epidermal cells. In bullous lesions, there is a typical sub-epidermal bulla while in maculopapular epidermis shows spongiosis and intra-epidermal edema.

Electron microscopy demonstrates the damaged basement membrane in the floor of the bulla, with a few ragged islands of epidermal cells showing some evidence of regeneration.

Differential Diagnosis

- In cases of bullae, you need to differentiate this condition from autoimmune bullous diseases, especially 'pemphigus' if mucous membrane involvement is prominent, and 'bullous pemphigoid' if lesions are small and erythema prominent at the periphery of the bulla. Pemphigus bullae develop on normal skin, and bullae in erythema multifome develop on erythematous areas. Nikolsky's sign and Tzanck test are positive for acantholysis in pemphigus bullae, whereas there is no acantholysis in erythema multiforme.

- Lupus erythematosus (LE) also needs to be differentiated from this condition. LE has butterfly lesions on the face, chronic infiltrated erythematous patches, follicular plugging and scarring.

- Kawasaki's disease may resemble erythema multiforme, but the characteristic red lips, strawberry tongue, red and swollen palms and soles, and the lymphadenopathy should permit a clinical diagnosis.

- Distinction between atypical erythema multiforme and urticarial vasculitis can be difficult.

ERYTHEMA NODOSUM

Erythema nodosum is a hypersensitivity reaction (to the various causes already listed above), characterised by inflammation of skin and subcutaneous tissue. It is common in children and young adults (especially women).

The eruptions are bilaterally symmetric, deep, red, tender nodules, 4 to 10 cm in diameter, occuring especially pretibially, and on the extensor surfaces of the lower, and rarely the upper limbs. The onset is acute, frequently associated with fever, malaise, leg edema, and arthralgias or arthritis (ankles are most commonly affected). On palpation, the lesions are slightly warm and very tender.

Initially the skin over the nodules is red, smooth, slightly elevated, and shiny. Over a few days, the lesions flatten, leaving a purple or bluish green color resembling a deep bruise. The natural history is for the nodules to last a few days or weeks, appearing in crops, and then slowly involute. ESR is usually elevated.

Differential Diagnosis

- Cellulitis also has a rapid onset with tenderness and warmth on palpation, but is differentiated from erythema nodosum, which has more than a single lesion, and is of several days duration.

- Superficial thrombophlebitis also occasionally mimics erythema nodosum but it is rarely, if ever, bilateral.

GYRATE ERYTHEMAS

These are characterized by clinical lesions that are annular or arcuate. The primary lesions are erythematous and slightly elevated. In some of these diseases the lesions are transient and migratory and in some cases they are fixed.

ERYTHEMA ANNULARE CENTRIFUGUM

It is the commonest gyrate erythema, characterized by polycyclic, erythematous lesions that grow eccentrically and slowly. Over several weeks the lesions break up and disappear, and are replaced by new lesions that follow a similar course. The lesions occur on the trunk, especially the buttocks and inner thighs. There is a characteristic trailing scale at the inner border of the annular erythema. The disease course is usually chronic and recurrent.

ERYTHEMA GYRATUM REPENS

It is a rare condition where there are undulating wavy bands of slightly elevated erythema over the entire body, with marked pruritus. Lesions spread rapidly and are characteristically concentric, with a trailing scale present. Eosinophilia is characteristic.

TOXIC ERYTHEMA

Here there are toxins reaching the skin that tend to produce an erythema. These toxins are either products of focal sepsis in the ear, nose, throat, teeth, intestines, urinary tract, etc.; products of digestion and metabolism, acute illness, fever, rheumatism, drugs, injections, etc. Children and young adults are more often affected.

Lesions here tend to occur symmetrically and are usually more widespread, large and confluent. The trunk, face and proximal extremities are generally affected. The erythema reduces on pressure. The condition lasts from days to weeks, depending upon the cause. The eruptions may be accompanied by mild constitutional disturbances like low-grade fever, headache and joint pains.

Differential Diagnosis

Pityriasis rosea, drug eruptions, miliaria, secondary syphilis and infectious fever must be ruled out.

Homeopathic Approach to Erythema

The above condition demonstrates typical multi-miasmatic evolution. The illness starts with constitutional symptoms like fever, malaise, etc. and then gradually develops edematous, erythematous macules of various shades especially red, crimson red, purplish red, bluish red, etc. Very rarely one develops bullous eruptions. The lesions usually disappear in a few weeks with a strong tendency to recurrence.

This clearly exhibits Psoric miasm (erythema), gradually progressing to Sycotic (bullous).

Important points to be noted during history

1. History of ingestion of drugs like barbiturates, phenolphthalein, sulphonamide, salicylates.
2. Every case to ba taken to locate septic focuses in the body especially in the nose and throat.
3. Since erythema multiforme is the result from sensitization of products of infections and drugs; it indicates disruption of the immune system. One should rule out any other associated condition, like allergic purpura, herpes simplex, infection, rheumatism, etc.
4. The most important point to consider is that it is a self limiting condition which usually disappears in few days to weeks, hence homeopathic treatment is aimed at recurrence of lesion and treating the septic focus if any.

The approach to the problem should be, carefully observing

1. The lesion (site, character, colour, duration, onset).
2. The associated constitutional symptoms.
3. The deriving miasmatic background from past history and family history.

In my view erythema multiforme falls under **tubercular miasm** chiefly because of:

1. Immune reaction.
2. Tendency to recurrence.

I would like to caution the treating physician that the bullous variety could on a few occasions be fatal; hence utmost precaution should be taken whilst treating the patient homeopathically.

Some Important Drugs for Erythematous Rashes

Agar, am-c, anac, ant-c, ant-t, apis, ars, aur, acon, ail, bell, bry, berb, calc, chlor, con, coff, graph, kali-bi, kali-c, kali-s, lach, lyc, mag-c, merc, mez, nit-ac, ph-ac, phos, rhus-t, sulph, sul-ac, stram, tab, thuj, tub.

REPERTORY

- **Skin, eruptions.**
    - Erythematous: ars, thuj.
- **Skin.**
    - Erythema: androc, antip, bell, bor-ac, grin, lat-h, mez, morg-p, narc-ps, physala-p, pic-ac, plan, plb-chr, prot, syc, ter, tub, urt-u.
- **Chest, discoloration, redness, erythematous:** apis.
- **Extremities, eruptions**
    - Erythematous: ars, thuj.
    - Eruptions, upper limbs, erythematous: bor-ac.
- Face, discoloration, red, erythema: gels, graph, syc.
- Male genitalia, eruptions, penis, erythematous: Petr, Samb, Sumb.

For Erythema nodosum

- **Skin, eruptions, erythema nodosum:** acon, apis, chinin-s, jug-c, kali-br, kali-i, led, narc-ps, phyt, rhus-t, rhus-v, sul-ac, tub.
- **Skin, discoloration, red spots, bluish red, nodules:** lyss.

Chapter-22

Urticaria

Synonym

Nettle rash; Hives; Weals.

Definition

Urticaria is a commonly seen clinical condition where there is a transient eruption of raised and circumscribed erythematous or oedematous swellings of the superficial dermis, associated with itching.

There are a variety of its *clinical variants* seen, two of which are:

- Angioedema (angioneurotic oedema, giant urticaria, Quinke's oedema) consists of transient swellings in the deeper dermal, subcutaneous and submucosal tissues. Urticaria and angioedema often occur together and for practical purposes are similar processes. However, the form of pure angioedema that is caused by C1 esterase inhibitor deficiency shows some differences clinically and in response to treatment.

- Systemic anaphylaxis is an acute life-threatening condition induced by an IgE-mediated allergic reaction. It consists of a combination of symptoms and signs including diffuse erythema, pruritus, urticaria, angioedema, hypotension and cardiac arrhythmias. A similar clinical picture from non-allergic causes is called a systemic anaphylactoid reaction.

Classification & Etiology

Urticaria can be broadly **classified** in terms of 'duration' or its 'trigger factors'.

1. In terms of duration, urticaria can be divided into acute and chronic forms. **Acute urticaria** is usually self-limited and the weals commonly resolve within 24 hours, but may last up to 4-6 weeks. In **chronic urticaria** the weals continue daily or on most days for longer than 6 weeks. Acute urticarias are more common in young adults of both sexes, whereas chronic urticarias are more commonly seen in women, in their fourth or fifth decades. A cause or trigger factor can be easily found in acute urticaria, as compared to the chronic form.

2. When classified in terms of trigger factors, it can be divided into:

    a. **Nonimmunologic or nonallergic or ordinary urticaria**: These are caused by degranulation of mast cells and histamine release by mechanisms not involving antigen-antibody reaction. The most commonly seen causative factors of nonallergic urticaria are:

    *   *Drugs:* Anesthetics, angiotensin converting enzyme inhibitors, aspirin and other non-steroidal anti-inflammatory drugs, codeine, morphine, penicillin, cephalosporins, sulfonamides and other antibiotics, diuretics, iodides, bromides, quinine, vancomycin, isoniazid and antiepileptic agents.

    *   *Foods:* Chocolates, eggs, fish, milk and milk products, nuts, pork, shellfish, strawberries, tomato, and yeast.

    *   *Food additives:* Hydroxybenzoates, salicylates, sulphites, and tartrazine.

    *   *Inhalants:* Animal danders, grass pollens, house dust, mould spores, new perfumes.

- *Infections:* Pharyngitis, gastrointestinal, genitourinary, respiratory, fungal (e.g., dermatophytosis), malaria, amebiasis, hepatitis, mononucleosis, coxsackie virus, mycoplasma, infestations (e.g., scabies), HIV, and parasitic infections (e.g., ascaris, strongyloides, schistosoma, and trichinella).

- *Systemic disorders:* Amyloidosis, carcinoma, hyperthyroidism, lymphoma, polycythemia vera, polymyositis, rheumatic arthritis (RA), and SLE

- *Physical:* Cold, exercise, friction, perspiration, pressure, and sunlight.

- Miscellaneous: Contact with nickel (e.g., cheap jewelry, jean stud buttons), latex, nail polish or rubber (e.g., gloves and elastic bands); emotional or physical stress; pregnancy (usually occurs in last trimester and typically resolves spontaneously soon after delivery); and recent use of new clothes, creams, detergents, or lotions.

b. **Immunologic or allergic or idiopathic or autoimmune urticaria**: Genes tend to play a role in a few urticarial conditions, where a strong personal or family history of atopic disorders can usually be found. Angioedema and a few rare urticarial variants can be of a hereditary type occurring due to a C1 esterase inhibitor deficiency.

Pathophysiology

Urticaria tends to occur due to a local release of histamine, bradykinin, kallikrein or acetylcholine from the granules of mast cells and basophils. This causes an intradermal edema due to capillary and arteriolar dilatation, and increased vascular permeability via H_1 and H_2 receptors on blood vessels, with occasional leukocyte infiltration.

Urticaria has 3 major mechanisms. Most commonly, it is a manifestation of acute IgE mediated (Type 1) hypersensitivity reaction, with histamine as its primary mediator released from mast cells. Sometimes urticaria can be a manifestation of immune complex reaction or complement-mediated reactions, specific drug reactions or due to an idiopathic cause.

Histopathology

The histology of an urticarial lesion is usually non-specific with vascular and lymphatic dilatation, dermal oedema with a variable perivascular cellular infiltrate consisting of helper T lymphocytes, monocytes, neutrophils and eosinophils. On electron microscopy, dermal mast cells show signs of degranulation. In angioedema the same process occurs in the deep dermis, subcutaneous and submucous regions.

Biopsies are generally performed if individual weals are persistent and may show features of delayed pressure urticaria or urticarial vasculitis. In delayed pressure urticaria, the infiltrate is denser with neutrophils often present in early weals, and eosinophils extending deep into the fat in early and late weals. Urticaria with histological evidence of vasculitis (venulitis) is defined as urticarial vasculitis.

Clinical Features

The urticarial lesions begin as itchy erythematous macules, which develop into weals consisting of pale-pink or red, oedematous, raised skin areas, of varying shapes and sizes, often with a surrounding flare. These usually transient and migratory lesions can form linear, annular (circular) or arcuate (serpiginous) patterns, and can occur anywhere on the body in variable numbers. These weals are generally very itchy, especially at night, but the patients tend to usually rub the part, rather than scratch and thus these lesions resolve leaving a normal skin surface, without any excoriation marks. In a number of cases, these weals are seen to get worse in the evenings or nights and also usually before menses. Urticarial vasculitis should be suspected if the lesions last for more than 24 hours.

Half the cases of urticaria are associated with angioedema, where large, non-pruritic or slightly itchy, non-pitting, pale or pink, diffuse swellings occur, especially on the face, affecting the eyelids, lips, tongue, pharynx and larynx, hands, feet, genitalia, ears, and neck. These lesions may last for several days.

In a few cases urticaria or angioedema can be associated with systemic symptoms like malaise, fever, headache, dizziness, nausea, vomiting, abdominal pain, diarrhea, arthralgia, feeling of a lump in the throat, hoarseness, wheezing, shortness of breath, and syncope, and in its most severe acute form with anaphylaxis.

Diagnosis

Specific laboratory studies are not generally indicated. Instead a detailed personal and family case history is taken in suspected clinical cases, especially as regards to previous attacks, and an attempt made to find out the trigger factors, though in more than half the cases no particular cause can be traced.

In a few cases a fluoroimmunoassay may help in detection of food allergies undetected by routine examination and testing.

Differential Diagnosis

• Anaphylaxis.

• Erythema multiforme.

Treatment

Education on avoidance of the suspected offending allergen is essential.

In cases of angioedema or anaphylaxis, timely emergency care needs to be taken in a hospital setting, with checking of vital statistics and checking for air flow in the respiratory passages, and if needed administering oxygen. In a few cases, intubation or even tracheostomy may be required, where there is laryngeal obstruction due to angioedema.

Homeopathic Approach to Urticaria

Homeopathy has maximum scope in the above condition, as modern medicine has nothing more to offer other than antihistaminics.

The following pattern should be observed most meticulously whilst treating the patient:

- Confirm whether the lesion fits into urticarial rash. The typical lesion should include a rosy-red, erythematous macule with edematous weals. The erythema fades on pressure.

- Time of aggravation. I have found a night aggravation more common.

- Does urticaria alternate with any other complaint? Especially asthma or rheumatism.

- Always ask whether urticaria is preceded by any other symptoms like nausea, chill, menses, etc.

- Inquire as to which season the patient develops urticaria and at what temperature e.g. hot room, cold room, open air, near the seashore, etc.

- The most important factor that helps us to eliminate majority of the drugs is the patient's feeling of wellbeing after an application of heat or cold.

- Try and find out which particular foodstuff aggravates the condition, especially shellfish, sweets, meat, chocolates, etc.

- Has the patient got any emotional stress?

- I have seen many patients of urticaria who have a history of worm infestation. Therefore one should inquire for any history of worms. Also history of insect bites or contact with any plants or ingestion of drugs like penicillin or salicylates.

- Sometimes physical factors especially exposure to sun, excessive physical exertion and exercise lead to urticaria.

All the above should be thoroughly scrutinized to get the maximum data. In very rare cases, patient may develop swelling of face with laryngeal obstruction. At that time the patient should be shifted to a homeopathic hospital and his airway should be kept clear with endotracheal intubation and oral drugs like chlorum, etc. should be administered

The treatment consists of not only giving the indicated homeopathic drugs, but to eliminate the offending agent e.g. eliminative diet, withdrawal of causative drug, treatment of parasitic infection, correction of the existing physical stress. During an acute attack the patient should be kept on a bland diet – alcohol, tea and coffee are preferably avoided. Finally reassurance should be given to the patients who have chronic urticaria.

Some Important Homeopathic Remedies and Certain Important Rubrics Helpful in Clinical Practice

Astacus fluviatilis, Bacillus proteus, Bombyx, Chloralum hydratum, Medusa, Santoninum, Tilia, Boletus luridus, Copaiva.

- Urticaria worse at night: Apis, Bov, Chlol, Cop.
- Urticaria alternating with asthma: Apis.
- Giant urticaria: Lyc, Stroph-h.
- Chronic urticaria: Hygroph-s.
- Urticaria during fever: Rhus-t.
- Extremely giant urticaria: Antip, Bacillus no. 7, Bol-lu, Santin.
- Urticaria associated with lot of Edema: Cortico.

Drugs for Acute Urticaria

Anthracokali: Urticaria increases with general sweat. There is intense itching, which is < night. The site of urticaria is hands, tibia, shoulders, and dorsum of feet. Eruptions always decrease with the full moon. Concomitant symptoms with urticaria are dropsy and intense thirst.

Antimonium crudum: Dirty, unhealthy skin. Urticaria with white lump with red areola which itch. The itching is not continuous, but seems to come and go. There is a marked aggravation after the ingestion of **meat** and when in bed. The itching makes the patient irritable, hot, and thirsty. Urticaria associated with gastric disorders, which is characterized by a thick white-coated tongue.

Antipyrinum: Chiefly between fingers and toes with troublesome itching and erythema. Urticaria appears and disappears quite suddenly and is often accompanied by internal coldness. Also angioneurotic edema with swelling about eyes and lachrymation is seen. Urticaria associated with tinnitus.

Apium graveolens: Stomach pains and shivering before the outbreak of urticaria. Urticaria with stinging itch, rapidly changing location.

Apis mellifica: Stinging and itching as if from bee stings < night. The urticaria may consist of isolated elevations, which are quite painful and tender to touch; these later become purple or livid. There is slight fever and heat of skin accompanying urticaria with burning pain. The urticaria is worse during chill and fever. The urticaria sometimes accompanies asthmatic trouble. Change of weather, warmth and exercise cause troublesome itching and burning urticaria. Generalized anasarca as a strong concomitant to urticaria. > Open air, uncovering cold bathing.

Arsenicum album: Urticaria with burning and restlessness. Useful for persistence of complaints during recession of urticaria. < Eating shell fish, < at seashore, < sea bathing.

Astacus fluviatilis: Short acting remedy having a special affinity for skin producing urticaria all over the body with violent pruritus. Liver affection with nettle rash. The urticarial rash is so violent that patient may go into a mild miliaria. < Fish or shellfish.

Belladonna: Violent sudden outbreaks of red, hot, painful urticaria, location – inner aspects of limbs, face. Urticaria associated with metrorrhagia.

Bombyx chrysorrhea: Hard large tubercles with a red areola. The tubercles are most marked near the joints. There is a sensation of a foreign body under the skin, with itching of the whole body.

The itching gets worse in the evening but is not relieved in any way. There is a burning heat everywhere.

Bovista lycoperdon: Urticaria covers nearly whole body. Itching and burning < by scratching, < night. Urticaria caused by tar. The itching is worse on getting warm. Urticaria with a disposition to diarrhea. Each stool is followed by tenesmus. The other concomitant symptoms are scorbutic gums, inflammation of eyes, metrorrhagia, various mental symptoms. Urticaria on excitement, with rheumatic lameness, palpitation and diarrhea. Urticaria < on waking in morning, < from bathing. Stupor, staring, even delirium with urticaria.

Chloralum hydratum: Characterized by its periodicity. It disappears by day and comes on by night with such intense itching as to prevent sleep. < Wine, spirituous liquors, hot drinks. Wheals come on from a chill > warmth. Red blotches with violent stinging itching all over the body. Erythema aggravated by alcoholic drinks with palpitation; causes pains in tendons and extensors. Emotional excitability; hallucinations.

Copaiva officinalis: Hives with fever and constipation. Chronic urticaria in children. Itching < at night and during fever. Urticaria over whole body with red face.

Skin dry and hot with violent itching. Severe headache with urticaria.

Dulcamara: Hives comes on at night, especially when nights are cool, with heavy dew, after a hot day or when weather changes from warm to cool and damp. Urticaria with violent cough and edema of glands. Feverish urticaria. Urticaria obliging one to scratch and burning after scratching, every eruption being preceded by sensation of pricking over whole body. Eruption of white, irregular blotches raised upon the skin, surrounded with red areola, appearing in warmth and disappearing in cold. Extremities, face, chest and back violently itching and burning after scratching. Headache, want of appetite, nausea, bitter taste, vomiting, intense aching in pit of stomach and precordial region, restlessness and sleeplessness, night sweats, turbid dark urine, diarrhea, pains in limbs. Urticaria from gastric disorders.

Ichthyolum: Chronic urticaria in patients of uric acid or tuberculous diathesis. Urticaria seen in alcoholics and especially in old people. Most important concomitant is intense appetite.

Medusa: Face, arms shoulders and breasts. Oedema – face, eyes, nose, ears and lips. Burning, pricking, itching sensation associated with urticaria.

REPERTORY

- **Skin, eruptions, urticaria:** acon, agra, all-c, alum-p, alum-sil, am-c, am-m, anac, ant-c, ant-t, anthraco, antip, ap-g, apis, arn, ars, ars-i, ars-s-f, arum-d, arum-dru, astac, aur, aur-ars, aur-s, bar-c, bar-m, bar-s, bell, benz-ac, bomb-pr, bov, bry, bufo, calad, calc, calc-s, carb-an, carb-v, carbn-s, caust, cham, chin, chinin-ar, chinin-s, chlol, chlor, cic, cimic, coca, cocc, con, cop, corn, crot-h, crot-t, cub, cupr, dulc, elat, ferr-i, ferr-s, frag, gal-ac, graph, helia, hep, hydr, ign, iod, ip, kali-ar, kali-br, kali-c, kali-i, kali-p, kali-s, kreos, lach, lat-k, led, linu-u, lipp, lyc, lycps-v, mag-c, med, medus, merc, mez, myric, nat-ar, nat-c, nat-m, nat-p, nit-ac, nux-v, pall, petr, ph-ac, phos, physala-p, podo, psor, puls, rhus-t, rhus-v, senec-abv, rob, rumx, ruta, sal-ac, sars, sec, sel, sep, sil, skook, sol-a, sol-o, staph, stram, sul-ac, sul-i, sulph, ter, tet, throsin, thuj, til, trios, urin, urt-u, ust, valer, verat, vesp, voes, zinc, zinc-p
  - Morning: bell.
  - Awakening on: bov.
  - Afternoon: chlol.
  - 4 p.m. and evening: hyper.
  - Evening: kreos, nux-v.
  - Night: apis, bov, chlol, cop, hydr, nux-v, puls.
  - Air cold aggravates: nit-ac, rhus-t, sep, caust, dulc, kali-br, nat-s, rumx.
  - Amel: calc, dulc.

- Alternating with.
    - Asthma: calad.
    - Rheumatism: urt-u.
- Ascarides, with: urt-u.
- Asthmatic troubles, in: apis.
- Bathing after: bov, phos, urt-u.
- Burning: cop, sep, urt-u, rhus-t.
- Catarrh with: dulc.
- Change of air and weather: apis.
- Children, chronic urticaria in: cop.
- Chill
    - Before: hep.
    - During: apis, ars, ign, nat-m, rhus-t.
    - After: apis, chlol, elat, hep.
- Chronic: anac, ant-c, antipyr, ars, astac, bov, calc-c, chloral, condur, cop, dulc, hep, ichth, lyc, mez, nat-m, petr, rhus-t, sep, stroph, sul, urt-u, ver.
- Climateric: morph, ust.
- Clothes, from pressure of: med.
- Cold bath, after: calc-p.
    - Amel: apis, dulc.
    - From taking: dulc.
- Constipation, fever with: cop.
- Croup, alternating: ars.
- Diarrhea, with: ars, apis, bov, puls.
- Drinking cold water, agg.: bell.
- Drinks.
    - Spirituous, from: chlorals.
    - Hot, amel: chloral.

- Edema with: apis, vesp.
- Emotions: anac, bov (excitement), ign, kali-br.
- Erosions on toes, with: sulph.
- Exercise.
  - After violent: con, nat-m, psor, urt-u.
  - Warmth of, amel: hep, sep.
- Exposure, from: chloral, dulc, rhus-t.
- Fever during: apis, chlor, cop, cub, ign, rhus-t, rhus-v, sulph.
  - Fever suppressed: elat.
- Flat plaques in: form, lob.
- Fish agg.: ars.
  - Shell: terb, urt-u.
  - Shellfish, roe: camph.
- Fruit, pork, buckwheat from: puls.
- Gastric derangement, from: ant-c, ars, carb-v, cop, dulc, nux-v, puls, robin, trios.
- Giant: apis, kali-i.
- Itching, burning after scratching, no fever: dulc.
- Itching without: uva.
- Liver symptoms, with: astac, myric, ptel.
- Livid: apis.
- Lying amel: urt-u.
- Meat, after: ant-c.
- Menses.
  - After: kreos.
  - Before: dulc, kali-c.
  - During: bell, bov, cimic, kali-c, mag-c, puls, sec.
  - Delayed, with: puls.
  - Profuse with: bov.
- Nausea, before the: sang.
- Nodular: agar, alum, ant-c, apis, bry, calc, carb-an, carb-v, caust, chel, chlol, cop, dulc, hep, iod, jug-c, kali-br, lach,

led, lyc, mag-c, mang, mez, nat-m, petr, puls, rhus-t, ruta, sec, sep, sil, staph, sulph, urt-u, verat.

- Rosy (erythema): androc, bell, bor-ac, grin, mez, morg-p, pic-ac, plan, prot, syc, ter, tub, urt-u.
- Open air in: nit-ac.
- Palpitation, with: bov.
- Periodically, every year, same season: urt-u.
- Perspiration, during: apis, rhus-t.
- Petechial disturbance or erysipelatous eruption: frag.
- Pressure where skin in: med.
- Purple: chin-s.
- Reading: stroph-h.
- Receding: stroph-h.
- Respiration, difficult, with: apis.
- Rheumatism, with: rhus-t, urt-u.
- Rheumatic lameness, palpitation, diarrhea: bov, dulc.
- Rubbing amel: elat.
- Scratching after: agar, alum, am-c, am-m, ant-c, ars, ars-s-f, bar-c, bry, calc, calc-sil, carb-an, carb-v, carbn-s, caust, chin, chinin-ar, cic, cocc, con, dulc, graph, hell, hep, ip, lach, led, lyc, mag-c, mag-m, mang, merc, mez, nat-c, nat-m, nit-ac, nux-v, olnd, petr, puls, rhus-t, ruta, sel, sep, sil, spig, staph, sulph, thuj, verat, zinc, zinc-p .
- Seaside at: ars, mag-m.
- Sequelae from suppressed hives: apis, urt-u.
- Shuddering with: ap-g.
- Spirituous liquors, after: chlol.
- Spring, every: rhus-t.
- Strawberries, from: bry.
- Suddenly, appearing and disappearing: antip.
- Syncope, sudden violent onset: camph.

- Tar from: bov.
- Tuberosa: anac, bol-lu.
- Undressing agg.: puls.
- Uterine trouble, from: apis, bell, kali-c, nat-m, puls, sep.
  - Walking in cold air, while: sep.
- Warmth and exercise: apis, bov, con, dulc, kali-i, led, lyc, nat-m, nit-ac, psor, puls, sulph, urt-u.
  - Amel: hep, sep.
- Wet from becoming: rhus-t.
- Wine from: chlol .
- White: nat-m.
  - Apex: ant-c, puls.

Location

- **Head:** agar .
- **Face:** am-c, anan, apis, ars, bell, calc, chel, chinin-s, chlol, cop, crot-t, dulc, gels, hep, hydr, kali-i, lach, led, mag-m, mez, nat-m, nit-ac, rhus-t, sep, sil, sulph, urt-u.
  - Morning: chin.
  - Air in open, amel: calc.
  - Symmetrical: crot-t .
  - Winter: kali-i.
- **External throat:** bamb-a, bry, kali-i.
- **Abdomen:** merc, nat-c, tub.
- **Male:** clem, cop, merc, nat-c.
- **Chest:** calad, hydrc, sars, sulph, tub, urt-u.
- **Back:** apis, cann-s, choc, lac-ac, lach, sulph.
  - Scratching after: lyc.
  - Cervical region: sil.
- **Extremities:** acon, ant-c, apis, bell, berb, calc, chin-s, chlol, cop, dulc, hydrc, hyper, indg, kali-br, kali-i, lach, lyc, merc, nat-m, rhus-t, rhus-v, sulph, tarax, urt-u.
  - Shoulder: lach.

- Elbow: aran.
- Forearm: am-c, calad, chin, clem, lyc, nat-m, sil.
  - Morning: chin.
  - Evening: lyc.
  - Heat during: calad.
  - Scratching after: calad, calc, chin.
- Wrist: hep, stann.
- Hand: apis, berb, bufo, carb-v, hep, hyper, nat-c, nat-m, nat-s, sars, sulph, urt-u.
  - Morning: chin.
  - Cool, when hands become: thuj.
  - Hand, back of: acon, apis, berb, cop, hyper, indg, sulph, thuj.
  - Palm: rhus-v, stram.
  - Red after rubbing: nat-m.
- Fingers: hep, thuj, urt-u.
  - Between the fingers: hyper, merc.
  - Cold, on becoming: thuj.
- Lower limbs: apis, calc, chlol, clem, kali-i, marb-w, merc, plan, sulph, zinc.
  - Scratching after: clem, spig, zinc.
- Nates: hydr, lyc.
- Thigh: all-c, caust, clem, iod, merc, sulph, zinc.
  - Itching: caust, dulc.
  - Scratching after: clem, zinc.
- Knee: zinc.
  - Hollow of: zinc.
- Leg: calc, chlor, marb-w, rhus-t, sulph.
  - Calf: carb-v.
- Foot: calc, sulph.

Chapter-23

Purpura

Definition

Purpura is a condition where there is a discoloration of the skin or mucous membranes due to bleeding and extravasation of red blood cells into it. The mucous membranes of the mouth, nose, gastrointestinal tract, uterus, and urinary tract are also affected.

Etiology

Localized purpura is due to localized injuries, sprains, blows, insect bites, needle punctures, etc.

Generalized or widespread purpura signifies severe damage to the blood vessels by internal toxins, allergens, and disturbance of the platelet or coagulatory mechanism (like thrombocytopenia or thrombocytopathy or primary disorders affecting the blood vessels).

A few of the common causes of purpura seen are:

Hereditary

Hemophilia, hereditary hemorrhagic thromboasthenia, and hereditary hemorrhagic telangiectasia.

Fevers

Meningitis, rheumatic fever, scarlet fever, smallpox, typhus.

Toxic

Septic focus, snake venom.

Drugs

Corticosteroids, phosphorus, arsenic and anaesthetics, benzol, sulphones (bone marrow depression), quinine, quinidine, salicylates, penicillin, sulphonamides, rifampicin, digoxin, streptomycin, alpha methyldopa, carbimazole, chloramphenicol, cyclosporins, tetracycline, phenylbutazone, etc.

Liver & Spleen disease

Acute yellow atrophy (including drugs, cirrhosis of the liver), splenomegaly.

Kidney disease

Chronic renal disease.

Bone Marrow & Platelet abnormalities

Thrombocytopenia (essential and idiopathic and symptomatic); thrombobasthenia; aplastic anemia; megaloblastic anemia; carcinomatosis, acute and chronic leukemia, lymphoma, myelofibrosis, multiple myeloma; pernicious anemia; myelodysplasia, drugs, alcohol.

Nutrition

Scurvy; Cachexia; Vit. K. deficiency.

Infections

Infectious mononucleosis, subacute bacterial endocarditis, viral and HIV infection.

Other causes

Cushing's syndrome, hypertension, old age, primary

amyloidosis, polycythemia vera, trauma, systemic lupus erythematosus, venous thrombosis, giant haemangioma, Schamberg's dermatosis, dysproteinemia, and vasculitis.

Clinical Features

Purpura presents as a circumscribed bleeding into the skin or mucous membrane, presenting as discolored macules or papules on the skin surface, which do not blanch on pressure (unlike erythema).

Petechiae are small, purpuric lesions up to 3mm across, often occurring in crops. Ecchymoses, hematoma or bruises are larger extravasations of blood.

Extravasated blood in the skin is usually broken down to various other pigments derived from haem within 2 or 3 weeks. This accounts for the characteristic colour changes, purple, orange, brown and even blue and green, which occur in many purpuric lesions. This discoloration disappears slowly in a couple of weeks.

Platelet count below 100,000/mm³ is designated as thrombocytopenia. At this level mild bleeding tendency may start, but bleeding becomes pronounced when the platelet count falls below 50,000/mm³. Severe bleeding occurs when platelets fall below 20,000/mm³. The severity of bleeding does not always correlate with the degree of thrombocytopenia. It may be spontaneous or may follow minor trauma.

Classification

- Coagulation defects usually present as large ecchymoses and external or internal bleeding but not petechiae. Capillary fragility is normal.

- Thrombocytopenia is often associated with petechiae but there may be external or internal hemorrhages and bruising.

- Inflammatory lesions of the vessels are seldom the cause of external bleeding or ecchymoses, and are the commonest cause of persistent and localized purpura. An erythematous inflammatory component is often present.

- External bleeding and large ecchymoses are due to coagulation or platelet defects or to diseases of connective tissue such as Ehlers-Danlos syndrome.

- Petechiae are due to platelet defects or capillary changes.

- Inflammatory purpuric lesions are due to vascular changes.

- Purpura on the legs of the elderly, in association with other skin diseases, is common and seldom requires extensive investigation.

- Splinter hemorrhages of the nails are due to purpura of the nail bed and are not diagnostic of any one condition.

Diagnosis

Platelet count

- A full blood count should always be undertaken in the investigation of purpura. The normal platelet count varies from $150-400 \times 10^9/l$. It varies greatly even in health from person to person, and from time to time in the same person. It may be affected by numerous external factors, hormonal factors and minor infections. Purpura due to thrombocytopenia seldom occurs with a platelet count above $50 \times 10^9/l$. Thrombocytosis may also be a cause of bleeding.

Capillary resistance

- If the pressure difference between the tissues and the capillaries is sufficiently increased, leakage of blood cells occurs. This is the basis of a variety of semiquantitative tests for capillary fragility.

Bleeding time

- This is the time taken for bleeding to cease after a standardized tiny incision in the skin. This type of bleeding normally ceases because of contraction of the small vessels aided by production of platelet thrombus. It is normal in disorders of coagulation. It is usually prolonged in thrombocytopenia below $80 \times 10^9/l$ and becomes progressively prolonged as the count falls, being

30min at counts less than $10 \times 10^9/l$. It is also often prolonged in von Willebrand's disease and some other disorders of platelet function.

Coagulation screen

- Major coagulation defects can be excluded by a clotting screen including prothrombin time, kaolin cephalin clotting time, thrombin clotting time and fibrinogen. Clinical considerations and the results of the screening tests may suggest further laboratory tests, including individual clotting factors.

Capillary microscope

- Direct microscopic examination of capillaries is disappointing in the elucidation of hemorrhagic and purpuric diseases. Purpura may at times be seen in the nailfold capillaries when not present elsewhere in the skin. It may also be possible to see the exact point in the capillary at which extravasation of blood occurs. This may occur at the junction of the precapillary arteriole with the capillary, at the tip of the capillary or more usually at the venous end.

Histology

- Histological examination of purpuric lesions is relatively unhelpful. When purpura is due to disease of the vessel wall, evidence of this may be found, but often there is no hint as to the underlying cause.

Differential Diagnosis

Purpura has to be distinguished from macular rash. The former does not blanch on pressure whereas the latter does.

HOMEOPATHIC APPROACH TO PURPURA

I have purposely discussed this topic of purpura with skin therapeutics as frequently patients visit a homeopath for the purpuric spots. Since there are multiple aetiologic factors for purpura, it is wise to wait till the exact cause of purpura is detected.

On first consultation, patient should be advised tests of platelet count, coagulation time, bleeding time, clot retraction time, prothrombin time. If the result of the above list is not confirmatory then one should advise more invasive methods like bone marrow investigation. I would like to mention in a table various homeopathic medicines indicated for specific etiology.

Etiology	Homeopathic Drugs
1. Hereditary Factor	Deep acting constitutional remedy.
2. Fever	Arn, Carb-v, Bapt.
3. Toxic	Carb-v, Lach, Crot-h.
4. Drugs	Ars, Carb-v, Sulph.
5. Liver disease	Lyc, Chin, Phos.
6. Spleen disease	Phos.
7. Bone marrow	Thyr, Phos.
8. Injury	Arn, Led.

While treating a case of purpura, the homeopathic improvement should be in liaison with the various parameters described above. Constant watch should also be kept for anemia, which is so common in this condition. Occasionally other constitutional medicines, sometimes we may have to prescribe drugs chiefly for the hemorrhagic cases if the purpura is very severe.

Some important homeopathic remedies

Arn, ars, carb-v, chlor, crot-h, ham, lach, merc, ph-ac, phos, rhus-v, sec, sal-ac, led, kali-i, sul-ac, ter.

REPERTORY

- **Skin, purpura:** acon, arn, ars, carb-v, chlol, cor-r, crot-h, ham, jug-r, kali-chl, lach, led, merc, ph-ac, phos, rhus-v, sal-ac, sec, sul-ac, tax.

- **Skin, ecchymosis:** aeth, allox, anth, arg-n, arn, ars, bad, bar-c, bar-m, bell, bry, calc, canth, carb-v, carc, cham, chin, chlol, cic, coca, con, crot-h, dulc, erig, euphr, ferr, ham, hep, hyper, iod, lach, laur, led, mill, nux-v, par, petr, ph-ac, phos, plb, puls, rhus-t, ruta, sec, sul-ac, sulph, tarent, ter

- **Mouth, bleeding, palate, oozing purpura:** crot-h, lach, phos, ter.
- **Nose, epistaxis, purpura hemorrhagica, with:** crot-h, ham, lach, phos, rhus-t, ter.
- **Sleep, sleepiness, purpura, after:** hell.

Location

- **Mouth:** crot-h, lach, phos, psor, ter.
- **Chest:** kali-i, phos.
- **Back, cervical region:** ars.
- **Extremities**
    - Upper limbs: lach, phos, sec, sul-ac, ter.
    - Hand, back of: lach, phos.
    - Lower limbs: kali-i, lach, phos, sec, sul-ac, ter.
    - Leg: kali-i, lach, phos, sec, ter.

■

Chapter-24

Diaper (Napkin) Rash

It is a common cutaneous disorder responsible for dermatitis in children, affecting the diaper area. The highest prevalence occurs between 6 and 12 months of age. It is also seen in elderly incontinent patients and children and adults with urinary or faecal incontinence from Hirschsprung's disease or genito urinary tract anomalies.

It is characterized by erythematous and papulovesicular dermatitis distributed over the lower abdomen, genitals, thighs, and the convex surfaces of the buttocks. The lesions may show superficial erosions in severe cases. Usually the flexures are not affected, since they are in direct contact with the diaper. This is contrary to what happens in intertrigo. The erythematous patches sometimes spread to the legs from contact with the wet diaper. In some infants spots of blood are seen on the diaper along with frequent urination. This occurs when the tip of the penis becomes irritated and crusting over the erosions.

Complications include punched out ulcers or erosions with elevated borders (Jacquet's erosive diaper dermatitis); pseudoverrucous papules and nodules; and 0.5 to 4.0 cm violaceous plaques and nodules (granuloma gluteale infantum).

Typical satellite pustules seen to occur at the periphery as the dermatitis spreads are due to secondary invasion by Candida albicans.

Etiology

Wet or soiled napkins, soap left in the napkins after washing, strong ammoniacal urine, and poor general health. Moist skin is more easily abraded by friction of the diaper as the child moves. Wet skin is more permeable to irritants such as ammonia. Skin wetness also allows the growth of the bacteria. Bacteria are responsible for increasing the local pH, thus leading to an increased activity of the fecal lipases and proteases.

Differential Diagnosis

It has to be made from other erythematous eruptions in this area, viz. *congenital syphilis* (it is accompanied by other syphilitic manifestations, rash on the palms and the soles, involvement of anal region, the lesions are erythematous or bullous); *thrush* (moist red areas with peeling at the edges, also thrush lesions in the mouth); *intertrigo* (confined to flexures only) and *tinea* (the lesions are characteristic, besides, tinea is rare in infancy).

HOMEOPATHIC APPROACH TO NAPKIN RASH

The primary area that is affected in napkin rash is the thigh, perineum and genitalia. The following signs and symptoms should be carefully noted:

- Erythema – its extent and color.
- Sensations – like burning, pricking, stinging,etc.
- Thermal and time modalities.

Since napkin rash occurs in infancy, it is difficult to get symptoms. Hence, the prescription has to be based on signs and observations.

If the irritation persists, then apply gently to the affected part mixture of Calendula and olive oil in the ratio 1:4.

Prophylaxis

Prevention is the best treatment. Part must be kept dry and exposed to fresh air as far as possible. Rubber and nylon panties should be avoided. Napkins should be changed as soon as they become wet and should be rinsed in clear water after being washed with soap. The general health of the patient should be improved. If the urine is strong, water should be given for drinking in between feeds.

Some Important Homeopathic Remedies

Apis mellifica: Appearance of rash is fiery red; child rubs the affected part with the fingers quite vigorously. This is due to stinging, burning, sticking, smarting sensation experienced by the child. < Evening, night, warm application. > Cold application. Affected part is swollen and has a bloated appearance. The part is very hot to touch. If the child is covered it becomes very uncomfortable. Child feels better in open air.

Cantharis vesicatoria: Small ulcerations with exudation of watery discharge and small blisters. Child is restless due to burning sensation and feels better when washed with cold water. Affected part is sensitive and the child will not allow anyone to touch.

Rhus toxicodendron: Tiny vesicles characterize erythematous rash, which tends to become crusty with itching and burning that is better by warm fermentation. Here the child likes parts to be covered, as the skin is sensitive to cold air. (Slightest exposure to damp. Rash is prone to suppuration and crust and then one gets vesicles with small abscesses.

Sulphur: The appearance of the rash is bright red with fine scales in between. The child is most uncomfortable at night in bed and while washing. Burning is sensitive to draft of air, wind and washing; voluptuous itching and child scratches violently. Rash alternates with other complaints, e.g. asthma.

REPERTORY

- **Extremities, eruptions, nates,**
    - Erythematous, infants in: med.
    - Between nates, rash in children, newborns; red: med.

INTERTRIGO

Clinical Features

Intertrigo is a superficial inflammatory dermatitis occurring where two skin surfaces are in apposition. As a result of friction (skin rubbing skin), heat and moisture, the affected fold becomes erythematous, macerated and secondarily infected. There may be erosions, fissures and exudation, with symptoms of burning and itching.

It is most frequently seen during hot and humid weather and chiefly in obese persons.

This type of dermatitis is seen to involve the retroauricular areas; the folds of the upper eyelids; the creases of the neck, axillae, antecubital areas; finger webs; inframammary area; umbilicus; inguinal, perineal and intergluteal areas; popliteal spaces; and toe webs.

As a result of the maceration, a secondary infection by bacteria (fungi) is induced. The inframammary area in obese women is most frequently the site of intertriginous candidiasis. The groins are also affected by fungal (yeast or dermatophyte) infection. Streptococci, staphylococci, pseudomonas or corynebacteria may cause bacterial infection.

Differential Diagnosis

It is generally with Seborrheic dermatitis, which typically involves the skin folds.

HOMEOPATHIC APPROACH TO INTERTRIGO

- The commonest cause of intertrigo in countries experiencing a tropical climate like India where the weather is sultry are obesity, poor hygiene. E.g. not to completely dry the body before wearing the clothes, wearing undergarments during sleep.
- Due to above conditions the skin needs proper circulation of

air esp. in the folds hence drying the skin properly after a bath will prevent moisture and dampness in the folds.

- Anti fungal ointments used commonly for these conditions is not of much help unless the person changes his habits and maintains a proper hygiene.

- It is important to keep in mind that a long-term use of anti fungal ointments is not advisable as they produce an excessive pigmentation around the affected area.

Keeping in mind the above factors the one needs to follow the following rules in order to get beneficial results in cases of intertrigo.

- Wear loose clothing.

- The underwear should be preferably a loose one, so that the length reaches about 6 inches above the knees. Avoid wearing underwear having a "V" shape as it acts as an exciting factor for the itching causing a source of constant irritation.

- The undergarments should preferably be of cotton, made of a thin material and whiten colour. Avoid the use of synthetic and coloured materials.

- The undergarments should be such that there is enough space for the air to circulate.

- On hot days one should change the undergarments atleast twice.

- The skin should be dried properly with a towel after a bath especially the folds of the axilla, inguinal region and in between the toes. These are the regions especially affected.

- The nails should be trimmed down properly. This is a must so that the patient does not aggravate the condition by scratching the lesion.

- One should take special care while changing the clothes, as this is the usual exciting factor to excite itching.

Some Important Homeopathic Remedies

Aethusa cynapium: Excoriations of thighs < walking. Itching eruptions around joints. Profuse perspiration. Surface of body cold and covered with clammy sweat. Lymphatic glands swollen. Eruptions itching when exposed to heat.

Agnus castus: Corrosive itching of different parts > by scratching but it soon returns. Gnawing or itching in various parts.

Arsenicum album: Skin papular, dry, rough, dirty looking, scaly < cold and scratching. Hot, itching and violent burning in skin – Itching, scratching, bleeding, icy coldness of body. Disease begins as red spot spreads like ringworm covered with Silvery scales. Parts painful when scratching.

Belladonna: Dry, hot, burning skin, swelling spreading suddenly. Alternate redness and paleness of skin. Tense, scarlet smooth and shiny, hot, itching, burning skin.

Borax venata: Intertrigo difficult to heal. Dry unhealthy skin. Every injury tends to ulcerate. Inflammation of skin with chilliness, followed by heaviness and pulsation in the head.

Calcarea carbonica: Burning and itching more in morning and in bed. Dry, rough, unhealthy skin; as if covered with a kind of miliary eruption. Skin excoriated in various places. Intertrigo of lenticular, red, raised spots with great heat. Skin sensitive to rubbing, must wash gently. Eruptions moist and scurfy thick scales.

Causticum: Soreness and violent itching in folds of skin, back of ears, between thighs, ulcerative vesicles. Skin prone to intertrigo during dentition.

Chamomilla: Eruptions with itching and nocturnal tickling. Unhealthy skin. Rash in infants during nursing and skin moist and burning hot with bruising and smarting pain.

Fagopyrum esculentum: General and excessive itching with or without eruption, most marked on pubis, pudenda, whiskers and hairy portions of body generally < afternoon 5 p.m. to 7 p.m. skin hot, swollen.

Graphites: Rough, hard, obstinate dryness and absence of perspiration, rawness in bends of limbs, groins, neck and behind ears, unhealthy skin, violent itching and burning. Eruptions oozing out a sticky exudation.

Juglans regia: Itching all over the body. Itching in folds, burning, soreness < after perspiring, severe redness with new vesicles with severe burning and itching. Greenish yellow secretions from eruptions. Glandular swelling and suppuration < when heated, < from over exertion.

Kalium bromatum: Moist eruption. Itching at night in bed and at a high temperature.

Lycopodium clavatum: Great dryness of skin. Intertrigo, raw places bleeding easily. Skin unhealthy, corrosive vesicles. Nocturnal itching. Intertrigo between thighs and labia forming flat, hard ulcer with inflamed edges. Eruptions first vesicular than dry. Itching violently, raw places bleed, covered with thick crust with fetid secretion beneath.

Mercurius solubilis: Itching so intolerable almost makes him crazy < warmth of bed > cold bed > cold air. Almost constantly moist, free perspiration, which gives no relief.

Mezereum: Violent itching < in bed < from touch, compelling to scratch until epidermis is removed and denuded part is covered with a scab or there is repeated exfoliation.

Oleander: Biting, itching < undressing, compelling him to scratch. Intense itching and unsupportable nocturnal burning after scratching. Slight friction causes soreness and chafing especially above the neck or between the scrotum and thigh – want of perspiration.

Oxalicum acidum: Exceedingly sensitive skin – aggravated from sweat, with smarting and soreness. Mottled, marked in circular patches, perspires easily.

Petroleum: Skin dry, constricted, very sensitive, rough and cracked, leathery. Itching sore, moist surfaces with redness and rawness. External hard pressure not painful but a soft touch is unbearable. Cracks bleed easily.

Psorinum: Dirty, dirty look. Scratching gives temporary relief. Itching when body becomes warm < aggravated in bed. Scratches until it bleeds.

Sulphuricum acidum: Livid skin, redness and itching blotches. Distressing, itching and tingling of skin with eruptions.

Sulphur: Dry, scaly, unhealthy skin. Itching spots, painful red and hot after scratching. Bleeds after scratching recurring every night in bed. Violent on thighs and legs. Skin painful for a long time after rubbing as if denuded and sore. Excoriation of folds. Itching, burning < scratching and washing.

Tuberculinum: Eruptions, itching, blotches all over body with exception of face and hand. Intense itching < at night.

REPERTORY

- **Skin:**

  - Intertrigo: acon, aeth, agar, alum, ambr, am-r, am-m, agn, ant-c, apis, arn, ars, ars-i, ars-s-f, aur, bapt, bamb-a, bar-c, bar-s, bell, borx, bry, bufo, cal-c, calc-s, calc-sil, canth, carb-an, carbn-v, carbn-s, caust, chan, chin, chin-s, clem, coff, colch, dros, echi, euphr, fl-ac, fago, graph, hep, hydr, ign, iod, kali-ar, kali-c, kali-chl, kali-m, kali-s, kreos, lyc, lach, laur, mag-m, mang, merc, merc-r, mez, mur-ac, nat-c, nat-m, nat-p, nit-ac, nat-s, nux-v, ol-an, olnd, op, petr, ph-ac, phos, plb, podo, psor, puls, pyrog, phyt, rhus-t, ruta, sabin, sanic, sars, scil, sel, sep, sil, spig, sul, sul-ac, tereb, syph, vinc, zinc.

  - Excoriation, scratching, after must scratch it raw: agar, alum, am-c, ant-c, arg-met, arn, bar-c, bov, calc, calc-sil, carbn-s, caust, chin, dros, graph, hep, kali-c, kali-sil, kreos, lach, lyc, mang, merc, olnd, petr, phos, plb, psor, puls, rhus-t, ruta, sabin, sep, sil, squil, sul-ac, sulph, tarax, til.

  - Excoriation, sensation as if excoriated: canth.
    - Touched when: ferr.

- Children: ant-c, bar-c, bell, calc, carb-v, cham, chin, ign, kreos, lyc, merc, puls, ruta, squil, sep, sil, sulph.
  - Boring into with fingers: arum-t (scarlatina).

- With bilious symptoms: nat-s.
- Dentition during: aust.
- Atrophy of infants: petr.
- Easily chafed from walking or riding: ruta.
- Discharges in every outlet of body, acrid, excoriating skin wherever they come in contact: sulph.
- Dries up, becomes brown and livid, and local eschar forms: anthr (leaves a scar).
- Dries and mummifies, new blisters form around: anthr.
- Flexures of joints: sep.
- Obstinate: hydr.
- Erosions: arum-m, fl-ac.
- Humid: bar-c, graph.
- Pain as if excoriated: par, plat.
- Prurigo: graph.
- Raw decayed meat like: como.
- Scab, if inclined to: kali-m.
- Tettery, oozing constantly and bleeding easily when scratched: merc.
- Walking or riding when: sul-ac.

Location

- **Abdomen, inguinal region:** ambr, ars, arum-t, bov, bry, graph, med, nux-v, ph-ac.
- **Rectum:** aesc, agar, agn, all-c, aloe, alum, am-c, am-m, apis, arg-met, ars, ars-s-f, asc-c, aur-m, bar-c, berb, calc, calc-s, carb-an, carb-v, carbn-s, caust, cham, coloc, dirc, ferr, gamb, graph, grat, hep, hydr, ign, kali-ar, kali-c, kali-s, lach, lyc, merc-c, mur-ac, nat-ar, nat-m, nat-p, nit-ac, nux-v, petr, phos, plan, podo, puls, sanic, sep, sulph, sumb, syph, thuj, tub, urt-u, zinc.
  - Acrid moisture from: carb-v, merc-c, thuj, zinc.
  - Riding, horseback, on: carb-an.

- Wagon, in a: psor.
- Rub anus until raw, must: agar, alum, am-c, arg-n, bor-c, calc, carb-v, carbn-s, caust, graph, kali-c, lyc, merc, petr, phos, puls, sep, sulph.
- Stools, from: aloe, apis, ars, arum-t, asc-c, bapt, coloc, dirc, kreos, mag-m, merc, mur-ac, nit-ac, nux-m, nux-v, rheum, sulph, rub.
- Nates, between: arg-met, arum-t, berb, calc, carb-v, carbn-s, graph, kreos, nat-m, nit-ac, puls, sang, sep, sulph.
- Walking from: arg-met, caust, graph, nat-m, nit-ac.
- Perineum of: alum, arum-t, aur-m, calc, carb-an, carb-v, caust, chan, graph, hep, ign, lyc, merc, petr, puls, rod, sep, sulph, thuj.

- **Male genitalia:** cham, hep, podo, sulph.
- Penis: cop, kali-i, nit-ac.
- Glans: alum-sil, anan, asc-t, cor-r, graph, merc, merc-i-r, nat-c, nat-m, nit-ac, sep, sulph, thuj.
- Prepuce: anan, carb-v, chin-b, hep, ign, merc, mez, mur-ac, nit-ac, psor, sep, thuj.
  - Coition after: calen.
  - Easy: nat-c.
  - Margin on the: cann-s, ign, mur-ac, nit-ac, nux-v, rumx.
- Scrotum: ars, calc-p, chel, hep, ph-ac, sulph, sumb, thuj.
  - Sides of: berb, sumb, thuj.
  - Thighs, between scrotum and: bar-c, caust, graph, hep, lyc, merc, nat-c, nat-m, nit-ac, petr, rhus-t, sulph, thuj.
- Female genitalia: agar, alum, am-c, ambr, ars, berb, calc, calc-s, carb-v, carb-s, caust, fl-ac, graph, hep, kali-c, kali-s, kreos, lac-c, lit-t, lyc, meph, merc, nat-c, nit-ac, petr, sabin, sep, sil, sulph, thuj, til.
  - Menses, during: all-c, am-c, bov, carb-v, caust, graph, hep, kali-c, kreos, nat-s, rhus-t, sars, sil, sulph.

- Old women: merc.
- Perineum: calc, carb-v, caust, graph, hep, lyc, med, merc, petr, sep, sulph, thuj.
- Vagina: alum, hydr, kali-bi, kali-c, merc, nit-ac.
  - Around: ign.
- Chest
  - Axilla: ars, aur, carb-v, con, graph, mez, sonic, sep, sulph, zinc.
  - Mammae, from rubbing: con.
  - Nipples: alumn, anan, arg-n, arn, calc, calc-p, calc-sil, castor-eq, caust, chan, crot-t, dulc, fl-ac, graph, han, hell, hyper, ign. lyc, merc, nit-ac, phos, phyt, puls, sang, sep, sil, sulph, zinc.
- Back, coccyx: arum-t.
- Extremities
  - Finger between: graph.
  - Joints, bends of: bell, caust, graph, lyc, mang, ol-an, petr, sep, squil, sulph.
  - Nates between: arg-met, ars-s-f, arum-t, bufo, carbn-s, graph, nat-m, nit-ac, puls, sep, sulph.
  - Thighs, between: aeth, am-c, ambr, anan, ars, ars-s-f, bar-c, bufo, calc, carbn-s, caust, cham, chin, chinin-ar, goss, graph, hep, iod, kali-ar, kali-c, kreos, lyc, merc, nat-ar, nat-c, nat-m, nit-ac, petr, phos, rhod, sang, sep, squil, sul-ac, sulph, zinc.
  - Left: lyc.
  - Dentition during: caust.
  - Leucorrhea, from: alum, ars, borx, carbn-s, caul, cham, ferr, ferr-ar, fl-ac, graph, kreos, lyc, merc, nit-ac, phos, puls, sep, sil.
  - Menses, during: am-c, carb-v, caust, graph, kali-ar, kali-c, kali-n, lac-c, lach, nat-s, nit-ac, rhus-t, sars, sil, stram, sulph.

- Riding, from: ruta.
- Walking, from: aeth, graph, ruta, sul-ac, sulph.
- Knee, bend of: ambr, sep.
- Leg: lach.
- Foot
  - Heels: all-c.
  - Soles: sil.
- Toes, between: aur-m, bamb-a, berb, carb-an, clem, fl-ac, gink-b, graph, hydrog, lach lyc, mang, merc-i-f, mez, nat-c, nat-m, nit-ac, ph-ac, ran-b, sep, sil, syph, zinc.
  - Walking from: carb-an.

■

Chapter-25

Disorders of
Pigmentation

Introduction

Our skin color is dependent on the percentage of hemoglobin, carotenoid and mainly the melanin pigment in our body.

'Melanin' is formed from tyrosine, via the action of tyrosinase, in the melanosomes of melanocytes. The melanosomes are transferred from a melanocyte to a group of keratinocytes called the epidermal melanin unit. There is a lot of racial and ethnic variation in the number, size, shape, distribution and degree of melanization of the melanosomes. There are two types of melanin pigmentation occurring in humans, of which the first is termed 'constitutive', since it is genetically determined, and the second is termed 'facultative', which is dependent on the exposure of the skin to UV rays of the sun, endocrinal causes (like the melanocyte-stimulating hormone secretion in pregnancy), combination of light and hormonal effect on body (as in melasma), and Addison's disease.

The 'carotenoids' are yellow pigments that are exogenously produced and can be obtained only from plants in the diet. These are to be found in the epidermis as well as in the subcutaneous fat.

The wide variety of skin colour occurring in humans can be objectively measured by reflectance spectrophotometry.

Pathogenesis

Disorders of melanin pigmentation can be divided into the following types:

- **Hypermelanosis:** There is an increased amount of melanin in the skin (dermis or epidermis), and,

- **Hypomelanosis:** There is a lack of the pigment melanin in the skin, due to which the skin appears white or lighter than normal.

- **Amelanosis:** There is total absence of the melanin pigment in the skin, making it look white.

Changes in pigmentation can arise in a number of ways and can be due to a variety of genetic and environmental factors.

Abnormalities may involve:

1. The formation of melanosomes in melanocytes.
2. The melanization of melanosomes.
3. The secretion of melanosomes into keratinocytes.
4. The transport of melanosomes in keratinocytes with and without degradation in lysosome-like organelles.

The pathogenesis of the disorder can be known by performing the light and electron microscopy studies. In quite a few cases, more than one of the biological processes may be affected and responsible for the pigmentary disorder.

HYPERMELANOSIS

Hypermelanosis can be seen in a large number of conditions, where it can be either widespread or of a localized type. It can be classified either on the basis of the color of the skin or on the basis of the causative factor (genetic and nevoid or acquired due to a variety of factors).

MELANISM

Here there is diffuse hyperpigmentation all over the body, due to the presence of an autosomal dominant gene. There is excessive pigmentation of the skin right from birth, which tends to increase upto the age of 5 to 6 years. The face and flexures are especially hyperpigmented, with dark hair, but the iris is normally not abnormally pigmented in this condition.

In a few cases there is an extensive distribution of the many melanocytic naevi, pointing towards neurocutaneous melanoblastosis

There is marked hypermelanosis of the skin around the eyes, especially the lower lids, around the time of puberty, due to an autosomal dominant gene.

LENTIGINOSIS

Lentigo is a benign and pigmented macule, which has numerous melanocytes. Lentiginosis is a condition where there is presence of excessive lentigines in large numbers or are distributed in a particular pattern. The following are the clinical syndromes that fall under this type.

GENERALIZED LENTIGINOSIS

Here there is distribution of a single or multiple lentigines in small crops at irregular intervals from infancy onwards. There is no particular cause known for this condition.

UNILATERAL LENTIGINOSIS

Here there is distribution of lentigines only on one side of the body, with no CNS abnormalities. These are naevoid in nature.

ERUPTIVE LENTIGINOSIS

Here the lentigines tend to increase in number with age, cropping up especially at the time of adolescence or early adulthood.

The lesions may be telangiectatic at first, but rapidly become pigmented and subsequently evolve as cellular melanocytic naevi.

MULTIPLE LENTIGINES SYNDROME
(LEOPARD SYNDROME)

Definition

This is a syndrome occurring due to an autosomal dominant gene, where there is a generalized lentiginosis with multiple lentigines, along with a wide range of developmental defects, especially cardiac abnormalities.

Histopathology

It shows an increase in melanin pigment in the epidermis, with an increased number of melanocytes, with excessive melanosomes. Macromelanosomes are a prominent feature of this syndrome.

Clinical Features

Lentigines are present right since birth or start to appear early in life and increase in number until puberty. They are distributed all over the body, but are especially marked around the neck and upper trunk.

Other symptoms seen frequently in these patients are – retarded growth, fibrillations and the various other conduction defects, pulmonary or subaortic stenosis, ocular hypertelorism, mild mandibular prognathism, sensorineural deafness, and in a few cases genital abnormalities.

It is termed as LEOPARD syndrome because:

L – Lentigines.

E – Electrocardiographic abnormalities.

O – Ocular hypertelorism.

P – Pulmonary stenosis.

A – Abnormal genitalia.

R – Retardation of growth.

D – Deafness.

CENTROFACIAL LENTIGINOSIS

This syndrome, occurring due to an autosomal dominant gene, presents itself as a small brown or black macules appearing during the first year of life and increasing in number up to the age of 8 or 10 years. They are distributed as a horizontal band across the centre of the face, with no mucous membrane involvement. There can be associated epilepsy, mental retardation, coalescence of the eyebrows, high-arched palate, absent upper median incisors, sacral hypertrichosis, spina bifida and scoliosis.

PEUTZ-JEGHERS SYNDROME

Synonym

Periorificial lentiginosis.

Definition

Here there are pigmented macules on and around lips, on buccal mucosa and on the hands and feet, along with intestinal polyposis.

Etiology

This syndrome occurs due to an autosomal dominant gene.

Pathology

Here the pigmented macules show excessive melanin deposition in the basal layer of the epidermis. Along with this there is a tendency to develop malignancy, especially in the gastrointestinal tract, usually in the form of polyps, which are predominant in the jejunum and ileum.

Clinical Features

Though this is a genetic defect, about 40% of the cases may have no family history of it, and are presumed to be new mutations. The pigmented macules can be present since birth, or can appear in infancy or early childhood, or in less frequent cases, may develop later in life.

The areas most frequently involved are:

- The mucous membranes, especially the buccal mucosa, tongue, gums, and genital mucosa; where the lesions are round or oval, brownish or black, and about 1-5 mm in diameter.

- The face, especially around the nose, mouth and lower lip, where the lesions are about 1 mm and more darker.

- The hands and feet can also be involved, where the lesions are much larger.

- In a few cases, the nails can be pigmented diffusely or in longitudinal bands.

The most common complaint with which the patient may present is a history of repeated attacks of abdominal pain, vomiting, rectal bleeding and hematemesis due to intestinal obstruction and polypi.

Associated features noted in a few cases are – anemia, breast cancer, clubbing of fingers, ovarian tumors, and early pubertal changes.

Diagnosis

The mucosal pigmentation is a characteristic feature, and a family history of the same will help diagnosis. Endoscopy of the upper gastrointestinal tract and of the whole colon, together with a barium study will help diagnosis.

Differential Diagnosis

- Addison's disease.

- **Freckles:** These occur especially in those of a fair complexion, and the macules are light-influenced, and are not around the mouth or in the oral mucosa, and do not involve the mucous membranes.

- In Cronkhite-Canada syndrome also, there are melanotic macules on the fingers and gastrointestinal polyposis, but along with that there is a generalized, uniform darkening of the skin, extensive alopecia, and onychodystrophy. Also it affects the person after the age of 30 years, and the polyps that occur are of a benign type, involving the whole GIT.

Classification

The very large number of conditions associated with widespread or localized hypermelanosis cannot be classified easily. The present classification is based on the colour of the skin and on various causative factors. The hypermelanosis may be due to genetic and nevoid factors or it is acquired and due to a variety of factors.

Genetic and naevoid factors

Brown colour

Hypermelanotic macules may be seen in patients with:

- **Albright's syndrome:** This includes polyostotic fibrous dysplasia, endocrine dysfunction and segmental hyperpigmentation.
- Multiple lentigines are seen in
  (i) Peutz-Jegher syndrome; and
  (ii) 'Leopard' syndrome.
- **Neurofibromatosis:** Cafe au lait macules with freckles in the axillae.
- Familial progressive hyperpigmentation (FPH):

This is characterized by patches of hyperpigmentation on the skin, present at birth, which increase in size and number with age. Later, hyperpigmentation appears in the conjunctivae and the buccal mucosa. Inheritance is believed to be of a dominant mode. FPH is differentiated from other hyperpigmentations mainly by the presence of bizarre, sharply marginated patterns of hyperpigmented skin.

Blue or slate-brown colour

Here hypermelanosis is seen as follows:

- Mongolian blue spot in sacral region of mongoloid and negroid babies.
- Naevus of Ota around eye.

- Naevus of Ito on scapular areas, with bluish naevi on the dorsum surface of the hands and feet.

- Incontinentia pigmenti (Bloch-Sulzberger type), seen to develop in the neonatal period with linear group of blisters, which are later followed by slate-brown streaks and whorls of hyperpigmentation. Problems with the teeth and eyes are also seen in this condition, which characteristically affects only the females.

Acquired Hypermelanosis

Pregnancy & Menopause

Women, who are pregnant, menopausal, or are taking hormones or OCP, can develop a brown, patchy, sharply demarcated hyperpigmentation on the face, especially over the malar prominences, forehead and chin. There is also a darkening of skin over the nipples, abdomen and anogenital areas. This type of hypermelanosis is called as 'melasma or Chloasma faciei'. It is seen to affect dark-complexioned women more frequently.

Discontinuing the use of contraceptives rarely clears the pigmentation, and it may last for many years after the discontinuation. Melasma of pregnancy usually clears within a few months of delivery.

Systemic diseases

- **Endocrine disorders:** Hyperpigmentation is seen in adrenal tumors (hyperpigmentation seen with hypertrichosis), diabetes ('Rubeosis' is seen, which is a rosy discoloration of the face in young patients with uncontrolled diabetes; this may be associated with a yellowish discoloration of the skin, giving a 'peach and cream' complexion), Cushing's syndrome and Addison's disease (marked melanosis especially in the palmar creases, buccal mucosa, nipples and genitals).

- **Metabolic disorders:** Chronic renal failure, jaundice-associated diffuse hypermelanosis in primary biliary cirrhosis (along with pruritis and xanthoma), and porphyria.

- Amyloidosis, hemochromatosis, kwashiorkor, malaria, pheochromocytoma, porphyria cutanea tarda, scurvy, syphilis, vitamin A and B$_2$ deficiency are some other conditions in which hyperpigmentation is seen.

Post-inflammatory Hypermelanosis

- Resolution of lesions of eczema, lichen planus, lupus erythematosus.
- Scleroderma.
- Phytophotodermatitis – Pigmentary reaction of the skin to light, potentiated by psoralens in plants.
- Berloque dermatitis due to perfumes that contain psoralens.
- Erythema dyschromicum perstans.
- Riehl's melanosis: Here there is a photosensitivity reaction to sun resulting in a phototoxic dermatitis, which was first described by Riehl. This occurs mostly in women on the sun-exposed areas, and it tends to start as pruritus, erythema, and a gradually spreading pigmentation, which becomes stationary after a certain point. In addition to the melanosis, there may be circumscribed telangiectasia and temporary hyperemia. Diffuse hyperkeratosis occurs, making the skin appear as if dusted with flour.

The pathogenesis of Riehl's melanosis is believed to be sun exposure following the use of some perfume or cream (a photocontact dermatitis). Riehl's melanosis has been reported in patients with AIDS and Sjogren's syndrome. All treatment methods are of no avail unless the cause of photosensitivity is determined. Eventually the hyperkeratosis and pigmentation disappear spontaneously.

Haemosiderin Hyperpigmentation

- Here there is a dark red or reddish brown pigmentation of the skin due to deposits of hemosiderin, along with added widespread hypermelanosis. It occurs especially in cases of purpura, hemochromatosis, hemorrhagic diseases, and stasis ulcers.

- DD includes Sickle-cell anaemia and congenital haemolytic anaemia (affecting the lower limbs), Schamberg's disease (affecting the legs and thighs), drug reactions (seen as small patches on the legs, thighs, buttocks), and allergic reaction to clothing (where patches occur at the flexures or the trunk).

Drugs

- Chlorpromazine and other related phenothiazines – gives a slate grey or purple discoloration of skin.

- Dinitrophenol, tetryl, picric acid, trinitrotoluene, santonin, and acriflavine – gives a yellowish discoloration to the skin.

- Pigmentation of the face may occur from the incorporation in cosmetics of derivatives of coal tar, petroleum, or picric acid, as well as mercury, lead, bismuth, or furocoumarins (psoralens).

- Medical interventions like chemical peels, dermabrasions, laser therapy, or liposuction can also cause hyperpigmentation.

Metallic & Industrial Hyperpigmentation

- *Argyria* (with silvery blue or slate-grey colored pigmentation of sun-exposed parts due to the presence of silver in the skin); *Arsenic* (areas of hypopigmentation may be scattered in the hyperpigmented areas, gives a 'raindrop' appearance to the skin, especially in the inguinal folds and the areolae. There is also a punctate keratoses on the palms and soles); *Bismuthia* (with a bluish grey pigmentation on exposed part, with a bluish line along the gums); *Chrysiasis* (it is induced by the parenteral administration of gold salts, usually for the treatment of rheumatoid arthritis. It presents as a mauve, golden blue, or greyish purple discoloration on the sun-exposed surface); *Mercury* (with a greyish brown pigmentation, with subcutaneous nodules); and *Lead* (pallor and lividity along with the bluish hue of the skin and a bluish line on the gums).

- Melanosis is an important feature in coal miners, tar and petroleum handlers, anthracene workers, and those in similar occupations. Here there is severe widespread itching followed by the appearance of reticular pigmentation, telangiectasis, and a shiny appearance of the skin. Small, dark, lichenoid, follicular papules become profuse on the extremities, particularly the forearms.

Tumours

- Acanthosis nigricans is often associated with internal malignancy.
- Metastatic melanoma may produce diffuse slate-blue colour.
- Mastocytosis.

Hemochromatosis (Bronze diabetes)

This condition is characterized by a gray or brown generalized mucocutaneous hyperpigmentation (especially on the face, extensor surfaces of the forearms, backs of the hands, and the genitocrural area) due to an increased basal-layer melanin and iron deposition around the blood vessels, sweat glands and within macrophages. This occurs along with diabetes mellitus and hepatomegaly. Other associated complaints include cirrhosis of the liver, heart disease, hypogonadism, koilonychia, localized ichthyosis, and alopecia. It is seen to affect males more than females, and that too especially in their late 60's.

Periorbital hyperpigmentation

Dark circles around the eyes are very commonly seen with many disorders and in certain families and dark-skinned individuals.

Treatment

Hypermelanosis, especially when affected exposed areas like the face, hands and legs, can cause considerable mental distress and low confidence levels. Thus treating the condition with consideration of this aspect of the illness is necessary. Also, the treatment of the condition depends on first establishing the exact cause of the illness and trying to reverse the condition causing it, if acquired. Also, since exposure to the ultraviolet rays of sunlight can aggravate the pigmentation, using the right kind of photoprotective cream may be necessary.

HYPOMELANOSIS

Classification

Genetic and naevoid disorders

A number of genetically determined or nevoid conditions are characterized by localized and/or generalized hypomelanosis of the skin.

ALBINISM

Definition

Albinism is a partial or complete congenital absence of the melanin pigment production in the skin, hair, iris and ocular fundi (oculocutaneous albinism), or only in the eyes (ocular albinism), inspite of a normal number of melanocytes in the skin. There are two types of albinism

- Tyrosinase-negative (type I), and,
- Tyrosinase-positive (type II).

Etiology & Types

OCULOCUTANEOUS ALBINISM

In this condition there is a partial or complete failure of melanin production in the skin, hair, and eyes. Melanocytes, inspite of being present in normal distribution, fail to synthesize melanin adequately.

Here there are nine distinct, clinical and genetic variants inherited as autosomal recessive disorders, and one rare type is an autosomal dominant.

Of the two types, 'tyrosinase-negative albinism' is characterized by failure of the hair bulbs to become dark after being plucked and incubated with tyrosine; whereas in 'tyrosinase-positive albinism', the hair bulbs do tend to darken. The latter type is more commonly seen.

OCULAR ALBINISM

In ocular albinism, only the eyes are clinically involved, although careful investigation of the melanocytes in the skin does show some changes. There are four different types, two are X-linked, one dominant and one recessive. In two types there is an associated deafness.

ALBINOIDISM

This term is applied to families who have some partial defect in melanin production in the skin and hair, but only minimal changes in the eyes. The condition appears to be inherited as an autosomal dominant, but in some families it is recessive. Slight tanning is reported and the hair-bulb test is positive. The eyes are usually normal, but there may be photophobia.

Clinical Features

In all races there is a marked dilution of the pigmentation of the skin, hair and eyes.

In the tyrosinase-negative type IA the skin is pink in colour, the hair is white and the patients show a prominent red reflex. It is the most severe form, with complete absence of tyrosinase activity and complete absence of melanin in the skin and eyes. Visual acuity is decreased to 20/400.

In the yellow mutant type IB, the tyrosinase activity is greatly reduced but not absent. Affected patients may show increase in skin, hair (which become yellow-red), and eye color with age, and can tan.

In the tyrosinase-positive type II, some pigment is formed and with increasing age is to be found in the iris, skin and hair, the latter often developing a pale yellow colour. These patients may also tan and the iris is less translucent.

In both types, the patients have photophobia, errors of refraction, horizontal or rotatory nystagmus with head nodding, abnormalities of the optic pathway, and a characteristic facial expression due to apparent squinting. In the tyrosinase-positive type, the visual acuity may improve as they get older and they may have less severe nystagmus. Foveal hypoplasia occurs in the tyrosinase-negative type.

Patients with this disease are photosensitive, and those living in the tropics tend to develop actinic keratoses, squamous cell carcinomas and, occasionally, melanomas in areas of skin exposed to the sun.

Treatment

Using the right kind of photoprotective preparations and avoidance of undue sun exposure are the two main steps to be taken by the patient. Also regular examination of all albinos for the early detection and treatment of premalignant and malignant conditions of the skin is advisable, especially in the tropics.

VITILIGO

Hindustani name is "phuleri".

Definition

It is an acquired idiopathic pigmentary anomaly of the skin manifested by depigmented white patches surrounded by a normal or a hyper-pigmented border. The depigmented skin lacks melanocytes and has markedly diminished capacity to react to topically applied sensitizing substances.

Incidence

Worldwide distribution. It is most common in India (Gujarat and Rajasthan), Egypt and other tropical countries. Affects all age groups with no predilection to either sex. Many cases start at the age of five, fifteen and at menopause.

Etiopathogenesis

Four possible mechanisms (which are not mutually exclusive) that explain the pathogenesis of vitiligo are autoimmunity, neurohumoral factors, autocytotoxicity and exogenous chemical exposure.

Autoimmunity

Patients with vitiligo have increased organ specific autoantibodies including antibodies against adrenal cytoplasm, thyroid cytoplasm, thyroglobulin, gastric parietal cells and pancreatic islet cells. Autoimmunity has been blamed but in reality, it is a reaction pattern to drugs, infections and toxin, but not a cause per se.

Neurohumoral

It suggests that a neurotoxic agent, possibly nor epinephrine or some other catecholamine, is released at peripheral nerve endings in the skin that may inhibit melanogenesis and could have a toxic effect on melanocytes. Due to disturbances of autonomic nervous system, this hypothesis best explains the segmental cases of vitiligo.

Auto toxicity

Also known as the Self-destruct theory of Lerner. It suggests that melanocytes destroy themselves due to a defect of a natural protective mechanism that removes toxic melanin precursors.

Exogenous chemical exposure

Thiols, phenolic compounds catechol, derivatives of catechol, mercaptoamines, several quinines produce depigmentation through inhibition of tyrosinase and a direct cytotoxic action on the melanocyte.

Etiology

Genetic predisposition

Inherited disease transmitted as an autosomal dominant characteristic with variable expressivity. About 35% of the patients with a family history of vertigo develop this disorder.

Important known causative factors are:

Nutritional

Defects in copper, proteins and vitamins in diet; digestive upsets like amebiasis, helminthes, chronic diarrhea, dysentery, etc.

Endocrines

Association with thyrotoxicosis, diabetes, hypothyroidism, and acromegaly.

Trophoneurosis and Sutonomic Imbalance

Emotional stress and strain.

Infections and toxic products

Enteric fever, ill health and focal sepsis.

Drugs and Chemicals

Quinines, guanofuracin, amylphenol, chlorthiazide, broad-spectrum antibiotics, betablaeteus and chloroquin.

Other Probable Factors

Food adulterants, industrial chemicals and dyes, contaminating water, and foods.

Vitiligo has also been reported in association with pernicious anemia, Down syndrome, biliary cirrhosis, dysgammaglobulinemia and carcinoma stomach.

Pathology

A defect in enzyme tyrosinase is held responsible for vitiligo. Melatonin, a substance secreted in nerve endings inhibits tyrosinase, thus interfering in pigment formation. There is a marked absence of melanocytes and melanin in the epidermis. Histochemical studies show a lack of dopa-positive melanocytes in the basal layer of the epidermis. In the epidermis of the areas around the margins of vitiligo are abnormalities of the keratinocytes as well as degenerating melanocytes. In active cases, mononuclear hugging at the junction of the lesion and normal skin is a prominent feature.

There is an increased cellularity of the dermis and occasional colloid amyloid bodies are found. In inflammatory vitiligo, where there is a raised erythematous border, there is an infiltrate of lymphocytes and histiocytes. This infiltrate is also found in the marginal areas of some biopsies.

Clinical Features

Vitiligo can begin at any age, but in 50% of cases it develops before the age of 20 years. The condition is slowly progressive.

Distribution

The amelanotic macules in vitiligo are found particularly in areas that are normally hyperpigmented, for example the face, axillae, groins, areolae and genitalia. Areas subjected to repeated friction and trauma are also likely to be affected for example the dorsa of hands, feet, elbows, knees and ankles. The distribution of the lesions is usually symmetrical, although sometimes it is unilateral and may have a dermatomal arrangement. Rarely, there is complete vitiligo, but a few pigmented areas always remain.

The pigment loss may be partial or complete or both may occur in the same areas (trichrome vitiligo).

Hypomelanotic macules are usually first noted on the sun-exposed areas of skin, on the face or dorsa of hands. These areas are prone to sunburn. Rarely, itching in the absence of sunburn may occur. Damage to the 'normal' skin frequently results in an area of depigmentation-an isomorphic or Köebner phenomenon.

Completely depigmented merciless and patches of varying sizes and shapes surrounded by a normal or hyper-pigmented border characterize it. Very rarely the patches may have a red inflammatory border. The hair in the vitiliginous area usually becomes white also. Patient's skin is susceptible to even minor trauma; it heals with depigmentation.

Early lesion may be pale white and ill defined. At this stage, Wood's lamp helps to confirm the diagnosis.

Onset is slow and *course* insidious. It may continue to increase slowly or come to a halt, and then increase again.

At times lesions develop along the distribution of a peripheral nerve (zosteriform vitiligo).

Occasionally, vitiligo develops around pigmented moles (Halonevus).

Vitiligo like leucoderma may occur in melanoma patients. Lesions tend to develop in trauma prone areas. A Koebner reaction may occur.

The white patches are hypersensitive to ultra violet light and burn readily when exposed to the sun. It is not unusual to note the onset of vitiligo after severe sunburn.

Four types have been described according to extent and distribution of involved areas:

a) Localized (including a linear or segmented pattern).

b) Generalized.

c) Universal.

d) Perinevic (halonevus).

Clinical Criteria for Classification of Vitiligo

(Stage of vitiligo – V)

- Active (V)
    - New lesions developing.
    - Lesion increasing in size.
    - Border ill defined.
- Quiescent/Stable (V2)
    - No new lesion developing.
    - Lesion stationary in size.
    - Border hyper-pigmented and well defined.
- Improving (V3)
    - Lesions decreasing in size.

- No new lesions developing.
- Border defined and signs of spontaneous repigmentation (follicular and peripheral).

- Zosteriformis/Segmental.
  - Unilateral distribution of lesions, preferably along the course of nerves.

A few researchers have found a high percentage of ocular abnormalities such as abnormal pigmentation in the fundus, idiopathic uveitis, and sensorineural hypoacusis in a few vitiligo cases.

Diagnosis

It is usually apparent. Wood's lamp is of great help in diagnosis.

Differential Diagnosis

- Morphoea in which the skin is ivory colored, shiny and adherent to the underlying tissue.
- Leprosy – In vitiligo texture and sensations are normal.
- Seborrhoeides and Pityriasis – Absence of scaling, crusting and itching in vitiligo.
- White anetoderma, in which lesions are small, well defined and depressed below the surface of the skin.
- Pinta and Syphilitic leuco-melanoderma with the help of serology and other clinical stigmata.
- Leucoderma following herpes zoster may be difficult to distinguish from vitiligo.

'Leucodermoid' is a term coined to describe leucoderma like lesions at an early stage when the features are not definite and observation is necessary to come to a conclusion.

Prognosis

Resistant Areas

1. Lips, over the joints, acral areas.

F- 33

2. Patches with depigmented hair.

3. Patches with thickened integument, scaly and tendency to fibrosis.

4. Pale patches with lack of vascularity (do not bleed easily).

Reasons for Poor Response to Treatment:

1. Poor nutrition and general health.

2. Emotional stress and strain.

3. Recurrent /intercurrent infections.

4. Prolonged/repeated antibiotic courses.

5. Bad digestion, diarrhea and dysentery.

6. Extensive, galloping variety.

7. Leucotrichia / Mucosal involvement.

8. Endemic areas.

9. Age above 60.

PIEBALDISM

Etiology

This condition is also termed as 'Partial albinism' or 'White spotting' and is inherited as an autosomal dominant disorder, affecting the differentiation and possibly the migration of melanoblasts.

Pathology

Ultrastructural studies have shown either an absence of melanocytes and melanosomes in the hypomelanotic areas or sometimes reduced numbers of abnormal, large melanocytes.

Clinical Features

Patches of skin totally devoid of pigment are present at birth, which usually remain unchanged throughout life.

Patient has a mesh of white hair (white forelock), which arises from a triangular or diamond-shaped midline white macule on the frontal scalp or center of the forehead. The medial portions of the eyebrows, and eyelashes, may be white. There may be circumscribed, and at times symmetrical, areas of hypomelanosis on the upper chest, abdomen, arms and legs. The hands and feet, as well as the back, remain normally pigmented. A characteristic feature of piebaldism is the presence of hyperpigmented macules within the areas of lack of pigmentation and also on normally pigmented skin.

Differential Diagnosis

- In vitiligo, the lesions tend to appear later in life and their distribution is quite different. In piebaldism, there is almost invariably a white forelock and the pattern of arrangement of the lesions is quite characteristic. Also the presence of islands of normal pigmented skin in the hypomelanotic areas is typical.

- If the interpupillary distance is increased or the patient is deaf, the diagnosis of Wardenburg's syndrome must be considered.

- The patterns of hypomelanosis as seen in the localized and systematized types of naevus depigmentosus differ from piebaldism. Microscopy of the skin in naevus depigmentosus reveals normal numbers of melanocytes with sometimes rather stubby dendrites.

PHENYLKETONURIA

It is an inborn error of metabolism in which phenylalanine accumulates and impairs the melanin biosynthesis. The skin and hair are fair and there is mental retardation.

TIETZ'S SYNDROME

Here there is a total absence of the melanin pigment in the skin and hair, with normal pigmentation of the eyes, complete deaf-mutism and hypoplasia of the eyebrows. An autosomal dominant gene could be responsible for it.

WARDENBURG'S SYNDROME

Definition

This condition manifests as a white forelock and cochlear deafness, and is determined by an autosomal dominant gene. Some abnormality of the development of neural crest derivatives is postulated.

Pathology

Ultrastructural studies on the amelanotic skin show an absence of melanocytes. In the pigmented areas, there are abnormalities of the melanocytes and melanosomes.

Clinical Features

The changes are present since birth. There is lateral displacement of the medial canthi with dystopia canthorum, hypertrophy of the nasal root, hyperplasia of the eyebrows and the brows may be confluent. In a few cases there is partial or total heterochromia of the iris; the hypopigmented and hypoplastic iris is light blue. Also there is perceptive deafness in a few cases with a white forelock, and piebaldism. Abnormal patterns of hair growth have been noted in several cases.

Hypomelanotic Macules of Tuberous Sclerosis

This is a neurocutaneous disorder, which presents as spasms in an infant with irregularly scattered, lance-ovate or ash-leaf shaped hypomelanotic macules, and is transmitted as an autosomal dominant trait. Electron microscopy of the macules shows the presence of melanocytes, which contain fewer and smaller melanosomes than normal.

Naevus Depigmentosus

This condition is also termed as 'Achromic Naevus'.

It presents as circumscribed areas of depigmentation right since birth, where the lesions are often single (but may be multiple), circumscribed, and either rounded, dermatomal or in bizarre whorls and streaks in a marble-like pattern. Ectodermal and neurological abnormalities are often present.

Incontinentia Pigmenti Achromians of ito

This condition is also termed as 'Hypomelanosis of Ito', and here there are characteristic whorl-shaped depigmented areas present all over the body since birth, and can gradually progressive. These spots can get repigmented. There are associative affection of the musculoskeletal system, teeth, eyes and central nervous system. Convulsions and mental deficiency are common accompaniment. In this condition there is no basal layer damage and no pigmentary incontinence.

VOGT-KOYANAGI SYNDROME

Synonym

Harada's syndrome, or Vogt-Koyanagi-Harada (VKHS) syndrome.

Etiology

This syndrome affects the skin, eyes, inner ears and meninges of patients in their third and fourth decades, though children may also be affected in a few cases. There is no attributable cause, except for an abnormal response to a virus and immunological mechanism noted.

Pathology

There is an absence of melanocytes, which seem to be replaced by Langerhans' cells and by indeterminate dendritic cells, as in vitiligo. Colloid-amyloid bodies are also found at the dermo-epidermal junction.

Clinical Features

Prodromal period includes fever and malaise, with encephalitic or meningitic symptoms (like headache, nausea, vomiting) and lymphocytosis of the cerebrospinal fluid. After a week or two after the above symptoms there is a rapidly occurring bilateral uveitis, choroiditis and optic neuritis, resulting in decreased visual acuity, blindness or photophobia, followed by deafness or diminished hearing and tinnitus. Then within the first 3 months, symmetrical vitiligo, poliosis (involving especially the brows, lashes and scalp) and alopecia may develop. Vision is usually lost due to uveitis, though the hearing is usually completely restored.

Diagnosis

The association of vitiligo with loss of pigment in brows and lashes and with the residual ocular defects should clearly differentiate this syndrome from any other. In Alezzandrini's syndrome, the loss of pigment is unilateral and is associated with retinal degeneration.

ALEZZANDRINI'S SYNDROME

This rare syndrome is characterized by a unilateral impairment of vision from a degenerative retinitis, followed after several months by vitiligo on the face with poliosis on the same side. Bilateral perceptive deafness may also develop.

HALO NAEVUS

Synonym

Sutton's naevus; Leukoderma acquisitum centrifugum.

Definition

In this condition there is a characteristic halo of hypopigmentation around a central cutaneous tumor, usually a benign melanocytic naevus, usually seen in children or young people. Multiple halo naevi may occur in patients with melanoma.

Etiology

It is usually seen in patients with certain organ-specific autoimmune disorders, and is often associated with vitiligo.

Pathology

A lymphocytic infiltration of the naevus and damaged constituent cells are seen. In the depigmented halo, there is an absence of melanocytes, but Langerhans' cells are present. Melanophages are often present in the dermis.

Clinical Features

Circular areas of hypomelanosis are seen around the pigmented naevi, especially on the trunk and head. The naevus tends to flatten and may disappear completely. The depigmented areas often persist, but may pigment after many years.

ACQUIRED HYPOMELANOSIS

Here disorders in which there is an acquired loss of melanin pigment are noted.

Chemical Depigmentation

A number of chemicals coming in contact with the skin, either due to occupational or therapeutic reasons, come under this classification. The most frequently seen chemicals known to cause depigmentation are substituted phenols like hydroquinone (occupational or due to use in the treatment of hypermelanosis), 4-Tertiary butylcatechol or butyl phenol (occupational). Experimental studies indicate that these substituted phenols have a selective lethal effect on functional melanocytes. The areas most frequently affected are the dorsal surface of the hands. The depigmented areas frequently enlarge, and new ones appear even after the patient is no longer in contact.

Post-inflammatory Depigmentation & Infections

In a few cases, areas of hypomelanosis are seen to occur after resolution of an eczematous or psoriatic patch. This is also the case in pityriasis lichenoides chronica, pityriasis rosea, leprosy, sarcoidosis, lupus erythematosus, herpes zoster, mycosis fungoides, scleroderma, lichen planus, and cutaneous T-cell lymphoma. In cases of pityriasis alba and tinea versicolor, white scaly hypopigmented macules are seen. In a few cases there are hyperpigmented patches along with the hypopigmented ones. In cases of syphilis, there is a leuko-melanoderma seen. There is a loss of functional melanocytes in most cases. Burns, scars, postdermabrasion, and intralesional steroid injections with depigmentation are other examples where hypopigmentation occurs.

IDIOPATHIC GUTTATE HYPOMELANOSIS

Synonym

Leukopathia symmetrica progressiva, disseminate lenticular leukoderma.

Clinical Features

It is a commonly seen condition in white people after the age of 40 years, especially affecting women more than men. It is caused by solar damage, and is often mistaken for vitiligo. The lesions present as small, irregularly shaped, porcelain-white macules, with well-defined edges, especially on the shins and forearms. They rarely become very numerous (a dozen or two at the most), and never occur on the trunk or face. Histologically, there is a decrease in the number of melanocytes, many of which lack mature melanosomes. The disorder results from an age-related somatic mutation of melanocytes.

Symmetrical Progressive Leukopathy

This condition is commonly seen in Japan and Brazil. It presents as punctate leukoderma in young adults, symmetrically on the front of the shins and on the extensor aspects of the arms, and less often on the abdomen and interscapular region.

Hypopigmentation due to endocrine disorders

This is especially seen in cases of hypopituitarism, Addison's disease, and thyroid disease.

Miscellaneous Disorders

Hypopigmentation of the skin can be seen in cases of kwashiorkor and chronic protein deficiency, and vitamin B12 deficiency.

HOMEOPATHIC APPROACH OF HYPERMELANOSIS

Although constitutional prescription would be the right method of approach, I can discuss some remedies that I have used successfully in my practice.

- *Berberis vulgaris* is a very useful remedy for circumscribed brown pigmentation following eczematous inflammation.

- A person who has a tendency to develop numerous moles and numerous pigmented nevi and excessive amount of lentigo requires *Carcinosinum*.

- *Nitricum acidum* patient may have typical pigmented warty spots on the forehead.

- In chloasma, remedies like *Lilium tig. Caulophyllum* and *Sepia* are useful.

- In *Sepia* one gets a typical saddle-like brown discoloration across the bridge of the nose or freckles or patchy pigmentation may be present over the cheeks or be scattered all over the body.

HOMEOPATHIC APPROACH TO VITILIGO

Miasmatically vitiligo of primary origin is basically *tubercular miasm* whereas post primary vitiligo, which is due to destruction of melanocytes secondary to eczema or cellulites or dermatitis or burns or chemical injury, signifies syphilitic miasm. In primary vitiligo we do not encounter any symptoms associated with it and hence this resembles one-sided disease as explained by Dr. Samuel Hahnemann in § 173 (§172-§184) of Organon of Medicine.

HOMEOPATHIC TREATMENT OF PRIMARY VITILIGO

In my experience I have encountered following causative factors where the vitiligo spots / depigmentation have started after certain emotions, e.g.

- A/F cares, worries.
- Mortification.
- Indignation.
- Grief.
- Emotional excitement.
- Anger suppressed.
- Death of near and dear ones.
- Divorce.
- Shock.
- Embarrassment.

At the physical level, the following history have been confirmed repeatedly, e.g. P/H of amoebic colitis, chronic diarrhea, tuberculosis, thyroid disorders, warts.

Associated physical conditions were seen in many vitiligo patients, e.g. worms, thyroid disorders, warts, moles.

Methodology

Ideally the case has to be studied trying to find out the deepest feeling of the patient and thereby trying to study the patient behind the vitiligo than the vitiligo itself. This means to find out a constitutional remedy. Once the remedy is selected which covers the mental symptoms along with physical generals, enough time should be given for the remedy to act. I prefer to start the medicine with a medium potency of 200 without repeating for at least 2 months. Once the response is there, it is advisable not to repeat. Once the response stops, I prefer to repeat the same potency and then if further no improvement, the repetition is more frequent. If however, the response is still not there, then it is advisable to confirm the symptoms once again and then either one should change the remedy or to step up the potency of the previous remedy. This you should continue till the results are achieved.

After years of experience, I have come to conclusion that vitiligo patients require frequent repetition. Also, some of the cases require not only frequent repetition, but also frequent change in the potency.

I would like to warn the readers, not to indiscriminately use nosodes like Thuja and Bacillinum without matching the symptoms as this only leads to drugging and suppression of the symptoms.

Diet and Regimen

I have not imposed any specific dietetic rules for vitiligo a patient other than that is required for homeopathic treatment.

Finally, I would like to summarize by stressing upon the fact that constitutional medicine is the main stay.

Some rare remedies, which I have used with successful results, are *Berberis vulgaris, Mica* and *Pituitaria posterior*.

SOME IMPORTANT HOMEOPATHIC REMEDIES

Alum, ant-t, ars, ars-s-f, amm-c, aur, bac, berb, calc, cob, cob-n, calc-f, calc-sil, carbo-an, graph, hydrc, ign, kreos, merc, mez, mica, nat-c, nat-m, nit-ac, nat-ar, phos, pitu, sep, sil, sulph, stann, thuj, tub.

Some Therapeutic Hints

My interest in homeopathy has attracted me to many homeopaths all over the world and I would like to share some of the hints;

1. *Psoralea cor.* Q applied on the skin, diluted in water with a proportion of 110. Also Psorlea Cor 30 can be used in a similar way. These hints come from my experience with Calcutta homeopaths.

2. Dr. Rashid Wadia, I have seen prescribing *Hydrocotyle asiatica* in higher potencies.

3. A physician from Muzzafarpur, Bihar, uses potentized *Mica* or *Mica* 30 on infrequent repetition prolonged usage with good results.

ICHTHYOSES

It constitutes a group of genetic and acquired disorders characterized by accumulation of scales on the skin surfaces. There is dryness, roughness and scaliness of the integument resulting from deficient secretions and abnormal keratinization.

This condition appearing at birth is known to get worse in the cold of winter and seems to clear of, as the weather becomes warmer.

Classification of Ichthyoses

Primary ichthyoses

1. Ichthyosis Vulgaris.
2. Recessive X-linked ichthyosis (RXLI).
3. Epidermolytic hyperkeratosis.
4. Autosomal recessive ichthyosis (lamellar ichthyosis and non-bullous congenital ichthyosiform erythroderma).

Related disorders of cornification

1. Ichthyosis linearis circumflexa.
2. Erythrokeratoderma variabilis.
3. Harlequin foetus.

Ichthyosiform syndromes

1. Chanarin syndrome (neutral storage disease).
2. Sjoren-Larsson syndrome.

3. Refsum's disease.

4. Rud's disease.

5. Trichothiodystrophy.

6. Keratitis-ichthyosis-deafness (KID) syndrome.

7. Ichthyosis hysterix (epidermal naevus syndrome).

Acquired ichthyoses

1. Drug induced ichthyosis.

2. Essential fatty acid deficiency induced ichthyosis.

3. Malignancy-associated ichthyosis.

4. Xerosis of hypothyroidism.

5. Environmental xerosis.

6. Ichthyosis associated with diseases like sarcoidosis and leprosy.

In the primary forms of genetic ichthyosis the manifestations are confined only to the skin. In addition, a variety of other disorders of cornification, characterized by multisystem involvement, with cutaneous manifestations forming a part component of symptomatology are termed 'Ichthyosiform Syndromes'.

Pathophysiology

The pathophysiology of ichthyoses is debatable. Lamellar ichthyosis and bullous ichthyosis (epidermolytic hyeprkeratosis) are characterized by an increase in the number of cells entering division and a reduced epidermal transit time. These abnormalities are similar to those observed in psoriatic epidermis. The scaling in these disorders is due to failure of desquamation to compensate for an enhanced rate of formation of stratum corneum. In ichthyosis vulgaris and recessive X-linked ichthyosis the mitotic indices and cell transit time are normal / decreased. The primary abnormality in these is greater than normal corneocyte cohesion resulting in a thicker stratum corneum and decrease in the normal rate of desquamation. Hence, these are also termed retention ichthyoses.

Clinical Presentation

Site of affection

- Extensor surfaces of the trunk and the extremities.
- The whole integument seems to exhibit some degree of dryness.

Features of primary ichthyosis are as follows:

1. Ichthyosis

Mode of inheritance: Autosomal dominant.

Age of onset: 14 years.

Histopathology: Normal epidermis; reduced or absent granular layer; sparse dermal infiltrate.

Epidermal transit: 14 days.

Clinical features: Small, white, pasted scales. Keratosis pilaris.

Distribution: Back and extensors spared.

Course: Spontaneous improvement with age.

Associations: Atopy.

2. X-linked ichthyosis

Mode of inheritance: X-linked recessive.

Age of onset: Early infancy.

Histopathology: Acanthosis; normal granular layer; dermal infiltrate.

Epidermal transit: 14 days.

Clinical features: Large dark brown scales.

Distribution: Front of trunk, scalp, sides of face, encroaches on flexures.

Course: Persistent.

Associations: Corneal opacity, deficient steroid sulfatase.

3. Lamellar ichthyosis

Mode of inheritance: Autosomal recessive.

Age of onset: At birth.

Histopathology: Slight epidermal thickening; marked hypergranulosis; and marked compact hyperkeratosis.

Epidermal transit: 4 days.

Clinical features: Polygonal, shield-like adherent scales, state grey or black in color.

Distribution: Entire skin surface.

Course: Persistent.

Associations: Collodion baby; Ectropion; Eclabion.

4. Nonbullous congenital ichthyosiform erythroderma

Mode of inheritance: Autosomal recessive.

Age of onset: At birth

Histopathology: Marked epidermal thickening; and parakeratosis.

Epidermal transit: 4 days.

Clinical features: Fine white scales. Marked erythema. Sparsity of scalp hair.

Distribution: Entire skin surface.

Course: Persistent.

Associations: CNS abnormalities; Immunological abnormalities.

5. Epidermolytic hyperkeratosis

Mode of inheritance: Autosomal dominant.

Age of onset: At birth or shortly after.

Histopathology: Acanthosis; Accentuations of rete ridges; Vacuolar degenerative changes in the upper segment of epidermis.

Nuclei appear pyknotic; Abnormal keratohyaline granules; Upper dermal edema; Dermal lympho-histiocytic infiltrate.

Epidermal transit: 4 days.

Clinical features: Generalized erythema, scaling and blister formation. Blistering resolves by 7-8 years. Erythema resolves by middle age. Hyperkeratosis persists throughout life.

Distribution: Trauma prone areas.

Course: Persistent.

Associations: Ectropion; Crumpled ears.

Ichthyosis is symptomless except for a dry uncomfortable feeling which becomes worse in winters due to reduction in normal sweating and when the skin needs extra lubrication.

There may be mild itching. The mental stress that occurs is attributed mainly to the appalling look of the skin especially in young females. There is no association with atopy.

Complication

Chronic folliculitis and eczemas is quiet common. Severe erythrodermic variety of ichthyosis is called Congenital Ichthyosiform Erythroderma.

Diagnosis

Typical cases hardly present any difficulty in diagnosis. Onset of the disease in adults warrants a through search for an acquired cause e.g. reticulosis, leprosy and drugs. It may be supplemented by histopathological examination.

Prognosis

The malady progresses to a certain degree till puberty when it becomes stationary. There is no spontaneous recovery. Though the condition cannot be cured it can be considerably helped.

Treatment

1. **Climate:** The patient should live in a warm climate, which is to a certain degree, humid.

2. The general health should be kept at an optimal level. Vitamin A in large doses helps some cases. Thyroid and injection pilocarpine may also benefit temporarily.

3. Local treatment ameliorates the condition considerably. It consists of:

    (a) A daily warm bath.

    (b) A warm oil or ghee massage as often as possible.

    (c) Superfatted soap only is to be used.

    (d) 10 p.c. Urea and 5p.c. Lactic acid ointment in eucerine or vaseline base or coconut oil.

    (e) Ichthyosis vulgaris and X-linked can be managed by daily application of emollients or 40 to 60% propylene glycol in water, applied under occlusion overnight, two or three times a week.

    (f) Lamellar ichthyosis requires topical application of retinoic acid.

    (g) Sunbaths and U.V.R. exposure may help some cases temporarily.

4. Patient must be advised regarding selection of suitable occupation in order to prevent the development of pyodermas and eczemas.

HOMEOPATHIC APPROACH TO ICHTHYOSIS

The treatment for this condition is purely constitutional.

In cases with a strong family history, Syphilinum in LM potency over a prolonged period of time has given me good results.

Many a times I advice the use of Arnica mother tincture diluted with water in the proportion of 2:8 to reduce the itching that arises due to dry skin.

REPERTORY

The rubric is seen under

SKIN - ERUPTIONS - scaly – ichthyosis – Phos, ars-i, ars, hydrc, nat-c, plb, anag, aur, calc, chin, clem, coloc, graph, hep, lac-c, lac-d, lyc, mez, ol-j, petr, pip-m, platan-or, plb, sep, sil, sulph, syph, thuj, thyr, v-a-b.

■

Chapter-26

Pemphigus Vulgaris

Diagnostic Hallmarks

1. *Distribution* – Oral mucus membranes and upper trunk.
2. *Lesions* – Large shallow erosions, which heal very slowly.
3. *Biopsy* – Acantholytic intraepidermal bulla.
4. *Immunofluorescent studies* -- IgG in a network around epidermal cells.

Epidemiology

Equal frequency in men and women.

Common age group of affection is 25-50 years, though in a few rare cases, children may also be affected.

Pathogenesis

Pemphigus is considered to be an autoimmune disease. IgG antibody and sometimes complement are deposited at the site of epidermal cell damage; these same antibodies are regularly found in women.

The antigens responsible for this autoimmune reaction are unknown but they appear to be located on the exterior surface of certain epithelial cells. Further evidence of an autoimmune etiology includes the frequent association of pemphigus with other autoimmune diseases and the occasional presence of a thymoma.

Drug induced pemphigus: Thiopronine, penicillin, captopral, rifampin.

Direct IF test is of great value in the early diagnosis of pemphigus vulgaris. Direct IF test remains positive for a long time and may still be positive many years after disease has subsided and treatment has been discontinued.

The pathologic changes are acantholysis, cleft and blister formation in the intraepidermal areas just above the basal cell layer, and the formation of acantholytic cells.

Clinical Features

Pemphigus vulgaris is characterized by thin walled, relatively flaccid, easily ruptured bullae appearing upon either apparently normal skin and mucus membranes or on erythematous bases. The fluid in the bullae is clear at first, but may become hemorrhagic or even seropurulent. The bullae soon rupture to form erosions, raw surfaces which ooze and bleed easily. The denuded areas soon become partially covered with crusts, with little or no tendency to heal, and enlarge by confluence. The healed lesions often leave hyperpigmented patches, however, there is no scarring. Lesions appear first in the mouth and next most commonly in the groin, scalp, face, neck, axillae or genitals. The nail folds maybe involved first, together with mouth lesions.

The *Nikolsky sign* is present; that is, there is an absence of cohesion in the epidermis, so that the upper layers are easily made to slip laterally by slight pressure or rubbing. This sign is variously elicited The upper layers of the epidermis may easily be removed by a twisting pressure with the fingertip, leaving a moist surface. The lack of cohesion of the skin layers may also be demonstrated with the 'bullae spread phenomenon' by pressure on an intact bulla, gently forcing the fluid to wander under the skin away from the pressure site *(the Asboe - Hansen sign)*.

Mouth lesions appear first in 60% of the cases; the short-lived bullae quickly rupture to involve most of the mucosa in a painful erosion. The lesions extend out onto the lips and form heavy, fissured crusts on the vermilion. Involvement of throat produces hoarseness and difficulty in swallowing. Mouth odour is offensive and penetratingly unpleasant. The resultant malnutrition contributes to increased debility.

Oesophagus may be involved with sloughing of its entire lining in the form of a cast (oesophagitis dissecans superficialis). Wood et al described a patient in whom hematemesis proved to be due to pemphigus of the oesophagus. The conjunctiva, nasal mucosa, vagina, penis and anus may also be involved.

The initial lesions are usually found on the upper trunk and back but since new lesions develop faster than old ones heal, there is gradual extension elsewhere with special predeliction for face, groin and axillae. The prominence of these crusted erosions often obscures the fact that the patient has infact a bullous disease.

The disease may be complicated by:

1. Secondary impetigo, ulceration and even gangrene.

2. A gastrointestinal upset and debility.

3. Lung complications like pneumonia.

Any of these complications may be combined with toxaemia and exhaustion, which may cause ultimate death.

Diagnosis

TZANCK TEST: It is carried out by lightly scrapping the floor of a bulla after the roof has been removed. The scraped material is spread on a slide, stained with Geimsa's stain and examined under a microscope for characteristic acantholytic cells. The test is positive in pemphigus vulgaris, foliaceus, vegetans and Senear-Usher Syndrome.

Differential Diagnosis

Pemphigus may be confused with dermatitis herpetiformis, erythema multiforme and pemphigoid. The following features will serve to distinguish them:

- In *Erythema Multiforme Bullosum*, besides bullae oedematous macules may be seen; lesions are usually bilaterally symmetrical and confined to extremities; the disease lasts for 3-4 weeks. Bullae develop on erythematous bases.

- A *Drug Eruption* resulting from the ingestion of phenobarbitone, penicillin, phenolphthalein, iodides and bromides may resemble pemphigus. History of ingestion of drug and disappearance of bullous drug rash when drug is withdrawn confirms the diagnosis.

- The lesion of pemphigus on the buccal mucosa may suggest *Diphtheria or Syphilis*. The demonstration of the bacilli in the former and positive serological tests in the latter, would confirm the diagnosis.

Course and Prognosis

Pemphigus begins most commonly in mid to late adult life. It is a chronic disease which, left untreated lead to severe debility and death. With vigorous early treatment the mortality rate is approximately 15%. Other autoimmune diseases are found with unexpected frequency in patients with pemphigus and a small but significant number of patients have thymomas and a variety of other internal malignancies.

HOMEOPATHIC APPROACH TO PEMPHIGUS VULGARIS

Whenever a homeopath is confronted with a bullous eruption, answers to the following questions must be sought:

(a) Is the eruption localized, regional or generalized?

(b) Has it symmetrical or asymmetrical distribution?

(c) Is it groove or discrete, polymorphous or monomorphous?

(d) Are the mucous membranes involved?

(e) Do the bullae occur as such or on erythematous bases?

(f) Are they tense or flaccid, with serous or purulent content?

(g) What are the shapes and sizes of bullae?

(h) Any Nikolsky's sign?

(i) Are there accompanying signs like itching or pain?

(j) Any accompanying crusting or scaling?

(k) What kind of surface does one see when the roof of the bullae is removed?

(l) How is the general health of the individual and are there any toxic symptoms?

Constitutional treatment and good nursing is very essential.

Locally, the bullae must not be ruptured and linen dipped in a mixture of *Calendula* external and water in the ratio of 1:4 should be applied to prevent secondary infection.

The patient must be protected from cold.

The diet must be nutritious.

When blisters are present in the mouth, the patient has difficulty in mastication and swallowing, so give bland fluids or semi-solid diet.

Whenever the skin around the eye is involved, the eye should be cleaned with dilute solution of *Euphrasia* preferably 130.

Some Important Homeopathic Remedies

Anacardium orientale: Great burning of skin with scarlet redness over the whole body. The body is covered with blisters from the size of a pinhead to pea. Presence of intense itching with mental irritability. It is worse in the evening and by application of hot water.

Antipyrinum: Erythema with intense itching. Bullae appear and disappear quite soon. Pemphigus affects the mucus membrane of the oral cavity which is characterized by burning of mouth and gums; ulceration of lips and tongue, with edema and puffiness of face.

Arsenicum album: Intense itching, burning and swelling due to bullous eruptions, which have a tendency to either suppurate or turn gangrenous. The burning and itching severely < cold application < scratching. The patient is extremely restless and develops early prostration in the sickness. Patient feels better with warm application. There is aggravation of all the complaints.

Arum triphyllum: Appearance of skin is scarlet red with raw bloody surface everywhere. The discharges that ooze from the bullae are very acrid and produce inflammation and destruction of surrounding tissues. Special affinity for mucus membrane of oral cavity where it produces mucosal lesion of pemphigus. Sore, raw, burning feeling in oral cavity. Corners of mouth sore and cracked. Throat is swollen burns and is extremely raw. The patient is hot and gets < in a warm room.

Bufo rana: Itching and burning sensation in bullae > bathing in cold water. The bullae tend to suppurate easily. Bullae, which open and leave a raw surface, exuding an ichorous fluid. Bullae on palms and soles. Marked Lymphangitis of the surrounding part.

Caltha palustris: Bullae surrounded by a ring and they itch greatly. On the 3rd day they are transformed into crusts. Much itching. Face is swollen especially around the eyes. Bullae have tendency to suppurate easily.

Cantharis vesicatoria: Presence of bullous eruptions showing excessive tendency to turn gangrenous. There is presence of burning sensation, which is relieved by cold application. There is ulcerative pain in the lesion whenever it is touched. There is generalized oversensitiveness, accompanied by excessive weakness. Urinary troubles can be important concomitants.

Causticum: Large bullae on the chest and back with sensation of soreness. Patient feels better in a warm room and warm weather. Sensation of burning, itching and rawness. Progressive weakness. Warts, long-standing worries and local paralysis are important concomitants.

Carboneum oxygenisatum: The whole skin is covered with large and small vesicles of pemphigus. Sleepiness and coldness on the surface, especially hands are icy cold.

Copaiva officinalis: First mucous membrane is affected and then the skin. Excessive fetid discharge. Past history of gonorrhea.

Crotalus horridus: Pemphigus with low typhoid like or septic condition. The contained fluid assumes a dark, bloody character, threatening gangrene. The eruptions are surrounded by purplish mottled skin and edema. Pemphigus may alternate with internal affections like diarrhoea.

Dulcamara: Face, genitalia and hands. A thick, brown yellowish discharge oozes out which later on turns into crust. There is presence of pruritis, which is worse in cold wet weather. Glands surrounding the pemphigus get enlarged and suppurated. Eruptions < during menses.

Juglans cinerea: Eruptions that start in the axilla and then spread to the back and chest. Presence of itching and burning, which is > scratching. GI concomitants are usually associated with pemphigus.

Lachesis mutus: Eruptions are bluish black, the fluid within the vesicles is hemorrhagic and individual bulla is surrounded by purplish blue discoloration. The eruption has tendency to develop gangrenous condition which later on turns into gangrenous ulcers. Presence of severe prostration, inflammation, fever, quick intermittent pulse, fainting, nausea, spasmodic and bilious vomiting, convulsions and cold sweat.

Mancinella: Very large blisters which, when ripe, turns into heavy brown crusts. The serum that oozes out from bullae is extremely sticky. Depressed mental state and pain in thumb.

Mercurius corrosivus: Burning and redness of skin with formation of bullae. The eruptions gradually lead to ulceration with swelling of gland. Past history of gonorrhea or bloody dysentery are important concomitants.

Ranunculus bulbosus: Constantly repeating eruptions or blisters, secreting an offensive gluey matter forming crust and healing from the center. The acrid discharge makes the surrounding part sore. Burning and itching < slightest touch. Skin is sensitive to cold air.

Ranunculus sceleratus: Large, isolated blisters, which burst and form an ulcer, are discharging acrid, ichor making the surrounding part sore. There is boring. and gnawing pain within the vesicle.

Rhus toxicodendron: Confluent blisters, containing a milky or watery fluid with peeling of skin. The skin appears red and swollen. The bullous eruption suppurates very easily. Burning and itching < scratching > local heat < night, weather wet > dry weather.

Scrophularia nodosa: In and about the ears, bullous eruption turns gangrenous.

Thuja occidentale: Bullous eruptions on covered parts. Extremely offensive discharge. Itching and burning < evening, night, after scratching, > touch

REPERTORY

- **Skin, eruptions,** pemphigus: acon, anac, antip, ars, arum-t, bry, bell, bufo, calc, calth, canth, carbn-o, caust, chin, chin-s, cop, chloral, crot-h, cur, dulc, gamb, hep, hydrc, jug-c, lach, lipp, lyc, manc, merc, merc-c, merc-s, nat-m, nat-s, nat-sal, nit-ac, ph-ac, phos, psor, ran-b, ran-s, raph, rhus-t, sars, scroph-xyz, sep, sil, sul-ac, sulph, syph, thuj, merc-pr-rub.

  - Each bulla with a red areola: rhus-t.

  - Benign: hydrocort.

  - Blisters constantly repeating, secreting a foul smelling, gluey material, forming crusts and healing from center: ran-b.

  - Blisters small and on highly inflamed surface (tonsillitis): lyc.

- Children, in (neonatorum): acon, bell, bry, calc, cham, dulc, merc, psor, ran-b, rhus-t, sulph.
- Blisters, two, three or four inches in diameter: Ran-b, sil.
- Infant: ran-s.
- Fever low, parts bluish and discharge scanty, tardy or dark fluid, unhealthy: crot.
- Foliaceous: ars, chin-ca, lach, lyc, phos, sep, thuj.
- Foliaceous, epidermis on one third of body and almost half of back raised as if by an enormous blister, serous fluid escapes through small openings: thuj.
- Large blisters burst and leave raw surfaces: ran-b.
- Looks like a pock, often confluent and persistently reappears: syph.
- Malignant: kali-p.
- Especially when painful: thuj.
- Prostration: ran-b.
- Restlessness: ran-b.
- Scarlet redness over whole body: anac.
- Squamous: sars.
- Typhoid condition, fluid assumes a dark or sanguinous character, or gangrenous threatens: crot-h.

Location

- **Mouth:** phos.
- **Extremities**
  - Upper limbs: sep, ter.
  - Wrist: sep.
  - Hand, back of: sep.
  - Fingers: lyc.
  - Thumb: lyc.

Chapter-27

Scabies

Definition

It is a common contagious skin condition, occurring due to infestation by the mite *Sarcoptes scabiei*, and is characterized by pruritic papular lesions and burrows, which house the female mite and her young.

Etiology

The itch mite Sarcoptes scabiei, of the order Acarina and class Arachnida, is the causative organism. It has an oval body and is flattened dorsoventrally. The adult female measures approximately 0.4 mm x 0.3 mm, and the smaller male 0.2 mm x 0.15mm. The body is creamy white and is marked by transverse corrugations, and on its dorsal surface by bristles and spines (denticles). There are four pairs of short legs the anterior two pairs end in elongated peduncles tipped with small suckers. In the female, the rear two pairs of legs end in long bristles (setae).

The condition is often contracted by close personal contact, and less often by common use of contaminated towels, bed linen and clothing. Predisposing factors include overcrowding, poverty and poor hygiene.

Lifecycle of the Mite

Copulation occurs in a small burrow excavated by the female in the stratum corneum. After copulation, the fertilized female enlarges the burrow and begins laying eggs, 2-3 a day, for almost 4-6 weeks. The burrow is not confined only to the stratum corneum, but is inclined downwards into the epidermis. Gradual penetration appears to occur as a result of the production of a lytic secretion by the mite, which then propels itself forward as the host tissue is dissolved. The burrow is lengthened by approximately 2-3mm daily. Eggs and mite faeces are deposited behind the female in the burrow.

The male dies after copulation, and the female dies after laying the eggs. The eggs then hatch into larvae within 4 days, and these become into nymphs and then into adults.

In the host, severe itching due to sensitization (to the parasite) begins about 2-4 weeks after the onset of infection. Re-infection of a previously cured individual, however, provokes immediate pruritus.

Histopathology

Epidermal spongiosis is seen, with intraepidermal microabscesses containing neutrophils and eosinophils, and a dermal perivascular infiltrate of eosinophils, histiocytes and lymphocytes.

In nodular lesions there is a dense, pleomorphic dermal infiltrate seen, which is composed of plasma cells, eosinophils, lymphocytes, histiocytes and reticulum cells.

T-lymphocytes are the predominant cells in the dermal infiltrate of both papular and nodular lesions.

Clinical Features

The characteristic burrows are the lesions, which appear as slightly raised, brownish or grayish, straight or tortuous lines or dots on the skin. At the point of entry of the mite, there is scale formation, and at the end of the burrow there is formation of a vesicle or pustule, adjacent to which is the female mite.

The most frequent complaint is that of persistent and intense itching, which begins 3-4 weeks after the initial infestation, and this itching tends to get worse at night and from warmth.

The sites most often infested are the finger webs, wrists, palms and soles, antecubital fossa, axilla, areola (especially in females), umbilical region, lower abdomen, genitals (especially in males), buttocks and medial aspect of the thighs. In adults, the scalp and face are usually spared, but in infants and immuno-compromised individuals, the lesions are present all over the cutaneous surface, especially on the face and scalp.

The type of infection may vary depending on the climate, the host's immune status and physical condition, and history of any previous treatment taken.

Dull red, indurated nodules, about 3-5 mm in diameter, may appear in active stages of the disease, especially on the axillae, scrotum, groins and penis. These may or may not be itchy, and may persist for weeks or months even after the scabies has been cured.

In patients who are clean and bathe frequently, the eruption is seldom pronounced, which usually makes the clinical diagnosis much more difficult. Bullous or crusted lesions are seen in individuals who are immunocompromised, malnourished, or have a very sensitive skin. In cases where the disease has been present since a long time, eczematization, lichenification, impetigo and furunculosis may be present.

Diagnosis

- The typical history of pruritus with nocturnal exacerbations, and the distribution of the eruption of inflammatory papules should suggest the diagnosis.

- Demonstration of the mite under the microscope after scraping the burrow with a scalpel and mounting the material in KOH or mineral oil, will confirm the diagnosis.

Differential Diagnosis

Lesions of pityriasis rosea, tinea versicolor, pediculosis corporis and lichen planus may simulate those of scabies, but are easily distinguishable with histological features.

Complications

- Secondary infection of the lesions can result in the formation of pyodermas like impetigo or folliculitis, severe urticaria, secondary exudative eczematisation, and constitutional symptoms like malaise, fever, loss of appetite and weight.

- In infants and young children an eczema closely resembling atopic eczema is seen affecting the face and legs.

- In a few cases, glomerulonephritis can occur.

Treatment

The patient and all his contacts including household members should be treated simultaneously. The patient should take a hot scrub bath with soap and water. All the used clothes and linen should be properly washed. In case of infected scabies, the secondary infection is treated prior to anti-scabitic therapy.

HOMEOPATHIC APPROACH TO SCABIES

Some Important Remedies for Scabies

Arsenicum album: Eruption appears on the bends of knees. The eruptions could be dry as well as full of small pustules. Burning and itching < at night, application of cold water > local application of warmth. Scabies has a tendency to alternate with bronchial asthma.

Anthracokali: Eruption with itching appearing during the night and disappearing during the daytime; also the eruption decreases during full moon. Eruptions present on scrotum, hands, tibia, and dorsum of feet. Intense thirst.

Carbo vegetabilis: Dry eruptions almost all over the body especially worse on extremities. Itching < after undressing at night.

Scabies can occur after abuse of mercurial salts. Concomitant symptoms like dyspepsia, belching, passing flatus. Once infection takes place – acrid, bloody, foul discharge. The pus smells like asa foetida. Presence of excessive burning in the lesion which is worse by local application of heat as well as cold.

Causticum: Scabies suppressed by local application of mercury and sulphur. Excessive itching of whole body at night, also when secondarily infected there is presence of humid vesicles oozing corroding pus. Extremely sensitive to cold air. Concomitants – yellowish skin, warts, involuntary urination when coughing, sneezing or walking.

Croton tiglium: Eruptions on genitals, vertex, temples, extremities, etc. Violent itching and burning in lesions and skin becomes sore if scratched > gentle rubbing. Gradually the eruption becomes pustular which burst and form crust.

Hepar sulphur: Eruptions that resemble scabies are present on folds of skin, hands and feet. Eruptions are pustular, crusty, oozing a foul, old cheese like discharge. Skin is extremely sensitive to cold air. The itching is worse at night > warm application. Presence of scabies in an individual where eruptions are suppressed by mercury.

Lycopodium clavatum: Eruptions on scalp, extremities, genitals and abdomen. Eruptions are yellowish, brown, moist, and purulent. Itching and burning < by warmth > cold application especially, itching while burning > local heat. GI concomitants like weak digestion, craving for sweets, flatulence should help one to prescribe the drug.

Mercurius solubilis: Bends of elbows, genitals, extremities etc. The appearance of skin is – dirty, yellow, rough and dry. Secondary infection sets in early and there is presence of pustules, which liberate bloody, corroding, tenacious, sticky, offensive pus. Violent voluptuous, itching over whole body, principally in evening or at night. It is worse by heat of bed and sometimes attended by burning after scratching. Itching is so severe that patient develops insomnia. General tendency to free perspiration but patient does not get relieved.

Psorinum: This nosode should be used in those cases of scabies where one has a repeated history of scabies in the past or scabies are suppressed with the help of conventional medicine resulting into internal affection of asthma, migraine, heart trouble, etc. The eruptions are present on bends of elbow. Scabies appear in every winter and disappear in summer. Violent itching < warmth of bed < scratching.

Rhus venenata: Vesicular eruption resembles erysipelas. The appearance of skin is dark red. Itching > hot water.

Sepia officinalis: Eruption is predisposed to crack and ulcerate as soon as it appears. Itching and burning sensation < evening, open-air > warm room. Scabies come periodically every spring. It is also useful in those cases of scabies previously treated by Sulphur.

Sulphur: It is one of the supreme remedy in homeopathy which is used for recurrent maltreated, obstinate, suppressed cases of scabies, as a result of irrational homeopathic treatment or when mercurial or Sulphur ointment are used to suppress the lesion. There is presence of voluptuous tingling and itching in the bends of joints in between fingers, < as soon as he gets warm in bed, <when undressing. Burning and soreness after scratching. Skin appears rough and scaly with formation of little vesicles and pustules.

REPERTORY

Aloe, ambr, ant-c, ant-t, anthraco, ars, aster, bar-m, bry, calc, canth, carb-ac, carb-an, carb-v, carbn-s, caust, chrysar, cic, clem, coloc, con, cop, crasp-v, crot-t, cupr, dulc, eppa-an, graph, guaj, gynu-ce, hep, kali-s, kreos, lach, led, lyc, m-ambo, maesa-t, mang, merc-i-f, merc, mez, mur-ac, nat-c, nat-s, nat-m, nat-c, nat-m, nux-v, ol-lav, olnd, petr, ph-ac, psor, puls, psor, raphis-g, rhus-v, sabad, sel, senec-fa, sep, sil, squil, staph, sul-ac, sulph, ter, tarax, sulph, tod-a, valer, verat, vinc, viol-t, zinc.

Location

- Face: Mez, sars.
- Abdomen: Nat-c.
- Penis
- Prepuce: Thuj.
- Extremities
  - Elbows, bends of elbow: Bry, merc.
  - Knees, hollow of knees: Ars, bry, merc.

Chapter-28

Hansen's Disease - Leprosy

Synonym

Hansen's disease, Hanseniasis, Elephantiasis grecorum.

Definition

Hansen's disease or Leprosy is a highly infectious, chronic granulomatous disease that is caused by *Mycobacterium leprae*, where the peripheral nerves and the skin are primarily affected. The disease is so named since the bacilli known to cause it was discovered by Hansen.

Etiology & Epidemiology

All cases of leprosy, both in human being and the animal kingdom, are caused by the acid-fast *Mycobacterium leprae*, which is classified separately from the other mycobacteria due to the inability to culture it in vitro. They are pleomorphic, straight or curved, acid-fast, rod-like bacteria occurring in clumps like bunches of cigars inside the phagocytes termed lepra cells. Man is regarded as the only natural host of the disease though wild armadillos may also be infected.

This disease condition, though on a decrease now, is known to be endemic in *tropical* and *developing counties* like Bangladesh, Burma, Brazil, India, Indonesia, Central Africa, South and Central America, the Pacific Islands, the Philippines and the Hawaii.

- It is a disease that is usually acquired through genetic susceptibility, where the rate of incidence is especially high in cases of monozygotic twins.

- It is also seen to spread easily in areas where the general susceptibility of the population is low, with a poor nutritional status, inadequate housing, and unsuitable sanitation.

- Prolonged and close contact is ideal for its transmission. The disease occurs due to droplet infection, which is spread through an infectious patient either through coughing or sneezing; or it results from direct exposure to carrier organisms like armadillo, cockroaches or mice. Children are apparently more easily infected in these situations than adults. Indirect transmission may occur through wearing an infective patient's clothes and from articles of daily use. The point of entry could be either through the skin, mucous membranes of the respiratory tract or the GIT.

- Decorative tattooing, a trend that seems to be picking up in different countries, is another mode of transmission of the infection.

- It is seen especially in male adults rather than female adults. The peak ages of affection are from 10-15 years or between 30-50 years of age.

- Incubation period varies from 2-5 years, but can be much longer, especially in cases of lepromatous leprosy, where the incubation period can go upto 8-12 years.

Pathogenesis

In a significant number of individuals, especially children, there is presence of *Mycobacterium leprae* in the skin, without giving rise to any clinical symptoms; and this stage is called the 'silent phase' of the infection. The host's immune reaction to the leprosy bacillus is an important factor in determining the outcome of the infection. The classification of this spectral disease is thus based on differences in the cell-mediated immunity of the individuals.

At one pole, individuals with a good immunity are known to develop the *tuberculoid* type of leprosy; and at the other pole there are individuals with a poor immune status who tend to develop the *lepromatous* type. Between these two poles, there are individuals with an intermediate level of immunity tend who to develop the *borderline* type (BB) of leprosy. In this group individuals showing features closer to lepromatous leprosy are labeled as 'borderline lepromatous' (BL), and those with features closer to tuberculoid leprosy are labeled as 'borderline tuberculoid' (BT) types. One should remember that although the cell-mediated immune response of lepromatous patients to *M. leprae* is reduced, these patients are not immune suppressed for other infectious agents.

Restricted spread and self-healing are characteristic features of the tuberculoid type, whereas borderline and lepromatous types are more progressive, with a slow and extensive bacillary spread, with antigen overload, occurring at the sites of the lesions in cases of lepromatous leprosy.

Lepra reactions that are immune-mediated reactions are commonly seen in borderline cases of leprosy. Type 1 reactions are reversible ones caused by a delayed hypersensitivity after recognition of M. leprae antigens in the skin and various nerve sites. Type 2 reactions, with the development of erythema nodosum, occur due to immune-complex deposition and occur in borderline lepromatous and lepromatous leprosy cases.

Tuberculoid patients have positive lepromin skin tests and lepromatous patients negative ones.

Histopathology

The organism *M. leprae* is known to affect primarily the peripheral nervous system, entering the nerve and affecting especially the Schwann cell via endoneural blood vessels. Abnormalities in nerve-conduction studies and a histological picture of small fibre loss are seen with segmental demyelination and remyelination.

Punch biopsies performed from the active border of typical lesions will be adequate for diagnosis.

TUBERCULOID LEPROSY

In this type of leprosy, histiocytes are turned into epithelioid cells. There is the presence of dermal tuberculoid granulomas forming foci around the nerves and skin appendages. The granulomas, along with an infiltrate of macrophages, lymphocytes and giant cells, tend to extend right up to the epidermis. No acid-fast bacilli are seen, but diagnosis is established by checking for selective destruction of nerve trunks or swollen cutaneous nerves.

LEPROMATOUS LEPROSY

Here there is thinning of the epidermis with the typical diffuse leproma in the deeper layer of the dermis, consisting of foamy macrophages (foamy lepra cells) with the addition of lymphocytes and plasma cells. Acid-fast bacilli are typically abundant. In cases of neuropathic affections in this type of leprosy, one finds asymptomatic bacillation, followed by foamy degeneration of the Schwann cells. There is a resultant demyelination, damage and destruction of the neural axis, followed by Wallerian degeneration, nerve fibrosis and hyalinization in later stages.

BORDERLINE LEPROSY

In *borderline tuberculoid (BT)* leprosy, the changes are similar to that seen in the tuberculoid type, except that the epithelioid cell granulomas is more diffuse and shows some vacuolation, and the acid-fast bacilli may be present. There is an uninvolved narrow, papillary zone that separates the inflammatory infiltrate from the overlying epidermis. Also, the dermal nerves are moderately swollen by cellular infiltrate or may show only Schwann-cell proliferation.

In *mid-borderline (BB)* leprosy, diffuse epithelioid granulomas are seen with very scanty lymphocytes with foamy cytoplasm, and absence of giant cells. The nerves are slightly swollen by cellular infiltrate, and acid-fast bacilli are present in moderate numbers.

In *borderline lepromatous (BL)* leprosy, foamy changes are seen with increased lymphocytes, which are dispersed diffusely within the small granulomas. The Schwann cells are full of bacilli and the resultant widespread nerve damage occurs due to acute neuritis. Oedema of the granuloma compresses on the remaining Schwann cells causing rapid functional loss in an already compromised nerve.

Clinical Features

The range of symptoms seen in Hansen's disease can be said to have two stable poles – the tuberculoid and the lepromatous types. The early or initial signs seen in this insidious condition are pretty indeterminate and can usually go unnoticed. They consist of an area of numbness or presence of solitary, mildly hypopigmented spots or rarely a red erythematous macular formation on the skin, with poorly defined margins. The areas that are usually affected are the cheeks, upper arms and thighs, buttocks or the trunk.

The earliest sensory changes are loss of sensation of cold and light touch, especially in the feet and hands. Peripheral nerves are not enlarged and there is no formation of plaques or nodules.

This state may persist for a few days, but the picture gradually evolves into either of the two poles or if the immunity of the individual is good, the condition may spontaneously be resolved with no signs or symptoms of leprosy.

Further discriminating or characteristic features of each type are as follows:

TUBERCULOID LEPROSY

In cases of this high-resistance form of leprosy, only a few solitary lesions tend to develop, which are well-defined, raised, erythematous, copper coloured or purple with a flattened and hypopigmented center, distributed asymmetrically. The lesions are seen most commonly on the face, limbs or the trunk. Neural involvement is early and prominent in tuberculoid leprosy and in quite a few cases, there may be no skin lesions, but only symptoms like pain and swelling of the affected nerve is seen followed by anesthesia, muscle weakness, muscle wasting and paralysis of the facial muscles and foot drop.

The damage to the nerves in the skin makes the lesion anesthetic while damage to the neighboring structures such as the hair, the sebaceous glands and the sweat glands causes loss of hair, dry scaly skin and anhidrosis, respectively.

Diagnosis

On examination, usually just beyond the outer edge of the lesion, there is a thickened or indurated sensory nerve or nerve trunk palpable, which may be tender to touch. A positive Lepromin skin test is diagnostic.

Prognosis

The prognosis is good with spontaneous remission occurring in quite a few cases, usually within three years of time, with or without treatment.

LEPROMATOUS LEPROSY

This highly bacillated form of leprosy occurs in those with a low immunity and is always slowly progressive.

Initially the patient may only present with coryza, noseblock, epistaxis or oedematous swelling of the hands and feet. Gradually one can see small and multiple lesions on the skin, which are bilaterally symmetrical, diffuse, and hypopigmented occurring in the form of macules, papules or nodules. In cases of macules, the lesions are small, ill-defined, multiple, shiny, slightly erythematous or hypopigmented. Papules and nodules (lepromas) are usually of skin-color or at times can be erythematous. The lesions can occur anywhere on the body, except for the scalp, axillae, groins and perineum (since these parts have a bit of a higher temperature). In a few cases diffuse plaques are seen with shiny, wrinkled and atrophic skin.

In the initial stages, there is not much of alopecia or loss of sensation occurring over the lesions, but gradually numbness and anesthesia starts to occur, especially over the hands and feet (called as bilateral 'glove and stocking' anesthesia). Gradually progressive fibrosis and thickening of the peripheral nerves occurs.

In untreated and chronic cases, the skin over the face (especially the forehead) becomes thick, and is thrown into wrinkles or convoluted folds, which gives it a lion-like appearance (leonine facies). There is loss of hair over the eyebrows and eyelashes, thickened earlobes, distorted or collapsed nose (due to septal perforation and a depressed nasal bridge), waxy shiny face, hoarseness of voice, and loss of upper incisors. Involvement of the bones and digits gives rise to their resorption and the very slow nerve involvement leads to the appearance of claw hands, wrist drop and foot drop.

Diagnosis

The Lepromin skin reaction is negative in this type.

Associated Features

• Affection of the nerves of the eye can cause lagophthalmos and anesthesia of the cornea and conjunctiva, resulting in dryness of the cornea and repetitive injury. This further results in avascular keratitis, corneal lepromas, pannus formation, corneal opacity, corneal ulceration and finally blindness. There is also a tendency to develop a painful red eye condition due to iridocyclitis.

- The neural involvement predisposes anesthesia of the part (with resultant complications like repetitive trauma, bruises, burns or cuts, trophic ulcers, cellulitis, etc.), muscular weakness and contracture, and autonomic dysfunction

- Deformities (crooked or short) of the hands and feet are also seen with thin and brittle nails. X-ray shows osteoporotic changes especially of the phalanges, small osteolytic cysts and often hairline or compression fractures.

- Except for the gastrointestinal tract, lungs, and brain most of the other organs can contain leprae bacilli. The most frequent complications seen are lymphadenopathy, bone marrow affection, hepatosplenomegaly, testicular atrophy, gynaecomastia and sterility or impotency can result.

Prognosis

It is a slowly progressive disease with a poor prognosis if left untreated, resulting usually in death due to recurrent infections, ulcerations, amyloidosis or renal failure. Also, the occurrence of 'lepra reactions' in this type of leprosy makes the prognosis grave.

BORDERLINE LEPROSY

In this group one can find a variable mixture of features of both the tuberculoid and the lepromatous types, depending on the position of the patient within the borderline spectrum of the two poles (tuberculoid or lepromatous). Borderline leprosy is the commonest type of disease encountered, with BT usually predominating in Africa and BL in Asia.

At the '*tuberculoid end*' of the spectrum (BT type), one finds very few, asymmetrical and dry lesions with a more pronounced alopecia, anhidrosis, anesthesia and fewer bacilli in smears. The lesions are similar to TT lesions, except that they are smaller and more numerous (usually three to ten) and satellite lesions around large macules or plaques are characteristic.

Towards the '*lepromatous end*' of the spectrum (BL type), one finds more of skin lesions and lesser nerve involvement, with abundant bacilli seen in smears. The skin lesions are symmetrical and numerous, and the patients usually do not show features like leonine facies, nasal ulceration, keratitis, etc., which are characteristic features of a pure lepromatous leprosy.

Typical lesions of a '*pure borderline leprosy*' (BB type) are more numerous, asymmetrical, red and irregularly shaped, with small satellite lesions surrounding larger plaques. The edges of the lesions are not as well-defined as those in the tuberculoid type, and also the anesthesia is only moderate in intensity.

Borderline leprosy is more of an unstable type, at times presenting initially with neural symptoms and then downgrades into a more lepromatous type with marked skin lesions if left untreated; or at times 'up-grades' towards a tuberculoid type. It is known to not cause much damage to structures other than the skin and nerves.

Prognosis

The prognosis in cases of borderline leprosy is good if the treatment is started off in the early stages of detection and diagnosis. In cases where it is left untreated, the borderline patients will downgrade towards the lepromatous end of the disease spectrum, which is followed by increased chances of complications and subsequent poor prognosis.

Also, borderline patients are at risk of developing Type 1 reactions, which may result in peripheral nerve damage and its sequelae.

PURE NEURITIC LEPROSY

Pure neuritic leprosy is a type where there is only neural involvement in the patient without any kind of skin lesions. Thus there is primarily only asymmetrical thickening of the peripheral nerves or nerve trunks seen here, with or without tenderness. There can be anesthetic changes of the skin with its complications like trophic ulcers, bony deformities, etc. There can also be signs and symptoms of paresis, claw hand, foot drop or wrist drop.

Reactions

Leprosy is a chronic illness running a long and slowly progressive course, which can have acute reactions in between that are called as 'lepra reactions', which occur especially after the start of an antibiotic treatment or occur during an intercurrent infection, after vaccination, during pregnancy or puerperium, or after consumption of iodides or bromide.

There are two types of these reactions seen – one is where there is an exacerbation of pre-existing lesions, called Type I reactions; another is where there is development of new nodular type of lesions, called as Type II reactions or erythema nodosum leprosum (ENL).

TYPE 1 REACTION

Type I reactions are those occurring due to a change (either a rise or a downfall) in the patients immunity, and these occur spontaneously in cases of borderline leprosy (BT, BL, BB).

The characteristic of this type of reaction is that there is an acute or subacute inflammation of the already existing lesions, which become oedematous, red and tender. There can occur sudden acute symptoms of neuritis (with marked swelling and tenderness of the peripheral nerves along with sudden loss of sensory and motor functions) and/or of skin lesions (erythematous or oedematous changes with desquamation or rarely ulceration). In this type there are very mild or no constitutional symptoms seen, but the nerve damage can make it an emergency condition.

TYPE 2 REACTIONS

Type II reactions occur due to circulation and deposition of immune complexes in the skin and other organs, and is not known to occur due or show any increase or decrease in the person's immunity. These occur spontaneously especially in cases of lepromatous leprosy or borderline lepromatous leprosy. This kind of reaction is usually acute in nature, but can recur a number of times and become chronic.

There are acute, painful, dusky-red, subcutaneous and dermal nodules that are widespread, especially on the face and extremities (usually the extensor surface of the arms and medial aspect of the thighs), which can become suppurative, ulcerative or indurated with time. There is always a multisystem involvement in this reaction type with associative features like – anorexia, fever, myalgia, uveitis, iridocyclitis, arthritis, peripheral nerve neuritis, cataract, glaucoma, lymphadenitis, myositis and epididymo-orchitis. In cases where these reactions continue to recur, there is poor prognosis, with resultant death usually due to some infection or amyloidosis.

Diagnosis

- Clinical features are diagnostic; especially the hypopigmented or erythematous lesions or nodule formation, the insensibility or aaesthetic changes, and the thickened and palpable peripheral nerves.

- Identification and demonstration of the acid-fast bacilli M. Leprae in slit-skin smears by modified ZN staining is diagnostic. The bacillary index is determined from it, which is the bacterial load of the infection. The morphological index changes sooner than the bacillary index and is an early indicator of efficacy of treatment.

- Skin biopsies from skin or nerve lesions, stained for the bacilli are also useful.

- Lepromin test is a non-specific test of not much value for diagnosis, but can help in the classification of the type of leprosy since it helps to determine the immunologic status of the patient with respect to the leprosy bacillus. Thus, it is strongly positive in tuberculoid leprosy, weakly positive in borderline tuberculoid leprosy and negative in pure borderline, borderline lepromatous and pure lepromatous leprosy, and variable and in-diagnostic in indeterminate leprosy.

Differential Diagnosis

Leprosy is more often than not overdiagnosed in tropical countries and underdiagnosed in western countries. One should consider the following conditions for differential diagnosis.

- Hyperpigmented birthmarks and hypopigmented patches of vitiligo, eczema, vitamin deficiency, tinea, etc. should be differentiated. Vitiligo patches are completely depigmented, while the leprosy lesions are just hypopigmented, not completely depigmented. Pityriasis alba or eczema cases with hypopigmentation are in comparison difficult to differentiate, but checking for the overlying scaly surface and absence of the leprae bacilli in the skin biopsy helps diagnosis. Cases of tinea with the hypopigmentation can be differentiated from leprosy by the demonstration of fungus in the scrapings.
- Granuloma multiform, sarcoidosis and cutaneous tuberculosis, may resemble tuberculoid leprosy, but they are not insensible, and the peripheral nerves are not always palpable. Also, the tuberculin and Kveim tests will help further differentiation of tuberculosis and sarcoidosis from leprosy.
- Also, conditions like cutaneous leishmaniasis can cause the formation of nodules, but these are not as numerous as those seen in leprosy and unlike lepromatous nodules, these tend to form crusts and then ulcerate after some weeks or months.

Treatment

Besides treating it homeopathically, we need to take precautions to prevent the complications and reactions from occurring. Also, educating the patient to cope with the anesthetic changes in the hands or feet is necessary, especially a daily inspection for injury, bruise, ulcer or blister formation in the parts should be checked for. Wearing gloves at work or during cooking is helpful to prevent the above; also wearing the right kind of footwear is also necessary, especially a well-fitting shoe with a firm outer sole and a soft shock-absorbent inner sole.

Weakness or paralysis requires regular physiotherapy; and patients with contractures need to be taught exercises to prevent fixation.

Monitoring sensation and muscle power in a patient's hands, feet and eyes should be part of the routine follow-up so that new nerve damage is detected early.

Rehabilitating the patient socially and psychologically is important, since it is a condition that suffers rejection by the community. Education, productive employment, confidence from family and friends helps better cure.

HOMEOPATHIC APPROACH TO HANSON'S DISEASE

My experience in the treatment of leprosy, to be honest, is not very wide as other homeopaths in India have. The following conclusions have been drawn from the cases seen so far.

1. Leprosy patients usually present with very scanty symptoms at the level of the skin as well as at the level of constitution. There are hardly any peculiar, queer or rare symptoms present. In the majority of the patients I have seen in my practice, suffering from leprosy, I have observed that most of them have had a history of some suppressed skin eruptions or suppressed upper respiratory tract allergies.

2. About 50% of the patients do not respond to the constitutional medicine prescribed, which is based on the Hahnemannian totality.

3. The dominating miasm in majority of these patients is syphilis or tubercular. However, the fundamental miasm is almost always tubercular.

During the development of leprosy most of the constitutional symptoms go into background and only the local presenting symptoms are on the surface. These local symptoms require either anti-syphilitic remedies or some nosode, e.g. *Tuberculinum* or *Bacillinum*.

The *Lepra reaction,* which is the hypersensitivity response to the proteins liberated by the lepra bacilli, is interpreted miasmatically as an acute exacerbation of the syphilitic miasm. Sometimes use of *Tuberculinum or Bacillinum* may prove necessary. Leprosy carries with it tremendous social stigma which leads to depression, hence this aspect has to be considered while selecting the remedy.

In conclusion, I would suggest that when a patient comes with leprosy, study the presenting totality and treat it appropriately with anti-miasmatic remedy.

Keenly observe any change in the symptoms or miasmatic phase; and accordingly change the medicine if required. *Continue treating the patient for a very long period with frequent repetition in low potency.*

REPERTORY

- **Skin, eruptions,**

  - Leprosy: alum, am-c, ambr, anac, ant-t, ars, bar-c, calc, carb-ac, carb-an, carb-v, carbn-s, caust, chaul, coloc, com, con, crot-h, cupr, daph, diphtox, drym-cor, elae, form, graph, hell, hura, hydrc, iod, iris, kali-i, lach, kali-ar, kali-c, mag-c, mang, maeso-f, merc-sul, meph, mitra-st, nat-c, nat-m, nit-ac, nuph, pentac-m, phos, psor, petr, pip-m, ricino-h, sec, sep, sil, strych-g, sulph, thyr, tub, vac, zinc
  - Tubercles, leprous: Nat-c, sil, phos.

Location

- Face: ant-t, alum, graph, mag-c, phos, sec.
- Chin, on: calc, hir.
- Upper limbs: meph, phos.
- Nates, annular spots: graph.
- Leg: graph, nat-c.
- Toes, leprous ulcers: graph.

Chapter-29

Tuberculosis of the Skin

Introduction

Tuberculosis of the skin, also called as cutaneous tuberculosis, is an infrequently seen form of extrapulmonary tuberculosis. The incidence of it was high in the developing countries, but with improved hygienic conditions and better nutritious status, it is a bit on the decline now.

Etiology

Mycobacterium tuberculosis and mycobacterium bovis are strains known to cause tuberculosis in both humans and animals. In humans, it is usually a droplet infection, entering the body usually through the respiratory tract; but it is also known to enter through the tonsils, intestine, skin, or mucous membranes through direct contact. From there it can spread to any part of the body, especially the lymph nodes, via the lymphatic vessels and the bloodstream.

Classification

There are different clinical presentations seen in cutaneous tuberculosis, depending upon the mode of infection, morphology of lesion, the individual's immunity or susceptibility, the age of the person and the site of affection. In a primary infection, the tuberculin test is negative, and in the remaining conditions, it is positive, though the degree of reactivity is variable.

There are four major categories of cutaneous tuberculosis:

• Inoculation from an *Exogenous source* (primary tuberculosis complex and tuberculosis verrucosa cutis).

• *Endogenous cutaneous spread* through physical contact or by autoinoculation (scrofuloderma, tuberculosis cutis orificialis).

• *Hematogenous spread* to the skin (acute generalized miliary tuberculosis; lupus vulgaris; and tuberculosis ulcer, gumma or abscess).

• *Tuberculids* (erythema induratum [Bazin's disease], papulonecrotic tuberculid, and lichen scrofulosorum) – These also represent hematogenous spread of tuberculosis, which is quickly controlled by the host, usually resulting in the absence of detectable organisms. They are differentiated from true tuberculosis by no sign of an obvious active tuberculous focus in the body, negative tuberculin test, lack of response to antituberculosis drugs, and its tendency to resolve spontaneously.

PRIMARY TUBERCULOSIS COMPLEX

Synonym

Primary inoculation tuberculosis; Tuberculous chancre.

Etiology & Incidence

This condition occurs in a previously tuberculous-free individual. The M. tuberculosis bacilli possibly enter the skin or mucosa through minor injuries or tears. It is also seen in cases of individuals who have got a tattoo or ear piercing done, or in those who have had a circumcision done, used inadequately sterilized syringes, or had a mouth-to-mouth artificial respiration.

It occurs especially in children, affecting usually the face or extremities. In adults it can be seen following a trauma or injury.

Histopathology

In the initial two weeks, there is a marked inflammatory response with increased neutrophils and numerous tubercle bacilli, along with necrosis. In the next two to three weeks, there are more granulomatous changes seen with increased lymphocytes and epithelioid cells, and caseation, coinciding with reduction in the number of the tubercle bacilli. Within 3-4 weeks of inoculation, there are distinct tubercles seen to develop at the site of inoculation and in the regional lymph nodes

Clinical Features

After 2-4 weeks of the inoculation, a painless brownish-red papule forms, which turns into an indurated nodule, which may break down to form a ragged ulcer with an undermined edge and a granular hemorrhagic base. Gradually, the edge becomes firmer and a thin adherent crust develops. This is called as the tuberculous chancre.

There is regional lymphadenopathy seen within 3-8 weeks of the infection, which completes the formation of the 'cutaneous complex'. In a few cases, cold, suppurative and oozing lesions can develop over the lymph nodes.

Spontaneous healing occurs within a year or so, leaving a scar at the site of the ulcer, and an enlarged and calcified regional lymph node. In a few cases, there is formation of cold abscesses and sinuses. There can be dissemination of the lesion or there can be a resultant delayed suppuration of the lymph node, which can develop into lupus vulgaris. Erythema nodosum and miliary tuberculosis may supervene the infection in a few cases.

Diagnosis

- The clinical finding of a painless, unilateral, localized glandular swelling in a child should arouse suspicion.

- The tuberculin test is negative.
- The tubercle bacilli can be demonstrated from the chancre, before the stage of adenitis occurs.

Differential Diagnosis

- Sporotrichosis, tularemia, or actinomycosis are a few conditions that need to be differentiated in the initial stages of the illness, when there are acid-fast bacilli demonstrated from the lesion.
- Cat-scratch fever and especially M. marinum infections closely resemble primary tuberculosis but are distinguished by their distribution or course, and cultural characteristics.
- Blastomycosis, histoplasmosis, coccidioidomycosis, syphilis, leishmaniasis, yaws, and atypical mycobacterial disease are a few other conditions that can be considered for differential diagnosis.

TUBERCULOSIS VERRUCOSA CUTIS

Synonym

Warty tuberculosis.

Etiology & Incidence

This condition occurs from an exogenous inoculation of the tubercle bacilli into the skin of a previously infected person, who usually has a moderate or high degree of immunity against M. tuberculosis.

There can be external infection from external sources, where usually the physicians, pathologists and post-mortem attendants are usually at risk. Another way that the inoculation can occur is through external or autoinoculation with the sputum, in a person with either an active tuberculosis or in those having a certain degree of sensitivity towards the organism.

It is commonly seen in the East, especially seen in Hong Kong and Vietnam; and rarely in Africa and other western countries.

Histopathology

In the epidermis, there is marked pseudo-epitheliomatous hyperplasia seen with hyperkeratosis. In the dermal layer, suppurative and granulomatous inflammation is seen with superficial abscess formation, which at times perforates through the epidermis. In this condition scanty tuberculosis foci, and very few acid-fast bacilli are detected.

Clinical Features

There is initially a small, painless, indurated, usually solitary, papule that comes up, which becomes hyperkeratotic, looking like a wart. The lesion occurs on those areas that are exposed to trauma, infected sputum or other tuberculous material. Thus it is especially seen on the dorsal surface of the fingers and hands in adults, and on the ankles, knees and buttocks in children.

This lesion then gradually spreads and expands in size, at times reaching several centimeters or more in diameter, forming a verrucose plaque, with irregular edges. There can be formation of a huge, brownish or reddish, papillomatous excrescence with a firm consistency. In a few cases there can be a fissure formation on the surface, which oozes out a purulent discharge.

Also, with these lesions, lymphadenitis is rare, but it can occur in a few cases due to a secondary bacterial infection.

Diagnosis

The tuberculin test is strongly positive.

Differential Diagnosis

- Lesions on the fingers, hands and the tongue need to be distinguished from warts and keratoses.
- Culture and sensitivity test will help differential warty tuberculosis from atypical mycobacteriosis caused by *M. marinum*.
- It also needs to be differentiated from blastomycosis, chro-

moblastomycosis, verrucosus epidermal nevus, iododerma, and bromoderma.

- Crusted lesions need to be distinguished from leishmaniasis.
- In cases of lesions where the central scarring is surrounded by a serpiginous edge, tertiary syphilis needs to be ruled out.
- Lupus vulgaris is not usually hyperkeratotic and shows apple-jelly nodules.

Prognosis

The condition tends to extend very slowly with the lesions remaining almost inactive for months or years. In a few cases there can be spontaneous clearing.

SCROFULODERMA

Etiology & Pathogenesis

This condition especially occurs due to direct extension, involvement and rupture of the skin over an active tuberculous focus, usually a caseating lymph gland, and at times an infected bone, joint or lachrymal gland or duct.

The face, neck and groins are the most common sites of affection.

Histopathology

The tuberculous process from the underlying lymph node, bone or joint is seen to extend through the deep dermis. Tuberculous granulation tissue is seen at the periphery with caseating necrosis in the deeper layers of the dermis, where there is the formation of a cavity filled with liquefied debris and polymorphonuclear leukocytes.

Clinical Features

It is a chronic disease, developing slowly over a period of months. There is the formation of a non-specific, chronic inflammation of the skin or there is a painless, skin-colored or bluish-red nodule formation over the infected gland, joint or bone. This nodule then suppurates, softens and breaks open to form an ulcer with irregular borders, pale undermined edges and a reddish granulating base, which oozes a purulent and bloody discharge. There is formation of numerous interconnecting fistulae or sinuses.

In adults between 30 and 50 years of age, chronic anal fistula formation is seen with anal strictures, infiltrated nodules, and involvement of the scrotum with swelling.

Scrofuloderma heals gradually with characteristic cordlike scars and formation of irregular adherent masses, which are thickly fibrous at some places and fluctuant and discharging pus at others.

There is puckering scarring of the skin over the site of infection.

Diagnosis

It is a relatively easily diagnosed condition with the known history of tuberculosis in the individual, and the isolation of the M. tuberculosis bacilli from the pus.

Differential Diagnosis

- Suppurative lymphadenitis, actinomycosis, hidradenitis suppurativa, and deep mycoses need to be differentiated, especially by checking for the type of spread and the location, and also be checking for the culture.

- Lymphogranuloma venereum favors the inguinal and perineal areas, and has positive serologic tests for LGV.

TUBERCULOSIS CUTIS ORIFICIALIS

Synonym

Orificial tuberculosis; acute tuberculous ulcer.

Definition & Incidence

In this condition there is tuberculous infection of the mucous membranes or skin adjoining the orifices in a patient with long-standing and advanced internal tuberculosis. Thus lesions are seen around and in the nose and mouth in the laryngeo-pulmonary types; and around the anus, urinary meatus and vagina in the gastrointestinal, genitourinary or anogenital types of tuberculosis.

Males are known to be more affected than women, especially those with a poor general health, poor nutritional status, and poor hygiene.

Etiology & Pathogenesis

It is a form of autoinoculation tuberculosis, though external sources of infection can be responsible. The lesions result from direct inoculation or by lymphatic or haematogenous spread around the orifices.

Histopathology

The base of the ulcer shows a lot of granulation tissue infiltrated with polymorphonuclear leukocytes. Acid-fast tuberculous bacilli are easily demonstrated.

Clinical Features

This condition, seen in patients with long-standing cases of tuberculosis, indicates a failing resistance to the disease. Initially there is the formation of small, oedematous red nodules at the site, which rapidly break down to form small, soft, punched out, very painful and tender, shallow ulcers with undermined bluish edges, and pale granulation formation at the base. These ulcers do not heal spontaneously, spread rapidly, becoming chronic, and are especially seen around the mouth, nose, anus, vagina or urinary meatus. Lesions around the mouth occur especially on the tongue, though a tooth socket can also be involved in cases of a dental extraction.

Diagnosis

With the clinical signs, especially of pain and ulceration at orifices, and past history of tuberculosis in the individual, the diagnosis is not so difficult. The diagnosis is confirmed bacteriologically. The tuberculin test is variable, but usually present, especially in the later stages.

MILIARY TUBERCULOSIS

Synonym

Disseminated tuberculosis.

Incidence

Miliary tuberculosis of the skin or other organs can be seen in cases of fulminating pulmonary or meningeal tuberculosis, especially in infants and children. It is also seen in cases of immunosuppressed patients with AIDS or in those who have had an infectious disease with resultant decreased immunity (e.g. measles).

Histopathology

Diffuse suppurative inflammation of the dermis is seen, with predominantly polymorphonuclear leukocytes. Vasculitis or abscesses may also be seen. Acid-fast bacilli are abundant.

Clinical Features

There is acute hematogenous spread of tuberculosis occurring in this fatal condition, with formation of numerous, generalized, bluish or erythematous rash in the form of maculo-papular, vesicular, pustular or hemorrhagic lesions. In a few cases erythematous subcutaneous nodules are found. The lesions can be very painful.

In subacute and less severe cases, the papules or vesicles may undergo necrosis, producing ulcers.

Diagnosis

- The biopsy of a skin lesion shows the acid-fast bacilli.
- A search should also be made for evidence of other complications of tuberculous, like a cold abscess.
- The tuberculin test is negative, since the spread is hematogenous.

LUPUS VULGARIS

Definition

This condition is a progressive form of cutaneous tuberculosis in a person with a moderate to high degree of immunity. The lesions consists of plaques, with nodules of an 'apple-jelly' color, extending irregularly in some areas. In some cases scarring occurs, which results in considerable tissue destruction over the years.

Incidence

The frequency of its occurrence has reduced considerably in the western countries, but is still a common complaint in India. It is seen more commonly in children and young adults, and that too especially in females rather than males. A cool, moist or dull climate tends to favor its occurrence.

Etiology & Pathogenesis

It occurs either by direct inoculation or by extension from underlying infected glands or joints. It is also known to occur via the lymphatic spread from infected mucous membranes of the nose or throat; very rarely does hematogenous spread result in its occurrence.

Histopathology

Classically there are typical tubercles seen in the upper dermis. There is caseation seen within the tubercles in half the cases. Epidermal layer is at times flattened, or is hypertrophic. There are numerous tubercle bacilli, though at times difficult to demonstrate. T-cell activation and langerhans' cell hyperplasia are prominent features.

Clinical Features

The lesions usually arise at the site of primary inoculation, in scrofuloderma scars or at the site of BCG vaccination, but it can occur on normal skin too. Most of the lesions are seen on the head, neck and face, especially around the nose; only a few are seen to occur on the trunk, arms and legs. The lesions are usually solitary, though several of them can also occur simultaneously. Most of these patients will also have evidence of tuberculosis elsewhere, which needs to be diagnosed after thorough evaluation.

There is usually a single plaque composed of tiny, reddish-brown, flat macules, of a soft or almost gelatinous, consistency, which makes it look like a freckle. These are embedded deeply and diffusely in the infiltrated dermis. This lesion then enlarges and becomes raised slowly over months and years to become a big patch with well-defined edges and a few shades more darkish brown. Adherent scales are seen over these lesions. There is then clear or pale brownish-yellow type of nodules seen at the edge of the lesion, which are very soft to touch and so are called as 'apple-jelly' nodules. The lesions tend to heal slowly in one area and progress in another, with formation of new papules. On healing, the scar looks like a wrinkled tissue paper. Lesions on the hands, feet, knees and buttocks become thickened and rough or at times wart-like.

The five usual forms of the disorder are:

PLAQUE FORM

There is hardly any central scarring and infiltration. Erythema can mask the distinctive color of the lesion. There is marked scaling, especially on the legs, which makes it look like a psoriatic lesion. The lesions consist of large plaques with serpiginous borders, which extend over wide areas of the body, and some cause marked scarring. The edge of the lesion becomes very thick and hyperkeratotic.

ULCERATIVE AND MUTILATING FORMS

Here there is more of scarring and ulceration, with areas of necrosis with crust formation. The deeper tissues and cartilages can get invaded with contractures and deformities of the joints.

VEGETATING FORMS

Here there is marked ulceration, with areas of necrosis and phagedena. Though there is extensive infiltration, the scarring is minimal. Mucous membranes are affected, but the cartilage is slowly invaded.

TUMOR-LIKE FORMS

Here there is slowly progressive, deep or extensive infiltration, with formation of soft, smooth nodules or reddish-yellow plaques, which may be hypertrophic. There is no scaling and scarring. In a few cases there is development of huge, soft tumors on the ear lobes. Lymphangitis, lymphadenitis and vascular dilatation are sometimes marked. Prognosis of this form is not too good.

PAPULAR AND NODULAR FORMS

These are multiple lesions occurring in disseminate forms.

Prognosis and Complications

- The onset of the condition can be in childhood, with the lesions persisting throughout a lifetime. Though the lesions are chronic and slowly progressive, if left untreated, it can spread obstinately later on despite start of treatment. Also, it is seen that the older the patient at the onset of the lesions, the more rapid is the spread.

- Spontaneous resolution may eventually occur, leaving thin white scars, which may break open or become keloidal. Active lupus vulgaris frequently reappears in scar tissue.

- In a few cases contractures, atrophy, scarring and tissue destruction is also seen, with defects in eyes, nose, ear tips and the mouth. The tip of the nose can become sharply pointed or the whole nose can be destroyed with only the orifices, posterior septum and turbinates visible. On the tongue, deep and irregular, painful fissures are seen, with a certain degree of microglossia.

- Ulcerations can get infected or in chronic cases, there can be development of squamous cell or basal cell carcinoma or sarcomas.

Diagnosis

- Clinically, chronic and persistent reddish-brown patch with dermal infiltration and the presence of apple-jelly nodules are characteristic features.

- Match-stick test is positive; i.e. The apple-jelly nodule has no resistance to pressure by a sharp matchstick.

- Tissue paper-like wrinkled scars.

- Long history extending over years.

- Tuberculin test positive, since the patients have a moderate to high immunity to tuberculosis.

- Miliary tubercles in a biopsy specimen.

Differential Diagnosis

- In the early stages, lupus can be confused with lymphocytoma, spitz naevus and lupus erythematosus. In lupus erythematosus the lesions on the face are in a butterfly pattern; the lesions are well-defined with adherent scales and follicular plugging; characteristic biopsy features, and the patient is usually past puberty.

- In elderly people, syphilis should be ruled out. The lesions in syphilis are pretty much hard and those in lupus are very soft. Also, the serological test will be positive in cases of syphilis.
- Dermal leishmaniasis can be differentiated by its noduloulcerative lesions, which are bluish red and indolent, with l.t. bodies demonstrated in the smear test, and a negative tuberculin test.
- Deep mycosis can resemble the vegetating and crusting lesions of lupus, but histological features and culture will help differentiation.
- Lesions on the face can be mistaken for acne rosacea, or for port-wine stain, but histological features will help differentiation.
- Leprosy and sarcoidosis, however, are much more difficult to differentiate. The nodules of leprosy are firmer and other signs like sensory changes are present. The nodules of sarcoidosis resemble grains of sand rather than 'apple-jelly'.
- The lesions of lupus with the scaling, can resemble psoriasis, but psoriatic lesions are more extensive and lupus lesions more solitary.

TUBERCULOUS GUMMA

Synonym
Metastatic tuberculous ulcer or abscess.

Definition
In this form of tuberculosis there is the formation of firm, non-tender erythematous nodules that soften, ulcerate and form sinuses. Individuals with this disorder may or may not have other foci of tuberculosis identified. It is the result of a haematogenous dissemination of mycobacteria from a primary focus during periods of bacillaemia and lowered resistance. It is seen particularly in children, especially those with a decreased immunity from malnutrition, infectious disease or an immunodeficiency state.

Histopathology

Features similar to a tuberculous granulation tissue and abscess formation is seen with numerous mycobacterium tuberculi demonstrated from the pus.

Clinical Features

This condition is a highly infectious one presenting either as a firm, subcutaneous nodule or an irregular, ill-defined fluctuant swelling or abscess, which gradually softens and forms into an ulcer with undermined edges, which then forms sinuses. The lesions are especially seen on the extremities than on the trunk. There is bluish discoloration of the skin around the lesion. There can be lymphatic spread resulting in secondary lesions.

Diagnosis

- The diagnosis is confirmed by culture of the acid-fast bacilli.

TUBERCULIDES

Definition

The tuberculides are a group of symmetrical and disseminated skin eruptions associated with an underlying tuberculous affection or silent focus in an internal organ, and clear up when antituberculous therapy is administered to the patient.

Etiology & Pathogenesis

These occur probably due to a haematogenous spread of the tubercle bacilli to the skin, in a person with a moderate to high degree of immunity. The strong immunity to tuberculosis results in rapid destruction of the bacilli and autoinvolution of individual lesions in many cases, but yet new lesions continue to occur due to hematogenous dissemination from the underlying focus.

The person may not necessarily have an active tuberculous focus in the body, and is usually in good general health otherwise.

F- 37

Types

The papular tuberculides comprise of the papulonecrotic tuberculides, lichen scrofulosorum, and some other less common conditions. The lesions are usually bilaterally symmetrical and result from hematogenous dissemination.

PAPULONECROTIC TUBERCULIDES

Definition

It is a chronic disorder where necrotizing papular eruptions occur almost symmetrically, especially on the extremities, which responds well to the antituberculosis therapy.

Incidence

It is seen especially in young adults, but is also seen in infants and children. It occurs more commonly in females than males.

Pathogenesis

In a few cases, besides a tuberculous focus in the body being responsible for the hematogenous spread, the eruptions are seen to also arise after a BCG vaccination. The tuberculin test is seen to be positive, and although bacilli may never be found, new lesions are seen to stop coming after the start of antituberculous therapy. Newer studies involving the polymerase chain reaction has allowed detection of the mycobacterial DNA in the papulonecrotic skin lesions.

Histopathology

The epidermis is ulcerated in well-developed lesions, with a large central zone of coagulation necrosis, surrounded by extensive inflammation, extending right into the dermis and at times into the subcutaneous tissues. Adjacent lymphatic and small blood vessels are also involved in the inflammation and necrosis, followed by thrombotic occlusion.

Clinical Features

In this condition there occurs symmetrically distributed, firm, discrete, red, deep-seated papules or nodules, which do not itch much, but keep cropping up recurrently for months or years. The lesions vary in size from 2-8 mm. The centers of these lesions heal slowly, undergoing necrosis to form pustules, which bursts open and forms into a crust or ulcer, leaving pitted, pale scars with a hyperpigmented border on the skin surface.

The sites most frequently affected are the face and the extensor surface of the extremities, esp. on the legs, knees, arms, elbows, hands and feet; though sites like the ears, buttocks and penis can also be involved.

Diagnosis

It is a bit difficult to diagnose considering the frequent absence of an obvious tuberculous focus in the body. Skin biopsy and performing the tuberculin test, which is strongly positive, will help diagnosing the condition. Polymerase chain reaction will help identify the mycobacterial DNA.

Differential Diagnosis

- Insect bites may simulate these eruptions, but can be differentiated by the itching, asymmetrical affection and the acute history of the bite.

- Conditions like prurigo and excoriated papules also tend to itch a lot.

LICHEN SCROFULOSUM

Synonym

Tuberculosis cutis lichenoides.

Definition

In this condition, groups of closely placed, minute, discrete, indolent, keratotic or lichenoid papules, which are often perifollicular occurs, especially in children, or adults with a history of systemic tuberculosis (especially of the bones or lymph nodes).

Pathogenesis

This condition, resulting from a hematological spread, is seen in association with caseous lymphatic glands, tuberculous foci in the bone (rarely in the lungs), or both.

Histopathology

The lesions show non-caseating tuberculoid granulomas in the superficial layer of the dermis, between the surrounding hair follicles and sweat ducts. Lymphocytes, epithelioid cells and giant cells can be seen. Usually the tubercle bacilli are not seen in the pathologic specimens, nor can they be cultured from the biopsy material.

Clinical Features

Discrete, tiny, firm, yellowish to reddish-brown papules, 0.5-3 mm in diameter occur in a group or in discoid patches. The eruptions itch very slightly and are usually indolent, flat-topped papules with central spines or scales, with a tiny pustule over them. The lesions occur especially on the shoulders and the trunk, and they tend to heal gradually over a period of months, without much scarring; but this is usually followed by recurrences.

Diagnosis

- The tuberculin reaction is always positive.

Differential Diagnosis

- Lichen nitidus is a condition where the lesions have a shiny appearance and are more peripherally distributed.
- Lesions in keratosis spinulosa are skin-colored and more follicular.
- Lichen planus, sarcoidosis, secondary syphilis and drug eruptions need also to be differentiated.

Treatment

Here the response to antituberculosis therapy is much more slower and less dramatic than with the other tuberculides.

ERYTHEMA INDURATUM

Synonym

Bazin's disease.

Definition

In this chronic condition there occurs persistent or recurrent nodular lesions secondary to a past or active tuberculous foci in some other part of the body. It is usually seen to affect primarily the young women and the lesions are localized to the posterior aspect of the legs, but rarely occur in other parts of the body too.

Etiology

There is no known cause of this condition, but acrocyanosis is the basic predisposing factor. Thus the condition tends to get worse in winters. Sensitivity to tubercle bacilli or its toxins and sarcoid are the two supposed causes.

Histopathology

Lobular panniculitis, necrosis of the subcutaneous fat and granulomatous infiltration are a few characteristic features. In a few cases, a mixed picture with nodular vasculitis, tuberculoid granulomas and giant cell reaction is seen, without any caseation.

Clinical Features

There are symmetrical, bluish-red, infiltrated and indolent plaques or nodules with ill-defined edges, affecting the posterior aspect of the lower legs in young or middle-aged women with an erythrocyanotic circulation. The center of the nodules may soften and form scars or shallow ulcers with ragged, irregular, and bluish edges. The lesions get worse during the winter, and may appear to heal in warmer weather, but again recur by the next winter.

Prognosis

The prognosis is not so good considering the chronicity of the condition and the underlying problem with the circulatory system.

Diagnosis

- The tuberculin skin test is positive.
- Acid-fast bacilli are not found on special stains or biopsy cultures.
- Polymerase chain reaction helps to confirm the diagnosis.

Differential Diagnosis

- Erythema nodosum is a condition with tender, scarlet red nodules, without ulceration and has a short duration, and occurs with rapid development, affecting especially the anterior part of the leg. Erythema induratum in turn affects the posterior part of the leg, and is not at all that painful, with the lesions occurring in crops.
- Polymerase chain reaction helps in differentiating erythema induratum from idiopathic nodular vasculitis.
- In cases of tertiary syphilis with gumma formation, the lesions are usually solitary and unilateral. The serological tests and histological studies will help in the differentiation with erythema induratum.
- Nodular vasculitis is clinically and histologically quite similar, but there is no associated tuberculous infection, and it does not respond to anti-tuberculous therapy.

HOMEOPATHIC APPROACH TO TUBERCULOSIS OF THE SKIN

In cases of tuberculosis of the skin, one has to always treat constitutionally, irrespective of whatever the local symptoms are.

- *Tuberculinum Koch's* and *Bacillinum* are the two remedies that are extremely useful as intercurrent nosodes for this condition.

- Whenever there is a strong sycotic background, one can think of remedies like *Thuja*.
- When there is a formation of typical tuberculous ulcer and a lupus wound, then one should think of *Hepar sulph.*
- Other remedies that have been useful for tuberculosis of the skin are *Arsenicum album, Arsenic iod., Aurum met., Calcarea iod, Cistus canadensis, Graphites, Hydrastis, Hydrocotyle, Kalium bich., Kali iod., Sulphur,* and *Thiosinaminum.*

REPERTORY

The condition has to be studied using the rubric

- **Skin, eruptions, tubercles:** agar, alum, am-c, am-m, anac, ang, ant-c, apis, aran, ars, aur, bar-c, bar-m, bar-s, bell, bry, calc-p, calc-s, calc, carb-an, carb-v, carbn-s, caust, cic, cocc, con, crot-h, dulc, fl-ac, graph, hell, hep, hydrc, kali-ar, kali-bi, kali-br, kali-c, kali-i, kali-n., kali-s, lach, led, lyc, mag-c, mag-m, mag-s, mang, merc-c, merc, mez, mur-ac, nat-ar, nat-c, nat-m, nit-ac, nux-v, olnd, petr, ph-ac, phos, rhus-t, sec, sel, sep, sil, stann, staph, sul-ac, sulph, syph, tarax, thuj, tub, valer, verat, zinc.

  - Burning: am-c, am-m, calc, carb-an, cocc, dulc, kali-i, mag-m, mag-s, mang, merc, mur-ac, nit-ac, nicc, phos, staph.
  - Desquamating tubercles: sang.
  - Drawing, painful: cham.
  - Erysipelatous: nat-c, phos, sil.
  - Gnawing pain: rhus-t.
  - Hard tubercles: am-c, am-m, ant-c, bar-c, bry, bov, con, lach, mag-c, mag-s, nat-m, phos, rhus-t, valer.
  - Humid tubercles: kali-n, sel, thuj.
  - Inflamed tubercles: am-m, rhus-t.
  - Itching tubercles: am-m, aur, canth, carb-an, cham, cocc, dulc, graph, kali-c, kali-n, lach, lyc, mag-c, mag-s, mur-ac, nat-m, nit-ac, op, rhus-t, staph, stram, stront-c, tub, zinc.

- Leprous tubercles: nat-c, phos, sil.

- Malignant tubercles: ars.

- Miliary tubercles: nat-m.

- Mucous tubercles: fl-ac, nit-ac, thuj.

- Painful tubercles: am-c, ars, bell, bov, lach, lyc, ph-ac, zinc.

- Painless tubercles: arn, bell, graph, ign, led, olnd, squil, verat.

- Purple tubercles: tub.

- Raised tubercles: olnd, rhus-v, valer.

- Red tubercles: am-c, berb, bov, carb-an, carb-v, dig, hep, lach, led, kali-chl, kali-i, mag-c, mag-m, merc, mur-ac, nat-m, nit-ac, op, ph-ac, puls, sep, spig, sulph, thuj, verat.

- Areola: cocc, dulc, ph-ac.

- Scratching, after: mang, zinc.

- Scurfy tubercles: dulph.

- Smooth tubercles: ph-ac.

- Soft tubercles: bell, crot-h, lach.

- Sore, painful, as if: ant-c, caust, nit-ac, ph-ac, sep.

- Stab wound, after: dep.

- Stinging pain in tubercles: calc, caust, dulc, kali-i, led, mag-c, phos, rhus-t, squil, stram.

- Summer in: kali-bi.

- Suppurating tubercles: am-c, bov, caust, fl-ac, kali-bi, nat-ar, nat-c, nit-ac, sil.

- Syphilitic tubercles: ars, ars-i, dulc, fl-ac, hep, kali-bi, kali-i, merc, nit-ac, phyt, sil, thuj.

- Tearing pain in tubercles: cham, con.

- Tensive tubercles: caust, mur-ac.

- Tuberous tubercles: kali-bi, nat-c, phos, sil, tub.

- Ulcerating tubercles: am-c, bov, caust, fl-ac, kali-i, nat-c, sec.
- Umbilicated tubercles: kali-bi, kali-br.
- Wart-shaped tubercles: lyc, thuj.
- Watery tubercles: graph, mag-c.
- White tubercles: ant-c, dulc, sep, sulph, valer.
- Yellow tubercles: ant-c, rhus-t.
- Winter: kali-br.

■

Sexually Transmitted Diseases

CHANCROID

Synonym

Soft chancre, Soft sore.

Definition

It is an infectious, contagious, ulcerative, sexually transmitted disease cause by the gram-negative bacillus *Haemophilus ducreyi* (the Ducreyi bacillus). It is seen less commonly than other venereal diseases like syphilis or gonorrhea.

Incidence

This condition is commonly seen in tropical countries and in people with lower socio-economic states and negligent of personal hygiene. Males are usually more frequently affected rather than females, who are known more to act as asymptomatic carriers of infection.

Etiology

Haemophilus ducreyi or the Ducreyi bacillus is the causative organism, which is a gram-negative strepto-bacillus, 1.5 ??by 0.5? found in small groups or chains, usually outside the cells.

The infection spreads by sexual contact in most of the cases, though accidental infection by infected material is also known to occur.

Pathology

There is a non-specific inflammatory infiltrate. Involvement of the walls of small blood vessels in the region leads to ulceration.

Clinical Features

The characteristic features of the condition are the occurrence of one or more superficial or deep ulcers on the genitalia, which may tend to suppurate, along with painful inguinal adenitis seen to occur in more than half the cases.

It begins as an inflammatory macule or pustule, usually within a day to a week's time after intercourse. The initial ulcerating papule is followed by similar lesions in adjacent and opposing sites. The regional glands enlarge, and may suppurate. In males, the lesions are especially seen on the distal penis or near the frenum (junction of the skin of the prepuce with the glans), the perianal area, the corona, the under surface of the prepuce, glans penis and on the external urinary meatus. In women, the lesions are seen on the vulva, cervix, labia, fold between the inner surface of the thigh and groin or the perianal area. However, many cases of extragenital infection on hands, eyelids, lips or breasts have also been reported. Autoinoculation leads to the formation of many more kissing lesions on the genitals due to contact, which present a rosette appearance.

This inflammatory pustule ruptures to form a shallow, punched-out or undermined ulcer with a ragged and irregular margin, surrounded by mild hyperemia. The ulcer is soft and lacks the induration characteristic of a chancre. The floor of the ulcer appears raw and pale red with inflammatory thickening, and is covered with a purulent, dirty exudate. The ulcer is very tender and bleeds freely on friction with clothes or on examination. The lesions may fuse with each other forming large ragged areas.

Other constitutional symptoms include occasional headaches, slight pyrexia, especially when superadded infection with pyogenic organisms takes place, which also results in spreading the local lesions. About half the cases tend to manifest with inguinal adenitis.

Clinical variants of this condition include granuloma inguinale-like giant ulcers, serpiginous ulcers, transient chancroid, and follicular and papular variants.

Complications

The clinical course may subside on its own in a few weeks, but in cases of secondary infection, constant local irritation or with a spread or progress in the infection, there can be further complications as follows:

- Inflammatory balanitis and phimosis, with subsequent edema of the prepuce is one of the complications.

- Swelling and suppuration of the inguinal lymph nodes (bubo) may occur early in the disease, which is usually unilateral, smooth, soft and tender to touch, which may rupture spontaneously with a single opening (differentiate from LGV bubo which has multiple openings). The ulcer has ragged margins and a dirty, sloughy base, which continues to discharge sero-sanguinous and purulent matter.

- The suppuration of the bubo if left untreated may further lead to the formation of gangrenous balanitis or phagedena. It results from secondary infection with microorganisms like Vincent spirilla and fusiform bacillus. It is characterized by formation of chronic, painful, ugly, destructive, foul smelling ulcers, which begin on the prepuce or glans and spread rapidly along the shaft of the penis, occasionally involving the scrotum or pubes. The granulating base of the ulcer tends to bleed easily and exudes a thick, purulent and dirty exudate. This type of a spreading and sloughing ulceration is a rare complication of chancre and chancroidal infections.

Diagnosis

1. The typical clinical features with history of exposure and the appearance of sores within the incubation period.

2. On histological investigation, the ulcer may include a superficial necrotic zone with an infiltrate consisting of neutrophils, lymphocytes and red blood cells. Deeper to this layer there is the new vessel formation, with vascular proliferation. Deeper still is an infiltrate of lymphocytes and plasma cells. The gram-negative bacilli Haemophilus ducreyi may or may not be seen in the sections.

3. Solid-media culture techniques now make definitive diagnosis possible, and permit sensitivity testing. Specimens for the culture are to be preferably taken from the purulent ulcer base and active border without extensive cleaning.

4. Smears are only diagnostic in 50% of cases and the smear examination material is preferably taken from the deeper parts of the margin of the ulcer and then stained with Gram's stain.

5. A recent combined polymerase chain reaction (PCR) technique allows the diagnosis of syphilis, herpes simplex, and chancroid from a single swab.

6. Repeated darkfield examinations for Treponema pallidum (spirochaetes of syphilis) are necessary even in a sore where the diagnosis of chancroid has been established. Also, serological tests for syphilis and HIV should form a routine diagnostic procedure to rule out any concomitant infection.

Differential Diagnosis

It needs to be differentiated from herpes progenitalis, which has a history of recurrent grouped vesicles at the same site.

Chancroid should also be differentiated from dermatitis resulting from irritants or medicines and traumatic ulcerations, which occur most commonly along the frenulum or occur as multiple erosions on the prepuce. Here though there is not much adenopathy and only a certain degree of phimosis is seen.

Chancroids also need to be differentiated from syphilitic chancres, which have a much longer incubation period. The repeated darkfield examinations and serologic tests can help further differentiation.

It may also be needed to differentiate chancroid from epithelioma, granuloma venereum and lymphogranuloma venereum.

In scabies, secondary pyoderma may produce boils and pyogenic ulcers, but features like nocturnal pruritis and burrows are obvious.

Homeopathic approach – kindly refer to syphilis

REPERTORY AND THERAPEUTICS OF CHANCRE

- **Skin, eruptions, chancre:** acet-ac, ail, apis, arg-n, asc-t, aur-m, cinnb, cor-r, crot-h, iodof, jac-c, jug-r, kali-i, lac-c, lach, merc, merc-act, merc-c, merc-i-f, merc-i-r, nit-ac, ph-ac, plat-m, sulph.
- **Skin, ulcers, chancre:** cinnb, protg.

Location

- **Female genitalia,** ulcers, chancre: kali-i, merc.
- **Male genitalia,** ulcers, chancre
    - Penis: anan, apis, arg-n, ars, ars-i, ars-met, asaf, aur-met, aur-ar, aur-m, aur-m-n, aur-s, borx, caust, cinnb, con, cor-r, dulc, graph, hep, iod, kali-bi, kali-chl, kali-i, kali-m, lac-c, lach, lyc, merc, merc-c, merc-i-f, merc-i-r, mygal, nit-ac, ph-ac, phos, phyt, plat, plat-m, rhus-t, sars, sep, sil, staph, still, sulph, syph, thuj, viol-t.
        - Burning: ars, ars-met, hep.
        - Elevated margins: ars, cinnb, hep, kali-bi, lyc, merc, nit-ac, ph-ac.
        - Phagedenic: ars, aur-m-n, caust, cinnb, hydr, kali-p, lach, merc-c, nit-ac, sil, sulph.
    - Scrotum: aur-m.

- **Urethra, ulcers:** alumn, arg-n, canth, hep, ip, kali-bi, merc, nit-ac, sabin, sulph, thuj.
  - Meatus: abrot, eucal, lac-c, merc-c, nit-ac.
    - Retained, with sensation as if urine was: canth
    - Sticking, with: nit-ac.

GRANULOMA VENEREUM

Synonym

Granuloma Inguinale; Donovanosis; Ulcerating granuloma of the pudenda.

Definition

This condition is a chronic, mildly contagious, granulomatous infection of the genitalia and the surrounding skin. It is a locally destructive disease, characterized by progressive, indolent, serpiginous ulcerations of the groins, pubes, genitalia and anus.

Etiology & Incidence

It is caused by the gram-negative bacterium *Calymmato-bacterium granulomatosis* (formerly known as *Donovani granulomatis*), which have encapsulated bodies and present mostly inside the mononuclear cells. It is mostly venereal in origin and gets transmitted mostly through sexual contact with an infected individual or by infected vectors. C. granulomatis probably requires direct inoculation through a break in the skin or mucosa to cause infection. Those affected are generally young adults.

Pathology

The histological changes are not specific. In the inflammatory reaction that infiltrates the cutis and subcutis, plasma cells and polymorphonuclear leukocytes pre-dominate. There are also some lymphocytes and large mononuclear cells containing Donovan bodies.

In chronic lesions, fibrosis and epithelial hyperplasia are also present to a variable degree.

Clinical Features

Incubation period may vary between 8-60 or 80 days, with a two to three week period being most common. Course of the disease is slow and prolonged.

The earliest lesion is a firm papule or nodule, which can be single or multiple, and which breaks open to form clean, sharply defined lesions or ulcers with overhanging edges. The ulcers are usually painless and there is no adenitis.

These lesions occur especially on the genitalia; in males the prepuce and glans penis and in females the labia. A few lesions may occur on the inguinal and anal region. Deep and rapidly extending ulceration is seen mainly in women. Serpiginous extension with or without vegetative epithelial changes occurs in the groins and other flexures. Most of the cases form a hypertrophic, papilomatous, vegetative granulation tissue, which is soft, bleeds easily and has a beefy-red appearance. A few cases develop ulcerative lesions with overhanging edges and a dry or moist floor. A membranous exudate may cover the floor of fine granulations, and the lesions are moderately painful. The lesions spread by autoinoculation and peripheral extension.

The lesions are not painful and produce only mild subjective symptoms.

Persisting sinuses and hypertrophic scars, devoid of pigment, are fairly characteristic of the disease. Pseudoelephantiasis of the genitals may also occur due to blockage of lymph channels in later stages, as a result of cicatrization. The mucus membranes and viscera are usually spared. The regional lymph nodes are not involved but pseudo-bubo may be seen.

Spreading can occur from the inguinal region by hematogenous or lymphatic routes, leading to involvement of liver, spleen, limbs, eyes, face (esp. nose and lips), larynx, chest, and rarely bones.

Healing may occur at any stage, or slow or rapid extension

may continue intermittently and irregularly for years. Secondary infection may be severe and may lead to adenitis.

When the lesions are extensive, cachexia may, after a long course of many years, predispose to death from intercurrent infection.

Diagnosis

1. On histological examination, the epidermis in the center of the lesion is found to be replaced by serum, fibrin and polymorphonuclear leucocytes; and at the periphery, there is epithelial thickening. In the dermis there is a dense granulomatous infiltration of plasma cells and histiocytes. Also, numerous small abscesses are scattered throughout, which contain polymorphonuclear leucocytes. In chronic lesions, fibrosis and epithelial hyperplasia are also present to a variable degree.

2. Rapid diagnosis can be established by staining the crushed smears of fresh biopsy material (taken esp. from the edge of the lesion) with Wright or Giemsa stain. This permits the demonstration of ovoid Donovan bodies, which measure 1 to 2 im. The parasitized histiocytes may measure upto 20 im or more in diameter. This organism cannot be cultured.

Differential Diagnosis

1. It may be confused with ulcerations of the groin caused by syphilis or carcinoma. Thus, biopsy examination, dark-ground examination and serological tests for syphilis should always be carried out to differentiate. Also, the long duration and slow course of granuloma inguinale helps in distinguishing it further from these illnesses.

2. Also, all patients with venereal diseases should be also checked for HIV infection.

3. Granuloma inguinale can be distinguished from lympho-granuloma venereum by the absence of a positive lymphogranuloma venereum complement-fixation test and the presence of Donovan bodies in the lesions.

LYMPHOGRANULOMA VENEREUM

Synonym

Lymphogranuloma inguinale; climatic bubo; nicholas favre disease.

It is a contagious venereal disease, differing from granuloma venereum due to its rapid involvement of the lymphatic system. It is characterized by suppurative inguinal adenitis with matted lymph nodes, inguinal bubo with secondary ulceration, and constitutional symptoms.

Etiology & Incidence

It is caused by *chlamydia trachomatis* organism (types 11, 12 and 13) of 0.25 x 0.5 in size. Humans are the only natural host.

Infection is transmitted by heterosexual or homosexual sexual intercourse. Medical practitioners, nurses and lab workers can accidentally pick up the disease by handling infected material.

Usually young adults are affected, but no age is exempt. Females are often asymptomatic carriers of the disease.

It occurs in all races, but is more common among the sexually active and in the tropical countries. Also, anorectal LGV is increasing in the homosexual population of the western countries.

Pathology

The lymphogranulomatous chancre usually shows no specific changes, but the necrotic area may be surrounded by epithelioid cells and a zone of granulation tissue rich in plasma cells.

The lymph nodes first show scattered foci of epithelioid cells, with occasional giant cells. These foci enlarge irregularly and undergo necrosis to form the stellate abscesses characteristic of the disease. The abscesses, which contain polymorphonuclear leukocytes and macrophages, are surrounded by epithelioid cells and chronic granulomatous tissue with numerous plasma cells.

In the later stages, very extensive fibrosis and large areas of coagulation necrosis are usual.

Clinical Features

The incubation period of this condition is about 3-20 days, after which a primary lesion develops, which is a 2-3 mm superficial, painless, small papulo-vesicle or erosion that lasts for a short while and then heals without scarring or forms a shallow ulceration. In males, the primary lesion is seen on the glans penis, prepuce, meatus or the corona; in females it occurs especially on the fourchette, posterior half of the labia majora, or the posterior wall of the vagina or cervix. The chancre is inconspicuous, heals rapidly and is often unnoticed.

The primary lesion can also manifest itself in the form of bacterial urethritis in a few cases. Often the primary lesions may go unnoticed, especially in females. Extragenital primary infections of LGV are rare, except that a few ulcerating lesions may appear on the fingers, lips or the tongue.

Two to three weeks after the primary lesion, there is enlargement and subacute inflammation of the regional lymph nodes, which is usually unilateral (but may be bilateral in one third of the cases). The subsequent course of the disease depends on which glands are involved and on the extent and severity of the constitutional disturbance. Some cases resolve spontaneously within a few months, but in the majority chronic symptoms persist, often with irregular acute episodes.

The *inguinal syndrome* is the most frequent manifestation in men, where to begin with, the inguinal glands are usually painful, tender, swollen and elastic. Soon they become matted and fuse together into a large mass and then begin to soften, developing small areas of fluctuation, followed by suppuration (bubo); some of which then break through the reddish purple overlying skin to form chronic sinuses and fistulous openings. The groin-fold frequently divides the glands characteristically into upper and lower groups, the sign of the groove. Less commonly, the adenitis becomes chronic and indolent. The pelvic and iliac glands may also be involved, but they rarely suppurate.

The *rectal syndrome* occurs mainly in women, in whom the primary lesion is often in the vagina. The pelvic glands are involved and periproctitis and proctitis (with the characteristic bloody, mucopurulent discharge) are followed by a rectal stricture usually between 5 and 10 cm from the anal margin, which fistulae frequently develop. Carcinoma is not uncommon later.

The *genital syndromes* occur in both sexes. Most characteristic is genital lymphoedema, which may develop a few weeks or many years after infection and gives rise to elephantiasis. The association of elephantiasis of the vulva with scarring and fistulae of the buttocks and thighs is known as 'esthiomene'. Occasionally, small abscesses develop along the course of the superficial lymphatics draining the primary lesion and break down to form ulcers.

The adenitis is accompanied by *systemic symptoms* of general malaise, joint pains and stiffness, headache, conjunctivitis, loss of appetite, weight loss, anemia and low-grade fever, which may persist for several weeks. The adenitis is followed later by chronic genital and anorectal manifestations produced by hyperplastic or ulcerative changes. Elephantiasis of the genitalia, hepatomegaly, splenomegaly, vaginal strictures, and chronic local ulceration are the common late effects. Erythema nodosum or erythema multiforme like rash may also occur in a few cases. The eyes, lids, tongue, lungs and the meningeal membrane of the brain are rarely involved.

Prognosis

LGV is a slowly progressive disease, resulting in considerable mutilation of the genitalia, anus and rectum and hence causes a great deal of misery. The untreated disease usually runs an average course of 6-8 weeks and may then resolve completely. Delay in treatment results in disfiguring and troublesome sequelae left by the healed lesions. Many cases are left with the sequelae of lymphatic obstruction and some show periodic recrudescences of activity for many years.

Diagnosis

It is confirmed by:

1. Demonstration of elementary bodies in the smears of bubo pus by Giemsa's stain.

2. Hyperglobinemia is a constant feature.

3. On examination, the characteristic changes in the lymph nodes consist of an infectious granuloma with the formation of stellate abscesses. There is an outer zone of epitheloid cells with a central necrotic core comprised of debris of lymphocytes and leucocytes. In lesions of long duration, plasma cells may be present.

4. The complement fixation test (a simple serologic test for detecting antibodies) is usually positive, especially four weeks after onset of the illness. A titre of 164 is highly suggestive.

5. A fluorescence antibody test is more specific for diagnosis.

6. Microhemagglutination inhibition assays are also available and not only confirm the diagnosis but also identify the strain.

7. Blood shows an increased level of serum globulin. An S.T.S should be done to exclude any concurrent infection with syphilis.

8. Culture is not practical. Biopsy of a lymph node or a smear of the bubo pus may be helpful.

Differential Diagnosis

1. The adenitis of infectious mononucleosis, syphilis, granuloma inguinale, Hodgkin's disease or leukemia is less acute and usually not painful.

2. In cases of a Chancroid bubo, the primary lesion is always present, whereas in Lymphogranuloma venereum, the primary lesions are either absent, go unnoticed or are healed. Also chancroids are known to have a quicker evolution than LGV. Also, with chancroid, a primary chancre or multiple chancroidal ulcers are present and may permit the demonstration of H.

ducreyi. The skin lesions are characteristic and usually much larger and more persistent than the primary lesion of LGV. Iliac adenopathy is absent in cases of chancroid, which is invariably present in cases of LGV.

3. In cases of Granuloma inguinale, Ducrey's bacilli may be demonstrated in the pus or scrapping from the wall of the abscess. Whereas, in cases of LGV, the pus is usually sterile, and the elementary bodies may be demonstrated by special staining. Also, inguinal adenitis is not characteristic in cases of Granuloma inguinale.

4. Also, finally well-developed primary lesions of syphilis may be confused with the primary lesions of syphilis. Here dark field examination for Treponema pallidum is diagnostic. Also, syphilitic inguinal adenitis shows small, hard, non-tender glands. The serologic tests for syphilis and complement fixation tests help further differentiation.

5. HIV should also be ruled out by getting its serologic testing done.

GONORRHEA

Gonorrhea is one of the commonest sexually transmitted diseases the world over. It is almost always acquired by a homosexual or heterosexual act.

(Though this condition doesn't specifically affect only the skin, it is mentioned here as a part of the sexually transmitted diseases)

Etiology & Incidence

This disease is caused by a gram-negative diplococcus, named *Neisseria gonorrhea*, which affects especially the non-cornified columnar and cuboidal epithelium of the urogenital tract, usually by attaching themselves to cells with the help of pili before initiating infection. These organisms are ingested by polymorphs and they survive within the cells for variable periods, being protected from adverse environment. Four types can be distinguished by cultural characteristics, of which, types T_1 and T_2 are known to be virulent whereas T_3 and T_4 are comparatively not harmful.

The common age group of those affected is 15-30 years, with about half of them presenting during the adolescent period. Individuals or groups with increased sexual exposure, esp. truck drivers, prostitutes and their clients, are understandably infected more frequently.

Females usually act as carriers and suffer from complications of the disease more frequently because of the non-specific or asymptomatic nature of the initial infection.

Pathology

Gonococci affect columnar and transitional epithelium mainly and infection is initiated in the urethra, rectum, conjunctiva, pharynx and endocervix. Pus is produced locally. Direct extension from the site of infection leads to complications such as endometritis, salpingitis, peritonitis and bartholinitis in females; and periurethral abscess, epididymoorchitis and prostatitis in males. Ocular conjunctiva is affected. Metastatic spread of the organisms leads to arthritis, dermatitis, endocarditis, meningitis, myocarditis and hepatitis.

Clinical Features

In the male the disease has a more acute onset than the female.

The incubation period of the disease is about one to five days.

GONORRHEA IN THE MALE

In the heterosexual male, the uncomplicated infection presents as urethritis, and less frequently as pharyngitis. In homosexual males it may present as proctitis or urethritis.

Urethritis (usually where the anterior wall is affected) can be diagnosed by symptoms like dysuria, constant burning sensation in the penis and urethral discharge, which is often of a purulent nature. At times patients may have mucoid discharge that makes it difficult to differentiate from non-gonococcal infections. Meatal inflammation and penile edema may also be noticed. A small percent may remain completely asymptomatic. Complication may result from spread of the infection to cause epididymitis, inflammation of the spermatic cord and testes and chronic prostatitis.

If left alone, the acute manifestations subside over a period of weeks or months even without treatment. Exacerbations occur frequently as a result of sexual indulgence, alcoholism or undue exertion. Chronic affections cause anterior and posterior urethral stricture formation. Periurethral abscess may develop, with fistulous openings, discharging urine from multiple sites (*water-can-scrotum*). In 10% of subjects the lesion may be asymptomatic and has to be detected by examination.

GONORRHEA IN THE FEMALE

In the heterosexual female, the uncomplicated infection presents as vulvo-vaginitis and cervicitis, and less frequently as pharyngitis. The pharyngeal infection is usually transmitted through oral sex.

Quite a few patients can be completely asymptomatic or suffer from non-specific symptoms. Vaginal discharge or leucorrhea, vaginal discomfort, dysuria, menstrual abnormalities and features of pelvic inflammation are the common symptoms.

Rectal lesions develop in about 40 % of affected women due to contamination by cervical discharges. The gonococci may pass up from the endocervix leading to salpingitis and oophoritis. Exacerbations occur during menstrual periods or one to two weeks thereafter. Gonococcal salpingo-oophoritis is a common cause of sterility.

RECTAL AND OROPHARYNGEAL INFECTION

Rectal gonorrhea may occur in homosexual males and heterosexual females as a result of ano-genital sex. In females this may also occur because of direct inoculation of the anal canal with discharge from genital infection. The symptoms vary from mild anal pruritis and mucopurulent discharge to symptoms of severe proctitis with rectal pain and tenesmus.

Pharyngitis and tonsillitis result from oro-genital sex and may be seen in either sex. In the majority of cases the symptoms are not severe enough to seek medical care. Strong clinical acumen and microbiological investigation may be required to make the diagnosis.

OCULAR GONORRHEA

Gonococcal involvement of the eye is rare in adults. In the newborn, ocular involvement is the result of infection acquired during passage through the infected maternal birth canal. The newborn may develop acute purulent conjunctivitis that may affect deeper structures of the eye and may occasionally result in panophthalmia and blindness. The infection may also disseminate to other tissues and result in arthritis in the newborn.

GONOCOCCAL DERMATITIS

Primary gonococcal dermatitis is a rare infection that occurs mostly as erosions that may be 2 to 20 mm in diameter. It may also affect the median raphe without urethritis or it may occur as pustular eruptions at the base of the fingers, which look like a herpetic whitlow. It may also occur as scalp abscesses in infants, secondary to direct fetal monitoring in mothers with gonorrhea.

GONOCOCCEMIA

Gonococcemia is characterized by hemorrhagic vesiculo-pustular eruptions (esp. on the extremities), fever and arthralgia. The skin lesions begin as tiny erythematous macules that evolve into tender vesicopustules on a deeply erythematous base or into purpuric macules that may be as much as 2 cm in diameter. These purpuric lesions occur especially on the palms and soles and over the joints. These lesions are accompanied by fever, chills, malaise, migratory polyarthralgia, myalgia and tenosynovitis. Involution of the lesions takes place in about 4 days.

Many patients seen are women with asymptomatic anogenital infections in whom dissemination occurs during pregnancy or menstruation. Liver function abnormalities, myocarditis, pericarditis, endocarditis, and meningitis may complicate this infection.

Diagnosis

- Gonorrhea should be suspected in all clinical situations where there is purulent urethral discharge, leucorrhea in women, a typical oropharyngeal ulceration, proctocolitis and ophthalmia neonatorum.

- Bacteriological diagnosis is established by demonstrating gram-negative diplococci inside polymorphonuclear cells in the exudates.

- The causative organism, Neisseria gonorrheae, can at times by demonstrated in the early skin lesion histologically, by smears, and by cultures. The Gonococci may be found in the blood, genitourinary tract, joints and skin.

- Culture of cervical discharge is required in women with late manifestations to establish the diagnosis.

- Fluorescent antibody techniques help in making quick diagnosis.

- Complement fixation test is useful in selected cases of chronic gonorrhea with systemic manifestations.

Complications

- In males, epididymitis is one of the commonest complications, which presents as unilateral painful and tender swelling. Other complications in males include inflammation of the spermatic cord and testes, periurethral abscesses and chronic prostatitis.

- In females, salpingo-oophoritis and pelvic inflammatory disease are common complications and present as lower abdominal pain and a tender pelvic mass palpated on per vaginal examination. Bartholinitis and sterility are other common complications.

- Gonococcal bacteremia may result in an acute arthritis-dermatitis syndrome also known as 'disseminated gonococcal infection'. Risk of dissemination depends on the type and virulence of the organism. Dissemination is more common from the silent foci in the pharynx, rectum or endocervix. It occurs in about 30% of the infected patients, of which, 80% are usually females. Manifestations include cutaneous lesions, septic arthritis, septicemia, endocarditis, myocarditis and rarely pericarditis or meningitis. The cutaneous lesions take the form of vesicles and necrotic pustules (especially on the skin of the distal parts of the extremities), which do not usually ulcerate.

Differential Diagnosis

The skin lesions of Gonococcemia may be identical to those seen in meningococcemia, nongonococcal bacterial endocarditis, rheumatoid arthritis, the rickettsial diseases, systemic lupus erythematosus, periarteritis nodosa, Haverhill fever and typhoid fever.

HOMEOPATHIC APPROACH TO GONORRHEA

Patients suffering from gonorrhea can present to a homeopath with multiple symptoms.

- Acute gonorrhea.
- Chronic gonorrhea (sycosis).
- Gonorrheal stricture.
- Gonorrheal prostatitis.
- Gonorrheal cystitis.
- Gonorrheal ophthalmia.
- Rheumatism.
- Chordee (gonococcal).
- Disseminated gonococcal infection.

It is essential to know the philosophy of chronic miasm before one handles serious illnesses like gonorrhea. After the disappearance of the discharge (under any non-homeopathic treatment) the disease is, in 90% of cases, not cured but remains latent, not merely locally but constitutionally, what we call as 'Sycotic constitution'. The ignorant patient remains in dark for quite a long time till the symptoms of sycosis come to the surface in the form of:

1. Poor health,
2. Sterility,
3. Rheumatic troubles,
4. Cauliflower-like excrescences, etc.

Whenever a patient comes to a homeopath with symptoms that resemble the Sycotic trait and there is a past history of gonorrhea, then he should be treated with anti-sycotic remedy, till the previous urethral discharge is restored, then only in the true sense we can label the person to be cured.

To achieve the right selection of antisycotic one has to jump two hurdles:

1. Recognition of the sycotic state by detailed case taking,
2. Interposing intercurrent remedy like Medorrhinum, Sycotic-co and Thuja rationally whenever the case demands.

Whilst taking the history, the following points should be paid attention to carefully:

1. Note down carefully the patients presenting symptoms chronologically and then evaluate the complication, chronicity and type of gonorrhea (disseminated genital, oro-pharyngeal) etc.

2. Review the previous investigation reports and confirm your clinical diagnosis.

3. Whilst noting the symptoms, stress should be on the following points:

a) Characteristic of discharge.

b) Local appearance of genitalia.

c) Sexual history including erections.

d) Symptoms related to testes.

e) History of previous treatment.

f) Special sensations in relation to urethra and bladder. E.g. drops running up and down the course of urethra; sensation of dryness in urethra, etc.

Some Important Remedies for Gonorrhea

Agave americana: Extremely painful erections. Great difficulty in passing urine, accompanied by heat, pain and tenesmus at neck of bladder. Chordee. Drawing in the spermatic cords and testicles, extending to thighs so violent that he wishes to die.

Agnus castus: Testicles cold, swollen, hard. Penis is small and flaccid. Impotence with gleet, especially in those who have frequently had gonorrhea. Yellow, purulent discharge from urethra especially in old sinners, or after inflammation has subsided. Disagreeable and uneasy feeling in back part of urethra sexual desire almost lost. Penis so relaxed that voluptuous fancies excite no erection. Emission of prostatic fluid when straining at stool; during micturition. Itching of the genitals.

Female: Transparent leucorrhea; parts very relaxed. Leucorrhea spotting the linen yellow.

Mind: Scare of approaching death; keeps repeating that she will soon die. Extreme absence of mind; finds it difficult to read or keep up the train of thought.

Argentum nitricum: Frequently indicated in acute gonorrhea. Ulcerative pain in the middle of the urethra as from a splinter. Urging to urinate; urine burns while passing, urethra feels swollen, with sensation as if the last drop remained behind, causing a sensation of internal sore swelling. Towards the end of urination, there is a sensation as if the urethra was knotted or closed. Itching in urethra.

Chordee; stricture of urethra. Impotence; erections fail when coition is attempted. Coition painful, urethra as if put on stretch or sensitive at on. Painful tension during erection. Bleeding from the urethra and a shooting pain in the urethra from behind forward. Pain in the testes and scrotum as from pins and needles.

Camphora officinalis: Gonorrhea with constant sticking together of meatus. Strangury from stricture. Urine passes in a thin stream and is very acrid. Burning pain during emission of urine. Chordee. Absence of sexual desire. Sudden laxness of the penis. On the left side of the root of the penis, while standing, there is a sensation of pressure outwards, as if a hernia would protrude.

Cannabis indica: Burning and scalding, or stinging pain in the urethra before, during and after urination. Urging to urinate with much straining, but cannot pass a drop, or has to wait for some time before urine flows. Profuse colorless urine. Urine dribbles out after the stream ceases. White glary mucus may be squeezed from urethra. Sharp pricking like needles, in urethra, so severe as to send a thrill to cheeks and hands. Priapism.

Cannabis sativa: Discharge from the urethra is thin, watery and of a disagreeable odor. Discharge of pus from the urethra. Burning when urinating, but especially just after. Stream of urine is forked. Emission drop by drop of a scanty and sanguineous nature. Burning pain in the urethra and bladder before and during emission of urine. Urethra inflamed and painful to touch. Dark redness of glans and prepuce. Great swelling of prepuce, phimosis. Meatus is painful touch. Penis sore as if burnt, when walking; walks with legs apart. Swelling of prostate. Pressing, dragging sensation in the testicles when standing. Genitals cold.

Females: cutting pain in labia during urination. Urethra plugged with pus. Threatened abortion, complicated with gonorrhea. Great excitement with sterility.

Cantharis vesicatoria: Sexual desire greatly increased with painful, frequent erections (with gonorrhea), of long continuance; as in priapism. Violent pains in the bladder with frequent urging, intolerable tenesmus. Violent burning, cutting pain in neck of bladder, extending to fossa navicularis; < before and after urinating. Fruitless effort to urinate. Constant burning, desire to urinate, passing only a few drops at a time, often mixed with blood. Yellow or bloody discharge. Retention of urine and tenesmus vesicae when discharge is suppressed by injections. Retention of urine with pain. There is a cutting pain in the urethra before, during and after urination.

Females: Burning heat of the external parts. Swelling of vulva and vagina with itching, burning and a thick white discharge (Carleton).

Capsicum annuum: Discharge from urethra is purulent, bloody. Urethra is painful to touch, with a cream-like discharge. Prepuce swollen. Burning, biting or cutting pains in urethra between acts of urination, most marked at the meatus. Strangury, tenesmus of neck of bladder; he has urging to frequent, almost ineffectual urination. Painful erection at night. Especially indicated in the fat and indolent with lax fibre. Impotence and coldness of genitals. Dwindling of testes. Trembling of whole body during amorous caresses.

Chimaphila umbellata: Stricture of the urethra; difficult urination. Urine contains large quantity of ropy mucus. Tenesmus of the bladder. Acute and chronic cystitis. Inability to pass urine without standing with feet widely separated. Acute inflammation of prostrate with sensation of swelling in perineum on sitting, as if a ball was pressing against it. Urine is highly colored with bloody, greenish or reddish sediment.

Cinnabaris: Gonorrhea on a Sycotic base or complicated with syphilis of very long-standing type, with much soreness and pain during micturition. Warts on the prepuce, bleeding from the slightest touch with swelling and itching, soreness on urinating. Violent itching of the corona glands with profuse secretion of pus. Sexual desire strongly excited with great inclination for coition and a great appetite for eating and drinking. Fetid and corrosive perspiration between the scrotum and the thighs when walking.

Clematis erecta: Painful, inflamed, swollen testicles. Induration of the testicles, which are as hard as stone. Right spermatic cord sensitive, testicles drawn up. Pain and burning while urinating, most severe at its commencement. Mucus in urine, but no pus. Secretion of urine diminished; the last drops cause violent burning. Contraction of urethra, with the urine stopping suddenly, or only flowing drop by drop; jerk-like tearing in the forepart of urethra in intervals. Aversion to sexual enjoyment, as after excessive indulgence.

Digitalis purpurea: Burning in urethra with purulent discharge, thick bright and yellow. Glans inflamed with copious secretion of thick pus over its surface. Inflammation of neck of bladder. In the right testicle the pain, as if contused. Chordee. Dropsical swelling of prepuce. Dropsical swelling of genitals with nymphomania. Retention of urine. Urgent and most futile inclination to micturate, with discharge of hot, burning and very scanty urine. Frequent emission of small quantities of water-colored urine. While in a recumbent position the urine can be retained for a long time.

Gelsemium sempervirens: At the very beginning of urethritis (Acon.) with great pain and scanty discharge or little pain with much heat, urine voided in sufficient quantities, rather frequent, with smarting at meatus, whitish discharge. Genitals cold relaxed; dragging in testicles, suppressed gonorrhea; followed by rheumatism or orchitis. Gleet with stricture of urethra sensation as if something remained behind while urinating, streams stops and commences again. Constant dribbling of urine from muscular weakness. Painful redness of urethra (secondary gonorrhea). Headache > frequent micturition.

Hydrastis canadensis: Acute or chronic form. In second stage, copious, persistent discharge without pain or soreness in urethra; discharge being thick, yellow, tenacious. Urine has thick ropy, mucus sediment. Gleet with copious, painless discharge and debility. Feeling of debility and faintness after stool. Dragging in right groin to testicle; thence to it testicle, thence to left groin.

F- 39

Kalium bichromicum: Gleet with profuse stringy or jelly-like discharge. Pain across back with red urine. After micturition, burning in back part of urethra, with sensation as if one drop had remained behind, with unsuccessful effort to void it. Perforating Sycotic ulcers about glans and prepuce. Constrictive pain at root of penis (morning on waking. Violent pain in os coccyges < when rising, after he sat long, to urinate. Sexual desire absent in fleshy people. Worse from coition.

Medorrhinum: Burning in the meatus during urination, feeling of soreness in urethra, and after urination feeling as if something remained in urethra; profuse, yellow, purulent discharge, most copious in morning gumming up orifice; frequent calls to urinate. Suppressed gonorrhea. Syncope after urination.

Mercurius solubilis: Gonorrhea with phimosis or chancroids. Greenish discharge < at night. Lips of meatus red and inflamed. Glans penis dark red and hot, with burning, stitching, itching pains in urethra. Strangury, tenesmus, painful erections. Pulling and tearing at the prepuce all the time. Glans and prepuce inflamed; phimosis aggravated from cold air. Gonorrheal Cystitis. Urine turbid.

Females: Inflammation of the vulva, which is swollen, red and hot.

Mezereum: A drop of gluey, albuminous liquid appears at times at the orifices of the urethra. Discharge of watery mucus, worse from exercise. Itching of prepuce. Heat, swelling and titillation along the course of the urethra. Perineum is tender to touch. Gleet with green discharge in the absence of any other remedy. Abundant secretion of smegma behind glans, like gonorrhea balani. Biting burning in fore part of urethra at close of micturition. After micturition, there is itchng at prepuce.

Natrium muriaticum: Chronic gonorrhea after infections of silver nitrate. Clear, sometimes yellowish discharge in gleet. Cutting pain in urethra after urination, with spasmodic contraction in abdomen. Strong fetid odor from genitals. Loss of hair from pubes. Pollutions after coition.

Nitricum acidum: Gonorrhea with chancres and warts. Small blisters on the orifice of urethra and inner surface of prepuce. Bloody mucus or purulent discharge. Pricking pain in urethra. While urinating, smarting, burning in urethra. Ulcers in urethra. Gleet, Phimosis. Urine offensive like horse's urine. Urine cold when it passes. Itching, swelling and burning in vulva and vagina. Micturition in thin stream, as from a stricture. Discharge of prostatic fluid after a difficult stool.

Pareira brava: Urethritis with prostatic disorders. Violent pain in urethra. Strangury; violent pain in the glans penis when straining for urine. Discharge of mucus from urethra. Almost cartilaginous induration of mucus membrane of bladder. Paroxysms of violent pain with the strangury; he cries out loud and can only emit urine when he goes on his knees, pressing his head firmly against the floor; remaining in this position for 10–20 minutes; perspiration breaks out and finally the urine begins to drop with interruptions, accompanied by tearing, burning pains in glans penis.

Pulsatilla nigricans: Discharge from urethra thick, muco-purulent, yellow or yellowish green. Gonorrheal rheumatism, orchitis and prostatitis. Ailments from suppressed gonorrhea. Itching, burning on inner and upper side of prepuce. Inflammatory swelling of the testes and spermatic cords (sometimes only on one side), with pressive and drawing pains, extending into abdomen and loins, redness and heat of scrotum (from suppressed gonorrhea), nausea and inclination to vomit.

Sarsaparilla officinalis: Rheumatism from suppressed gonorrhea. Gonorrhea checked by cold wet weather or by mercury. Severe pain at the end of urination. Severe tenesmus of bladder and discharge of while and turbid matter mixed with mucus. Can pass urine only when standing. Burning in urethra with incontinence of urine < in daytime <when urine is high colored; < after drinking beer. Old dry sycotic warts remaining after mercurial treatment for gouty pains.

Sepia officinalis: Gleet; no pain; discharge only during the night, a drop or so staining the linen yellowish. Urine is turbid and offensive. Condylomata from suppressing gonorrhea with astringent injection. Chronic cystitis. Urine is so offensive that it must be removed at once. Fetid urine with reddish clay colored sediment adhering to the chamber. Smarting in urethra when urinating.

Sulphur: Burning in urethral orifice during micturition. Bright redness and inflammation of urethral orifice. Discharge thick and purulent or thin and watery. Phimosis with discharge of fetid pus. Phimosis; prepuce inflamed and indurated. (*Digitalis* prepuce not indurated with deep cracks, burning and redness.) Secondary gonorrhea. Small and intermittent stream of urine. Escape of prostatic fluid chiefly when urinating and while at stool.

Terebinthina oleum: Gonorrhea with strangury, tenesmus of bladder, smarting in urethra; chordee painful; urination every 10 minutes > by micturition. Haematuria. Gonorrheal rheumatism. Stricture of urethra. Spasmodic and incisive drawings in the testes and spermatic cords.

Thuja occidentalis: Painful spermatic cords from suppressed gonorrhea. Condylomata on glans and prepuce, moist, itching and suppurating especially when the moon is increasing. Red excrescences on the inner side of the prepuce, like fig-warts. Many red pedunculated condylomata surrounding the glans. Fig-warts smell like old cheese or brine. Prostatic affections from suppressed or badly treated gonorrhea. Gonorrhea; scalding when urinating, urethra swollen. Urine stream forked as if drop remained behind. Discharge is yellowish-green, watery. Warts and red erosions on glans; subacute and chronic cases; especially when injections have been used and the prostate has been involved. Gonorrhea with a soft lump, having an abrasion on it, on the left side of frenum preputial; the lump is small and painless. Renewed gonorrhea offer coitus. Jerking and voluptuous formication in fossa navicularis. After urination, sensation as if a drop remained behind; titillation as though a drop of urine was passing along urethra; urging to urinate frequently and hastily, stream interrupted. Perspiration on the genitals, especially the scrotum smells sweet like honey. Checked gonorrhea causes prostatitis. Impotence. Paresis-like weakness in the extremities. Hairfall. Urine clear when passed, but becomes cloudy on standing.

REPERTORY

- **URETHRA, discharge, gonorrheal:** acon, agav-a, agn, aloe, alum, alum-p, alumn; aur-m, anag, ant-c, apis, arg-met, ars, ars-s-f, aur, aur-m, bar-m, benz-ac, bism, borx, cajan, calad, calc, calc-p, calc-s, camph, cann-i, cann-s, canth, caps, caust, cedr, cham, chel, chim, chin-b, clem, cob, coc-c, coch, cop, crot-h, cub, cupr-ar, dig, dor, epiph, equis-h, erech, erig, ery-a, eucal, euph-pi, fab, ferr, ferr-i, ferr-p, ferr-s, fl-ac, frag, gels, hedy, hep, hib-sa, hydr, hydrc, hygroph-aur, ichth, jac-c, jac-g, kali-c, kali-chl, kali-i, kali-s, lac-c, lact-v, lant-t, lappa, led, lup, lyc, med, merc, merc-c, merc-n, nat-m, nat-s, nit-ac, nux-v, oci-car, oci-g, ol-an, ol-sant, petr, petros, ph-ac, phos, phyt, pin-c, pip-m, plb, polyg-xyz, psor, pub, rat, rhod, rumx-ab, sabad, sabal, sabin, sal-n, salol, sars, senec, sep, sil, sil-mar, still, sul-i, sulph, tarent, ter, thlas, thuj, trad, tus-p.

- **Acute inflammatory stage:** acon, arg-n, atrop, cann-s, canth, caps, gels, petros.

- **Adernutus Lymphangitis:** acon, apis, bell, hep, merc.

- **Bubo:** aur-m-n, bad, bufo, carb-an, lac-c, lach, merc, merc-c, nit-ac, phyt, syph.

- **Burning during urination:** carb-an.

- **Chordee:** acon, agar, anac, arg-n, aur-m, bell, berb, bry, camph, camph-br, cann-i, cann-s, canth, caps, clem, cop, chlol, cub, cur, dig, ery-a, fl-ac, hep, hyos, jac-c, kali-br, kali-m, kali-chl, kali-i, merc, mygale, merc-c, nat-c, nit-ac, nux-v, oena, ol-sant, petr, phos, pic-ac, pip-m, pip-n, puls, sabad, sal-n, sep, stram, still, ter, tussil, thuj, yohimb, zinc, zing.

  - Chordee can only be subdued in cold water: caps.
  - Chordee with frequent priapism: petr.
  - Chordee in 2nd stage: kali-m.

- Chordee: burning in urethra with: calc-p.
- Chordee, sensitiveness of urethra, with extreme: caps.
- **Chronic subacute stage:** arg-n, cann-s, cop, cub, erig, hep, hydr, kali-s, merc-c, merc, naph, nat-s, ol-sant, pin-c, psor, rhod, sabal, sep, sil, stigm, sulph, thuj.
- **Coition, renewed by:** thuj.
- **Cowperitis:** acon, cann-s, hep, merc-c, petros, pichi, sabal, sil.
- **Constitution in anaemic persons,** chronic: calc-p.
  - in blonde men of light temperament: puls.
  - in dark irritable vindictive men: nit-ac.
  - in elderly men, difficult urination: agro.
  - in gleet of old sinners: agn.
  - sanguine, full blodded: acon.
  - with scrofula: hep.
  - in strong men, particularly of hydrogenoid constitution: nat-s.
  - in timid, nervous men, acute: gels.
- **Discharge.**
  - Night: merc, merc-c, sep.
    - Night only: sep.
  - Chronic: alum, alumn, arg-m, brom, calc, calc-p, calc-s, chim, chlor, cinnb, colch, cub, cupr, ferr, hydr, kali-s, med, mygal, myric, nat-m, nat-s, petr, petros, plb, psor, sep, sil, sulph, thuj.
  - Acrid, excoriating: arg-n, aur-mur, caps, cop, gels, hydr, kreos, merc-c, sars, thuj.
  - Albuminous, yellow: petros.
  - Black: nat-m.
  - Bloody: ant-c, calc-s, canth, caps, ham, merc-c, nit-ac, puls.
    - Watery, shine: mill.
    - Mucus: nit-ac.

- Clear, transparent: mez, nat-m, ph-ac.
- Constant: ars-s-f.
- Copious: ars-s-f.
- Cream like: caps.
- Fetid: benz-ac, carb-v, puls, sil.
- Free & mucoid: merc-i-r.
- Green: cam-s, merc, merc-c, nit-ac, thuja.
  - Painless: merc.
  - Purulent, worse at night: merc.
- Yellowish, green.
  - Thick: nat-s.
  - With frequent obstructions: cub.
  - Indolent in character: arg-n.
- Lumpy: calc-s.
  - Increase after having decreased: bry, sep, sulph, thuj.
- Milky: cop, lach, petros.
  - Glairy mucus: cann-i, cann-s, cop, cupr-ar, graph, hydr.
- Mucous: caps, ferr, kali-bi, nat-m, petr, puls, sep.
- Muco purulent: benz-ac.
  - Yellowish green: agn, alum, arg-n, cann-s, canth, caps, cob, cop, cub, dig, hep, hydr, jac-c, kali-i, kali-s, merc, merc-c, nat-m, nat-s, ol-sant, pub, sep, sil, sulph-n, thuj, tus-fr, zing.
  - Painless: cann-s.
- Profuse: arg-n, cann-i.
  - Inflammation very high: petr.
  - Pus like, after two months: cub.
  - Scalding urine: cub.
  - Yellow, purulent, most copious in morning: med.
  - Yellowish white: sep.

- Purulent: agn, bar-c, cann-s, caps, chel, con, cop, nat-m, phos, ph-ac.
  - Yellow mucus or greenish: kali-s.
- Of pus: chel, sil.
- Glutinous: cub.
- Pus, like bloody: sil.
- Variable as to quantity: cupr.
- Scanty: coch.
  - Thick: rhus-t.
- Slight, shreddy: sil.
- Thick: calc-s, cann-s.
  - Greenish: kali-i.
  - Worse at night: merc.
  - With frequent obstruction of urethra: cub.
  - Of thick, pus: clem, cub.
  - Thick after six weeks: cub.
  - At first thin, afterwards thick: merc-c.
- Thin, transparent, mixed with opaque whitish mucus, which stains the linen yellow: med.
- Watery: cann-s, fl-ac, mez, nat-m, sep, sulph, thuj.
  - Mucus: cann-s, fl-ac, mez, nat-m, thuj.
  - Transparent, but acrid, and abundant, mixed with creamy liquid stains linen yellow brown: med.
- Whitish: gels.
- Yellow: agn, ars-s-f, calc-s, canth, caps, cop, hep, nat-m, nit-ac, sars, thuja.
  - Worse at night: merc.
  - Stains shirt light yellow, not profuse: tarent.
  - Thick yellow or yellowgreen: puls.
  - After six weeks: cub.

- Yellowish or bloody: nit-ac.
- Yellowish white: cann-i.
- Drugs, after abuse of copaiva and cubebs, thin discharge, with burning on urination and frequent urging for stool: nux-v.
- Dry: canth.
- Eruptions following suppressed gonorrhea: clem.
- Fever, febrile disturbance during inflammatory stage: acon, cop, gels.
- First stage (inflammatory): acon, cann-s, cop, ferr-p, gels.
- Gleet: agn, alum-p, bar-m, benz-ac, bov, calad, cann-i, cann-s, cinnb, cub, dor, erig, ery-a, graph, hydroph, kali-s, mez, mill, nat-m, petrol, petros, phyt, sabin, sel, sep, still, sulph, tereb, thuja, zinc-mur, zinc.

SYPHILIS

Definition

Syphilis is an infectious disease caused by the spirochete *Treponema pallidum*, which is acquired either sexually or through blood transfusion (Acquired syphilis), or in utero via an infected mother (Congenital syphilis).

Acquired syphilis is now classified as 'early' and 'late' syphilis. *Early syphilis* includes primary, secondary and early latent (arbitrarily defined as more than one year post-infection) syphilis, and *late syphilis* includes late latent (defined as more than one year post-infection) and tertiary syphilis.

Pathophysiology

The spiral bacterium, T. pallidum, penetrates abraded skin or intact mucous membranes easily through direct contact and disseminates rapidly via the blood and lymph circulation.

These bacteria cause vascular changes like those seen in endarteritis and periarteritis. The initial lesion of 'primary syphilis' develops at the site of transmission after an incubation period of about 10 days to 3 months, and then heals spontaneously within 3-8 weeks. Even before the appearance of the lesion, the organisms have disseminated all over the body.

'Secondary syphilis' may superimpose on a primary lesion or may occur 4-10 weeks after its appearance, and this stage has a wide range of presentation, predominantly affecting the skin, mucous membranes and lymph nodes. Symptomatic secondary syphilis usually resolves even without treatment and the disease then enters a latent stage which may be divided into early and late latent syphilis.

'Early latent syphilis' encompasses the first 1-2 years of the disease and is marked by occasional relapses of active secondary lesions. During 'late latent syphilis', the patient remains asymptomatic and generally noninfectious.

About one-third of untreated patients will develop 'tertiary syphilis', which may develop after years to decades of latency and manifests as gummatous, cardiovascular or neurosyphilis. Tertiary syphilis is associated with serious illness and disability; death may result in approximately 20% of untreated patients.

Incidence

Males have a higher incidence than females, and the condition is especially common during the years of peak sexual activity.

Clinical Features

A careful clinic history with the duration and detailed description of all symptoms and lesions should be looked into, in suspected cases. A complete sexual history including information about the use of condoms and the number and symptomatology of all partners should also be looked into.

Primary Syphilis

- Here one usually finds a solitary (and in rare cases multiple) genital chancre, which is a primary lesion. This starts as a painless red macule, which evolves into a papule, and then rapidly becomes eroded into a superficial hard ulcer, with indurated edges and base, and is tender on palpation. This chancre is usually located on the penis in heterosexual men, but in homosexual men may be found in the anal canal, mouth or external genitalia. Common primary sites in women include the cervix and labia. Extragenital lesions on the lips, nipple and other sites likely to come in contact with infected secretions may occasionally occur.

- Inguinal lymphadenopathy is always associated with the primary lesion; and is discrete, firm, mobile, non-tender and painless without overlying skin changes.

Secondary Syphilis

- This stage is usually asymptomatic, but can have the following systemic manifestations like malaise, sore throat, headache, anorexia, fever, myalgias and arthralgias, with diffuse mucocutaneous rash and generalized, non-tender lymphadenopathy.

- Typical early lesions are round, discrete, non-pruritic and bilaterally symmetric macules, papules or nodules; distributed on the trunk, face and proximal extremities. The lesions are almost never vesicular. The lesions in this stage heal either with hyper- or hypo-pigmentation or without any residue. Palmar and plantar hyperpigmentary lesions are characteristic and may at times be scaly.

- Superficial, moist, indurated, painless, and ulcerated or intact flat papules or nodules known as 'moist papules' or 'condylomata lata' may develop on the tongue, oral mucosa, lips, vulva, vagina, penis, around the anus and at skin folds. These are highly infectious lesions. These lesions in the mouth are usually flat-topped, greyish-white patches with a red halo, which become confluent to form the characteristic 'snail-track ulcers'.

- Patchy and non-patchy on-cicatricial alopecia may also occur.
- Lymphadenopathy is of a generalized or bilaterally symmetrical, asymptomatic, discrete, non-tender and non-adherent type, involving especially the posterior cervical, epitrochlear and suboccipital lymph nodes.
- In a few cases hepatosplenomegaly, meningitis, nephropathy, proctitis, arthritis and optic neuritis may also be seen.

Latent Syphilis

- The only evidence of syphilis in these patients is a positive blood serology.
- This stage can last forever or be cut short by the appearance of relapsed lesions of secondary syphilis or appearance of lesions of late tertiary syphilis.

Tertiary Syphilis

- In this stage there is a chronic, progressive inflammatory process that eventually produces clinical symptoms years to decades after the initial infection.
- The characteristic lesion is a granulomatous infiltrate called a 'gumma'. These manifest as asymmetrical, indurated and painless, coalescent granulomatous lesions that usually affect the skin, bone and mucous membranes, but may involve any organ system. The lesions often cause local destruction of the affected organ system.
- The lesions start as a painless subcutaneous nodule with involvement of the overlying skin. These break down to form punched-out ulcers, which heal at the center with an atrophic tissue-paper scar and spreads peripherally. The base of the gumma is dull red with a 'wash-leather' type of appearance. The sites predominantly affected are the presternal region, sternoclavicular joints, shins and scalp. Mucosal lesions may also occur and their extension into submucous tissues can affect

the soft or hard palate or the nasal septum, causing a clean and punched out perforation; uvula if involved, gets completely destroyed. The tongue becomes swollen, bald and furrowed and may show leukoplakic patches. Laryngeal involvement results in hoarseness of voice. Bones show periosteitis and layers of new osseous tissue can be seen. Destructive osteitis may occur in flat bones such as those of the skull.

- In cases of cardiovascular affection, the lesions are largely confined to the aorta, aortic ring, cusps of the aortic valve and ostia of the coronary arteries. There is thus endarteritis of the aorta, subsequent medial necrosis, aortitis, aneurysm of the aorta or aortic incompetence and the symptoms depend upon the nature of involvement.

- Affection of the CNS can give rise to symptoms like syphilitic meningitis, meningovascular syphilis or parenchymatous neurosyphilis; but in a few cases there are no symptoms seen, but the cerebrospinal fluid shows pleocytosis, elevated protein, decreased glucose or a reactive CSF VDRL.

- 'Syphilitic meningitis' usually develops several years after the initial infection, typical symptoms of headache, nausea, vomiting and photophobia but characteristically there is no fever. There can be cranial nerve abnormalities.

- 'Meningovascular syphilis' manifests about 5-10 years after the initial infection, due to endarteritis, which affects small blood vessels of the meninges, brain and spinal cord. Patients present with CNS vascular insufficiency or outright stroke.

- 'Parenchymatous neurosyphilis' results from direct parenchymal CNS invasion by T. pallidum and is usually a late development (15-20 years). Patients present with ataxia, incontinence, paresthesias and loss of position, vibratory, pain and temperature sensation. Paresis and dementia with changes in personality and intellect may develop.

- Tabes dorsalis, dementia paralytica, optic atrophy and pupillary abnormalities such as Argyll-Robertson pupil are also seen.

Diagnosis

- Serology and dark-ground microscopy or immunofluorescent staining makes the diagnosis of syphilis. A positive *Venereal Disease Research Laboratory* (VDRL) or *Rapid Plasma Reagin* (RPR) test should be quantified and titers followed at regular intervals after treatment. Unfortunately, the specificities of these are only fair. Though most patients will have nonreactive nontreponemal tests within several years of successful treatment for syphilis, a significant number will yet have persistently positive tests and are said to be serofast. False positives may also result after immunizations, in acute viral or bacterial infection or during pregnancy.

- Patients with a reactive VDRL or RPR should have the result confirmed by specific *treponemal antigen testing,* like fluorescent treponemal antibody absorption (FTA-ABS) and the microhemagglutination assay for T. pallidum (TPHA). The advantage with the non-treponemal tests is that these could give an indication about the effect of treatment on the disease.

- A complete blood count (CBC), electrolytes, erythrocyte sedimentation rate, blood cultures and other laboratory studies may be appropriate depending on the presentation of the patient.

- Evaluation of neurosyphilis requires a lumbar puncture and evaluation of the cerebral spinal fluid.

Differential Diagnosis

- Carcinoma.
- Chancroid.
- Condyloma acuminata.
- Genital warts.
- Granuloma inguinale.
- Herpes simplex – primary and recurrent.
- Lichen planus.
- Lymphogranuloma venereum.

- Mycotic infection.
- Pityriasis rosea.
- Psoriasis.
- Stevens-Johnson syndrome.
- Traumatic superinfected lesions.

Prevention

- Promotion of safe sex practices, by using condoms.

Complications

- Cardiovascular disease.
- CNS disease.
- Membranous glomerulonephritis.
- Paroxysmal cold hemoglobinemia.
- Irreversible end-organ damage.
- Jarisch-Herxheimer reaction.

Prognosis

The prognosis in primary and secondary syphilis is excellent, but the prognosis in tertiary syphilis is not so good. Therapy of the lesions may prevent progression but cannot reverse the damage already caused.

HOMEOPATHIC APPROACH TO SYPHILIS

I have personally very little experience as far as treatment of syphilis is concerned, since with the introduction of sex education, media publicity and use of condoms, the incidence of syphilis has drastically reduced in the last two decades. It is very important that we do not mix up the treatment of a disease with a syphilitic miasm with the treatment of actual syphilis.

From the few cases of syphilis that I have seen in my life, I have learnt that to treat it, one has to have a good understanding of the *syphilitic miasm*, with a sound knowledge of its treatment, from the Organon, the medicine and the chronic disease. This is a very basic step that one has to know before he starts treatment of syphilis.

Let us start with the treatment of *'primary syphilis'* where the chancre occurs anywhere between 3-8 weeks. As you know the incubation period of syphilis is anywhere between 3 weeks to 3 months, but after the incubation period, when the bacteria has spread through the lymphatic system, and if the susceptibility of the person is very good, the disease tries to localize in a form of a chancre, which is nothing but an oval, ulcerated, indurated, red and painless lesion, secreting a serous fluid, with localized adenopathy. Here it is very important that one *does not treat this disease locally* with some local remedies. Materia medica and therapeutics are loaded with local remedies for syphilitic ulcers and chancre. Treating such disease with a local remedy or giving some local application on top of the ulcer is trying to suppress the syphilis, which at a later stage can remain hidden for some weeks, months or years and then burst out in the form of a volcano in a very bad way. Hence, the approach is always to be *very constitutional* trying to understand the miasms (the fundamental miasm or the predisposing miasm), trying to understand the past history of the person, trying to understand the generals of the case, trying to analyze the mind of the person, and then select the constitutional medicine. Here, *susceptibility being good*, one has to select the remedy in a *high potency*. It may not require a lot of repetition of doses, but in a high potency, about 3-4 doses should be repeated and then you need to observe the case.

Here observation is very important. Mostly, the primary symptoms or the chancre tries to disappear and that should not be the basis that the remedy has acted in a positive way, as chancre otherwise also disappears on its own within 2-3 weeks. Hence, one has to consider the generals and any other new symptom that has come after the remedy. One has to observe the patient very closely for the next 6 months as to what is happening to the system.

Many times I have seen that when a new set of skin symptoms come out, or a new set of general symptoms come out, there may be change in the menstrual cycle, there may be a change in the desires and aversions of the person, there may be a change in the sleeping pattern of the person, there may be an altogether a new malady at a different level of the body. Initially when chancre was there, it was there at the level of what was known as the skin, but now you may get what is known as asthma. So this type of situation has to be very carefully studied, because it is very clearly mentioned in the chronic disease that syphilis can many times gets complicated with either psora or sycosis. Hence, one has to use *anti-psoric or anti-sycotic* remedies to have a complete and a proper cure of syphilis. So it is very important that one has to observe the symptoms in that particular direction.

Secondly, if you get a patient who has *already been treated for chancre with some local application*, here also the basic approach has to be purely constitutional. The only difference over here is that, in such a case, I prefer starting with a very *low potency* and give very *frequent repetition* till some reaction is produced. I usually wait for such a reaction and once it is produced, I stop repeating the remedy and then I start observing the patient.

So this is the marked difference between the two. A patient who has chancre and gets himself locally treated and then comes for homeopathy, and, a patient with chancre, who comes directly for homeopathy, without taking any local treatment.

Let us go through the *'secondary stage'* of syphilis, which can occur anytime within 2 months to 3 years. This is characterized by localized sub-cutaneous lesions, mostly painless, could be in the form of condylomata or lesions at the mucocutaneous junctions like anus, genitals or mouth. Systemic involvement could be in the form of periostitis of the bones and joints; visceral involvement could be in the form of hepatitis, splenitis, nephritis, meningitis, etc. Here, the situation is very bad, the *susceptibility is not so strong,* but the approach still remains *constitutional,* and hence, in this case I would prefer to start with a *medium potency.* I will not repeat the medicine so frequently which has been constitutionally selected and this is the stage where you will see that a lot of new things will come one after another as you start treating the patient.

F- 40

For example, a patient may come with some skin lesions, let's say papillomatous skin lesion on the palms, you take the biopsy of the lesion and syphilis is positive. Otherwise the patient enjoys a good health. You start with a medium potency with infrequent repetition and you will see that after sometime the person may develop some problem with the vision and the doctor diagnoses this stage as uveitis and then you treat uveitis and after sometime the patient may develop papilloedema. So such type of changing patterns are observed a lot in such cases. This is the situation, where, instead of giving the constitutional medicine on symptom similarity it is very important that one tries to pay importance to the miasmatic background of the case, and here, the remedy, which has helped me, along with the anti-syphilitic remedy, is *Tuberculinum*. I have repeated Tuberculinum as an intercurrent remedy many times in cases of secondary syphilis.

As far as the third stage of syphilis is concerned, what you call as the *'tertiary stage'*, which can occur anytime between 5 to 20 years. This is the stage that I have really not seen in my practice, and hence I cannot comment much on the homeopathic treatment of it, but I may only say that the approach remains the same. The susceptibility being very poor, the medicine has to be started in a *very low potency* and should be given *very infrequently* and try to treat one layer after another. This means, that when you give a remedy and the symptoms disappear, allow the body to react and bring out the second set of symptoms and then you may think of the second set of remedy. This should be supported with an *intercurrent nosode*.

It is very essential for a homeopathic physician to know that homeopathy can cure syphilis only in its initial stages i.e. primary and early secondary stage. The congenital and latent variety cannot be cured because in such cases irreversible, structural changes have taken place. Hence such cases can only be palliated. Also while treating a case of primary syphilis, all sexual contacts made by the patient in the last four eight weeks must be identified, examined and investigated, since the incubation period is about 4 weeks. A person whose morals are too low and who frequently has illicit intercourse should be advised to wear condom during, and to wash his genitalia with calendula soap and water after, every intercourse.

Whilst treating a case of syphilis homeopathically, a homeopath is strictly advised to assess the case clinically with the parameters given below:

- Rendering the contagious lesion into non-contagious lesions.

- All cases of syphilis should be watched regularly for at least 2-3 years. During this period, the blood serological examination should be performed once in 3 months for one year and once in 6 months for 2 years.

- A CSF examination should be performed in 6 months, and then again in two years after finishing the therapy.

Some Important Homeopathic Remedies

Anacardium orientale: Syphilitic patients who often suffer from an impaired memory, depression and irritability, usually a diminution of the senses of smell, sight and hearing is also observed. There is a severe of burning in glans penis during and after urination. The patient has tremendous sexual desire with dribbling of the prostatic fluid during stool.

Arsenicum album: Phagedenic chancres, usually a livid hue in color with an intense burning. And occasionally even sloughing chancres after mercury with very florid granulations. Margins of the ulcers are hard and bleed at the least touch. Such ulcers exude a thin offensive discharge. The inguinal glands are swollen, indurated and very painful. There is an indescribable feeling of weakness, occasionally accompanied with dropsy and malignant ulceration.

Asafoetida: Tertiary syphilis, especially after the abuse of mercury. Ulcers, especially when affecting the bones, discharging an ichorous, fetid, thin pus and extremely sensitive to touch. Syphilitic caries and necrosis with fetid and bloody discharge. Patients with hysterical and hypochondriacal manifestation, intolerably nervous and oversensitive.

Aurum metallicum: Infantile and secondary syphilis, especially after the abuse of mercury and the potassium salts. Iritis with a tense feeling and much pain around the eye as if in the bones. The pain extends from without inward and is much worse < touch. Boring pains in the mastoid process with caries of nasal bones. Skull bones are painful while lying on them. There is a putrid smell from mouth with caries of palate along with offensive and ichorous discharge. Syphilitic cerebral or meningeal tumors. Great melancholia and sleeplessness due to excessive pain. All pains better in open air. Self-destruction.

Aurum muriaticum: Chancre on the prepuce and scrotum; bubo in left groin. Snuffles of children suffering from hereditary syphilis, with flat ulcers on the scrotum secreting a fetid ichor; secondary syphilis with exostoses and bone pains in both shinbones. Melancholy with diminished vitality. Vaginitis and gonorrheal discharge with swelling of both groins.

Badiaga: Syphilis of infants who present themselves with glandular enlargements. The patient develops bubos and chancres with violent burning pain at night. In cases where chancre has been suppressed by mercurial ointments leaving elevated discolored cicatrices. The patient is emaciated and his skin is full of freckles and rhagades. Also it is indicated in those cases of cancer especially of breast, who in the past, had a water maltreated syphilis.

Belladonna: Syphilitic buboes that are large and painful with an intense inflammation of the integuments. These present with a deep red hue extend over large surfaces. Eruptions are very painful. Phlegmonous phimosis or paraphimosis; erysipelatous balanitis.

Benzoicum acidum: Syphilitic spots and marks. Syphilitic rheumatism with very painful nodes. Warts around the anus, appearing after suppression of a chancrous gonorrhea. Urine usually repulsively offensive.

Carbo animalis: Constitutional or tertiary syphilis. Coppery-red blotches on the skin, especially on face. Glands enlarge slowly and painfully and become indurated. Bubo, which is hard as a stone, especially if maltreated, opened or cauterized soon. They present with large, terrible ulcers with callous edges and secrete an offensive ichor. Buboes are usually on the left side, indurated with lancinating and cutting pains. When they begin to suppurate, they are extremely sensitive to touch. Nasal syphilis.

Carbo vegetabilis: Syphilitic ulcers with high edges. These ulcers tend to become more irritable after some local treatment. Sores with sharp, ragged and undermined margin, with a thin acrid and offensive discharge. They are painful and liable to bleed very freely when touched. Vesicles and blisters on prepuce; burning pains of labia.

Causticum: Vesicles under the prepuce, which change into suppurating ulcers. Watery, greenish corroding discharge with jerking pains. Chancres with fungus excrescences. Even buboes secrete an acrid, corrosive ichor, with various systemic complications, such as scurvy or gout.

Cinnabaris: Chancres that are indurated or neglected. They appear fiery red, inflamed, swollen, hard, discharging thin pus. The chancre is not so sensitive to touch or pressure. When Merc-Sol apparently well indicated fails. It is also a good drug for syphilitic iritis. The important concomitants are – (1) corner of the mouth chapped, (2) small fiery red ulcers on roof of mouth and on tip of tongue.

Corallium rubrum: It is prepared from red coral. The syphilitic ulcers resemble the coral. Presence of red, flat ulcers on glans of inner surface and prepuce with profuse, yellow, ichorous discharge, which emits an offensive odor. The ulcers are extremely sensitive to touch. Concomitant is presence of constant trickling of mucus from posterior nares into fences and smooth, copper colored spots on palms of hands and fingers.

Fluoricum acidum: It has signs and symptoms suggestive of congenital syphilis accompanied by ulcerations in mouth and throat. The bones are prone to caries, the one that are affected the most are temporal and mastoid, the pain is characterized by burning and boring sensation the discharge from the caries is thin, acrid and corrosive. Psychologically patient has tremendous desire for sex and is extremely ill humored and fault finding, full of imaginary fears.

Hepar sulphur: Chancres extremely sensitive to touch with splinter like pain. Disposed to bleed easily the margins of the ulcer are elevated and spongy looking without granulations in their center. Buboes are extremely painful and prone to easy suppuration; when it ruptures, it liberates cheesy offensive matter. Bones especially of nose, face and skull area are inflamed and necrosed. As a result, nose is flattened or destroyed; with offensive ozaena.

Jacaranda caroba: The chancre is surrounded by itching pimples. Prepuce is painful and swollen. It is indicated in syphilitic arthritis with morning stiffness and soreness of muscles.

Kalium bichromicum: Syphilitic ulcers affecting the root and glans penis. Margins are indurated and they perforate quite deep. The edges are punched out. The ulcer secretes thick jelly like yellow discharge. Constrictive pain at root of penis < at night. Depressed round scars after healing of the syphilitic ulcers. Syphilitic coryza affecting mucus membranes of the mouth, nose and throat. Perforating ulcers in mouth and throat. Offensive and destructive ozaena with thick, yellow nasal discharge.

Kalium iodatum: Ulcers on the genitalia, which secrete acrid, thick, foul discharge. Exostosis in skull and tibia. Syphilitic rheumatism especially phalanges of fingers and toes. Excoriating syphilitic coryza which forms blisters on nostrils and mouth. Boring pain < local application of heat, night, after abuse of mercury. Extremely useful for syphilitic headache.

Kreosotum: Congenital syphilis: fall of hair, hot acrid smarting tears, deafness, chronic catarrh from the nose, very rapid decay of teeth with putrid odor from mouth, foul breath.

Chapter-31

Tumors of the Skin

Termed as a localized multiplication and proliferation of cells, which are of the same cell type and which tends to display a degree of autonomous control of growth, with normal differentiation. 'Hamartomas' are benign tumors where more than one cell type involvement is seen. An 'in situ tumour' is a collection of morphologically malignant cells of the same cell type, but these have not yet acquired the capacity to invade through a basement membrane. Finally, a 'malignant tumour' is one with the full capacity to metastasize to lymph nodes and other parts of the body, and is thus of poor prognostic value.

BENIGN TUMORS

FIBROMAS

Definition

These are well-defined benign neoplasms of the connective tissue, composed of connective tissue cells and fibres.

Pathology

There is a marked proliferation of connective tissue cells.

Clinical Features

These are single or multiple tumors, of a soft to hard consistency, usually pedunculated, and are of varying sizes, occurring anywhere in the body. They are usually skin-colored, but may have a smooth, pinkish or reddish surface. They usually tend to keep enlarging continuously and do not necessarily occur at the site of trauma.

DERMATOFIBROMA

Synonym

Histiocytoma Cutis; Subepidermal Nodular Fibrosis; Sclerosing Hemangioma; Fibroma Durum; Nodulus Cutaneus; Dermatofibroma Lenticulare.

Definition

These are benign, hard, but small papules or nodules originating from the dermal layer.

Etiology

There is no known cause for this condition, though a few cases are reported with lesions occurring after injuries to the skin, like insect bites or blunt trauma. It is seen usually in middle-aged adults, rarely in children.

Pathology

There is a pseudoepitheliomatous hyperplasia and acanthosis of the overlying epidermis. The dermal mass is composed of dense whorls of fibrous tissue in which are numerous cells with large nuclei rich in chromatin, epithelioid cells or elongated spindle cells. The cells have features of fibroblasts and myofibroblasts.

Clinical Features

The lesion is a single, firm, palpable, round or ovoid papule or nodule about 1 cm in diameter, which is reddish brown, occasionally with a yellowish hue. The nodule is adherent to the overlying epidermis, which becomes indented when squeezed. This depression created over the dermatofibroma when the overlying epidermis is squeezed is termed as the 'Dimple Sign'. These nodules are freely movable over the deeper tissue. The lesions occur especially on the lower limbs, but may occur around the elbows or on the sides of the trunk.

In a few cases giant lesions, greater than 5 cm are seen.

Differential Diagnosis

The lesions need to be differentiated from clear cell acanthoma, granular cell tumor, and dermatofibrosis lenticularis disseminata, with the help of biopsy.

CUTANEOUS TAGS

Synonym

Skin Tags; Fibroma Fruste; Fibroma Pendulum; Fibroma Molluscum; Soft Warts; Acrochordon; Papilloma Colli; Cutaneous Papilloma; Templeton's Skin Tags.

Definition

This is a commonly seen, harmless, benign condition where there are multiple, small, pin-head to lentil-sized, skin-colored or dark brown, fibroepithelial, sessile and pedunculated polyps or soft fibromas, seen especially on the eyelids, neck, axillae and rarely in the other major flexures.

Incidence

These occur especially in women especially at or after menopause. The incidence of it occurring increases when the person is gaining weight or during pregnancy.

Pathology

The dermal layer consists of loose, fibrous tissue and collagen fibers. The epidermis is thin, flattened and often hyper-pigmented. There is no proliferation of the melanocytic or naevus cells seen.

Clinical Features

The lesions vary in size, but are usually very small, round, soft, sessile or usually pedunculated with a long stalk. The lesions are usually skin-colored, but may be hyperpigmented. They occur especially on the eyelids, neck, and axillae; and rarely on the trunk, face and in the other major flexures (groins). They are usually seen to occur in association with small seborrhoeic keratoses.

Complications

When the lesions are twisted very often out of habit, they tend to become inflamed, tender or even gangrenous.

Diagnosis

The lesions are easy to diagnose with their very small size and other characteristic features.

The lesions are unmistakable. They are smaller than the average pedunculated melanocytic naevus or the lesions of neurofibromatosis.

KELOIDS & HYPERTROPHIC SCARS

Definition

Keloids and hypertrophic scars are benign, firm, irregular and well-demarcated lesions of fibrous tissue overgrowth, occurring due to an excessive connective tissue response to an injury, which may be very trivial. The difference lies in the fact that a keloid extend beyond the margins of the original lesion or injury, invading the surrounding normal skin; whereas a hypertrophic scar remains within the margins of the original defect, and tends to resolve with time.

Etiology & Incidence

They are known to usually occur following some kind of trauma, inflammatory skin lesion (like acne) or at sites of bites, burns, ear piercing or operational scars; but they can arise spontaneously also. There is no definite cause known as yet.

Keloids are known to occur especially after puberty upto the age of about 30 years; they are rare in infant and the aged.

Keloids are especially seen in the black Africans, Mongoloids, the Chinese and the Japanese. Women are more likely to be affected, with the lesions occurring or getting worse during pregnancy.

Pathology

There is increased cellularity seen in both the conditions.

In keloids of recent onset, endothelial proliferation is surrounded by increased numbers of myofibroblasts and collagen in the dermis, which form large, irregular nodules or whorls of collagenous fibers with a peripheral capsule-like band. Scanning electron microscopy of keloids shows more haphazard organization of collagen bundles than in normal skin or mature scars. The collagen filaments are about half the diameter of those of normal skin.

In hypertrophic scars, there is an increase in the mast cells.

The epidermis is normal, or thinned by the underlying lesion.

Biochemical studies confirm that collagen and proteoglycan synthesis is increased in keloids and hypertrophic scars.

Immunohistochemical studies have shown that neuropeptide-containing nerves are present in hypertrophic scars but not in non-hypertrophic scars, and these may contribute to the symptoms of discomfort and itching in such scars.

Clinical Features

They can occur anywhere on the body, but are usually seen on the limbs, earlobes, neck, shoulders, upper back or chest. Spontaneous keloids usually develop on the presternal region or upper chest. Keloids are often multiple, varying in size and number.

In both the conditions the lesions become firm, pink or red, elevated and thickened within 3-4 weeks of the stimulus. These may keep growing for months or years, with the keloids usually assuming a 'dumb-bell' shaped contour or an irregular lesion with claw-like projections. The skin surface over the lesion is smooth, shiny and thinned from pressure.

A hypertrophic scar tends to reduce in size with time and gradually resolves after a few months; whereas, a keloid becomes smoother, rounder and tends to keep increasing in size growing beyond the margins of the initial lesion. Keloids may regress after several years or never at all.

The lesion in both the conditions often becomes itchy, irritable and hypersensitive, but the keloidal lesions tend to frequently become tender or painful.

Diagnosis

Diagnosis is easy with the biopsy and the history of trauma or an inflammatory skin lesion.

Differential diagnosis

A few carcinomatous lesions may be confused with keloids in the initial stages. E.g. sclerotic basal cell carcinoma, scar sarcoid or malignancy developing in a scar, and dermatofibrosarcoma.

Prognosis

The prognosis is good in cases of hypertrophic scars and small keloids; but poor in cases of large or multiple keloids.

Treatment

Individuals who are susceptible to the formation of keloids should be wary of any suspicious wound or burn and get it treated properly. Also unwanted surgery should be avoided in order to prevent the occurrence of scar formation.

LIPOMA

Definition

These benign tumours are slowly growing, well-defined, soft, rounded, lobulated, and mobile nodules composed of mature fat cells, arising from the adipose tissue in the subcutaneous layer of the skin.

Etiology & Incidence

There is no particular cause known.

Histopathology

The lesion consists of lobulated groups of normal fat cells held together by strands of connective tissue, which are enclosed within a capsule of connective tissue. Occasionally, eccrine sweat glands may be associated and then they are called as 'adenolipomas'.

Clinical Features

Lipomas are soft, lobulated, subcutaneous nodules, varying in size and number. These grow very slowly and are generally not adherent to the overlying epidermis and can thus be moved freely on the underlying structures on palpation. They are usually asymptomatic, but can become painful in cases of them causing pressure over the nerves.

These tend to occur anywhere on the body, but are usually seen on the neck, limbs, back and shoulders.

Diagnosis

These lesions are easy to diagnose with its typical clinical presentation and it typically slipping away from the palpating fingers on examination. In doubtful cases, a biopsy will confirm the diagnosis.

Differential Diagnosis

An epidermoid cyst can resemble a lipoma, but the presence of the central punctum helps make the correct diagnosis.

Angiolipomas are encapsulated, lobulated benign tumours differing histologically from a lipoma with its excessive degree of vascular proliferation, and it being usually painful and tender to touch.

NEUROMA

Definition

Here the lesion develops from the nerve or ganglion cells, nerve fibres or the perineural sheath.

Pathology

These lesions do not have a capsule and are composed of spindle cells with characteristically wavy nuclei.

Clinical Features

The lesions in this condition are usually solitary, slow-growing tumours, occurring along a nerve. They are skin-colored or with a slight red hue. The patient usually complains of a radiating pain.

Differential Diagnosis

Neurofibromatosis is a condition that mimics neuroma, but the histopathology exhibits numerous bundles of myelinated nerves in the dermis surrounded by fibrous tissue.

GLOMUS TUMOR

Synonym

Glomangioma.

Definition

The solitary glomus, a vascular nail bed tumor, arises from a normal glomus (neuromyoarterial organ surrounding the arterio-venous junction which is supposed to regulate blood pressure and temperature).

Histopathology

The glomus tumor contains numerous vascular channels lined by a single layer of flattened endothelial cells, peripheral to which, many layers of cuboidal glomus cells are seen. Myelinated and non-myelinated nerves are found.

Clinical Features

The lesion is a skin-colored or slightly dusky blue, single, small, well-defined, firm nodule, about 1-20 mm in diameter, which is usually extremely tender to touch. The pain is paroxysmal and sharp, radiating to various parts. The lesions seen are usually small subungual ones, though lesions can occur on the fingers and arms. Progressive growth may lead to ulceration.

In a few cases multiple glomangiomas tend to occur, which are usually non-tender and widely distributed over the body.

Diagnosis

In almost half the cases, a depression of the underlying phalanx is seen. MRI will detect the exact limits of the tumor.

Biopsy is diagnostic.

SEBORRHOEIC KERATOSIS

Synonym

Seborrhoeic Wart; Senile Wart; Basal Cell Papilloma.

Definition

These pigmented benign tumours are composed of epidermal keratinocytes, seen especially in the elderly, with the face and upper trunk being the usual sites of affection.

Etiology & Incidence

There is a familial predisposition seen, with an autosomal dominant mode of inheritance. They are especially common in the white races; rarely seen among the black or dark skinned individuals.

Males are more frequently affected than females, especially in the fourth or fifth decade.

Pathology

There is a gradual build-up of keratinocytes between the basal layer and the keratinizing surface of the epidermis. Proliferation of the melanocytes then takes place among these keratinocytes, which gives rise to the pigmentation. There is focal keratinization occurring in the immature cells, which give rise to the formation of small horn pseudocysts. There are no mitotic cells, and dermal infiltration is absent.

Clinical Features

The condition usually presents as multiple, oval, slightly raised, hyperpigmented lesions, which are of a soft consistency and slightly itchy. They occur anywhere on the body, but are seen more often on the face, neck and the upper trunk. The palms and soles are spared. They have a smooth, lusterless, verrucous and granular surface, with well-defined margins. They increase slowly in size and number.

Lesions on the eyelids and flexures are pedunculated and less keratotic. Irritation or infection causes swelling, bleeding, oozing and crusting, and an increased pigmentation.

Differential Diagnosis

In a few cases there can be difficulty in differentiating a malignant melanoma from an inflamed solitary seborrhoeic keratosis, though melanomas are usually smooth-surfaced. Biopsy will help confirm the diagnosis.

Actinic keratosis is usually more red, rough and slightly scaly, occurring especially on sun-exposed surfaces like the face and back of hands.

KERATO-ACANTHOMA

Synonym

Molluscum Sebaceum.

Definition

It is a rapidly evolving solitary tumour of the skin, composed of keratinizing squamous cells, which resolves spontaneously if left untreated.

Etiology & Incidence

This condition is especially seen in the light-skinned persons, and is uncommon in dark-skinned people. Males are more commonly affected than females, especially in the middle-aged or elderly ones.

A few studies have shown that there is an increased frequency of this condition with too much exposure to the sun, contact with tar and mineral oils. In a few cases the lesions occur after injury to the skin, or it is seen to occur in association with internal malignancies or in those with a poor immunity status.

Histopathology

In the early stages, the lesion consists of rapidly multiplying squamous cells. The marginal cells rapidly spreads into the surrounding dermis, while those that are centrally located tend to keratinize to form a branched pattern of accumulated keratin and inflammatory exudate, extending all the way to the surface. This tends to dilate the central pore and the epidermal lips recede from the center and the lesion opens like a flower bud. The horn is then shed off and the irregular epithelium beneath it is reproduced, which then forms a scar with papillomatous tags at the margin. In cases of chronic lesions, there is collection of leukocyte microabscesses at the base.

Clinical Features

This condition usually presents as a solitary lesion, though in a few cases multiple lesions are also seen. Initially there is evidence of a small, firm, hemispherical, dome-shaped, skin-colored or reddish nodule or keratotic lesion, which then rapidly grows to become 10-20 mm in diameter in 3-6 weeks. There is telangiectases just beneath the lesion and the epidermis over it is thin, smooth and shiny. The center of the lesion consists of a horny keratinous plug or a crust situated over a keratin-filled crater. The accumulated keratin then gradually projects like a horn or softens up and breaks down. Gradually, in a few months, the horny core is shed off spontaneously, revealing an irregular and puckered scar. Recurrence is known to occur after the spontaneous resolution.

The sites that are most frequently affected are the face, head, back of hand, arm, wrist and forearm. The buttocks, thighs, chest, buccal mucosa, ears and penis are less often affected. Subungual keratoacanthomas are tender, have a destructive crateriform center, and often cause damage to the terminal phalanx. These do not regress spontaneously and cause early bony destruction.

Differential Diagnosis

- Since keratoacanthoma simulates initial stages of squamous cell carcinoma, a biopsy would be necessary to confirm the diagnosis, though features like the keratotic plug, undamaged surrounding skin and spontaneous healing go in favor of keratoacanthoma.

- Conditions like cutaneous horn, hypertrophic solar keratosis, viral wart, molluscum contagiosum, pseudoepitheliomatous hyperplasia and granulomas of various types may need to be differentiated from it.

CYSTIC TUMORS

These include the following:

- Dermoid Cyst.
- Pilonidal Cyst.
- Epithelial Cyst.
- Pilar Cyst.
- Milium.

DERMOID CYST

Definition

It is a congenital cystic tumor containing hair, hair follicles, sebaceous glands, etc. and arising above the mylohyoid muscle in the midline of the neck.

Etiology

It develops due to improper embryologic development, where there is inclusion of epidermal structures in the subcutaneous tissue.

Histopathology

The cyst is located in the subcutaneous layer and is often adherent to periosteum, at times invading or eroding the underlying bone. The cysts are lined with stratified squamous epithelium containing hair follicles, sebaceous and sweat glands, lipid, keratin and lanugo hair.

Clinical Features

Though this is a congenital condition, it tends to usually become obvious after 5-10 years of age. They appear as small, soft, elastic, oval or hemispherical, subcutaneous nodules, about 0.5-5 cm in diameter, with a doughy feel on palpation. In children, they are often seen on the scalp, around the eyes, midline or root of the nose, floor of the mouth, neck and the anterior chest wall. In adults, they are usually seen in the genital and post-anal areas.

They are generally not attached to the skin and are freely movable. In cases of an intracranial extension there is a rim of bone surrounding the base of the cyst.

They tend to become infected recurrently, causing pain and tenderness of the part.

Complications

- Osteomyelitis, meningitis and pressure erosion of bone may occur.
- Visual impairment can also occur due to the extension into the orbit.

Diagnosis & Differential Diagnosis

- Lesions on the neck need to be differentiated from a thyroglossal cyst and an ectopic thyroid gland. A CT or MRI scan or high-resolution ultrasound will help make the diagnosis, along with the thyroid function tests.
- Lesions on the bridge of the nose should be distinguished from nasal gliomas, which appear as firm, reddish tumors, present since birth.

PILONIDAL CYST

Synonym

Pilonidal Sinus.

Clinical Features

The pilonidal cyst is an embryogenic defect, comprising of a midline hairy patch or pit near the tip of the coccyx below the sacral region, with a sinus orifice in the bottom or a cyst beneath it, in which hair is growing. It becomes clinically obvious during adolescence, when it can become infected and form an abscess.

EPITHELIAL CYST & SINUSES

Synonym

Epidermal Cyst; Epidermoid Cyst; Sebaceous Cyst; Keratin Cyst; Steatoma.

Definition

It is a commonly seen clinical condition where there is the development of a fluctuant, tense cystic swelling, which consists of keratin and its breakdown products lined by an epidermoid wall.

Etiology & Incidence

Young and middle-aged adults are especially affected.

Most of the epithelial cysts arise due to inflammation around a pilosebaceous follicle, and are especially common in persons presenting with a severe form of acne vulgaris.

In a few cases, accidental deep implantation of a fragment of the epidermis into the underlying tissue after some penetrating injury or trauma to the part can give rise to it. (These can also be termed as *Implantation cyst* or *Traumatic Cyst*).

Histopathology

It is a unilocular, spherical cyst situated within the dermal layer of the skin, the pasty contents of which comprise of macerated keratin, keratohyalin granules and cheesy, fatty material. The cyst is lined by a stratified squamous epithelium.

Clinical Features

An epithelial or epidermoid cyst is a firm, elastic or fluctuant, well-defined, spherical or irregular shaped, skin-colored swelling situated in the dermis. It occurs in different sizes and is attached to the skin but is mobile over the deeper structures. The surface of the overlying skin is usually smooth and shiny due to the upward pressure. These grow gradually in size and are usually painless, except when they become infected and inflamed. Suppuration may occur as a complication.

The sites that are usually affected are the face, neck, trunk, scalp, shoulders and the scrotum. Lesions are commonly multiple, but may be solitary.

Diagnosis

An uncomplicated and uninfected cyst can usually be diagnosed with ease. Other benign and rounded dermal tumours may be mistaken for epidermoid cysts, but can be differentiated with the help of a biopsy.

TRICHILEMMAL CYST

Synonym

Pilar Cyst; Wen.

Definition

These are similar to the epithelial cysts, but the location is different; these tend to occur on the scalp, and its wall resembles the external hair root sheath.

Etiology & Incidence

This condition is seen in women more often than men. It is seen mainly during middle age and is inherited as an autosomal dominant trait.

Pathology

Trichilemmal cysts differ from epidermoid cysts in the way the lining cells mature. They do not flatten and form a granular layer like in the epithelial cyst, but they have a wall lined by keratinizing epithelium. In a few cases, the cyst may rupture and proliferate, with an increase in the granulation tissue.

Clinical Features

These cysts occur mainly on the scalp, and are smooth, mobile, firm and rounded in shape, though a few of them may be lobulated.

Pain or tenderness occurs in cases where the cyst has become infected. The cyst wall may fuse with the epidermis to form a crypt, which can occasionally terminate by discharging its contents and healing spontaneously. In contrast, the contents may protrude above the surface to form a soft, cutaneous horn.

MILIA

Definition

These are small, white, subepidermal, keratinous cysts occurring especially on the face, usually on the eyelids or below the eyes. They are considered to be simple epithelial retention cysts or represent the encysted retention of sebum and hair cells.

Etiology & Incidence

They occur with increasing frequency in women, though they can occur at any age, even in infancy.

There is no particular cause known of the condition.

'Primary milia' are said to occur as a predisposition; whereas 'secondary milia' occur in inflammatory conditions and on the traumatous areas or scars of skin diseases like epidermolysis bullosa, pemphigus, porphyria cutanea tarda, herpes zoster, contact dermatitis, bullous lichen planus, etc. They also occur frequently after trauma or burns, or after prolonged use of non-steroidal anti-inflammatory drugs.

Pathology

The white milium body is composed of lamellated keratin.

Clinical Features

These small, uniform, smooth, spherical, lesions occur in multiple numbers, and are usually of pinhead size, rarely more than 1 or 2 mm in diameter. They are usually pearly-white or yellowish in colour, and appear to be immediately beneath the epidermis. Besides causing cosmetic problems, they are otherwise asymptomatic. When punctured, a whitish substance is expelled resembling the kernel of rice.

They occur especially on the face, usually on the eyelids or below the eyes; rarely they are seen on the genitals.

HOMEOPATHIC APPROACH TOWARDS BENIGN TUMORS OF THE SKIN

Homeopathic management of fibromas, dermatofibromas, cutaneous tags, lipoma, and all the other benign growths come under the sycotic miasm. Abundant use of anti-sycotic and intercurrent remedies like Thuja, Sycotic-co, Graphites, Calcarea fluor., Calcarea carb., Lapis albus, Silicea, Epihysterinum, Aurum mur. natronatum, Carcinosinum, Vaccininum have been very useful to me for the same.

Remembering the fact that the choice of selection was purely on symptom similarity and not using them empirically, the above diseases sometimes are difficult to treat with homeopathy and I had my fair share of failures as diseases like skin tags, dermatofibroma, etc. may sometimes take years to improve. Also, patients who suffer from skin tags should always be investigated for diabetes as within ten years of developing the skin tags, half of them become diabetic.

Majority of homeopaths give some local application to which I strongly disagree. Here too, like any other sycotic disease, the remedy has to be repeated frequently. It is safe to start on a LM scale, then gradually going higher till you reach the highest potency. Around 40% to 50% of cases of cutaneous skin tags come under my failures.

Paradoxically, fibromas respond very well to homeopathy where the success rate is as high as 80%.

As far as lipoma is concerned, my results have not been too satisfactory in my 23 years of practice of classical homeopathy. Multiple lipomas all over the body should never be accepted for homeopathic treatment, as you cannot resolve all the lipomas. Also don't give a false guarantee that after homeopathic treatment, one may not develop new lipomas. I have seen so many homeopaths who encourage this, but ultimately they spoil the name of the science. Lipomas should not be considered 100% benign always, as sarcomatous changes in benign lipomas are known, especially if located in the region of the thighs. Two rare medicines found most useful in lipoma are *Bacillus No.* 10, a bowel nosode and *Uricum acidum.*

MALIGNANT TUMORS

SQUAMOUS CELL CARCINOMA

Synonym

Prickle Cell Carcinoma; Epidermoid Carcinoma.

Definition

Squamous cell carcinoma is a malignant tumour arising from the proliferation of keratinocytes of the epidermis and the surrounding mucous membrane.

Etiology & Incidence

It is especially common in light-skinned people, especially in males as compared to females, with the chances of its occurrence increasing with age.

The predisposing factors to this condition especially include prolonged or strong exposure to sunlight; or in cases of those coming in contact with industrial or chemical carcinogenic agents like tars and hydrocarbon oils. In a few cases radiant heat, thermal injury or burn from hot metal fragments, hot coal or tar can give rise to a tumor after a few weeks or months.

It can also occur as a complication to other skin conditions like chronic granulomas, syphilis, chronic ulcers or scars, lupus erythematosus, chronic infections like lupus vulgaris, osteomyelitis sinuses, old burn scars, xeroderma pigmentosum, albinism and hidradenitis suppurativa. It can also occur in areas irradiated by X-rays, grenz rays and gamma rays.

Human papillomavirus (HPV) is associated with squamous cell carcinoma

Histopathology

There is hyperplasia seen with irregular nests of atypical keratinocytes from the epidermal layer invading the dermis to varying degrees. The epidermal cells show abundant mitoses. The cells of squamous carcinoma vary from large, well-differentiated, polygonal cells to completely anaplastic cells with basophilic cytoplasm. The degree of cell differentiation has been used to grade squamous cell carcinoma. The greater the differentiation, the less the invasive tendency and the better the prognosis. In cases of poor differentiation or anaplastic cells (with rounded or spindle shaped cell outlines), the prognosis is very poor.

Clinical Features

There is a skin-coloured or dull red erythematous, firm, hard, nodule or plaque, with a smooth, verrucous or papillomatous surface. This lesion tends to then indurate and form rolled borders, becoming deeply nodular. Later on, as the lesion grows, there is early ulceration occurring at its center, and inflammation of the tissue around it. The edge of the ulcer is elevated, everted and indurated, whereas its base appears granular, papillomatous or even fungating and with a tendency to bleed easily or there is crust formation over it.

The sites that are usually affected are the backs of the hands and forearms, the face, pinna, the muco-cutaneous junctions and the mucous membranes of the mouth and the genitalia (especially in cases of chimney sweepers). In a few tropical cases, there are lesions occurring especially on the lower legs, due to the frequency of ulceration and scars in the area.

The course of the disease is pretty rapid, with local destruction of structures like the eyes, cartilages or the bones taking place too. The regional lymph glands may show enlargement due to infection or metastases, which usually occurs within 6-12 months. The nodes may feel harder, more irregular and may become fixed to the adjacent tissues.

Complications

Metastasis is common in this condition with the spread taking place usually by the blood or the lymphatic route. Studies have shown that squamous cell carcinoma occurring in areas due to ultraviolet rays of the sun have a low rate of metastasis as compared to those occurring on the mucocutaneous surfaces or those due to burns or ulcers.

Other malignancies commonly seen to occur following squamous cell carcinoma are:

- Cancer of the buccal mucosa or pharynx.
- Cancers of the respiratory tract.
- Non-Hodgkin's Lymphoma.
- Leukemia

Diagnosis

The diagnosis of squamous cell carcinoma is based on the following factors:

- An indurated, fast-growing lesion in a person past middle-age, especially in areas of the skin that is damaged by sunlight or other predisposing factors.
- An ulcer with an indurated border, everted margins and a granular base that bleeds easily.
- Biopsy and histopathological findings.

Differential Diagnosis

This condition tends to simulate the following:

- The pearly white lesions of basal cell epithelioma are absent in this condition. Also the disease progress is much more rapid in squamous cell carcinoma as compared to basal cell epithelioma. Biopsy report with its histological findings will confirm the diagnosis.

- Keratoacanthoma progresses at a much faster rate as compared to squamous cell carcinoma; plus the rolled border of the lesion with a keratotic central plug is characteristic of keratoacanthoma. Histological findings will confirm the diagnosis.

- It is difficult to distinguish squamous cell carcinoma, in its early stages, from 'hypertrophic actinic keratosis'. Here biopsy becomes necessary.

- Warty lesions such as viral warts or seborrheic keratoses are not indurated, and are frequently multiple.

- Lupus vulgaris is differentiated with its characteristic onset occurring in childhood, its typical reddish patch with apple jelly nodules, and tendency to heal with a wrinkled tissue paper scar.

- Tertiary syphilis has a rapid and much bigger ulceration with a punched out ulcer and is easily distinguishable by a positive serology test.

BASAL CELL CARCINOMA

Synonym

Basal Cell Epithelioma; Basalioma; Rodent Carcinoma; Rodent Ulcer; Jacobi's Ulcer.

Definition

Basal cell carcinoma is a malignant tumour arising from the basal cells of the epidermis and its appendages. It is usually only locally malignant, without any tendency to metastasize.

Etiology & Incidence

It is a common skin malignancy seen in fair-complexioned persons, with rates of affection higher those seen in squamous cell carcinoma.

The predisposing factors for this condition is again exposure to ultraviolet rays of the sunlight; though it is known to occur following exposure to ionizing radiation, scars of burns or old vaccination.

It is known to affect males more commonly than females, especially after their middle age. It is seen to affect younger individuals who are immunosuppressed.

Histopathology

There is downward projection and budding of the cells from the basal layer of the epidermis and its appendages, into the dermis. The compactly arranged cells appear columnar with a large nucleus that stains darkly as compared to its cytoplasm. The cell margins are indistinct with adjacent cells connected by bridges. The dermal stroma is an integral and important part of the basal cell carcinoma. A few mitoses are present and cysts may form. The interlacing strands of tumor cells may present a meshy or web-like pattern.

There is a round-cell inflammatory reaction occurring to some degree, with ulceration. There is increase in the presence of mast cells and Langerhans' cells within and around the tumor.

Histochemical and electron microscopy investigations show little evidence of differentiation of the tumour cells.

Clinical Features

The initial lesion may present as a small, firm papule, which grows slowly into a semitranslucent nodule or a flat, raised plaque. A depression then forms in the center of this lesion, which then breaks down to form an ulcer or crust, which may or may not bleed. The lesion is telangiectatic and has a rolled border with pearly papules or nodules at its periphery. Gradually there is a crust formation over the ulcer, which if peeled off, tends to bleed easily without any pain. This ulcer gradually enlarges, invading and destroying surrounding structures and the subcutaneous tissue, bone or cartilage in the process.

The site that is usually affected is the face, especially at the inner canthus of the eye, nose and behind the ears; the head and neck is also affected in a few cases. The hands and the trunk are less commonly affected, except that there are lesions on the legs commonly seen in females.

Course & Prognosis

The course of this condition is usually slowly progressive, extending over a few years time. Prognosis is better than in squamous cell carcinoma with its low rates of metastasis. Recurrences or relapses are seen in cases of an improperly done surgery, where the removal of the cancerous lesion is incomplete. In cases left untreated, the prognosis is poor.

Diagnosis

The diagnosis of basal cell carcinoma is based on the following factors:

- The typical site on the face, especially around the nose or inner canthi of eyes.

- The chronic, slowly progressive history of the lesion.

- The typical pearly or semi-translucent nodule or the ulcer with rolled edges.

- The biopsy and histopathological findings.

Differential Diagnosis

Basal cell carcinoma needs to be differentiated from the following conditions:

- Keratoacanthoma tends to grow rapidly and has a keratinous crater.

- Squamous cell carcinoma also grows rapidly and the lesions are dome shaped, elevated, hard and infiltrated with everted ulcers.

- Lupus vulgaris is differentiated with its characteristic onset occurring in childhood, its typical reddish patch with apple jelly nodules, and tendency to heal with a wrinkled tissue paper scar. Here there are no pearly nodules.

- Malignant melanoma is usually dusky greyish brown and lacks the characteristic ulceration with its rolled, telangiectatic border and pearly nodules as seen in basal cell carcinoma.

- Tertiary syphilis has a rapid and much bigger ulceration with a punched out ulcer and is easily distinguishable by a positive serology test.

- The superficial basal cell carcinoma is easily mistaken for psoriasis or eczema, which needs to be ruled out with the help of careful examination and histological finding.

- In the initial stages, basal cell carcinoma may simulate a melanocytic naevus, especially if pigmented. Here the distinguishing feature is the hair growing from the surface in cases of a naevus, which is absent in basal cell carcinoma.

- In both molluscum contagiosum and senile sebaceous hyperplasia there is the presence of a central keratin-filled pit, which helps differentiating it from basal cell carcinoma in the initial stages.

BOWEN'S DISEASE

Synonym

Intra-epidermal epithelioma.

Definition

Bowen's disease is a slowly growing, persistent, intraepidermal squamous cell carcinoma, where the lesions are characteristically non-elevated, red, scaly or crusted.

Etiology & Incidence

Chronic exposure to the sun and chronic arsenism are the commonest causes. Arsenic salts, besides being present in industrial processes, are also present in fungicides, weed killer or pesticides, and thus can be accidentally consumed by farmers.

It is usually seen in light-skinned men, who are well beyond their middle ages.

Histopathology

Atypical squamous cells proliferate through the whole thickness of the epidermis. There is hyperkeratosis, parakeratosis, acanthosis and thickening of the interpapillary ridges in the epidermis, with retention of a distinct dermo-epidermal junction and an intact basement membrane. The upper dermis shows a chronic inflammatory infiltrate. Arsenical Bowen's disease is characterized by the presence of numerous vacuolated atypical cells.

Clinical Features

Initial lesion presents itself as a small, firm, slightly red papule, which develops into a scaly or crusted, well-defined patch. On removal of the crust or the scale, there is a moist red surface, which is granular or papillomatous. As the lesion grows gradually, there is spontaneous cicatrisation taking place in parts. In cases where the intraepithelial growth becomes invasive, there is nodular infiltration of the lesion with ulceration.

The vulva, vagina, nasal mucosa, conjunctiva and larynx are also frequently the sites of affection.

Course & Prognosis

The tumor cells grow sidewards and upwards remaining within the epidermis for years, and may later on develop into a basal or squamous cell epithelioma. It is thus considered as a precancerous dermatosis.

Diagnosis

- Bowen's disease needs to be differentiated from psoriasis, eczema, lichen simplex, seborrheic keratosis and arsenical dermatosis.

- Differentiation from superficial basal cell carcinoma can be difficult in the initial stages, but the rolled edges and thread-like margin go in favor of basal cell carcinoma. The biopsy report will help further differentiation.

MALIGNANT MELANOMA

Definition

It is the most malignant tumour of the skin, arising from the melanocytes at the epidermal-dermal junction or the mucosal epithelium, or from pre-existing naevi cells, or rarely from melanocytes in visceral sites.

Etiology & Incidence

It is especially common in the light-skinned individuals chronically or excessively exposed to ultraviolet rays of the sun, with its peak incidence in the elderly age group. Long-term use of oral contraceptives is also linked as a predisposing factor in a few cases.

Other factors that are known to increase the risk of developing this disorder are – obesity, smoking, people with a sensitive skin, freckles and red or fair hair.

Studies have shown that it is a prevalent disorder in individuals coming from a high socio-economic status, though the mortality rate is definitely higher in those of a lower socio-economic class.

Histopathology

There is the presence of cytologically atypical, immature, malignant melanocytic cells invading the dermis, the dermo-epidermal junction and the upper layers of the epidermis. There is also ulceration and lymphocytic infiltrate seen in the part. The cytological characteristics of malignancy are a high nuclear to cytoplasmic ratio, intense nuclear staining, variation between adjacent cells and the presence of abnormal mitotic figures.

The tumour thickness and invasive level into the deeper layers of the skin is the most valuable prognostic guide. The presence of ulceration in the part and proliferation of tumour cells into the blood vessels are poor prognostic signs associated with a risk of both local and distant spread.

Clinical Features

The characteristic features to look for in cases of malignancy in a mole are –a recent increase in size of the mole (usually more than 6 mm), its asymmetrical growth, deepening or change of its color, its irregular border, induration or itching of the part, whether it bleeds easily on pressure, and also to check for any radiating lines of pigmentation in the lymphatics. Malignant melanomas metastasize rapidly first to the regional lymph glands, and later, to other parts of the skin, liver, lungs and brain.

The various clinical types commonly seen are as follows:

Superficial spreading or Pagetoid Melanoma

This is the commonest type, comprising over 70% of the melanomas seen clinically. The sites usually affected are the upper back in a male and the leg in cases of a female, with no preference for sun-damaged skin. It presents initially as an irregularly shaped, elevated, hyperkeratotic, and pigmented (brownish, bluish black or blackish) lesion. This may then have signs of increased growth in size (usually more than 6 mm), altered sensation or itching. It may become palpable (due to its vertical growth) and there is slight inflammation of the peripheral skin. This elevated nodule with the easy bleeding or serosanguinous oozing should arouse suspicion, especially when associated with erosion or ulceration.

Nodular Melanoma

This sub-type is especially common in males, with the lesion presenting usually on the head, neck or trunk. The prognosis is poor since these lesions tend to grow and spread rapidly. They usually present as an elevated, dome-shaped, papule or nodule, 1-4 mm wide, with a reddish or greyish brown pigmentation, that is not as marked as is seen in the 'superficial spreading type of melanoma' (due to a lack of the melanin pigment in this type). These lesions may grow larger and become papillary, fungoid, or ulcerated. Bleeding from these lesions occur in the later stages.

Acral Lentiginous Melanoma

This sub-type is especially seen to occur more frequently in the Asians rather than the light-skinned individuals. They present as a large, macular, lentiginous pigmented area around an invasive raised tumour. These lesions occur especially on the soles and palms. Mucosal and Subungual lesions are classified within this sub-type

Mucosal Melanoma It is a rare condition, occurring either in the mouth, nasal mucosa, upper jaw, lip or the vulva. If in the mouth, it is usually pigmented and ulcerated. The tumor in the nose looks like a polyp. Lesion on the lip looks like an indolent ulcer. Vulval lesions are often diagnosed late, after they have ulcerated.

Subungual Melanoma Here there is pigmentation of the nail, the nail bed and the nail fold. As the lesion continues to grow, the nail is destroyed.

Lentigo Maligna (Melanoma in Situ, Noninvasive Melanoma)

This condition occurs equally in men and women in their late sixties or seventies in chronically sun-damaged skin, especially on the face. The lesions occur especially on the face, with a characteristic horizontal spread on the skin rather than a deeper dermal spread into the skin. Initially the lesion appears as a flat, irregular, brownish or blackish macule, which grows very slowly, over years, into a nodule and then spreads deeper (vertically) into the dermis.

Amelanotic Melanoma

Here the lesion is pink, erythematous or skin-colored, and is characterized by a lack of pigment. It is especially seen in the albinos.

Prognosis

The prognosis of malignant melanoma is usually always grave, especially due to the rapid spread and metastases. If diagnosed early, before the vertical spread takes place, the prognosis is better.

Differential Diagnosis

- Angioma, histiocytoma or pigmented basal cell carcinoma need to be differentiated from nodular melanoma. Here an excision biopsy becomes necessary.

- Nevi are differentiated from melanomas by the latter's tendency for later onset, steady growth, slow change in color and its mottling.

- In the initial stages, a subungual melanoma can be easily confused with a benign melanocytic lesion, a traumatic haemorrhage under the nail, persistent paronychia, a fungal infection, or even a subungual wart. Thus one needs to perform a thorough clinical examination.

- Pigmented actinic keratoses and seborrheic keratoses need to be differentiated from early lesions of lentigo maligna melanoma.

- Amelanotic melanoma needs to be differentiated from granuloma pyogenicum.

PAGET'S DISEASE

Definition

It is an unilateral, intra-epidermal and intra-ductal epithelioma affecting the nipple and areola of females usually, though it is also seen in males, and can affect other organs like the genitals and the umbilicus.

Incidence

It is a condition seen most commonly in females in their late 50's or 60's. It is usually associated with intra-ductal type of carcinoma of the breast.

Histopathology

The epidermis is thickened with enlargement of the interpapillary ridges and hyperkeratosis or parakeratosis on the surface. There is characteristically Paget cells found in the epidermis, which are large, round, pale-staining cells with a large nucleus, and a high nuclear/cytoplasmic ratio. A layer of basal cells separates the Paget cells from the dermis. Acanthosis is usually present. There is also a chronic inflammatory reaction seen in the upper dermis.

Clinical Features

In the early stages of this condition there is a small, dry, scaly or crusted patch seen on the nipple, which in a few days progresses into a marginated, well-defined erythema and eczematous scaling or oozing of serosanguinous fluid from the part. There is associated complaint of itching, pricking and burning in the part, and at times a bloody discharge from the nipple. In a few cases a lump can be palpable in the breast. The change is confined to one nipple. Gradually the part becomes indurated, infiltrated, and ulcerated with retraction of the nipple.

Besides the nipple, the other sites usually involved in cases of Paget's disease are the vulva, perianal area, penis, scrotum, umbilicus and the groin. These are frequently associated with an underlying glandular adnexal carcinoma or a regional internal carcinoma with or without metastasis.

Since the rate of spread of this malignancy is very slow, the patient comes to seek advice at a later stage, by which time there is already infiltration and enlargement of the regional lymph nodes. The change may occasionally involve not only the skin of the breast but also spread onto the chest wall.

Diagnosis

The condition presents itself as a unilateral eczema of the nipple with sharply-defined, raised, red, crusty or moist, indurated lesion. In cases where the nipple is retracted, the diagnosis is easy. The biopsy report usually helps confirm the diagnosis.

Differential Diagnosis

- Nummular eczema, contact dermatitis or atopic dermatitis usually presents as a bilateral, chronic condition, occurring at any age, and running an irregular course with periods of complete remission. Also the lesions in cases of dermatitis or eczema are ill-defined and lack the raised rounded margin and the superficial induration seen in cases of Paget's disease.

- Hyperkeratosis of the nipple and areola can present as a unilateral affection, but histological findings reveal the diagnosis.

- Superficial basal cell carcinoma, perianal Bowen's disease and superficial malignant melanoma can be differentiated by site of affection and the histopathological findings.

Prognosis

The prognosis of it depends upon the stage at which the diagnosis is made. Also, studies reveal that its prognosis in men is poorer than that in women.

KAPOSI'S SARCOMA

Definition

It is a multifocal neoplasm arising from both the vascular and lymphatic dermal endothelium.

Pathology

Early lesions show a chronic inflammatory or granulomatous tissue change with new and dilated blood vessels, edema, hemorrhage and marked lymphocytic inflammatory reaction and macrophages around them. Here is proliferation of the abnormal or jagged vascular endothelial cells in the upper dermis, which tend to anastomose. Then in the later stages there is spindle cell proliferation.

Clinical Features

Initial lesions consist of a small pinkish-red or bluish-black macules and patches occurring especially on the toes or the soles, though hands, ears, face, genitals, trunk and soft palate can also be affected. The lesions gradually grow and become painful and itchy, these then coalesce into a plaque or nodule, which bleeds on trauma. The lesions may involute to leave pigmented scars, or become eroded, ulcerated or fungating. New lesions can appear along the course of superficial veins and there can be associated lymphedema due to lymphatic involvement.

There are four different clinical sub-types of this condition seen Sporadic, endemic, associated with non-HIV immunosuppression and finally one related to HIV infection.

- Sporadic cases are found especially in elderly males. These lesions very slowly start to occur around the ankle and then spread up the leg insidiously. The prognosis is rarely very grave.

- Endemic cases are seen in both male adults and in children, especially in tropical Africa. There are crops of vascular lesions on the skin, with marked oedema. These have a locally aggressive but systemically indolent course. Visceral lesions can also occur, in which case the prognosis is poor.

- Kaposi's sarcoma associated with non-HIV induced immunosuppression is seen especially in young patients who have undergone a transplant. Here, early diagnosis can be missed out because of small and few lesions scattered over the body resembling slight areas of trauma or a simple bruise. Then both systemic and cutaneous involvement takes place aggressively, causing the prognosis to be grave in these patients.

- Kaposi's sarcoma in HIV infected individuals presents itself in the later stages of the disease. Initially there can be only a few flat macules seen on the skin, but gradually the lesions spread and occur anywhere on the body. There is a fulminant, progressive course with nodal and systemic involvement. The prognosis is poor.

Extracutaneous involvement occurs in the small intestines, lungs, heart, conjunctiva, adrenal glands and the lymph nodes of the abdomen. Bone or skeletal involvement is an indication that the disease is wide-spread in the body, making the prognosis grave.

Differential Diagnosis

- Early lesions of Kaposi's sarcoma can be confused with a benign vascular proliferation or histiocytoma, though its evolution from a macular lesion and its characteristic colour, slow development and multifocal distribution make the diagnosis likely in most instances. Histological examination will help confirm the diagnosis.

- In a few cases, where there is prolonged venous hypertension of the lower legs, nodules can be confused with Kaposi's sarcoma, but here a lack of progression and no spindle-cell proliferation in the histological sections confirm the diagnosis.

- A venous dermatitis on the lower legs can simulate an early lesion of Kaposi's sarcoma but histological examination will confirm the diagnosis.

MYCOSIS FUNGOIDES

Definition

It is the commonest type of cutaneous T-cell lymphoma, which is associated with a chronic and indolent clinical course.

Incidence

The condition is twice as common in males than females, especially in the elderly age group.

Histopathology

Initially there is a non-specific lymphocytic infiltration in the papillary layer of the dermis. The small lymphoid cells line up just below the dermo-epidermal junction. There is then a selective colonization of the epidermis by the large and atypical lymphocytes, which is termed as Pautrier's microabscesses. There is papillary dermal fibrosis with bundles of collagen arranged haphazardly.

Clinical Features

The condition is a chronic, slowly progressive one, with initial symptoms consisting of non-specific lesions, which makes diagnosis difficult in the early stages.

The three stages through which this condition is known to pass are as follows:

1. **The premycotic or non-specific stage:** Here the symptoms consist of itchy, scaly, erythematous, round or oval plaques (simulating those seen in eczema, psoriasis, pityriasis or erythema multiforme), varying in size from 1-5 cm or more. The eruption may be generalized or begin localized to one area and then spread. These occur on the covered parts of the body, especially the breast, trunk, upper thighs and the buttocks. In dark-skinned individuals, the lesions appear as hypopigmented spots.

2. **The infiltrative stage:** The earlier lesions of the premycotic stage get infiltrated, becoming widespread, markedly red, and are associated with intense itching of the part. The lesions may form nodules, which then ulcerate. The mucous membranes are also affected.

3. **The tumour stage:** The earlier infiltrated lesions gradually increase in size or coalesce, and then form nodules or tumors, with rolled edges. Also, deep ulceration can take place in these tumors, the base of which is covered by a dull greyish crust.

Along with the above symptoms, there can be lymphadenopathy, where the lymph nodes are non-tender, firm and freely movable. Organs connected with the reticular system (i.e. liver, spleen and lymph nodes), lung, bone or kidneys may also be secondarily involved; wherein the prognosis becomes very poor.

Prognosis

In the initial stages, the condition has a good prognosis, which becomes poor in cases of widespread cutaneous or extracutaneous spread, with the patient usually dying of septicemia.

Diagnosis

With the non-specific histological and clinical findings, diagnosis becomes difficult, but it should be suspected in the elderly age group.

Differential Diagnosis

- This condition needs to be differentiated from eczema, dermatitis, pityriasis rosea, fungal infection, and psoriasis in its initial stages. One needs to confirm the diagnosis after making several biopsies from different lesions.

- Lymphomatous drug reactions may simulate mycosis fungoides in the initial stages, but the perivascular infiltration in the histopathology report will help confirm the diagnosis.

LEUKEMIA CUTIS

Definition

This is a condition where specific cutaneous eruptions are seen in patients suffering from leukemia, especially in the acute lymphocytic leukemia, chronic myelogenous leukemia and chronic lymphocytic leukemia.

Clinical Features

The lesions especially include multiple, skin-colored or erythematous or plum colored, papules or nodules or infiltrated plaques, which seem rubbery on palpation. In a few cases, non-specific lesions like leukemids, ecchymoses, subcutaneous nodules, petechiae, urticaria, bullae or ulcerations may be present. In a few patients, hypertrophy and bleeding of the gums is seen.

Prognosis

Leukemic patients presenting with leukemia cutis have a poor prognosis.

CUTANEOUS METASTASIS

Definition

Here there is metastatic dissemination to the skin of infiltrates from primary carcinomas situated in the systemic organs, either through the lymphatic or the hematogenous route.

Incidence

About 5-10 percent of the patients with systemic cancer develop metastases to the skin, especially those with carcinomas in the breast, liver, prostate, gastro-intestinal tract, and melanomas. Adults over the age of 40 are especially prone.

Clinical Features

It presents as solitary or numerous, discrete, firm, hard, painless, rubbery papules or nodules, especially on the chest, abdomen, or scalp. Involvement of the skin is likely to be near the area of the primary tumor. The lesions can be skin-colored, or can be red, brown or black in color. They are freely movable in the initial stages, and become fixed to the underlying tissues within a few weeks time.

Prognosis

Prognosis is usually poor since metastasis to the skin is an indication of terminal stage of cancer.

HOMEOPATHIC APPROACH TOWARDS
MALIGNANT TUMORS OF THE SKIN

In cancerous affections of the skin, I personally have seen very few cases. My approach is purely classical, trying to avoid as much as possible, to treat any local symptoms. I try to take the deeper constitutional symptoms to prescribe in such cases.

Many patients with cancer of the skin present with radiation burns or many patients with cancer of the skin are exposed to a lot of X-rays and other radiation, having to suffer their complications. The drugs of choice in such patients are – potentized *X-ray (Radium Bromide), Cobaltum, Kali ars.,* etc.

Also, I many a times advocate the use of Iscador Therapy along with my homeopathic prescription, in the cases of cancer of the skin.

REPERTORY

One refer the following rubrics:

- **Generals, tumors; cystic:** bar-c, calc, graph, phos.
- **Skin,**

    - Excrescences: calc, caust, graph, lyco, nit-ac, staph, thuj.
    - Keloid: graph, nit-ac, sil.
    - Nevi: acet-ac, fl-ac, phos.

Chapter-32

Disorders of Sebaceous Glands

The sebaceous gland is holocrine as the secretion being formed by the complete disintegration of the glandular cells. The cells are replaced by cell division at the periphery of the lobes or acini of the glands, with the consequence that differentiating cells are displaced towards the centers of each acinus. The average transit time of the cells, from formation to discharge, has been given as 7.4 days in the human gland.

Sebaceous glands occur over much of the body, although not normally on the palms or soles, and only sparsely on the dorsal surfaces of the hand and foot. Sebaceous glands are largest and most numerous in the midline of the back, on the forehead and face in the external auditory meatus and on the anogenital surfaces.

In a number of sites, sebaceous glands open directly to the surface of the skin, and not by way of a hair follicle. Examples of such glands are the Meibomian glands of the eyelids and Tyson's glands of the prepuce.

Sebum, the discharge from the sebaceous glands, is complex mixture of lipids. The function of sebum is both to control moisture loss from the epidermis and protect the skin from fungal and bacterial infection.

There has been an established connection between the activity of the sebaceous gland and the endocrine system. Androgens are responsible for the development and maintenance of sebum secretion in both sexes. The sebaceous glands regress to become minute during the prepubertal period, but undergo vast enlargement at puberty, when the sebum output of males increases more than fivefold. Adrenal androgens increase sebum production but appear to require conversion to testosterone within the sebaceous gland. The effect of progesterone on sebaceous glands has been a matter of dispute. Progesterone administration can produce acne, and when given to elderly women it increases sebum production, but no such effect could be demonstrated in young women. The pituitary has a major effect on sebaceous gland activity. The pituitary acts indirectly through its various target glands and as a result of a direct action by some of its hormones on sebaceous glands. Gonadotrophins stimulate sebum secretion in the human male, but probably do not have any direct independent action on the sebaceous gland. Thyrotrophic hormone has a similar action. ACTH has an effect through adrenal androgens. Patients with hypopituitarism and those with isolated growth hormone deficiency have low levels of sebum, while patients with acromegaly show increased sebum secretion. Oestrogens undoubtedly depress sebaceous activity. It has been suggested that oestrogens may act by reducing endogenous androgen production.

ACNE VULGARIS

Synonym

Pimples; in Hindustani Kee, Muhase.

Introduction

Acne is a chronic inflammatory disease of the pilosebaceous follicles. It is characterized by the formation of comedones, erythematous papules and pustules, less frequently by nodules or pseudocysts and, in some cases, is accompanied by scarring.

The pathogenesis involves four major factors

1. Increased sebum production.
2. An abnormality of the microbial flora.
3. Cornification of the pilosebaceous duct.
4. Production of inflammation.

Incidence

The condition usually starts in adolescence and frequently resolves by the mid-twenties. The increased incidence during puberty is due to the increased sebaceous activity. Acne develops earlier in females than in males, which may reflect the earlier onset of puberty, but it usually is somewhat severer in boys. In the twenties, it gradually decreases and is again seen especially in women after the age of 28 or so (post adolescent acne), since they usually stop producing children (family planning) and periods may become scanty at that age. Several studies have shown that genetic factor influence susceptibility to acne.

Etiology

Increased sebum production presents to the patient as a seborrhea (greasy skin). Active sebaceous glands are a prerequisite for the development of acne. Acne patients, male and female, excrete on average more sebum than normal subjects, and the level of secretion correlates reasonably well with the severity of the acne.

Hormones

Common occurrence of acne at puberty is because of increased production of sex hormones, which makes the sebaceous glands hyperactive. Sebaceous activity is predominantly dependent on androgenic sex hormones of gonadal or adrenal origin. Abnormally high levels of sebum secretion could thus result from high overall androgen production or increased availability of free androgen, because of a deficiency in sex-hormone-binding globulin (SHBG). Androgen and progesterone are responsible for hyperplasia of the oil glands (Eunuchs do not have oily skins). There is general agreement that plasma testosterone levels are not abnormally high in males with acne.

Diet

The possible effect of nutrition on the age of puberty may be relevant, as acne is more likely after the start of sexual development, and this occurs when the body weight attains about 48kg. Diet rich in fat and starches may be a contributing factor.

Hereditary factor

Several members of the same family may be affected with severe scarring acne.

Premenstrual flare

About 70% of women complain of a flare 2-7 days premenstrually. It is unlikely that any possible variation in sebum excretion during the menstrual cycle could be substantial enough to explain the flare. Possibly it is related to a premenstrual change in the hydration of the pilosebaceous epithelium. Progesterone and oestrogen also have both pro- and anti-inflammatory effects.

Sweating

Up to 15% of acne patients notice that sweating causes a deterioration in their acne, especially if they live or work in a hot humid environment, for example as a cook. Ductal hydration may be the responsible factor.

UV Radiation

Patients and doctors alike accept that natural sunlight often improves acne, but there is no scientific evidence that it does. The cosmetic effect may be the entire explanation. Artificial UV radiation appears to be less satisfactory than natural radiation, and psoralen and UVA (PUVA) have been reported to induce acne lesions. Furthermore, UV radiation may enhance the comedogenicity of sebum.

Psychogenic stress

Particularly the habit of picking pimples makes them worse. Questionnaire studies have shown that many acne patients experience shame (70%), embarrassment and anxiety (63%), lack of confidence (67%), impaired social contact (57%) and a significant problem with unemployment. Severe acne may be related to increased anger and anxiety.

Occupation

Hydration of the ductal stratum corneum may induce acne in such occupations as catering. Patients dealing with oil undoubtedly develop an acneiform oil folliculitis, particularly on their trunks and limbs.

Besides this constipation, sedentary life, excessive use of greasy cosmetics, pomade, detergents and mechanical rubbing are seen to have considerable effect.

Pathogenesis

Ductal Hypercornification

Acne patients show ductal hypercornification, which presents histologically as micro-comedones, and clinically as blackheads and whiteheads. There is a significant correlation between the severity of acne and the number and size of follicular casts, the presence of which is a measure of comedogenesis. Comedones represent the retention of hyperproliferating ductal keratinocytes in the duct. Several factors have been implicated in the induction of hyperproliferation, and include sebaceous lipid composition, androgens, local cytokine production and bacteria.

The change in the process of keratinization of the sebaceous follicle produces an increased adherence of the horn cells resulting in retention hyperkeratosis. This leads to a disruption of the follicular epithelium, permitting discharge of the follicular contents into the dermis.

F- 43

Bacterial Colonization

Acne is not infectious. Bacterial colonization of the sebaceous follicle may contribute in the pathogenesis of acne. The three major organisms isolated from the surface of the skin and the duct of patients with acne are Propionibacterium acnes, Staphylococcus epidermidis and Malassezia furfur. They colonize the follicle and produce lipases. Bacterial lipase acts on the entrapped sebum to produce free fatty acids, which contribute to follicular hyperkeratosis.

This in turn causes the formation of inflammatory papules, pustules and nodulocystic lesions. Also biologically active substances produced by P. Acnes seep into the dermis and attract neutrophils and activate compliment.

Mediation of Inflammation

It probably results from biologically active mediators that diffuse from the follicle where they are produced by P. acnes.

Clinical Features

Location

Acne is a polymorphic disease, which occurs predominantly on the face, most frequently on the cheeks and in lesser degree on the nose, forehead and chin.

Ears: Large comedones in the concha, cysts in the lobes and sometimes retroauricular comedones and cysts.

Neck: Large cystic areas may predominate which may later become keloidal.

Upper part of the chest, shoulder and back.

Occasionally seen on the thighs and buttocks.

Distribution

It is usually bilaterally symmetrical.

The primary lesion of acne is the *comedone;* it signifies a plug composed of dried sebum, epithelial cells and keratinous scales; it fills the pilosebaceous canal.

The first stage is erythema, which surrounds or engulfs the comedone and a papule develops: *acne papulosa*. Most of these papules gradually involute leaving no trace; others suppurate to form pustules resulting from the action of secondary invading microorganism's chiefly staphylococci – *acne pustulosa*. *Acne indurata* – firm perifollicular nodules of bluish red colour. They persist for a long time. Many of them eventually become completely or partially absorbed, others transform into cysts – *acne_cystica*. They, however, also tend to persist, discharging from time to time a thin, purulent fluid.

Scarring

Scarring, usually pitted, is a common sequel of acne. In acne conglobata the suppurating cystic lesions predominate and severe scarring results. Sometimes the pits are closely aggregated giving rise to a worm-eaten appearance.

Non-inflamed Lesions (comedones Grade I)

They are more frequent in the younger patients and consist of blackheads (open comedones), in which the black colour is due to melanin not dirt, whiteheads (closed comedones), in which the black colour is due to melanin not dirt, whiteheads (closed comedones) and the so-called intermediate non-inflamed lesions, which show features of both blackheads and whiteheads. Whitehead appears as a slightly elevated white dot. With the passage of time the Sulphur constituent of sebum soon gets converted into Sulphide turning the whitehead into a black dot, called a blackhead.

Inflammatory Lesions (Grade II)

They may be superficial or deep, and many arise from non-inflamed lesions. The superficial lesions are usually papules and pustules (5mm or less in diameter), and the deep lesions are deep pustules and nodules.

For many years, up to and including now, the term nodulocystic or cystic acne has been extensively used. The term is a misnomer. Acne 'cysts' are not true cysts as they are not lined by an epithelium. Perhaps it is more appropriate to describe such lesions as nodules.

Nodules more frequently occur in males and, if exudative or haemorrhagic, are particularly disfiguring. Nodules may extend over areas of a few to many centimetres, and may be remarkably deep with very little surface involvement. Sinus formation between nodules may also occur, with devastating cosmetic effects. Such lesions can be very tender. Itching is a rare symptom of acne. Pyogenic granulomas develop very infrequently. The deeper inflammatory lesions are often associated with *scarring (Grade III)*, but scarring can occur with superficial lesions.

A common feature of darkly pigmented skin is the relatively persistent post-inflammatory pigmentation, which may be more disabling than the original disease.

Special varieties of acne are:

ACNE EXCORIÉE

This variant occurs predominantly in females. Two subgroups exist those with some primary inflammatory acne lesions, and those with virtually none. Both groups usually consist of females who 'fiddle' with the skin to exacerbate even the smallest lesions. Because of this chronic picking minor acne lesions are kept inflamed and active for weeks or even months at a time. There is often some personality or psychological problem.

DRUG-INDUCED ACNE/ACNEIFORM ERUPTIONS

The use of certain drugs, particularly iodides and bromides (No comedones develop and the eruption is frequently associated with mild pruritis), ACTH, androgens and anabolic hormones (Unconnected with comedones, but frequently accompanied by hypertrichosis). Such cases are often seen in women who receive high doses of testosterone propionate for CA of the breast and

ACTH for rheumatoid arthritis. Administration of phenytoin cohlartin to individuals already prone to acne has an adverse effect on the severity and duration of the disease.

'ENDOCRINE' ACNE

The role of the endocrine system in the aetiology of acne is discussed above. Majority of female patients have no evidence of virilism and require no further investigation. The term 'endocrine acne' should be reserved for cases of clinically manifest endocrine disease such as Cushing's disease, adrenogenital syndrome and the polycystic ovarian syndrome, which is the commonest cause of 'endocrine' acne.

EXTERNALLY INDUCED ACNE

The various types are:

Cosmetic Acne

Caused due to the greater use of potentially comedogenic cosmetics.

Pomade Acne

Pomades are greasy preparations used to 'defrizz' curly Negroid hair. The rash is similar to cosmetic acne but consists of non-inflamed lesions around the forehead and other areas where greasy pomades may extend onto the hairless skin.

Occupational Acne Sue to Oils and Tars

This uncommon acneiform eruption occurs in areas in contact with oils and crude tars. Not surprisingly, men are more often affected than women. The skin may show conspicuous comedones and only occasionally do frank inflammatory lesions arise; these are usually superficial.

Chloracne

This variant is part of a syndrome that follows exposure to

certain toxic, chlorinated hydrocarbons. Chloracne lesions consist of multiple comedones; inflammatory lesions are infrequent.

Mechanical Acne syn. Acne Mechanica

This term covers a mixed group of disorders in which the acne occurs at the site of physical trauma, as indicated by the pattern of the lesions. Examples are so-called fiddler's neck, which occurs on the neck of violin players, and is also characterized by the presence of lichenification and pigmentation. Headbands (as worn by sports-people and hippies) and tight bra straps are other causes.

Detergent Acne

This uncommon form of acne develops in patients who wash many times each day, in the mistaken hope of improving their existing acne. Pustular and papular lesions are most noticeable. Several bacteriostatic soaps contain weak acnegenic compounds, such as hexachlorophene.

Tropical Acne (Hydration Acne)

Certain occupations may aggravate pre-existing acne, for example workers in a hot, humid environment, such as cooks and pressers, are at risk. It is characterized by (a) their sudden developments among white people visiting the tropic (b) a severe eruption of large pustules and abscesses, which leave disfiguring scars. (c) Affection of the chest, back, buttocks and thighs – (face is comparatively clear). (d) The eruption subsides dramatically when the patient leaves the tropics.

Infantile and Juvenile Acne

It is confined to the face. The main lesions are comedones with only a few papules and pustules (probably caused by maternal harmones). Oily substances applied to the scalp and face can also produce grouped comedones in children.

Acne in the Aged

Single or grouped comedones are frequently seen in elderly

people. The main seat of involvement is the temporal and peri occular region.

Severe varieties of acne are:

Acne Conglobata

This is a most uncommon but severe form of acne, found particularly in males; the lesions usually occur on most of the trunk, face and limbs. The individual lesions are big, fluctuating, dark red cysts like abscesses, which persist for a long time. Nodules are characteristic and frequently fuse to form multiple draining sinuses. Others become ulcerated resembling scrofuloderma. They leave hypertrophic, often bridged scars. Multiple double ended comedones in skin adjacent to cysts. Sometimes associated with fever, leucocytosis and arthralgia.

Acne Fulminans

This was originally described as acute febrile ulcerative acne conglobata. It is an uncommon, immunologically induced, systemic disease in which the offending antigen is P. acnes. The patients are predominantly young males, who quite suddenly develop extensive inflammatory lesions, especially on the trunk. Associated features are fever, polyarthropathy, marked leukocytosis (even a leukaemoid reaction), weight loss, anorexia and general malaise Painful splenomegaly, erythema nodosum and bone pain due to aseptic osteolysis have also been reported.

Gram-negative Folliculitis

This is a complication of long-term treatment of acne with antibiotics. It presents either as a sudden eruption of multiple, small follicular pustules or with nodular lesions.

Pyoderma Faciale

Synonym - Rosacea fulminans.

This was initially believed to be a variant of acne but evidence is in favour of it being related to rosacea. It is uncommon, and occurs in patients who usually have mild disease, which suddenly erupts producing many pustules and nodules especially on the face. It mainly affects post-adolescent women (aged 20-40 years), often following a period of stress. Comedones are rare and facial flushing frequently precedes the acute illness. In the beginning, flushing appears under certain circumstances such as emotional stress, exposure to intensive cold, heat, the sun's rays or after alcoholic drinks. In due course the hyperemia state tends to persist and eventually becomes permanent. The telangiectasia presents an important feature of the disease. In acne rosacea, infiltration and hypertrophy may increase considerably, particularly on the nose. In men a clinical picture develops which is called rhinophyma. The nose is enormously enlarged and often lobulated. The pores are widened and oily masses can be readily expressed. In contrast to acne fulminans, there are usually no systemic symptoms. The reason for the sudden flare is unknown. Recurrence does occasionally occur. Rosacea fulminans has been reported in association with Crohn's disease-the significant of which is unclear.

Prognosis

It is a chronic disease with tendency to progressive aggravation. Response to treatment is not very satisfactory.

Treatment

- Foods like hot tea, coffee, alcohol and spicy foods, which cause flushing of the face, should be strictly avoided.
- Vegetarian food is encouraged.
- Exposure to sudden alterations in temperature should be minimized.
- Every effort should be made to relieve nervous tension.

Differential Diagnosis

Acne is rarely misdiagnosed. The commonest mistaken diagnosis is *rosacea*, which occurs in an older group and lacks comedones, nodules, cysts or scarring. Occasionally, patients may have both rosacea and acne. Rosacea patients may also have ocular involvement, but rarely truncal lesions.

Whiteheads may be confused with *milia*. Milia are predominantly infraorbital and are whiter. They can occur in association with, although they are unrelated to, acne.

Course and Prognosis

Generally the peak activity of acne is in the mid or late teen years with steady improvement starting around age 20. However, occasionally, disease activity continues into the fourth decade. Women seem particularly prone to this long lasting form of acne.

Acne in general seems to be more severe in men. Cystic lesions, which are common in men, are only rarely found in women. In women a monthly peak of acne activity often occurs during the week prior to their menses. Acne tends to improve during the 3rd to 9th month of pregnancy but rebound worsening sometimes occurs following parturition and cessation of lactation. It is difficult to predict the future severity of acne at the time a young patient is first seen. The presence of cysts and a F/H of scarring acne are however bad prognostic signs.

When acne is untreated, individual small papules and pustules resolve spontaneously in 7 to 10 days. Resolution of these lesions does not result in scarring even when some degree of picking is carried out. Large papules and cysts require several weeks to resolve and even then post inflammatory colour changes may persist for months. Scarring is occasionally found at the site of deep-seated papules and is almost invariably present following resolution of fluctuant cysts.

HOMEOPATHIC APPROACH TO ACNE

Acne vulgaris can be considered as one of the common diagnoses brought forward by the patient to a homeopath. The problem should never be tackled with superficial, local acting remedies. Instead, deep acting constitutional remedies should be prescribed judiciously as soon as the complete totality is available.

Whilst treating acne, inquire about the following points:

- Exact type of acne acne rosacea, vulgaris.

- The site is extremely helpful to select the appropriate drug e.g. I am able to prescribe *Carbo-veg.* on many occasions when no other symptoms are available only its characteristic site of affection that is back (Refer – Kent Repertory. Back eruptions – acne, Carbo-veg.).

- Ascertain whether:

  - Is patient symptomatic and has come to take preventive measures for recurrence of acne.

  - Is it Pustular and cystic variety where pain is the presenting symptom?

  - When patient presents with lots of scarring and disfigurement of skin due to acne.

The above differentiation is a must as the course progresses and the line of treatment is quite different.

Acne from the homeopathic standpoint has known to be caused by various causative factors e.g.

  - Menstruation and pregnancy.

  - Masturbation.

  - Food habits and allergies.

  - Emotions.

A sincere attempt to find the cause pays rich dividends. The following additional causes have been frequently observed in my practice. They are:

  - during stressful situations, especially amongst teenagers,

  - after abuse of various cosmetics,

  - occupational that is exposure to various organic and inorganic chemicals.

- The aggravating and ameliorating factors should be noted, e.g. acne aggravated during summer – Bovista.

- Concomitant symptoms that are usually associated with acne should be noted. We have frequently observed that amongst the concomitant symptoms, constipation and GI upset are two of the commonest out of the lot.

  Guidelines given:

- Patient should be strictly advised not to apply any local medicaments on acne as this does not help in overcoming the tendency to develop acne. Instead patients should be encouraged to clean the face, preferably with hot water at least 6-8 times a day without using any soap. This helps to removal dust particles and the bacteria.

- The patient should be advised to have proper timing for their diet and to omit from the diet

  - Highly seasoned food and pungent food.

  - Foods that is rich in fats.

  - High carbohydrates: Mithais, sweets, chocolates. Patient should be encouraged to eat plenty of green leafy vegetables and fresh fruits.

  - Exercise in fresh open air adds a feather to the cap of treatment.

- The recent trend to be on long-term antibiotics to subside the acne should be discouraged.

- When the patient is passing through stressful situation psychotherapy is often of tremendous help to cope up with the situation.

  Acne is a very disfiguring disease owing to the fact that it selects the face by preference as its location. The non-professional man than any other skin affection often mistakes it for syphilis.

  Acne tends to be chronic, and is obstinately resistant to treatment. Moreover, it is subject to periods of amelioration and aggravation without treatment of any kind. With proper diet and attention to hygiene, together with the homeopathic remedy it yields to treatment in course of a few weeks to a few months.

It is an inflammatory structural disorder of the sebaceous glands or follicles of the skin. Dirt plugs the outlet of many of the follicles, forming 'black heads', or comedones. According to Unna, however, the uniform blackening of these outlets is due to a pigmentary staining. It may be both, but it certainly is chiefly the former. Retention of the natural secretion or sebum causes irritation of the follicles and congestion of the surrounding tissue. Pressure of the skin with the finger nails squeezes out the secretion in little cylinders, generally regarded by the laity as worms. Some points suppurate and some intermediate follicles inflame, and pimples, as well as hardened masses, appear. It is a complete spoiler of a fine complexion and hence dreaded by the fair sex.

The cases that suppurate are those that become infected with some variety of the staphylococcus pyogenes or pus germ. The variety described above is the acne simplex. A more formidable kind is the acne rosacea, characterized by hypertrophy, redness, dilatation of the blood vessels and even neoplastic tubercles.

Acne simplex is the form most frequently met with. It is more common about the time of puberty. The direct causes are said to be local irritants, cosmetics, uncleanliness, exposure to heat, cold and wind, and the entrance of pus germs into the gland. The general causes are inappropriate food, too rich or too nitrogenous, masturbation, sexual excesses, uterine derangements, and debilitating diseases generally. It is most intimately connected with derangements, overactivity, etc., of the sexual organs, which accounts for its frequent occurrence at the time of puberty. At this age the hair follicles and the sebaceous glands are very active, and many changes are taking place in the developing individual.

Certain drugs produce acne-like eruption of the face – namely, Tar, Potassium bromide (forehead) and Potassium iodide. The habitual use of alcohol, especially in excess, is responsible for a good number of cases.

SOME IMPORTANT HOMEOPATHIC REMEDIES

Antimonium crudum: Cheeks and chin. Simple acne that turn into pustules and then gradually develop into boils. Pimples associated with gastric derangement. Burning and itching sensation in acne < night. Tendency to develop cracks and warts. Acne in drunkards (Led., Nux-v.).

Berberis aquifolium: The acne eruptions come in blotches. The rest of the skin is dry and scaly. Pimples extend from face towards the neck. It is an age-old remedy to clear the complexion of the face. Acne associated with menstrual irregularity.

Bovista lycoperdon: A/F cosmetics. Acne with indurated papules.

Bromium: Acne in scrofulous individuals with glandular enlargements (Calc-s., Merc-s.). Acne with indurated papules.

Carbo animalis: Acne rosacea with burning and rawness. Skin has a tendency to develop ulcers with indurated glands, especially neck, axilla and groins. Acne with unsightly scars (Kali-br.). Indurated papules.

Chrysarobinum: Acne rosacea that leads to easy formation of crusts. Acne is associated with violent itching.

Calcarea phosphorica: Face is pale, yellowish, earthy, and full of pimples. They ulcerate very easily and form deep scars. Also they tend to suppurate easily. Acne vulgaris in individuals who are tall, lean, anemic with glandular enlargement; with vertex headache and flatulent dyspepia > by eating.

Calcarea sulphurica: Tendency to suppuration after the pus has found its vent, comes within the range of this remedy. The face is full of pimples and pustules. The discharge is thick, yellow, lumpy and bloody. Obstinate pimples that refuse to heal early. Even though a hot patient, Calc-sulph. patient feels better by local heat.

Carbo vegetabilis: Pimples with mottled cheeks and red nose. They are fat, sluggish, old, lazy, lifeless individuals with pimples that suppurate and have an offensive odor. Acne associated with gastric derangements.

Cimicifuga racemosa: Pimples with facial blemishes in young women. Pimples associated with ovarian and uterine complaints. Acne in nervous, depressed and oversensitive individuals. Acne associated with gastric derangements.

Conium maculatum: Pimples, small, red, burning appear with scanty menses and disappear when menses are over. Pustular acne on the face that itch violently. The skin is discolored red. Pustules rupture and form thick crusts. Acne alternates with internal symptoms e.g. diarrhea. Acne with indurated papules.

Eugenia jambosia: It is specially indicated for indurated and painful acne along with comedones. The pimples are painful for some distance around. It is also useful for acne rosacea. Skin cracks about toes. Fissures between toes and nightly cramp in soles of feet become important concomitants. Acne associated with menstrual irregularities.

Graphites: Acne that exudes gluey moisture, but bleeds easily and has a tendency to develop thick crusts. Acne vulgaris before the menses. Skin symptoms alternate with digestive complaints.

Juglans regia: Comedones and acne of the face that itch violently. When the acne bursts, it forms thick crusts. Acne that is associated with menstrual irregularities.

Kalium bromatum: Face has a blotchy red appearance with multiple indurated acne in fleshy young people with coarse habits, especially during puberty. Acne developing in individuals after sexual excess. Bluish red pustules on face, chest and shoulders. Acne with unsightly scars and menstrual irregularities.

Kalium arsenicosum: Pustular acne worse during menses. The skin is dry, scaly, wilted. Intolerable itching that is worse from warmth.

Ledum palustre: Red pimples on forehead and cheeks, stinging when touched. Pimples develop in individuals after suppressed discharges or after excess of alcohol (Nux-v., Rhus-t., Ant-c., Bar-c.). Acne with rheumatism (Rhus-t.).

Medorrhinum: Acne and pustules come out in blotches of reddish colour during menses; worse after menses. Discharge from the acne has a fishy odour. H/O sycoses.

Nux vomica: A/F cheese, excessive use of liquor. Pimples associated with gastric derangements.

Phosphoricum acidum: Acne from onanism (Aur.). Acne that gradually turns into small painful boils with stinking pustular discharge. Acne with loss of hair from beard.

Psorinum: Acne rosacea with dirty, rough, scabby, greasy skin.

Robinia pseudacacia: Acne with indurated papules and gastric derangement.

Sarsaparilla officinalis: Acne with menstrual irregularities. Acne during pregnancy (Sep., Bel.l, Sabina).

Sulphur: Pale sickly face with bright red lips with multiple painful acne. Acne with dry rough wrinkled scaly skin. There is burning and itching sensation in acne < at night in bed. Acne alternates with other complaints like asthma.

Sulphuricum acidum: Acne rosacea with obstinate constipation.

REPERTORY

- **Female genitalia, menses, scanty, acne, with:** sang.
- **Perspiration, oily:** agar, arg-met, arn, ars, aur, bry, bufo, calc, chin, fl-ac, lyc, mag-c, med, merc, nat-m, nux-v, ol-j, petr, plb, psor, rhus-t, rob, sel, stram, sumb, thuj, thyr.
    - Daytime: bry.
    - Morning: bry, chin.
    - Night: agar, bry, croc, mag-c, merc.

Location

- Nose, nodosities, surrounded by red swelling like acne rosacea: cann-s.

- **Face**
  - Discoloration, black spots, acne; from, suppressed: glycyrg.
  - Eruptions, acne: abrot, agar, ail, ambr, ant-c, ant-s-aur, ant-t, anthraci, arist-cl, ars, ars-br, ars-i, ars-s-f, ars-s-r, asim, aster, aur-met, aur-m, aur-s, bar-c, bar-s, bell, bell-p, berb, berb-a, brom, bov, bry, bufo, calc, calc-f, calc-p, calc-pic, calc-s, calc-sil, carb-ac, carb-an, carb-v, carbn-s, carc, caust, chel, chim, chlorpr, cic, con, cop, cortico, crot-h, dig, dios, dros, dulc, echi-p, eug, fl-ac, foll, graph, hep, hir, hydrc, ign, thuj, tub, uran-met, uran-n, zinc
  - Cachexia, in: ars, carb-v, nat-m, sil.
  - Cheese, from: nux-v.
  - Chin: hydr, ichth, jug-r, prot, sanic, sulfa, thuj, verat, violt.
  - Chronic: merc.
  - Comedones: abrot, ant-c, ars, aster, aur-met, aur-ar, aur-s. bar-c, bell, brom, bry, calc, calc-sil, carb-v, carbn-s, chel, dig, dros, eug, graph, grat, hep, hydr, jug-r, kali-br, lach, lyc, mez, nat-ar, nat-c, nat-m, nit-ac, petr, plb, psor, sabad, sabin, sel, sep, sil, sul-i, sulph, sumb, thuj, tub
    - Chin: dros, jug-r, tub.
      - And upper lip: sulph.
    - Forehead: sulph.
    - Nose: dros, graph, mez, nit-ac, sabin, sel, sulph, sumb, tub.
    - Ulcerating: dig, sel, tub.
  - Constipation, with: calc-sil, nux-v.
  - Cosmetics, from: bov.
  - Cystic: nit-ac.
  - Delivery; after: sep.
  - Drunkards, in: ant-c, ars, bar-c, carbn-s, kreos, lach, led, nux-v, puls, rhus-t, sulph.

- Fire, near a: ant-c.
- Forehead: ant-c, aur, aur-ar, bar-c, bell, calc, calc-pic, caps, carb-an, carb-v, carbn-s, caust, clem, cic, clem, hep, hydr, kali-bi, kali-br, kreos, led, nat-m, nit-ac, nux-v, ph-ac, psor, rhus-t, sep, sil, sulph.
- Girls, in anaemic: ars-br, aster, bar-c, calc, graph, hep, kali-c, nat-c, nat-m, sabin, sel, sulph, thuj.
- Glands, with swelling of: arom, calc-s, merc-sul.
- Heated, becoming, agg.: caust.
- Kalium iodide; from abuse of: aur.
- Masturbation, from: crot-h, ph-ac.
- Menses
  - After: med.
  - Before: graph, mag-m, pitu-a, psor, sep.
  - Delayed: crot-h.
  - During: cycl, dulc, kali-br, mag-m, med, psor.
  - Irregular: aur-m-n, bell, bell-p, berb, berb-a, calc, cimic, con, eug, graph, kali-br, kali-c, kreos, nat-m, psor, puls, sang, sars, thuj, verat.
  - Scanty: sang.
- Mercury, from abuse of: kali-i, mez, nit-ac.
- Papules, with indurated: agar, arn, ars-i, berb, bov, brom, carb-an, cic, cob, con, eug, iod, kali-br, kali-i, nat-br, nit-ac, rob, sulph, thuj.
- Persistent: hir.
- Pregnancy, during: bell, sabin, sars, sep.
- Puberty, at: podo.
  - Girls with vertex headache and flatulent indigestion, eating amel; in anemic: calc-p.
- Punctate acne: kali-br, sulph-i.
- Pustular: kali-ar, kali-br, merc.

F- 44

- Rheumatism, with: led, rhus-t.

- Rosacea: agar, ars, ars-br, ars-i, aur, aur-ar, aur-m, aur-s, bell, bufo, calc, calc-p, calc-sil, cann-s, canth, caps, carb-ac, carb-an, carb-v, carbn-s, caust, chel, chrys-ac, cic, clem, cortico, eug, guare, hep, hydr-ac, hydrc, iris, kali-bi, kali-br, kali-i, kreos, lach, led, mez, morg-p, nux-v, ov, petr, plb, psor, rad-br, rad-met, rhus-r, rhus-t, ruta, sars, sep, sil, sul-ac, sul-i, sul-ac, sulph, syc, tub, verat, viol-o, viol-t.

  - Bluish: lach, sulph.

  - Groups, in: caust.

  - Nose, on: ars-br, calc-p, calc-pic, cann-s, carb-an, caust, kali-i, psor, rhust-t, sars.

- Scars, with unsightly: carb-an, kali-br, merc, sil, thuj.

  - Red: bell.

- Scrofulous persons; in: bar-c, brom, calc, calc-p, con, iod, merc-sul, mez, sil, sulph.

- Sexual excesses, with: aur, calc, eug, kali-br, ph-ac, rhus-t, sep, thuj.

- Stomach complaints, with: ant-c, carb-v, cimic, lyc, nux-v, puls, rob.

- Symmetrical distribution, with a: arn.

- Syphilis, from: aur, kali-i, merc-sul, nit-ac.

- Tubercular children, in: tub.

- Young people; in fleshy coarse habits and bluish, red pustules on face, chest and shoulders; with: kali-br.

- **Eruptions, papular:** aur, borx, calc, carb-v, crot-h, cub, dig, dulc, galeoc-c-h, gels, hydrc, kali-c, kali-i, lyc, ol-an, petr, pic-ac, sabal, sep, sil, sulfa, syph, zinc.

  - Cheeks: borx.

  - Chin: borx, calc, caust, crot-h, lyc, merc, nit-ac, sars.

  - Forehead: cycl, mur-ac.

- ˙ Lip, upper: zinc.
- Nostril, right, inside: chen-a.
- Painful: calc.
- **Eruptions, pimples:** agar, agath-a, aids, alum, alum-p, am-m, ambr, anac, anan, ant-c, apis, arg-met, ars, ars-i, ars-s-f, arum-t, aster, aur, aur-ar, aur·i, aur-s, bar-c, bar-i, bar-m, bar-s, bell, berb, borx, bov, calc, calc-p, calc-s, calc-sil, caps, carb-an, carb-v, carbn-s, caust, chel, cic, clem, cocc, coli, coloc, con, crot-h, cub, cycl, cystein-l, dros, eug, fuma-ac, gels, ger-i, glon, graph, hep, hir, hura, hydrc, idgn, iod, jug-r, kali-ar, kali-c, kali-chl, kali-m, kali-n, kali-s, kali-sil, kreos, lac-d, lach, led, lyc, lyss, mag-c, mag-m, meny, meph, merc, mosch, mur-ac, nat-ar, nat-c, nat-m, nat-p, nat-s, nit-ac, nux-v, ol-an, pall, pant-ac, par, petr, ph-ac, phos, psor, puls, rhus-t, sabin, sanic, sars, sep, sil, sol-t-ae, stann, staph, suis-hep, sul-ac, sul-i, sulph, tarax, tarent, tell, tere-la, thuj, til, verat, vero-o, vinc, zinc, zinc-p.
- Bluish: lyss.
- Burning: aphis, cic, graph, kali-c, nat-c, sars.
    - Touched when: coloc, nat-s.
- Chin: alum, ambr, amp, ant-c, arg-n, aster, borx, calc, caust, chel, clem, cloi, con, crot-h, dulc, ferr-m, fuma-ac, hep, kali-chl, lyc, mag-c, mag-m, merc, nat-c, nat-pyru, nat-s, nit-ac, nux-v, par, ph-ac, psor, rhus-t, sars, sep, sil, succ-ac, suis-hep, thuj, zinc.
- Cold air agg.: ars.
- Confluent: cic, psor, tarent.
- Copper coloured: kali-i.
- Elevated margins: verat.
- Forehead: acon-ac, agar, alum, alum-p, am-c, am-m, ambr, anac, ars, aur, aur-ar, aur-s, bell, berb, bov, bry, calc, calc-p, canth, carb-v, chel, chin, cic, clem, con, cycl, ferr-m, gels, gran, hep, hura, hyper, indg, kali-bi, kali-br, kali-chl, kreos, lac-d, lac-h, lach, lachn, led, mag-m, meph, mez,

mur-ac, nat-c, nat-m, nat-p, nat-sil, nit-ac, nux-v, olnd, par, ph-ac, phos, positr, psor, puls, rhod, rhus-v, sabin, sep, sol-ni, suis-hep, sulph, suprar, tab, tarent, zinc, zinc-p, zing, ziz.

- Burning: ars, bell, canth, cic.
- Itching: alum, calc, mag-m, sulph, ziz.
- Painful: ambr, clem, indg, sep, staph, sulph.
- Red: ambr, anac, bell, carb-v, led, nat-c, nat-m, nux-v, sep, sol-ni.
- Rubbing agg.: mag-m.
- Sore to touch: ambr, hell, led, ph-ac, zinc.
- Stinging on rubbing: sulph.
- Washed, smarting when: nux-v.
- White: carb-v, kali-br, sulph, zinc.
- Wine after: zinc.

- Greenish: cupr.
- Inflamed: bry, chel, nat-sil, sars, stann, sulph.
- Insects, pimples as from: ant-c.
- Itching: agar, ant-c, asc-t, calc, caust, clem, con, dulc, ephi-si, graph, hep, mur-ac, ol-an, pall, psor, sars, sep, stann, staph, til, zinc.
- Jaws, lower: ars, coli, lac-lup, meph, par, sil.
- Lips: agar, am-m, arn, aur, bell, berb, borx, bov, bufo, calc, caps, carb-v, chin, dulc, ferr-m, graph, guaj, hep, hyos, ip, kali-c, kali-chl, kali-p, mag-m, merc, mur-ac, nat-c, nit-ac, nux-v, pall, par, petr, ph-ac, positr, rhus-t, ruta, sep, spig, spong, staph, thuj.
  - Burning: aur, hep, ph-ac, staph.
  - Itching: am-m, kali-c, nit-ac, thuj.
  - Inside: mag-m.

- Lower: bell, bry, calc, caps, caust, ign, kali-chl, mang, merc, mur-ac, nat-c, nicc, nit-ac, pall, rhus-t, samb, sil, spig, sulph, teucr, zinc.

- Upper: acon, am-m, amph, ant-c, arn, bell, bufo, calc, caps, carb-v, caust, cench, clem, dig, kali-c, led, lyc, mag-m, mang, nat-c, nat-sil, nux-v, par, positr, rhus-t, sars, sep, sil, spig, squil, staph, stront-c, thuj, zinc.

  - Burning: aphis, graph.

  - Itching: graph, lyc.

  - Red: positr, zinc.

  - Sore to touch: zinc.

- Liver spot, on: con.

- Menses

  - Before, agg.: dulc, mag-m, sol-ecl.

  - During: dulc, eug, graph, kali-c.

- Moist after scratching: graph.

- Mouth around: agar, bar-c, bov, calc, dulc, kali-c, mag-c, mur-ac, phos, rhus-t, sep, sil, zinc.

  - Corners of: ant-c, arg-n, bar-c, bell, calc, canth, caust, coloc, lyc, mag-m, mang, merc, mur-ac, nat-c, nat-m, petr, phos, rhod, rhus-t, sil, tarax, verat.

- Night agg.: mag-m.

- Nose: agar, alum, am-c, anac, ant-c, arum-d, asc-t, aur, bar-c, bell, berb, borx, bov, brom, calc, cann-s, cath, caps, carb-an, carb-v, caust, clem, cob, coc-c, cocc, coli, con, dulc, euph, euphr, fl-ac, graph, guaj, kali-c, kali-i, kali-n, lach, led, lyc, m-arct, mag-m, mag-s, mang, merc, nat-c, nat-m, nicc, ol-an, ox-ac, pall, petr, ph-ac, phos, plan, plb, podo, psor, rat, rhus-t, sars, sel, sep, sil, stram, stront-c, suis-hep, sul-ac, sulph, syph, teucr, thuj, zinc.

  - About nose: carb-v, nat-m, pall, par, plan, sep, tarax.

  - Below nose: caps, dig, oxal-a, par.

- Burning: alum, aphis, canth, kali-n, ol-an.
- Corners, in: dulc, rhus-g, tarax.
- Dorsum, with inflamed base; on: fl-ac.
- Inside: arn, calad, calc, carb-an, chin, graph, guaj, kali-c, ox-ac, petr, phos, rat, sep, sil, tub.
- Nostrils: chin, sep.
    - Left: acon-ac, calc, dulc, graph, kali-c.
    - Right: aphis, ox-ac, phos, rat.
    - Painful only when muscles of face and nose are moved: calc.
- Oozing: ol-an.
- Red: ant-c, aur, calc-p, ph-ac, plan, sulph.
- Root: bell, caust, cench, clem, led.
- Septum: arg-n, asc-t, calad, chin, nat-m, ol-an, teucr.
    - Oozing: ol-an.
    - Below: nat-m.
- Side: aster, sil.
    - Left: caps, nat-c.
    - Right: alum, euphr, lach, ox-ac, sars.
    - Small and hard: agar.
- Tip: am-c, asaf, caust, cench, clem, coc-c, cund, lyc, nit-ac, pall, ph-ac, spong.
    - Bleeding when pressed: pall.
    - Sore: lyc.
- White: carb-v, kali-c, nat-c, nat-m.
- Wings: anac, bar-c, chel, chin, nat-m, phos, tarax, zing.
    - left: gl-ac.
    - perforation, size of a pea: fl-ac.
- Painful to touch: petr.

- Purplish halo, with: merc.
- Red: aids, coli, ephe-si, kreos, lach, ph-ac, phos, zinc.
- Scratching after: alum.
- Stitching: staph.
- Temples: arg-met, carb-v, cocc, mur-ac, nit-ac.
- Warm, when: ant-c, coc, til.
- Warm room, agg.: mag-m.
- Washing agg.: nux-v, sulph.
- Whiskers: agar, ambr, calc, calc-s, graph, lach, nit-ac, pall, sulph.
- White: agath-a, aids, coloc, graph, mag-m, sinus, zinc.

- Eruptions, pustules: am-c, anac, ant-c, ant-t, arn, ars, ars-i, ars-s-f, aur, aur-ar, aur-s, bell, bov, calc, calc-p, calc-s, carb-v, carbn-s, caust, chel, cic, cimic, clem, con, crot-t, cund, cycl, dros, dulc, eug, eup-per, graph, grat, grin, hep, hydr, hyos, ind, iris, jug-c, kali-bi, kali-br, kali-c, kali-i, kali-n, kreos, lach, lyc, mag-c, mag-m, mag-s, merc, mez, morg-p, nat-c, nat-p, nit-ac, nux-m, pall, petr, ph-ac, phos, propl, psor, puls, rhus-t, sars, sulph, syph, tarax, thuj, tub, verat, viol-t, zinc.

- Eruptions, suppurating: ant-c, cic, lyc, psor, rhus-t.

- Eruptions, tubercles: alum, ant-c, ars, asaf, bar-c, calc, carb-v, cic, con, dulc, fl-ac, graph, hep, kali-bi, kali-c, kali-i, kali-n, lach, led, lyc, mag-c, mag-m, merc, nat-c, nit-ac, olnd, phyt, puls, sil, sumb, syph, thuj, zinc.

    - Chin: carb-an, euph, hep, mag-m, olnd.
    - Forehead: ant-c, fl-ac, led, lyc, olnd, sep, sulph.
    - Itching: kali-n.
    - Jaws, lower: graph, nat-c, staph, verat.
    - Mouth, about: ars, bar-c, bry, caust, con, mag-m, sep, sil, sulph.

- Corners: mag-c.
- Nose.
  - Root of; painless tubercle at: sep.
  - Side of; painless tubercle at right: nat-c.
  - Wings of: hippoz.
- Painful: sep.
- Suppurating: fl-ac, nat-c, sil.
- Greasy: agar, apis, arg-n, ars, aspar, aur, aur-m-n, bar-c, bry, bufo, calc, carc, card-m, caust, chin, con, cortico, des-ac, ferr-ar, hydr, iod, lyc, mag-c, mand, med, merc, merc-c, nat-m, olnd, phos, plb, psor, rhus-t, sel, sep, sil, stram, sulph, syc, thuj, tub.
- Forehead: hydr, psor.
- lips: am-m.
- Chest: amph, bar-c, carc.
- Back: amph, carb-v, carc, morg-p, ros-d, rumx, sulph, tub-r.
- Cervical region: amph, jug-r, pitu-a.

Chapter-33

Diseases of the Hair

Hair has no vital function in humans, yet its psychological functions are extremely important, especially in women. In all mammals, including humans, but with the possible exception of the merino sheep and the poodle dog, hair follicles show intermittent activity. Thus, each hair grows to a maximum length, is retained for a time without further growth, and is eventually shed and replaced.

ALOPECIA AREATA

It is a condition characterized by rapid and complete loss of hair in one, or more often, several round or oval patches, usually on the scalp, beard area and other hairy areas of the body.

Incidence

The sexes are approximately equally affected, and that the onset occurs at any age, with a peak decade lying at some point between the ages of 20 and 50 years.

Alopecia areata is seen disproportionately commonly among Japanese in Hawaii.

Etiology

There is no particular cause that can be attributed to this condition. There is considerable evidence pointing towards an autoimmune etiology. Studies have shown abnormal cell-mediated immune factors in alopecia areata. Genetic influence seems to be an important contributory factor, with 25-30% of the patients having a positive family history.

Patients with the more severe forms of alopecia areata are rather likely to have autoantibodies directed against thyroid.

Finally, recent immunofluorescent studies, which are as yet inconclusive, have shown the occasional deposition of immuno-globulins at the site of affected follicles.

Emotional stress also plays an important role, although it is often difficult to decide whether it is a cause or a result of the disease. Attempts at objective evaluation using standard psychiatric procedures such as the Rorschach test showed over 90% of patients with AA to be psychologically abnormal and up to 29% to have psychological factors and family situations that may have affected the onset or course of the disease.

Pathology

Alopecia areata progresses as a wave of follicles that enter the telogen phase prematurely. Anagen/telogen ratios vary considerably with the stage and duration of the disease process. Biopsy specimens taken early in the course of the disease show the majority of follicles in telogen or late catagen. Some anagen hair bulbs are situated at a higher level in the dermis than normal; a *dense peribulbar and intrafollicular lymphocytic infiltrate* is seen, especially in the early lesions; the infiltrate consists predominantly of helper T-cell infiltrate, with increased numbers of Langerhans' cells. The infiltrate disappears during regrowth but the sequence of events is unknown.

'Exclamation-mark hairs' may be present, which are club hairs of normal caliber and pigmentation, but the distal ends are ragged

and frayed. Below their broken tips they taper towards a small but otherwise normal club.

Eosinophils are said to be common in all stages of alopecia areata, both within the peribulbar infiltrate and within the fibrous tracts.

An electron-microscopic study of alopecia areata showed the lesional anagen follicles to have evidence of non-specific injury to matrix cells around the upper pole of the dermal papilla. There was also the presence of degenerative changes in the suprapapillary matrix. The presence of HLA-DR antigen in cells of the precortical matrix provided evidence that this site could be of fundamental importance in the pathogenesis of AA and may be the primary target for the disease process.

Types

There are four types of alopecia areata categorized by Ikeda:

Type 1

The 'common' type accounted for 83% of patients. It occurred mainly between the ages of 20 and 40 years, and usually ran a total course of less than 3 years. Individual patches tended to regrow in less than 6 months, and alopecia totalis developed in only 6%.

Type 2

The 'atopic' type accounted for 10% of patients. The onset was usually in childhood and the disease ran a lengthy course in excess of 10 years. Individual patches tended to persist for a year and alopecia totalis developed in 75%.

Type 3

The 'prehypertensive' type (4%) occurred mainly in young adults and ran a rapid course with an incidence of alopecia totalis in 39% of patients.

Type 4

The 'combined' type (5%) occurred mainly in patients over 40 years and ran a prolonged course, but resulted in alopecia totalis in only 10% of patients.

There has been little support for Ikeda's prehypertensive type, but most authors agree that the presence of atopy confers a poor prognosis and slow rate of remission.

Clinical Features

The characteristic initial lesion of this condition is commonly a circumscribed, totally bald, smooth patch, which is often noticed by chance by a parent, hairdresser or a friend. Usually, rapid and complete loss of hair in several round or oval patches is seen, usually on the scalp, beard, eyebrows, eyelashes and less commonly on other hairy areas on the body. The patches vary from 1-5 cm in diameter. The hair loss is usually patchy in distribution, though a diffused pattern can also be seen. There are loose hairs around the margins of the patches, which break off easily, leaving short stumps with exclamation-mark hairs.

The initial patch may regrow within a few months, or further patches may appear after an interval of 3-6 weeks and then in a cyclical fashion. These intervals are of varying duration. A succession of discrete patches may rapidly become confluent by the diffuse loss of remaining hair. Diffuse hair loss may occur over part or the whole of the scalp without the development of bald areas. Regrowth is often at first fine and unpigmented, but usually the hairs gradually resume their normal caliber and color. Regrowth in one region of the scalp may occur while the alopecia is extending in others.

The scalp is the first affected site in over 60% of cases. The eyebrows and eyelashes are lost in many cases of alopecia areata and may be the only sites. The extension of alopecia along the scalp margin is known as ophiasis. Alopecia areata strictly confined to one-half of the body has been reported after a head injury.

Though alopecia areata usually occurs without associated disease, there is a higher incidence of it occurring in those suffering from atopic dermatitis, Down's syndrome, lichen planus, and such autoimmune diseases as SLE, thyroiditis, myasthenia gravis and vitiligo.

Course & Prognosis

Patients destined to undergo complete remission generally develop only a few small patches, which grow quickly to a maximum size of 2 to 3 cm and then remain stable in appearance for about 6 to 12 months. Thereafter new hairs, which are often initially white in color, begin to re-grow. By 18 months, the process heals up completely.

Patients developing alopecia areata before puberty have a poorer prognosis than those developing it after puberty. Also, patients with larger or more numerous patches of alopecia have a poorer prognosis. Individual patches of alopecia may expand centrifugally for many months before undergoing stabilization.

Also, alopecia areata of the atopic type has a poorer prognosis, and if hair loss is total before puberty it is unlikely to regrow permanently.

Unfortunately some patients continue to keep having new bald patches, until there is a total baldness (alopecia totalis). Patients with alopecia areata who have obtained complete remission have about 25% chance of developing one or more subsequent episodes later in life. When hair over the entire body is lost, it is termed as 'alopecia universalis'.

Complications

In about 7 to 66% of the cases, there is a nail involvement, which varies from marked alteration of the nails to diffuse or uniform fine pitting that may from transverse or longitudinal lines. There may also be shedding or atrophy of the nails. Trachyonychia, onychomadesis and red or spotted lunulae occur but less commonly.

There are many reports of cataracts in association with alopecia totalis. Horner's syndrome, ectopia of the pupil, iris atrophy or tortuosity of the fundal vessels have also been reported with alopecia areata.

Differential Diagnosis

- **Tinea capitis**: This condition is usually seen among boys and occurs due to the different species of fungi. The occipital & temporal regions are the regions most frequently affected. The hair is broken off at, or close to, the surface of the skin, resulting in the presence of fine stubble, which is visible as a series of black dots within the patch of alopecia. The patches are also characterized by their sharp margination and their confinement precisely to the area of scalp disease. Confirmation of a suspected instance of tinea capitis depends on performance of KOH preparations & fungal cultures. Treatment of tinea capitis is almost always accompanied by complete re-growth of hair.

- **Early lupus erythematosus**: Discoid lupus erythematosus of the scalp is associated with very sharply localized hair loss. The center of these lesions are hypopigmented and scarred and may appear at first glance as if scalp disease is not present, but a careful examination of margins will reveal the annular active erythematosus border, which is distinctive of the disease. These scalp lesions rarely occur alone, but are usually associated with the presence of typical facial lesions.

- **Syphilis:** Patients with secondary syphilis of many months duration often develop a patchy moth-eaten alopecia, which can easily be differentiated from alopecia areata by the large number of patches, their smaller size & their indistinct margins. The hair loss is transient; re-growth occurs following adequate homeopathic therapy.

- **Congenital triangular alopecia, Alopecia neoplastica**, and **Trichotilomania** should also be kept in mind when alopecia areata is considered.

TELOGEN EFFLUVIUM

Introduction & Etiology

Telogen effluvium is a condition usually occurring due to disturbance in the hair cycle.

In the normal young adult scalp, 80-90% of follicles are in the anagen phase of the hair cycle, although there is some variation with age, sex, race and site. Kligman introduced the term 'telogen effluvium' to describe an early, diffuse and excessive shedding of normal club hair from normal resting follicles in the scalp, which follows the premature precipitation of anagen follicles (of the growing phase of the hair growth cycle) into telogen (of the resting phase of the cycle), a process that may be regarded as the common response of the follicles to many different types of 'stress'. Here the follicle itself is not diseased and the inflammation is absent.

The causative factors leading to stress include: Fever, parturition, prolonged and difficult childbirth, surgical operations, hemorrhage (including blood donation), drugs, sudden severe reduction of food intake (starvation or 'crash' dieting) and emotional stress, those suffering from kwashiorkor. Hypothyroidism and renal dialysis with secondary hypervitaminosis A are other possible causes. It can also be seen in cases when the contraceptive pill is discontinued after it has been taken continuously for some time.

The severity of the condition depends partly on the duration and severity of the precipitating cause and partly on unexplained individual variation in susceptibility.

Incidence

Mostly seen in those between 30-60 years of age.

Pathology

Histological examination shows no abnormality other than an increase in the proportion of follicles in telogen. The shed hair are normal 'club' hair.

Clinical Features

The patient usually presents to the physician with the complaint that there is an increased loss of hair, which tend to shed out by the roots, on brushing or combing or shampooing. This hair loss is usually of a diffuse type and will rarely cause visible thinning or baldness of the hair.

An individual tends to loose only about 100-150 hair daily, but in telogen effluvium, there can be a loss varying from about 150 to more than 1000. If the lower rates of shedding are continued for only a short period there may be no obvious baldness in the previously normal scalp, because loss of over 25% of the total complement of hair is never attained. If shedding occurs at higher rates, or is long continued, obvious diffuse baldness is produced. It may be severe but is seldom, if ever, total.

It is seen more commonly in women and frequently found in postpartum state and following the discontinuation of oral contraceptive pills. These observations suggest that hormonal factors play a role in pathogenesis. However, the process is also seen following physiologic or psychologic stress (the causes as mentioned earlier) suggesting that other unknown factors may also be important.

'Postpartum telogen effluvium' has been found to begin between 2-6 months postpartum. Often the hair loss is first noted over the anterior one-third of the scalp, although the loss is diffuse. The hair loss may continue for some 2-6 months or longer.

'Postnatal telogen effluvium' of infants may occur between birth and the first 4 months of age. Usually regrowth occurs by six months of age.

'Drug-induced telogen effluvium' has been noted with the use of amphetamines, aminosalicyclic acid, bromocriptine, captopril, coumarin, carbamazepine, cimetidine, danazol, enalapril, etretinate, lithium carbonate, levodopa, metyrapone, propranolol, pyridostigmine, and trimethadione.

Course & Prognosis

Patients with telogen effluvium rarely, if ever progress to clinically significant baldness. Unless the 'stress' is repeated, most instances of telogen effluvium resolve spontaneously, with complete regrowth taking place almost invariably in about 6 to 12 months time. The prognosis is good if a specific causative factor is found, but usually a chronic form of the condition may occur. Exceptionally, prolonged or high fevers, such as typhoid, may destroy some follicles completely so that only partial recovery is possible. If postpartum effluvium is severe and recurs after successive pregnancies, regrowth may ultimately be incomplete.

Diagnosis

- The diagnosis is usually simple. Increased shedding of hair is clearly related to the stressful episode that preceded it by 6-16 weeks. Plucked hairs show a large proportion of normal club hair until the shedding is complete.

- The diagnosis is usually estimated by the 'pull test' – Grasp a bunch of 40 to 50 hair firmly between the thumb and the forefinger, and then slowly pull them, which cause a mild discomfort to the patient. If there is a hair loss of more than 4-6 club hair, it is a sign positive for this condition, but the results may come in false negative due to shampooing (where the club hair loss may be only about 2-3), combing and the phase of telogen effluvium (whether resolving or entering a chronic phase).

- The 'clip test' may also be useful, where 25-30 hair are cut just above the scalp surface and mounted. Telogen hair are distinguished by their being short and of a smaller diameter. One should also note that androgenic alopecia also results in miniaturization of hair, and coexistent androgenetic change may influence the count.

- In other cases the patient may be instructed to collect and count the hair daily, making sure to collect all small hairs and even those lost in washing and on the bed. The daily hair shed counts are not needed when the pull test is positive.

F- 45

- High telogen counts on horizontal sections of 4 mm punch scalp biopsies is seen, with more than 12-15% of the terminal follicles in telogen. This indicates a significant shift from anagen to telogen, which is a non-inflammatory change without any dystrophic changes in the inner sheath.

Differential Diagnosis

- The alopecia induced by heparin is very similar to this condition, but the time interval is often shorter.

- Alopecia areata of very rapid onset is usually patchy at first but may become total within a week. Telogen effluvium is always diffuse and never total.

- Acute syphilitic alopecia is patchy.

- Increased shedding of club hair is, of course a variable but often very obvious symptom of early androgenetic alopecia.

- Loose anagen hair syndrome can be differentiated by root microscopy.

ANDROGENETIC ALOPECIA

Synonym

Androgenetic alopecia is widely referred to as **male-pattern alopecia** or male-pattern baldness (common baldness), but this term is too restrictive and leads to missed diagnoses, especially in females.

Incidence

This condition or process may begin at any age after puberty, but usually becomes clinically apparent by the age of 20 years in a male and by early 30's in a female. In women it assumes more often a sort of a diffuse form.

Etiology

Genetic factors

Hormonal influence with the effect of androgens on the hair follicle is also an important contributory factor to this condition, esp. in males.

In a general sort of way there is a correlation between the age at which onset begins and severity of eventual loss.

Pathology

One of the earliest histological features seen in this condition is a focal perivascular basophilic degeneration in the lower layers of the connective tissue sheath of the anagen follicles. There is then a perifollicular lympho-histiocytic infiltrate at the level of the sebaceous duct. The sclerotic remains of the basophils in the connective tissue sheath are viewed as 'streamers'. The destruction of the connective tissue sheath may account for the irreversibility of hair loss.

The development of baldness is associated with shortening of the anagen phase of the hair growth cycle and a lengthening of the telogen phase, consequently with an increase in the proportion of telogen hairs. The shorter the anagen phase, the shorter is the hair growth. Terminal follicles are progressively transformed into 'vellus' follicles, i.e. a 'miniaturization' process. Eventually there is a reduction in the size of the affected follicles, which become short and small (an essential histological feature of androgenetic alopecia), and these then results in a reduction in the diameter of the hair they produce. This reduction is said to be greater in women than in men.

Clinical Features

The presence of 'whisker hair' at the temples may be the first sign of this condition. The follicles produce finer, shorter and lighter or virtually unpigmented terminal hair, until a complete cessation of terminal hair growth results. Miniaturized hairs become increasingly evident, replacing coarser intermediate or terminal hair.

In males, the replacement of terminal by smaller hair occurs in a distinctive pattern that spares the posterior and lateral scalp margins, even in the most advanced cases and in old age. There is a recession of the anterior and bitemporal hairline, so that the forehead becomes high, followed by balding of the vertex. The loss is thus most noticeable at the vertex and in the bitemporal regions of the scalp. The rate of hair loss varies from person to person, depending on the heredity factors.

In females, the early stages of this condition may not conform to the 'male pattern' type of baldness. Here the follicles first affected are the ones that are widely distributed over the frontovertical region, especially along the line of the hair partition. As a result, many secondary vellus hairs are interspersed with hairs that are still normal and others only slightly reduced in diameter. Partial baldness is usually first apparent and is restricted in the area of the vertex, but there is usually a sort of a diffuse alopecia. It is seen that there is an acceleration of the hair loss with the classical 'male type' baldness seen with increasing frequency after the menopause.

Course & Prognosis

There is usually a fluctuation seen with the alopecia either remaining the same for years, or usually gradually getting progressively worse, especially after the menopausal period.

In the absence of a precise cause, no specific treatment is found to be useful.

Complications & Differential Diagnosis

- It is necessary to take a full medical history and do a complete physical examination, especially along with endocrinological investigation in a few cases, especially in women with androgenetic alopecia of rapid onset.

- In women with baldness of gradual onset but accompanied by menstrual disturbance, we need to rule out hirsutism or recrudescence of acne. More extensive baldness is usually always accompanied by hirsutism.

- Diffuse hair loss in women can also be a form of chronic telogen effluvium, which needs to be ruled out by performing horizontal sections of a 4-mm punch biopsy. Histologically, although there may be a slight increase in telogen hair, the major feature distinguishing the condition from androgenetic alopecia is the relative absence of vellus hair in chronic telogen effluvium and their abundance in androgenetic alopecia.

TRICHOTILLOMANIA

Introduction

It is a neurotic practice of plucking or breaking the hair from the scalp or eyelashes, seen especially seen in girls under the age of 10 years, but it may be seen in boys or adults too.

Clinical Features

This condition is usually of a localized type, where a few areas of alopecia are seen, which characteristically contains hair of varying length. The hair is of a rough texture due to the short remnants of broken-off hairs. This condition is a manifestation of an obsessive-compulsive disorder but may be associated with depression or anxiety. Thus the treatment of the underlying condition, especially with psychotherapy or behavioral therapy is necessary.

Diagnosis

- The clinician can ask the child how the removal of hair is done, in order to establish the diagnosis.
- Shave a 3 x 3 cm area in the involved part of the scalp and watch the hair regrow normally as the hair in this area will be too short for plucking.
- A horizontal biopsy will confirm the diagnosis because of the high number of catagen hairs, pigmentary defects and casts., trichomalacia, and haemorrhage.

CONGENITAL ALOPECIA

Synonym

Total alopecia; Atrichia congenita.

Introduction & Etiology

It occurs either as a total or partial loss of hair or a lack of initial growth, accompanied usually by other ectodermal defects of the nails, teeth and bone.

This condition is usually determined by an autosomal recessive gene. Dominant or irregular dominant inheritance has occurred in some families. The two genotypes seem to be phenotypically indistinguishable, but detailed investigation would probably reveal differences. The term 'total' is relative, but if any hair are present they are extremely few.

Pathology

The hair follicles are absent in adult life, even when the fetal hair coat has been normal. Sebaceous glands are smaller than normal. When a few stray hair have survived, the structure of the shaft appears to be normal.

Clinical Features

The scalp hair is often normal at birth but is shed between the first and sixth months, after which no further growth occurs. The hair is light and sparse, and grows slowly. In some cases the scalp has been totally hairless at birth and has remained so.

Eyebrows, eyelashes and body hair may also be absent, but more often there are a few pubic and axillary hairs seen with scanty eyebrows and eyelashes.

With associated defects

Total or almost total alopecia is unusual in hereditary syndromes.

Progeria

- Scalp and body hair is totally deficient.

Hydrotic ectodermal dysplasia

- Total or almost total alopecia is associated with palmoplantar keratoderma and thickened discolored nails. Any hairs that are present are structurally normal but are often finer than the average.

Moynahan's syndrome

- This autosomal recessive syndrome, reported in male siblings, is associated with mental retardation, epilepsy and total baldness of the scalp; the hair may regrow in childhood between 2 and 4 years of age.

Baraitser's syndrome

- This autosomal recessive syndrome presents as almost total alopecia following the loss of some downy scalp hair present at birth. Three cases are reported in an inbred family all had almost total alopecia of all sites, including eyebrows and lashes. There were occasional isolated hairs. Mental and physical retardation were associated.

ALOPECIA OF NUTRITIONAL ORIGIN

In cases of malnutrition with the resultant protein-calorie deficiency affect, in the initial stages itself, the structure and colour of the hair. There is atrophy of the bulb (to one-third its size) and loss of internal and external root sheaths, so the hair is fine, dry, lusterless, brittle and fall of or break easily; but there is no changes seen in the anagen/telogen ratio, atleast in the initial stages. The hair that were normally black may assume a reddish tinge. Many hair shafts may show constrictions, which increase their vulnerability to trauma.

In those who suffer from iron deficiency, there is occasionally a diffuse alopecia noted, inspite of them not being frankly anemic.

Also, in cases of zinc deficiency, there is alopecia with a few cutaneous changes seen. This kind of a deficiency (of zinc with essential fatty acids), especially seen in cases where from prolonged parenteral alimentation, results in erythema, scaling of the scalp and eyebrows, bullae, dry and unruly hair with diffuse alopecia. Topical application of safflower oil tends to reverse this process.

In cases of homocystinuria, where there is an inborn error in the metabolic pathways of methionine, the hair tends to become sparse, fine and lighter in shade. It appears normal on microscopy but shows an orange-red fluorescence when stained with acridine orange and examined under UV light. Affected children are mentally retarded, have a shuffling, duck-like gait, a malar flush and a wide variety of skeletal defects.

COSMETIC ALOPECIA

With differences in religion and its customs and with increased awareness of the different styles in fashion and different hairdressing techniques, there is an increased degree and wide variety of physical stresses that our hair has to go through.

Pathology

The two commonly seen processes responsible for most of the pathological changes observed are as follows. Hair, tends to get weak by the various chemical applications and there is constant wear and tear occurring due to the different styles experimented on the hair, which break off by friction or tension. Prolonged tension is known to induce follicular inflammatory changes that may eventually cause scarring. Telogen hair are known to be weaker and more readily subjected to wear and tear as compared to the anagen hair.

A few commonly occurring 'clinical syndromes' are as listed below:

TRAUMATIC, TRACTION OR MARGINAL ALOPECIA

Traumatic or traction alopecia occurs from prolonged tension on the hair either from pulling or wearing the hair tightly braided or in a ponytail, or in conditions where the kinky hair is pulled in order to straighten it or is rolled into curlers that are too tight. This condition also occurs in persons (esp. young Sikh boys) who have the habit of twisting their hair with their fingers.

Here one tends to especially find short, broken hairs with folliculitis and some scarring in circumscribed patches at the margins of the scalp. Itching and crusting may also be seen.

Libyan women tend to complain of a frontal hair loss from wearing a tight scarf. Tight braiding along with the wooden combs used by the people in Sudan could be contributory factors of traction alopecia occurring in that region. Tight braiding of hair into cane rows by the Afro-Caribbean people tend to cause marginal alopecia and central alopecia with widening of the partings.

BRUSH ROLLER ALOPECIA

Individuals who tend to make frequent or vigorous use of brush rollers may develop irregular patches or diffuse type of alopecia, which is usually surrounded by an erythematous area with broken hair.

HOT-COMB ALOPECIA

In the earlier days, esp. the African women, would use hot combs to straighten their kinky hair. This would cause progressive alopecia, extending from the vertex to the sides. This condition is seen rarely nowadays since there is not much usage of hot combs now.

BRUSH OR MASSAGE ALOPECIA

Vigorous brushing or massaging of the scalp can cause significant damage to hair that is already fragile, frizzy or curly. The brushes that have square bristles made of synthetic fibres or those with angular tips tend to be particularly traumatic.

ALOPECIA SECONDARY TO HAIR WEAVING

There is a patchy loss of hair reported in cases where there is weaving of extra hair done to persistent terminal hair in order to hide the alopecia that the person has.

PRESSURE ALOPECIA

This occurs especially in the occipital region in a few babies who are kept lying on their backs all the time. In adults it is seen in cases where there is prolonged pressure on the scalp, like when the person is given general anesthesia, after major surgeries or in chronically ill and bed-ridden patients. It could be due to pressure-induced ischaemia.

DIFFUSE ALOPECIA OF ENDOCRINE ORIGIN

HYPOPITUITARY STATES

The dwarf-like individual suffering from a hypopituitary state is usually absolutely bald. In cases of a deficiency in the pituitary levels, which starts occurring after puberty, there is a gradual loss of hair from the scalp, and the pubic and axillary hair are totally lost. There is also a yellowish discoloration of the skin with dryness and lack of turgidity.

HYPOTHYROIDISM

Persons suffering from hypothyroidism usually complain that the hair tends to become coarse, dry, brittle and sparse. There is a diffuse sort of hair loss, especially from the scalp, though there is loss of hair even from the eyebrows and the axillae. The hair roots seem to be in the telogen phase to an abnormally high degree, suggesting either prolonged telogen or premature catagen, or both. When the hypothyroidism is controlled, there is regrowth of the hair, but it may be incomplete. The diagnosis is established with the help of clinical assessment, along with the estimation of the thyroxine and thyroid-stimulating hormone (TSH) levels.

HYPERTHYROIDISM

Here the hair tends to become extremely fine and sparse. There is diffuse alopecia seen to occur in women with moderate to severe hyperthyroidism, but here the case is usually reversible if 'miniaturization' is not extreme. The mechanism through which this occurs is unknown but it seems unlikely that it is directly related to serum levels of thyroid hormone since replacement, while preventing further loss, fails to reverse the process. Alopecia areata and vitiligo occur with increased frequency in severe cases.

HYPOPARATHYROIDISM

In cases of hypoparathyroidism, there is dryness, coarseness and loss of the scalp hair, which tend to be shed easily by the slightest of trauma. The loss of hair thus appears irregularly patchy.

DIABETES MELLITUS

There are quite a few cases of diffuse alopecia reported in cases of poorly controlled diabetes.

ORAL CONTRACEPTIVES

There are a few cases of diffuse alopecia seen to occur in women on oral contraceptives. There was a fluctuating response seen in the anagen-telogen count study – some women showed a temporary and some a more prolonged increase in telogen ratio, and in others no change was observed.

ALOPECIA OF CHEMICAL ORIGIN

THALLIUM

Thallium salts, banned from pharmaceutical use in most countries, are unfortunately still used as pesticides in a few places, with serious outbreaks of poisoning have followed the contamination of grain stores and other food. These salts, being tasteless, are used for homicidal and suicidal purposes.

This chemical is rapidly taken up by anagen follicles and is known to disturb keratinization. The hair tends to break within the follicle, with irregularity of the dark keratogenous zone and air bubbles within the shaft near the tip. Many other follicles enter catagen prematurely. Alopecia is the commonest symptom seen, even in cases of a mild poisoning, with diffuse loss of anagen hairs that may rapidly become complete or may be followed by the gradual shedding of club hairs over a period of 3 or 4 months. The diagnosis may be suspected on clinical grounds but can be confirmed only by the detection of thallium in the urine and faeces in which it may continue to be excreted for 4 or 5 months.

THYROID ANTAGONISTS

Few cases of thyrotoxicosis treated with thiouracil or carbimazole tend to develop diffuse alopecia. Also a long continued administration of iodides is known to induce hypothyroid alopecia.

ANTICOAGULANTS

All anticoagulant drugs (heparin, heparinoids and coumarins) tend to induce alopecia, the degree of which is dependent on the dosage level, rather than the duration of exposure. Apparently normal club hairs are shed some 2-3 months after the effective blood level is achieved. There is usually a diffuse sort of a hair loss, without obvious alopecia, but in cases of exposure to high dosage of the anticoagulant medicines can give rise to moderate or severe alopecia, but full recovery is known to follow the cessation of the drug.

HYPERTRICHOSIS

This is a condition where there is an overgrowth of hair that is not localized to the androgen-dependent areas of the skin. There are various forms/types of this disorder, which are as follows:

CONGENITAL HYPERTRICHOSIS LANUGINOSA

Synonym

Hypertrichosis Universalis Congenital; Generalized Congenital Hypertrichosis.

Etiology

Studies suggest that this condition is most likely the result of an autosomal dominant inheritance. It is said to be due to an X-linked dominant trait.

Clinical features

This rare condition is where the child is noticed to be excessively hairy at birth, which gradually lengthens and by early childhood, the entire body of the child (except the palms and soles) is covered with fine, silky vellus hairs that is about 2-10 cm or more long. The scalp hair appears to be normal, but the long eyelashes and thick, bushy eyebrows are characteristic features. Individuals with these features of hairiness have been thus labeled as dog-faced boy, human werewolf, bear man, etc. This condition, once established, tends to be of a permanent type, except in a few cases that tend to have a reduction of the hair on the trunk and limbs by late childhood. By puberty, the axillary, pubic and beard hairs tend to be more of a fuzzy, soft and silky or wooly type.

Associated features

This condition may be associated with dental abnormalities (hypodontia or anodontia), deformities of the external ear and gingival hyperplasia or fibromatosis, but otherwise the physical and mental development of most patients is usually normal.

ACQUIRED HYPERTRICHOSIS LANUGINOSA

Etiology

This condition is rarely seen in its severe forms. It is usually seen as an accompaniment to a serious or fatal illness, especially in cases of an internal malignancy (usually of the gastrointestinal tract, bronchus, breast, gall bladder, uterus, or bladder) or occur secondary to drug intake. The presence of hypertrichosis may infact be a preceding sign to the diagnosis of a neoplasm by quite a few years.

Clinical Features

In this condition there is fine, light-colored, wooly hair with lanugo characteristics that rapidly replaces normal hair all over the body.

In its earlier stages or milder forms the hair growth is limited to the face, esp. over the nose and eyelids. As the disease progresses, the hair continues to grow in other areas, ultimately involving the whole body, except the area over the palms and soles. Terminal hair over the scalp, beard area and pubic region are not necessarily replaced by lanugo hair. Cases have been reported where, even in cases of a previously bald scalp, hair may start to grow abundantly in those with this condition. On an average the hair growth can at times be more than 10 cm long.

UNIVERSAL HYPERTRICHOSIS

In this condition the hair growth pattern is normal, but the hair tends to be a bit larger and coarser than is usually seen. Thus even the eyebrows may appear to be of a thick bushy type. It is usually attributed to an autosomal dominant gene. These cases are especially seen in dark-skinned Mediterranean and Middle Eastern subjects.

OTHER VARIETIES & CAUSES OF HYPERTRICHOSIS

- Dermal tumors, like melanocytic nevi, meningioma or Becker's nevi, can be associated with excessive terminal hair growth that is abnormal for the age and site, esp. as regards its length, shaft diameter and color. This condition can be termed as *naevoid hypertrichosis.*

- Repeated irritation, trauma, eczematous states, use of topical steroid, lymphedema with filariasis are conditions where there is a localized increase in hair growth.

- *Hereditary disorders: Porphyria,* where there is localized hypertrichosis of the exposed skin (esp. the forehead, cheeks and chin), esp. seen frequently in cases of porphyria variegata or porphyria cutanea tarda, where there is also increased pigmentation with the downy hair on the face. *Epidermolysis Bullosa* is another condition where there is a rare association of gross hypertrichosis of the face and limbs, which is especially of a diffuse or generalized type. In cases of *Hurler's syndrome* and other mucopolysaccharidoses, marked hypertrichosis is usually seen to exist from early childhood on the face, trunk and limbs, with bushy and confluent eyebrows. Profuse hypertrichosis of the trunk, limbs and lower face is also seen to occur in cases of children with *congenital macrogingivae,* having markedly acromegaloid features. Generalized hypertrichosis of variable degree is seen to occur in cases of patients with Trisomy 18 or in those diagnosed with Cornelia de Lange syndrome.

- *Endocrine disturbances:* In cases of those with *hypothyroidism,* there is a profuse growth of hair seen to occur on the back and the extensor aspects of the limbs. There is increased growth of coarse hair over the pretibial region in cases of those suffering from **hyperthyroidism**. Severe generalized hypertrichosis is seen to occur in young children after head injuries, after encephalitis and after mumps followed by the sudden onset of obesity. This is attributed to possible diencephalic or pituitary disturbance.

- *Malnutrition:* Gross malnutrition can cause profuse generalized hypertrichosis in children. An increased growth of fine, downy hair on face, trunk and arms is also seen in those suffering from anorexia nervosa.

- *Dermatomyositis:* Excessive hair growth is noted, esp. over the forearms, legs and temples, in children suffering from dermatomyositis.

- *Trauma:* Repeated or chronic inflammatory changes in the dermis, results in scarring, which results in growth of long and coarse hair at the site. E.g. There are circumscribed patches of hypertrichosis on the left shoulder in cases of people frequently carrying heavy sacks. There is a patch of hypertrichosis seen on one of the forearms, esp. in those who are mental retarded, due to the habit they have acquired of chewing this site. At times there is hypertrichosis of only a few follicles at the site of an accidental wound, a vaccination scar, burn, recurrent thrombophlebitis, or at the site of excision of warts. There are cases of hypertrichosis known to occur from occlusion of a limb in a plaster of Paris cast, esp. in cases of children. The hair returns to normal within a few weeks of removal of the plaster.

HIRSUTISM

Introduction

In this condition there is an excessive, male-pattern growth of terminal hair in women, of areas involving the upper lip, cheeks, chin, central chest, breasts, lower abdomen and groin. This may be associated with other signs like changes in the voice (that becomes deeper), temporal balding, clitoral hypertrophy, amenorrhea and acne.

Incidence

Racial and cultural variation is seen in both the severity of the hirsuties and in the degree of its social acceptance. There is an increased hair growth over the face, abdomen and thighs of white women; whereas Asians and black people have less of facial and body hair.

Etiology & Characteristic Features

Stress, with an inability to cope it, is considered to be one of the main etiological factors for and also an effect of hirsutism.

It is also seen that most of the hirsute women tend to be obese and have menstrual irregularities; here studies have shown that when these individuals work towards losing weight, their menses tends to get regular and there is a noted reduction in body hair growth.

Hirsutism results either from excessive secretion of androgens from either the ovary or the adrenal glands. It is also known to result from an increased stimulation by a pituitary tumor. The increased secretion is either due to functional excesses or from a neoplastic cause.

Ovarian causes

Polycystic ovarian syndrome

- Here there is obesity, amenorrhea, hirsutism and infertility associated with enlarged polycystic ovaries. There can be associated acne, acanthosis nigricans or menorrhagia. Diagnosis is established by checking out for elevated levels of LH, increased LH/FSH (follicle-stimulating hormone) ratio, and an increase in the testosterone, androstenedione and oestradiol levels. Also, USG of ovary shows multiple peripheral ovarian cysts around a dense central core.

Ovarian tumors (both benign and malignant)

- Hirsutism is a very common syndrome seen in cases of virilizing ovarian tumors. Amenorrhea or oligomenorrhea develop in all premenopausal patients, and alopecia, cliteromegaly, deepening of the voice and a male habitus develop in about half of the patients. Diagnosis is established by checking out for raised plasma testosterone levels.

Adrenal causes

Congenital Adrenal Hyperplasia

- 21-hydroxylase deficiency is the commonest defect associated with late-onset CAH. Women with late-onset congenital adrenal hyperplasia (CAH) may have normal menstrual cycles, but approximately 80% will have polycystic ovaries. This makes it a bit difficult to differentiate CAH from PCOS.

Adrenal tumors (adrenal adenomas and carcinomas)

• These usually present with abdominal swelling or pain, but about 10% of these cases can also present with isolated virilization.

Pituitary causes

Cushing's Disease

• In cases where the woman presents with virilization along with Cushing's syndrome, it is strongly suggestive of presence of a carcinoma. One needs to check the testosterone levels in such cases.

Acromegaly and Prolactin-secreting Adenomas

• Due to a possible effect of prolactin on adrenal androgen production or due to PCOS, there is an increased incidence of hirsuties in the amenorrhea-galactorrhea syndrome (almost 30-60%).

Other causes are hypothyroidism, phenothiazines intake and hepatorenal failure.

Other Causes

Exogenous intake of androgens, certain high-progesterone birth control pills and drugs (like glucocorticoid or anabolic steroids and other drugs used to enhance athletic performance).

Diagnosis

• A thorough history (esp. about the onset, progression, virilization, menstrual history and family/racial background) with cutaneous (to check for pattern and severity of hair growth) and general physical examination (to check for signs of Cushing's disease or acromegaly, distribution of fat and muscle mass, acne, androgenetic alopecia, acanthosis nigricans, deepening of the voice, galactorrhea, hypertension and cliteromegaly) is essential.

- Total Testosterone level and Dehydroepiandrosterone sulfate level should be checked for in women with mild hirsutism, who have no history or signs of virilism, menstrual irregularity or infertility.

- Pelvic ultrasonography is also useful to check for ovarian tumors or polycystic ovaries.

- In cases of rapid onset or progressive hirsutism, dexamethasone suppression test is useful to screen for Cushing's disease.

- In patients with galactorrhea, the Prolactin levels will help screen for prolactin secreting tumors.

- An LH/FSH ratio is useful to check for polycystic ovarian disease.

- A 17-hydroxyprogesterone and ACTH stimulation test will screen for late onset congenital adrenal hyperplasia.

Differential Diagnosis

On phylogenetic grounds, and on the basis of its specific androgenic induction, the growth in the female of coarse terminal hair in the male adult sexual pattern should be differentiated clearly from the numerous other forms of excessive hair growth of widely varying etiology. The term hirsutism will be restricted to androgen-dependent hair patterns and the term hypertrichosis will be applied to other patterns of excessive hair growth.

HOMEOPATHIC APPROACH TO HIRSUITISM

In cases of hirsutism, as you know, identifying and treating the cause medically, is of utmost importance. Polycystic ovarian disease is one of the commonest causes of hirsutism seen in my practice, and again I am stressing that specific remedies like *Thiosinaminum* are utterly useless and harmful. Similarly artificial measures to pluck the hair and do laser treatment can further worsen the case. Instead intercurrent remedies like *Thyroidinum, Thuja, Carcinosin, Medorrhinum, Syphilinum*, etc. are very useful. It is worthwhile to remember that the results in these cases are very slow and thus you need to convince the patients the necessity to continue treatment for a long time (3-5 years). For the first 3-6 months, there will a slow response inspite of the remedy being correct. Repetition should be frequent in low potency to avoid medicinal aggravation or the best bet is to use the medicine in an LM scale.

PRURITIC DISORDERS OF THE SCALP

Incidence

Pruritis of the scalp is commonly seen in the middle-aged or especially in elderly individuals.

Etiology

The cause of this condition is usually unknown.

Clinical Features

The pruritis and itching is of a spasmodic type and can be pretty intense, with frequent exacerbations, especially in relation to some stress or to general fatigue.

Differential Diagnosis

- Pruritis, being a predominant manifestation also of acne necrotica, needs to be differentiated from it by checking for scattered vesicles followed by the small crusts.

- Lichen simplex is a common cause of pruritus occurring in the occipital region and the nape of the neck in women. Here the lesion on the affected part of the scalp is thickened and scaly.

- Severe irritation of the scalp is sometimes the initial symptom of a sensitization reaction, either to hair dyes, medications applied on the scalp, strong shampoos or to other hair cosmetics. A severe form of it can result in localized dermatitis or eczema.

- Seborrheic, atopic dermatitis and other inflammatory disorders may be pruritic, but they have other associated features too, which help differentiate them.

- In women and children, pediculosis should be suspected and ruled out.
- In infants, in old age and in the immunosuppressed, scabies may cause scalp irritation.

TINEA CAPITIS

Synonym

Scalp Ringworm.

Incidence

Tinea capitis is an infectious disease seen especially in schoolchildren, with a lower incidence among infants and the elderly. It is more frequently seen in boys because boys have shorter hair; visit barbers more often and they tend to play about with each other's caps habitually.

Etiology

The causative fungi were known to be the different species of microsporum & trichophyton. Infection seems to take place from both affected human beings and animals.

Clinical Features

This condition can present itself in two clinical types: inflammatory or non-inflammatory lesions. Occipital and temporal regions are known to be the sites of choice. The lesions consist of sharply localized patches of alopecia, where the characteristic feature of the hair loss is that the hair is broken off at, or close to, the surface of the skin. The result is the presence of a fine stubble which if too short to palpate is sometimes visible as a series of black dots within the patch of alopecia. In cases of an associated scalp disease, there is a sharply marginated scaling plaque seen, characterized be varying degrees of inflammation.

Diagnosis

- Small areas of scaling with dull broken hair shafts (seen under the microscope, if not clinically visible) are typical of *Microsporum* ringworm.

- Also, diagnosis can be established by the wood's lamp illumination test, where only the microsporum infections are seen to show fluoresce.

- Using KOH preparations and making fungal cultures do help in confirmation of the diagnosis of the tinea capitis lesions.

Differential Diagnosis

- A nervous hair-pulling tic may result in twisted and broken hairs of normal texture in a patch of post-inflammatory scaling.

- Profuse, adherent silvery scale could also suggest pityriasis amiantacea, which needs to be ruled out.

PITYRIASIS (TINEA) AMIANTACEA

Introduction

Pityriasis amiantacea is a condition where there is a formation of thick crusts as a result of a sort of an inflammatory reaction and thus the condition tends to resemble psoriasis and seborrheic dermatitis to quite an extent.

Etiology

The cause is probably a secondary infection occurring as a complication of conditions like seborrheic dermatitis, psoriasis or lichen simplex.

Pathology

Biopsy results show signs of spongiosis, parakeratosis, migration of lymphocytes into the epidermis, and a variable degree of acanthosis. Diffuse hyperkeratosis and parakeratosis together with follicular keratosis (surrounding each hair with a sheath of horn) are responsible for the asbestos-like scaling features of this condition.

Clinical Features

Clinically, in this condition, one can observe thick asbestos-like (amiantaceous), shiny, silvery white or dull gray scales or crusts, overlapping each other, and adherent in layers to the shafts of the hair, which they surround. The disease is usually localized and remains confined to small areas of the scalp, but it can also be very extensive, spreading diffusely over the entire scalp. The proximal parts of the hair are matted together by the laminated crusts. The underlying scalp may be red and moist or may show simple erythema and scaling, or the features of psoriasis, seborrheic dermatitis or of lichen simplex. Most of the patients notice some hair loss in areas of severe scaling. The hair regrows when the scaling is effectively treated.

Diagnosis

Usually, the distinctive clinical appearance makes the diagnosis easy, but the identification of the underlying disease or cause may not be so easy, and in some cases no sure diagnosis is given.

HOMEOPATHIC APPROACH TO HAIR CONDITIONS

Hairfall

Hair falling is a universal complaint experienced by a majority of patients. As a doctor, one needs to always examine the scalp to rule out any atrophy or scaring of the scalp skin; atrophy of the scalp is seen as wrinkling, thinning and loss of elasticity of the skin surface, whereas . . . ring produces a thickened, shining scalp surface, with wrinkling and loss of elasticity. One needs to also remember that in cicatricial cases of the scalp, hair growth is unlikely to occur. Thus it becomes necessary for you to check for the cause of hairfall and only then start the treatment. Improvement of general health condition along with proper care of the hair should always be taught, and the principles of governing a healthy balanced diet with appropriate nourishment should be explained to the patient.

Advice to the patient –

* Avoid repeated and too frequent combing & shampooing.
* Avoid frequent changing of the brand of shampoo or soap used.
* Avoid excessive and overzealous use of oil & oily preparations especially in cases of seborrheic individuals.

Hairfall due to any infections of the scalp comes under tubercular miasm, whereas hairfall due to severe destruction of the hair root, as occurs in psoriasis and pyoderma, is purely syphilitic. Whereas hairfall due to seborrhea comes under sycotic miasm. Hairfall that precedes male pattern baldness is almost always syphilitic, whereas hairfall that precedes alopecia areata is tubercular. The reason why such miasmatic dimensions are important is since it helps one to select an intercurrent remedy.

Never should hairfall be treated symptomatically by giving specific remedy like *Wiesbaden, Phosphorus* and *Thallium*. By doing this one can get temporary results, but definitely tendency for hairfall can never be treated as the susceptibility never improves.

It is best to select a constitutional remedy and treat it accordingly. The following are a few practical hints that I would like to share:

* When a patient has only hairfall as a problem with no other systemic disorder – give a constitutional remedy in a high potency, single dose, taking care not to repeat it too frequently.
* While in cases of hairfall due to secondary disorders like anemia, diabetes, infections of the scalp, dandruff, etc. – one requires constitutional treatment, with frequent repetitions.
* Also when using intercurrent remedies, one needs to repeat nosodes repeatedly in high potencies, especially in cases of male-pattern baldness and alopecia areata.
* A remedy that has helped me in my very initial years of practice for cases of alopecia areata was *X-ray*; later on I started using *Leprominium* (a remedy prepared from potentized lepra bacilli); and very recently *Methotrexate* and *Adrenomycin*.

TINEA

Tinea is due to infection and thus it falls under the tubercular miasm. The approach still remains constitutional but intercurrent use of nosodes will always help you to speed up the cure.

TRICHOTILLOMANIA

This condition is basically a mental disorder, which strongly comes under the Sycotic miasm. Psychoanalysis and psychotherapy are essentially important along with the constitutional homeopathic treatment. The key factor to check for in these people is to understand the frustration and stress in their lives, and then accordingly help them resolve the same.

SOME IMPORTANT HOMEOPATHIC REMEDIES FOR HAIR CONDITION

Aloe socotrina: Hair come out in lumps, leaving bare patches eye lashes also fall out with frequent frontal headache.

Ammonium muriaticum: Large accumulation of bran like scales, with falling of the hair, which has a deadened and lusterless appearance with great itching of scalp.

Antimonium crudum: Losing hair from nervous headache.

Arsenicum album: Touching the hair is painful, bald patches at or near the forehead. The scalp is covered with dry scales & scales, looking rough and dirty, extending sometimes even to forehad, face & ears.

Aurum metallicum: Syphilitic alopecia.

Anantherum muricatum: Falling of hair from beard & eyebrows.

Baryta carbonica: Baldness especially of the crown. In young people the scalp is very sensitive to touch.

Borax venenata: Hair is rough & horny, cannot be combed smooth. Hair tangled at the tip and stick together.

Calcarea carbonica: Hair falls out especially when combing. Dryness of hair, great sensitiveness of scalp, with yellowish or white scales on scalp. Sensation of coldness on outer head.

Cantharis vesicatoria: Hair fall out when combing, esp. during confinement and lactation. There is presence of enormous dandruff with scales on the scalp.

Carbo vegetabilis: Falling of hair, after severe disease or abuse of mercury, with great sensitiveness of scalp to pressure. Hairfall out more from the back of head, after severe illness or parturition.

Cinchona officinalis: Hair sweats much and fall out.

Fluoricum acidum: Large patches entirely denuded of hair. The new hair is dry and lusterless and breaks off easily. The patient must comb the hair often. Therefore it matts at the end. Itching of the head with falling of hair. Falling of hair therefore of syphilis.

Graphites: Falling of beard & eyebrows.

Helleborus niger: Losing hairs from eyebrows or pudenda.

Hepar sulphur: Hair fall out here & there with bald spots.

Hypericum perforatum: Alopecia from headaches caused by concussion of brain.

Kalium carbonicum: Alopecia after fever, dry hair repeatedly falling off with dandruff.

Lycopodium clavatum: Hair become grey early. Hair-fall off after abdominal disease, after parturition with burning, scalding and itching of the scalp, especially on getting warm from exercise during the day.

Manicnella: Losing hair after severe acute diseases.

Mercurius solubilis: Fall out on sides & temples without any headaches.

Natrium muriaticum: Hair fall out if touched mostly on forepart of head, temples & beard. Scalp is very sensitive. Face is shiny as if greasy.

Nitricum acidum: Profuse falling of hair esp. of vertex with eruption. It may be due to syphilis, nervous headaches, debility or emaciation. The scalp is sensitive.

Petroleum: Itching of scalp with severe dandruff & falling of hair.

Phosphoricum acidum: Gnawing grief changes hair of the young.

Phosphorus: Round patches of scalp, completely deprived of hair, falling off of the hair in large bundles on the forehead and on the sides above the ears, the roots of the hair seems to be dry, the denuded scalp looks clear, white & smooth. There is presence of copious dandruff.

Plumbum metallicum: Great dryness of hair. It falls off even from the beard.

Sarsaparilla officinalis: Mercuro-syphilitic affections of the head with sensitiveness of scalp with falling off of hair.

Selenium metallicum: Hair fall off when combing; also hair fall from eyebrow, whiskers & genitals. Tingling & itching (S) on the scalp which feels tense and contracted.

Sepia officinalis: Losing hair after chronic headache.

Silicea terra: Premature baldness. Itching of the scalp before menses.

Sphingurus martini: Falling of hair, esp. from beard & whiskers.

Staphysagria: Hair falls off mostly from occiput and around the ears, with humid fetid eruption or dandruff on the scalp.

Sulphur: Hair is very unruly – sandy, hard and lusterless, growing in all directions. The scalp is sore to touch. Violent itching of the scalp, which is worse by getting warm in bed.

Thuja occidentalis: White scaly dandruff with dry hair.

Vinca minor: Hair falls out in single spots and white hair grow there. The skin of the scalp oozes moisture with matting of hair. There is irresistible desire to scratch.

Wiesbaden aqua: By the use of this remedy hair will grow rapidly & darker.

REPERTORY

- **Head, hair, baldness:** abrot, all-s, ambr, anac, apis, arn, aur, bar-c, fl-ac, graph, hell, hep, lyc, med, morg-p, nat-m, phos, pix, rosm, sep, sil, sulph, syc, syph, thal, vinc, zinc.
    - Gonorrhea, after: kali-s.
    - Patches: apis, ars, calc, calc-p, carb-an, cupr-s, fl- ac, graph, hep, kali-p, kali-s, lyc, morg-p, phos, psor, sep, tell, tub, vinc.
    - Young people: arund, bac, bar-c, lyc, sil, tub.
- **Head, hair, falling:** abrot, ail, all-c, alum, alum-p, am-c, am-m, ambr, ant-c, ant-t, anthraco, apis, arn, ars, ars-i, ars-s-f, art-v, arund, asc-t, aur, aur-ar, aur-m, aur-m-n, aur-s, bac, bar-c, bar-s, bell, bov, bry, bufo, calc, calc-i, calc-p, calc-s, calc-sil, canth, carb-an, carb-v, carbn-s, carl, caust, cean, cere-b, chel, chin, chlol, chrysar, cinch, colch, con, cop, crot-c, crot-h, cupr-s, des-ac, dulc, elaps, ferr, ferr-ar, ferr-m, ferr-ma, ferr-p, fl-ac, form, glon, graph, hell, hell-f, hep, hipp, hippoz, hyper, ign, iod, jab, kali-ar, kali-bi, kali-c, kali-i, kali-n, kali-p, kali-s, kali-sil, kreos, lach, mag-c, manc, med, merc, merc-c, mez, morg-p, naja, nat-c, nat-m, nat-p, nat-sil, nit-ac, nuph, oena, ol-j, op, osm, par, ped, petr, ph-ac, phos, pilo, pitu-p, pix, plb, psor, rein, rhus-t, rhus-v, rosm, sabin, sanic, sars, sec, sel, sep, sil, sphing, spira, staph, streptoc, stry-ar, sul-ac, sul-i, sulph, syc, syph, tab, tax, tep, thal, thal-act, thal-met, thuj, thyr, tub, ust, vesp, vinc, weis, zinc, zinc-p.
    - Combing the hair; when: canth.
    - Delivery; after: calc, canth, carb-v, hep, lyc, nat-m, nit-ac, sep, sil, sulph.
    - Disease; after
        - Abdominal: lyc.
        - Acute exhausting disease; following: carb-v, manc, thal.

- Forehead: ars, bell, hep, merc, nat-m, phos, sil.
- Grief; from: caust, graph, ign, lach, lyc, nat-m, ph-ac, staph.
- Handfuls, in: carb-v, lyc, mez, phos, rein, sulph, syph, thal.
- Injury; from: hyper.
- Lactation; during: nat-m.
- Menopause: lyc, phos, sep.
- Occiput, on: calc, carb-v, chel, hep, merc, petr, phos, sep, sil, staph, sulph.
- Pain in head, with: ant-c, nit-ac, sep, sil, syph, thuj.
- Pregnancy, during: lach.
- Sides: ars, bov, calc, graph, kali-c, merc, ph-ac, phos, staph, zinc.
- Spots, in: alum, apis, ars, bac, calc, calc-p, canth, carb-an, chin-b, cortiso, fl-ac, graph, hep, ign, iod, kali-p, lepr, lyc, nat-m, petr, phos, psor, syph, tell, tub.
  - Emotions, after suppressed: staph.
  - Grief, after: ign, staph.
  - Replaced by; and is gray / white / wooly hair: vinc.
- Temples: Calc, croc, graph, kali-c, lyc, merc, nat-m, par, sabin.
- Vertex, from: bar-c, graph, lyc, thuj.
- **Eye, hair falling,** eyelashes, from: alum, apis, ars, aur, aur-ar, bufo, calc-s, chel, chlol, euphr, kali-c, lepr, med, merc, nat-m, petr, ph-ac, psor, rhus-t, sel, sep, sil, staph, sulph.
- **Chest, hair falling:** ph-ac.
- **Face, hair, falling**
  - Beard: psor, tub.
  - Eyebrows: agar, ail, alum, anan, aur-m, bell, borx, caust, hell, kali-c, merc, mill, nit-ac, par, ph-ac, plb, pl-act, sanic, sel, sil, sulph.
    - Lateral half: lach, thuj.

- Mustache: bar-c, kali-c, nat-m, plb, sel, tub.
  - Left side: tub.
- Whiskers: agar, alum, ambr, anan, aur-m, calc, carb-an, graph, kali-c, nat-c, nat-m, ph-ac, plb, sanic, sel, sil.
  - Grief, after: ph-ac.
- Male genitalia, hair falling off: alum, bell, hell, merc, nat-c, nat-m, nit-ac, ph-ac, rhus-t, sars, sel, zinc.
- Female genitalia, hair falling out: alum, hell, nat-m, nit-ac, ph-ac, rhus-t, sel, sulph, zinc.
  - Delivery; after: nat-m.
  - Leucorrhea, due to: alum, graph, lyc, nat-m, phos, sulph.
- Skin, hair, falling out: alum, ars, calc, carb-an, carb-v, graph, hell, hist, kali-c, lach, lat-m, nat-m, op, phos, sabin, sec, sel, sulph, tub.
- Generals, hair falling: alum, ph-ac, sel.

■

Chapter-34

Diseases of the Nails

The study of the nails includes examination of shape, contour, colour, glossiness, translucency, consistency, deformities and structure. The latter should include a study of the nail folds (both the posterior and lateral), the nail bed, and the plate consisting of the root, lunula and the body proper.

It is important for clinicians to understand and accurately describe nail findings if they are to communicate accurately with their colleagues and avoid the vagueness that often surrounds nail pathology. Signs fall into categories of shape, surface and color.

ABNORMALITIES OF SHAPE

CLUBBING

Etiology

Clubbing is divided into two types Idiopathic and acquired (or secondary). '*Idiopathic clubbing*' is either of the isolated dominantly inherited type or of the pachydermoperiostosis type with its associated findings. '*Secondary (acquired) clubbing*' is usually a consequence of pathological conditions of the pulmonary (bronchogenic carcinoma, lung abscess, interstitial fibrosis, bronchiectasis, tuberculosis with secondary infection, etc.), cardiac (infective endocarditis, congenital cyanotic heart disease, etc.), hepatic (biliary cirrhosis), gastrointestinal systems (inflammatory bowel disease) or thyroid acropathy. Typically, there is periostitis, with periosteal new bone formation in the phalanges, metacarpals, and distal ulna and radius. In forms associated with bronchiectasis or neoplasm (bronchogenic carcinoma), prominent inflammatory joint signs may also be seen, resulting in hypertrophic pulmonary osteoarthropathy.

Unilateral or asymmetrical clubbing is reported in a few cases of Takayasu's arteritis and sarcoidosis. Solitary clubbing can be seen in cases of a digital mucous cyst.

Clinical Features

Clubbing is a condition where there is a bulbous enlargement of the distal segment of a digit due to soft tissue proliferation, and the nails tend to bulge and are curved in a convex arc in both transverse and longitudinal directions. There is a softening and sponginess of the nail bed.

Pathology

Clubbing is a condition that appears to be related to increased blood flow through the vasodilated plexus of the nail unit vasculature, more than to vessel hyperplasia.

Diagnosis

There are three forms of geometric assessment that can be performed:

- The junction between the nail plate and the dorsal surface of the distal phalanx forms an angle (*Lovibond's angle*), which is normally less than 160°; however this is altered to over 180° in clubbing.

- Also, *Curth's angle* at the distal inter-phalangeal joint, which is normally about 180°, is diminished to less than 160° in clubbing.

- *Schamroth's window* is seen when the dorsal aspects of two fingers from opposite hands are apposed, revealing a window of light, bordered laterally by the Lovibond angles. As this angle is obliterated in clubbing, the window closes.

Differential Diagnosis

- In a few cases of bronchiectasis, there is shell-nail syndrome seen, which is a variant of clubbing, distinguished from it by the presence of atrophy of underlying bone and nail bed

KOILONYCHIA

Synonym

Spoon Nails.

Etiology

- The majority of adults with koilonychia demonstrate a familial pattern, an autosomal dominant trait. This condition may also result from faulty iron metabolism or can be an associated feature of Plummer-Vinson syndrome or hemochromatosis.

- It is also seen in cases of coronary disease, syphilis, polycythemia, acanthosis nigricans, psoriasis, lichen planus, Raynaud's disease, scleroderma, acromegaly, hypothyroidism and hyperthyroidism, Monilethrix, palmar hyperkeratosis, and steatocystoma multiplex.

- A significant number of cases are idiopathic.

- Manual trauma in combination with cold exposure may result in seasonal disease.

Clinical Features

Koilonychia (Greek *Koilos*-hollow, *onyx* – nail) is a condition where there is a reverse curvature of the nail in the transverse and longitudinal axis, giving a concave dorsal aspect to it. The nails may be thickened, thinned, softened or unchanged in quality, but have edges everted in such a way that it looks like a spoon, and if a drop of water were placed on the nail it would not run off.

F- 47

Both the finger and toenails may be affected, but the condition is most evident on the thumb and the great toe.

Differential Diagnosis

Psoriasis, lichen planus, Raynaud's disease, scleroderma, acromegaly, hypo and hyperthyroidism.

MACRONYCHIA & MICRONYCHIA

Macronychia is a condition where a nail is considered too large in comparison to other nails. Similarly, micronychia is a condition where the nail is too small in comparison with other nails on nearby digits.

ANONYCHIA

Etiology

- This condition can result either as a result of a congenital ectodermal defect, or as a sequel of Stevens-Johnson syndrome, or in association with congenital developmental abnormalities such as microcephaly and wide-spaced teeth, or Cooks syndrome.
- It can also be a result of or an association with ichthyosis, severe infection, severe allergic contact dermatitis, self-inflicted trauma, Raynaud's phenomenon, lichen planus, or severe exfoliative diseases.

Clinical Features

- Anonychia is a rare anomaly where there is absence of all or part of one or usually several nails. The term implies a permanent state, which may be associated with underlying bony changes.
- In cases where there is a residual nail matrix, there may be some vestigial nail or hyperkeratosis.
- Temporary anonychia may arise from onychomadesis (nail loss) associated with transient local or systemic upset.

ABNORMALITIES OF NAIL ATTACHMENT

NAIL SHEDDING

Shedding of nails can occur from any of the following mechanisms:

- Periodic complete loss of the nail plate can occur due to an idiopathic shedding of the nail beginning at its proximal end. This condition is termed as 'onychomadesis' and it results either from a systemic disorder (where there is a temporary loss of all nails) or can be a result of penicillin allergy, neurologic disorders, peritoneal dialysis and fungal infections

- Dermatoses, lichen planus, pustular psoriasis and paronychia may also cause nail loss.

- Trauma is a common cause of recurrent nail loss (along with an underlying haemorrhage) and it usually reflects the cause; e.g. when playing football, due to some bad footwear or injury to the toes or finger.

- Cases of a traumatic, familial, non-inflammatory nail loss are reported, where they are usually associated with a dental abnormality.

ONYCHOLYSIS & ONYCHOMYCOSIS

'Onycholysis' is a spontaneous distal and/or lateral separation of the nail from the nail bed, usually beginning at the free margin and progressing proximally (except in cases of psoriasis, where the lesion occurs as an oval spot in the meddle portion of the nail).

The nail itself is smooth and firm with no inflammatory reaction. Pain occurs only if there is further extension as a result of trauma or if active infection supervenes. Areas of separation appear white or yellow due to air beneath the nail along with sequestered debris and glycoprotein exudate, along with an accumulation of bacteria. At the border of onycholysis, the nail bed is usually reddish-brown, reflecting the underlying psoriatic inflammatory changes. If the condition persists for several months, the nail bed becomes dark and irregularly thickened.

This condition is especially seen in women, considering the fact that it usually occurs 'secondary to' traumatically induced separation, with rapid secondary infection with the most commonly isolated pathogens being Candida albicans or Pseudomonas pyocyanea. The longer the infection lasts the less likely it is for the nail to become reattached, due to keratinization of the exposed nailbed.

There is infection occurring also due to Trichophyton rubrum, leading to *'onychomycosis'* (or tinea ungium) (infection of the nail by fungus). Here there is a build up of soft yellow keratin in the space created by the onycholysis or separation of nail plate from the nail bed. Then the entire nail plate is lifted and nail becomes misshaped, thick and yellow in appearance, which becomes painful due to constant pressure from wearing fitting shoes.

Onychomycosis affects the great toes more often and is more commonly seen in adults and that too especially in males.

Etiology

Besides infection by the organisms, 'idiopathic' cases are also known where no particular cause can be pointed out.

Some other common 'causes' known to lead to these two conditions are –

- *Trauma:* Overzealous or persistent manicure, foreign-body implantation, frequent wetting and use of strong cosmetic 'solvents' or soaps. A trauma to the tips of the digits, leading to subungual hematoma, especially in people who keep their nails abnormally long, can also be another cause.

- *Dermatological conditions:* Psoriasis being the most common, followed by fungal infections, atopic dermatitis, lichen planus and eczema.

- *Systemic Causes:* Poor peripheral circulation, hypothyroidism, hyperthyroidism, pregnancy, porphyria, pellagra, syphilis, viral (herpes) infections, yellow-nail syndrome and shell-nail syndrome.

- *Drug or chemical induced conditions* may result from the use of antibiotics, solvents, nail base coat, or formalin derivatives to harden the nail, etc.

- *Hereditary forms* are also known, inherited in an autosomal dominant fashion.

Treatment

The affected part of the nail should be clipped away and further trauma to the nail should be absolutely avoided. The nail bed should be kept completely dry in order to avoid further spread of the fungal infection.

PTERYGIUM UNGUIS

Pterygium unguis is a condition where there is a wing-shaped appearance of the nail with a central fibrotic band dividing the nail proximally into two parts.

There is an inflammatory destructive process that precedes the pterygium formation, where the nail matrix is destroyed by the inflammation and replaced by fibrosis. This fibrosis causes a fusion between the proximal nail fold and its underlying nail bed, which then obstructs normal nail growth.

Etiology

This condition is especially seen in cases of:

- Trauma.
- Lichen planus.
- Hansen's Disease (leprosy).
- Idiopathic atrophy of the nail.
- Peripheral circulatory disturbances.
- Sarcoidosis.

VENTRAL PTERYGIUM

Ventral pterygium or Pterygium inversum unguis occurs on the distal portion of the nail bed, which adheres to the ventral surface of the nail plate. Here there is a forward extension of the nail-bed epithelium, which eventually leads to an extension of the hyponychium to a more ventral and distal position, mimicking the clawnail. The overlying nail may be normal, but adjacent soft tissues can be painful, especially when manipulating small objects, typing or when manicuring.

Etiology

This condition can be hereditary and present since birth; or is usually of an acquired type, caused either due to trauma, systemic sclerosis, systemic lupus erythematosus or Raynaud's phenomenon.

SUBUNGUAL HYPERKERATOSIS

Here there is hyperkeratosis of the nail bed and the hyponychium resulting in thickening of the nail plate with other variable changes. The overlying nail prevents simple loss of the excessive squamous debris from the nail bed epithelium, which then gets compacted into a layer of debris. The only route of loss is by emerging distally with the growing nail. Thus there is dry, white or yellowish material crumbling away from the overhanging nail.

This condition can be a result of onychomycosis, wart virus infection, psoriasis, pityriasis rubra pilaris, eczema, scabies, etc.

HANGNAILS

These are overextensions of the cuticle of the nail, which tends to split and peel off from the proximal or lateral nail fold. They tend to be pretty annoying and painful due to accidental brushing or trauma to the part, to avoid which the patient tends to frequently try and bite the cuticle off. The best way to allow the part to heal is by allowing it to grow a bit and then trimming the part with a scissor or nail cutter.

NAIL THICKENING

Thickening of the nail is usually associated with a yellowish discoloration, due to the obscuration of nail bed vasculature, and an alteration of the shape of the nail, depending on the cause.

Some of the common causes leading to this condition are psoriasis, eczema, trauma and onychomycosis.

'Onychauxis' is a condition where there is a simply hypertrophy and thickening of the nails without any deformity. This is seen to occur because of trauma, acromegaly, Darier's disease, psoriasis, or pityriasis rubra pilaris. Periodic partial or total debridement of the thickened nail plate by mechanical means may help.

'Onychogryphosis' is a condition, usually seen in the elderly, where the nails resemble claws or a ram's horn. It can be caused by trauma or peripheral vascular disorders, but is usually due to neglect and failure to cut nails for a long time.

'Onychophosis' is also a common finding seen in the elderly, where there is a localized or diffuse hyperkeratotic tissue that develops on the lateral or proximal nail folds, within the space between the nail folds and the nail plate, esp. of the first and fifth toes. Use of comfortable shoes should relieve the distress.

ONYCHOCRYPTOSIS OR INGROWING TOENAIL

Synonym

Unguis Incarnatus; Ingrowing Toenail.

Etiology

Wearing ill-fitting or tight shoes are usually the most frequently seen causes of this condition. Also, incorrect or too deep cutting of the nails, especially at the lateral edges (esp. when trying to give shape to the nail) can cause the anterior portion of the nail to pierce the flesh as the nail grows distally and thus cause a lot of pain.

Clinical Features

This painful condition occurs especially on the great toe, where the nail tends to immoderately extend laterally into nail fold, causing a red, painful and inflammatory state of the part. The lateral margin of the nail acts as a foreign body and may cause exuberant granulation tissue.

Bacterial infection usually tends to occur in the paronychial tissue traumatized by the presence of an ingrown nail.

CHANGES OF NAIL SURFACE

Longitudinal Grooves

Longitudinal grooves are narrow furrows that cut through the thickness of the nail fully or partially, and which can either be a small slit or a long one that covers the whole length of the nail. The thumb is the most commonly affected nail, and the affection tends to be usually symmetrical. The nail may become normal after a few months or years, but it usually tends to form a ridge at the site of the original defect, where a relapse of a groove is likely to appear.

The most commonly seen form of groove is the *'Median Nail Dystrophy'*, where there is a longitudinal splitting or almost a canal-like formation in the midline of the nail. The split is such that it almost resembles a fir tree.

Etiology

History of trauma is usually given by the patient, which thus seems to be the commonest cause of this condition; but hereditary cases have also been recorded.

Other conditions that tend to cause or be associated with the formation of grooves are:

- Lichen planus.
- Tumors, papillomas, cysts can press on the matrix and produce a longitudinal groove.
- Darier's disease.

- Peripheral vascular disease.
- Rheumatoid arthritis.
- Old age.
- Taking oral retinoids.

TRANSVERSE GROOVES AND BEAU'S LINES

'Transverse grooves' can also cut through the thickness of the nail fully or partially, but as the term suggests they occur transversely across the nail. The distance of the groove from the nail fold is related to the time since the onset of growth disturbance. The depth and width of the groove may be related to the severity and duration of disturbance, respectively.

These transverse grooves can occur either on a few isolated digits, or it can be of a generalized type. When of an isolated type, the causes are usually trauma, inflammation or neurological events. When of a generalized type, systemic causes such as coronary artery disease, measles, mumps or pneumonia are more common.

Etiology

They can occur due exogenous causes (e.g. after a manicure or after too much of washing) or endogenous ones. When due to exogenous causes, there are multiple transverse grooves, the margins of which match the proximal nail fold. When due to an endogenous cause, they have a curved margin matching the crescent-shaped white lunula at the base of the fingernail. These are usually referred to as 'Beau's lines'.

Beau's lines are 1 mm wide transverse or horizontal depressions in the nail plate, ascribed to the temporary arrest of the functioning of the nail matrix, and are usually found to have a bilateral and simultaneous affection of all the nails. The various causative factors for the formation of Beau's lines are episodes of significant physiologic stress like childbirth, dramatic illnesses, drug reactions, measles, paronychia, acute febrile illnesses, severe malnutrition, major injuries (e.g. a broken hip) or fractures and systemic illnesses.

PITTED NAILS (STIPPLED NAILS)

Here one finds tiny, dot-like, shallow or deep, pinpoint depressions or punctate erosions distributed randomly on the surface of an otherwise normal nail.

Pathology

Histologically, pits represent foci of parakeratosis, reflecting isolated nail malformation.

Etiology

Pitting can be seen in the following conditions:

* Psoriasis (esp. in the early stages).
* Alopecia areata.
* Early stages of lichen planus.
* Psoriatic or rheumatoid arthritis.
* Chronic eczema or dermatitis.
* Perforating granuloma annulare.
* In a few cases no cause is found.

Differential Diagnosis

In cases of psoriasis or Reiter's syndrome, the pits are usually more of an irregular form, and are deeper and broader than those seen in cases of alopecia areata, which are shallower and more of a regular type.

TRACHYONYCHIA

This condition is also called as 'Twenty-nail dystrophy', where all the twenty nails become dull, opalescent, greyish, thin, fragile, rough and longitudinally ridged. It is seen in children as well as adults.

Etiology

It can be idiopathic or caused by or be associated with conditions like alopecia areata, psoriasis, lichen planus, atopic dermatitis, ichthyosis vulgaris, or other inflammatory dermatoses. Familial forms of this condition are also known to exist. It is also known to be associated with autoimmune processes such as selective IgA deficiency, vitiligo, and graft-versus-host disease.

Histology

Spongiosis and a lymphocytic infiltrate of the nail matrix is seen.

Prognosis

It may be a self-limiting condition with childhood cases resolving spontaneously by the time the patient is 20 to 25 years of age.

ONYCHOSCHIZIA

Synonym

Splitting of nails.

Etiology

The dysadhesion between the layers of keratin could occur due to dehydration. Though there is no particular cause attributed to it, it has been associated with polycythemia in a few cases.

Clinical Features

Onychoschizia, also known as lamellar dystrophy, is a condition where there is transverse splitting of the distal nail plate into layers, at or near the free edge, especially in cases of women and infants. There can be a resultant discoloration of the nail due to the collection of debris between the layers. Longitudinal splits may also occur. This condition usually gets worse with aging.

Frequent washing in water and application of nail polish can make the condition of the nails worse.

ONYCHORRHEXIS (BRITTLE NAILS)

Brittleness of the nails with its subsequent breakage usually tends to result from use of strong soaps and frequent immersion of the hands in water. It can also result from the use of a nail polish remover; from conditions like hypothyroidism, iron deficiency anaemia and impaired peripheral circulation; or after oral retinoid therapy.

Brittle nails are usually associated with onychoschizia, and thus a diet rich in vitamin B complex (egg yolk, liver, yeast, etc.) tends to usually be of help.

BEADING AND RIDGING

Beading and ridging of the nails are common signs seen in old age, since here the rate of the nail growth tends to slow down. Both these conditions are also seen to occur in a few cases or rheumatoid arthritis.

CHANGES IN COLOR

Alteration in nail colour may arise through changes affecting the dorsal nail surface, the substance of the nail plate, the undersurface of the nail or the nail bed.

EXOGENOUS PIGMENT

There can be pigmentation occurring on the dorsal surface of the nail due to exogenous causes. These are easy to demonstrate by scraping the surface of the nail. There will usually be a narrow proximal margin of unstained nail, which will grow wider with time (and as the nail grows). This can especially be seen in chronic smokers, who have now given up smoking.

In cases where there is exogenous pigmentation on the undersurface of the nails, the needs to be avulsed in order to check for it. There are transverse green stripes of the fingernails produced by paronychial infection with *Pseudomonas aeruginosa*. This may or may not be associated with onycholysis.

NAIL-PLATE CHANGES

There can be changes in the nail plate, either in terms of the color or in terms of its clarity or transparency. There can be a brownish streak formation or pigmentation of the nail plate due to melanin deposition. There are also cases of staining reported due to nicotine, chemicals, dyes (hair dyes, nail polishes and their removers), drugs, heavy metals, etc.

There can also be a disruption in the normal nail-plate formation either due to disease, chemotherapy, poisons or trauma, which can result in small splits between the cells within the nail, with loss of the normal lucency.

Scraping the surface of the nail plate several times firmly with a scalpel blade will help distinguish the nail plate staining from exogenous causes, which frequently scrape off completely. Also, if the stain follows the curvature of the lunulae, the cause is probably endogenous; if it follows the curvature of the proximal and lateral nail folds, the cause is probably exogenous.

MELANONYCHIA AND OTHER NAIL-BED CHANGES

'Melanonychia' is a condition where there is a blackish or brownish pigmentation of the normal nail plate, usually in the form of vertical or horizontal bands. These are seen commonly among Africans, or it can occur as a result of trauma to the nail, or it can be an effect of some drug intake (usually chemotherapy, antimalarials, minocycline or gold) or may occur as an associated feature of lichen planus, some systemic disorders, acanthosis Nigricans, Addison's disease, vitamin B_{12} deficiency,

Other nail bed changes include those due to nail bed 'tumors' (pyogenic granuloma, fibromas, nevi, myxoid or epidermoid cysts and angiofibromas, subungual melanoma) or those resulting from 'splinter hemorrhages'. The 'splinter hemorrhages' are usually longitudinal, thin, dark red lines, 1 to 3 mm in length, which occur due to rupture of subungual vessels at the junction of the nail plate and the nail bed. These hemorrhages are carried outward to the distal tip of the finger as the nail grows. Besides trauma, they are also found in cases of psoriasis, dermatitis, bacterial endocarditis, trichinosis and fungal infection of the nails.

LEUKONYCHIA OR WHITE NAILS

There are four forms of white nails recognized so far – leukonychia punctata, leukonychia striata, leukonychia partialis, and leukonychia totalis.

Cases of '*leukonychia punctata*' are commonly seen even in normal persons with otherwise normal nails. They present as white spots of 1 to 3 mm in diameter and are usually attributed to minor trauma to the nail matrix (e.g. as in the case of manicure) or can be an associated feature with alopecia areata. The pattern and number of spots may change as the nail grows. Symmetrical affection is seen to occur following a current episode of traumatic leukonychia.

'*Leukonychia striata*', where there are transverse or longitudinal white bands of 1 to 2 mm width. It may be a hereditary finding or it can be traumatic or systemic in origin (e.g. in cases of chemotherapy or poisoning).

'*Leukonychia partialis*', with usually the proximal two-thirds of the nail discolored as white, is seen to occur in association with any of the following – tuberculosis, nephritis, Hodgkin's disease, chilblains, metastatic carcinoma, or leprosy. Idiopathic cases are also noted.

'*Leukonychia totalis*' is usually a hereditary disorder of a simple autosomal dominant type, where the nails are of a milky porcelain white color. It can also present in cases of typhoid fever, leprosy, cirrhosis, ulcerative colitis, trichinosis, in those who tend to bite their nails, and in those using emetine.

There is also a condition termed as '*apparent leukonychia*', where the changes in the nail bed are responsible for the whitish appearance of the nail. Nail-bed pallor can, for example, be a non-specific sign of anaemia, oedema or vascular impairment.

TERRY'S NAIL

In this condition, due to changes in the nail bed, there is a whitish appearance of the nail at the proximal end or the entire nail plate, except for a normal pinkish color in the distal 1-2 mm of the nail. These changes are especially seen in patients suffering from cirrhosis, congestive cardiac failure, and adult-onset diabetes mellitus and is also a feature noted in the elderly.

Differential Diagnosis

Half and half nails, a condition where there is whitish appearance of the proximal portion of the nail and red, pink, or brown distal half, with a sharp line of demarcation between the two. It is especially seen in patients with some renal disorder along with azotemia.

MUEHRCKE'S BANDS

Here there are narrow paired white bands that occur parallel to the lunula in the nail bed, with a pinkish appearance of the 'nail between the two white lines. A disturbance in the nail bed, where due to edema there is a slight separation of the normally adherent nail from its bed, seems to be a likely cause. This condition is especially seen in association with hypoalbuminaemia, and when the serum albumin is raised or brought to normal, the lines are lost and the nails appear normal. These lines are also seen in those taking chemotherapy.

Differential Diagnosis

Mees' lines, a condition where there are single or multiple white bands, positioned transversely, usually seen in cases of inorganic arsenic poisoning, thallium poisoning, septicemia, dissecting aortic aneurysm, parasitic infections, chemotherapy, and in both acute and chronic renal failure.

YELLOW-NAIL SYNDROME

The characteristic feature of this condition is a yellowish (or yellowish green) discoloration of the nails, which are markedly thickened. The nails are markedly curved both transversely and longitudinally, with loss of cuticle and an indistinguishable lunula. Also, the nails in this condition tend to grow every slowly.

This condition is usually seen in adults and is especially in those with complaints of lymphedema, respiratory disorder (chronic sinusitis, chronic bronchitis, bronchiectasis, recurrent pleural effusion, etc.) or nephritic syndrome. Histologically, in the nail bed and matrix, dense fibrous tissue is found replacing subungual stroma, which could lead to obstruction of the lymphatic flow in the fingers.

The condition of the nails may revert back to normal on its own, or it may need treatment with vitamin E or zinc, and it is also necessary to treat the cause or chronic condition triggering the syndrome.

DISCOLORATION OF THE LUNULAE

Red lunulae is a condition where there is dusky erythema of the lunula area, especially of the thumbs. It is less intense in the distal part of the lunula, where it merges with the nail bed or is demarcated by a pale line. This condition is usually seen to occur in association with alopecia areata or in patients who are on oral prednisone, or in those with a history of psoriasis, cardiac failure, cirrhosis, lymphogranuloma venereum, psoriasis, vitiligo, chronic urticaria, lichen sclerosus, carbon monoxide poisoning, chronic obstructive pulmonary disease, twenty-nail dystrophy, and reticulosarcoma.

A bluish discoloration of the lunula is also seen in those suffering from Wilson's disease (hepatolenticular degeneration), in cases of subungual hematoma and melanocytic whitlow.

Color Changes Due to Drugs

There are a few allopathic drugs that can lead to or cause change in the nail color. A few of them are described below:

- Temporary yellowish discoloration of the nail occurs in prolonged tetracycline therapy.
- A violet-bluish discoloration is seen in those on chemotherapeutic drugs or those on mepacrine.
- A dark bluish black pigmentation of the nail bed is seen in those on chloroquine or other anti-malarial drugs.
- Transverse white stripes occur across the nail in cases of ingestion of inorganic arsenic.

HOMEOPATHIC APPROACH TO NAIL DISORDERS

In cases of homeopathic treatment, emphasis should be made on prescribing a constitutional and deep acting remedy. Local treatments in such cases are rather unsatisfactory.

Amongst all the diseases of the nails, the most common that I see in my practice are fungal infections. Let me be very honest with you, it is the most difficult disease to treat with homeopathy as even a small improvement is quite a time-consuming job, at times taking months or years to show an improvement; this specifically in relation to the cases of chronic infection. Hence one is to explain to the patient about the duration of treatment. However, let me tell you that all acute infections of the nail can be controlled in 24 hours.

Along with the constitutional medicine, sometimes I do advocate local treatment like dipping hands and nails in warm water, which contains *Hydrastis* mother tincture. The solution is prepared in a concentration of 2:8 with water.

Another thing worth mentioning is that constitutional medicine, when selected, needs frequent repetition over a prolonged period.

Deformities and discoloration of nails are two presenting symptoms in fungal infection. Deformity is the first symptom that starts showing improvement much faster than the discoloration.

Removal of the nail or surgical intervention in cases of fungal infections is never the answer, since the next generation of nail that comes up will be equally affected with fungus. Hence one needs to improve the immunity of the person. One has to use intercurrent remedies like *Sycotic-co, Thuja, Tuberculinum*, and *Psorinum*, which are extremely useful. Certain rare remedies like *Castor Equi* and *X-ray* have also been very useful to me. On rare occasions, for ingrowing toenails, the *South Pole of the Magnet* has been used by me successfully in my practice.

Whitlow is usually a manifestation of tubercular miasm, whereas conditions like tinea ungum, etc., where the nail is distorted, ridged and thickened, the sycotic miasm is more dominant.

General health of the patient must be improved by taking a healthy, balanced diet, along with fresh fruits that would help supply enough vitamins.

Also before treatment, one needs to examine all the nails, both of the fingers and the toes and check for the following:

- Whether the affection is more at the proximal or distal end.

- Whether there is a unilateral affection or just a single nail or a few nails are involved randomly. Single nail involvement is usually due to some local cause; unilateral involvement could be due to a neurological or circulatory cause; while bilaterally symmetrical involvement occurs usually due to a systemic cause or due to generalized dermatosis.

- Take a detailed history and try and find a cause, followed by a complete physical examination - dermatological, systemic, nutritional, etc. One needs to also check for any signs of trauma, manicuring, etc. that may provide clues to the cause and diagnosis.

Some Important Homeopathic Remedies

Alumina: Panaritium with brittle nails, lancinating pains and tendency to ulceration of the finger tips; gnawing beneath the fingernails with crawling along the arm as far as the clavicle; nails brittle or thick, spots on nails. Ingrowing toe nails, white spots on nails.

Anthracinum: Violent burning pain in panaritium; absorption of pus into the blood-gangrenous destruction; cerebral symptoms.

Antimonium crudum: Deficient growth of nails, split nails, growing cracked and thick split hoot in horses) thick, horny, callosities of skin.

Apis mellifica: Burning, stinging, throbbing panaritium which is hard and has a white sickly bleached out appearance, characteristic of the bee sting; very sensitive to touch; the fingers swell rapidly with tense glossy red surface extending up to forearm.

Arnica montana: Ulceration around root of nails with painful soreness of the ends of the fingers.

Asafoetida: Whitlow, with violent nightly pains and threatening necrosis of phalanx.

Berberis vulgaris: Pain under finger nails with coldness of feet, extending up to ankles & swelling of some of the finger joints.

Bryonia alba: Tight compressed feeling with pressing out sensation, as if the finger needed more room, dark, congested, part chilly feelings at times, but dry heat and burning, tearing, shooting pains more prominent, at first cold applications pleasant, later moist hot poultices more agreeable; dry mouth without thirst or great thirst; bitter taste; dry stool; dry skin; pulse fast; frequent & strong.

Bufo rana: Bluish black swelling around nail, followed by suppuration; pains run in streaks up the arm to axilla; after slight confusion, tearing pain, with redness along whole arm, following lymphatic vessels into armpit, causing painful glandular swellings.

Dioscorea villosa: Disposition to felons; frequent sharp pains in bones of fingers, one finger at a time, as of a brier in the middle finger of each hand with throbbing, darting, stinging pain next to the bone and very tender to pressure; nails brittle; jumping; darting pains in corns. Brittle nails.

Fluoricum acidum: Bone felons with offensive discharge > from cold applications; phalanges swollen far above their natural size, on dorsum of finger an opening discharges ichorous pus; panaritium also simple onychia with ulceration; sharp, sticking pain at root of right thumb nail. Nails grow more rapidly, crumpled or longitudinal ridges in them; soreness b/w toes, soreness of all the corns. It promotes expulsion of necrotic bones. In growing toe nails.

Graphites: Ingrowing toe nail; sides & roots of the finger and toe nails become sore, ulcerate and smell, they are exceedingly painful, violently burning and throbbing, then suppuration & proud flesh. Given at the beginning it absorbs the ailment in a few hours, hypertrophy of nails.

Hepar sulphur: Superficial erysipelatous onychia around the root of the nail; (before suppuration – Hep.) (after it suppurates – Lach.) thumb livid, violent throbbing, cutting, burning pain, lymphatics inflamed, lump in axilla; patient sensitive to touch & cold; subject to it every winter; decided yellow colour of the skin; pulse can be plainly felt, and the patient cannot bear the weight or pressure of a poultice though > warmth generally. Exfoliation of nails.

Hypericum perforatum: Panaritium; injuries of parts rich in sentient nerves, esp. fingers & toes & matrices of nails; pain severe and of long duration; mechanical injuries by splinters or needless under nails; squeezing or hammering of toes & fingers.

Lachesis mutus: Maltreated cases of long standing. When gangrene is threatening or has already set in, emitting an intolerable odor (Ars.); pricking in ends of the fingers.

Ledum palustre: Consequent to injuries, but only in first stage, as by pulling off abruptly a hang nail, during sewing; nightly itching of feet.

Lycopodium clavatum: Inflammation extending over whole hand; dark red swelling, belching, bloated abdomen, emptiness in stomach, with yawning.

Mercurius solubilis: Inflammation in the cellular tissue beneath the cuts, in the sinews, their facial and their phalangeal joints, pains not violent, more throbbing than shooting; patient extremely sensitive to heat or cold.

Natrium sulphuricum: Living in damp dwelling or workshops, pale appearance, lassitude and dull headache in the morning, chilly and feverish in the evening. A blister on the ungular phalarix, followed by deep red swelling; festering at root of nail; great pains, more bearable outdoors than in the room.

Nux vomica: Suppuration in palmar surface of finger or thumb throbbing or burning pain < warmth or by letting the hand down, in the evening after sunset – more comfortable in bed.

Rhus toxicodendron: Slow local development, frequent remission; dark red erysipelatous with little blisters or edema; pain running up the armpit.

Sepia officinalis: Itching with throbbing, shooting and burning at intervals or alternately; part dark red and pus visible. White spots on nails.

Silicea terra: Affection of periosteum; moderate redness or heat, deep seated inflammation, violent shooting pain deep in the finger, worse in the warm bed, sleepless at night, pain being unbearable, with great restlessness, irritability even unto convulsive jerks; opening with a surrounding wall of proud flesh, pus malignant discolored; it promotes expulsion of necrotic bones; ingrowing toenail, tearing pains as if the bones would be actually torn out, preventing all sleep. Frequent crops of boils; chronic fetid foot sweats, slightest draught unbearable. Nails are corrugated, distorted, thick or brittle and falling out, white spots on nails.

Sulphur: Hangnails; complementary to Apis in panaritium. Ingrowing toenails; thick nails; falling of nails, exfoliation of nails; brittle fingernails.

Thuja occidentalis: Fingers nails distorted, crumbling, soft, discolored (Graph., Nit-ac., Sil.), toe nails brittle and distorted; ingrowing toe nails. White spots on nails.

REPERTORY

- **Nail affections in general:** am-m, ant-t, ars, aur, bar-c, bell, borx, bov, calc, caust, chin, coch, colch, con, dig, dros, graph, hell, hep, iod, kali-c, lach, lyc, mag-s, merc, mosch, mur-ac, nat-m, nit-ac, nux-v, par, petr, ph-ac, plat, puls, ran-b, rhus-t, ruta, sabad, scil, sec, sep, sil, sul-ac, thuj.

   - Around: calc-p.

   - Black: crot-h, graph.

   - Blue: aur, chel, chin, colch, dig, dros, ip, lyc, manc, nat-m, nux-v, petr, plb, sil, verat-v.

   - Brittle: alum, ars, calc, calc-f, graph, lept, merc, nat-m, sabad, sep, sil, thuj.

   - Burning, as of: aaust, con, elaps, nit-ac, sars, vinc.

   - Burrowing: caust.

   - Crawling under: lach.

   - Crumbling: merc, sil, thuj.

   - Deformed, thickened, etc.: alum, ant-c, ars, calc-f, caust, ferr, graph, merc, sabad, sep, sil, sulph, thuj.

   - Discolored: ant-c, ars, caust, ferr, graph, mur-ac, nit-ac, sil, sulph, thuj.

   - Exfoliating: ferr, graph, merc.

   - Falling off: ant-c, ars, bor, canth, chloral, croc, form, graph, hell, merc, sec, sil, sul, thuj, ust.

   - Sensation: apis, pyrog.

   - Growing slowly: ant-c, sil.

   - Hang nails: calc, lyc, nat-m, rhus-t, sang, stann, sulph.

   - Horny growths under: ant-c, graph.

   - Ingrown: coloc, graph, kali-c, merc, sil, sulph, sul-i. ·

   - Needles under as if: led.

   - Numb and tingle: colch.

   - Pain under: carb-v, caust, fl-ac, hep, kali-c, merc, sil.

- Painful: am-m, ant-t, bell, caust, graph, hep, kali-c, mag-s, merc, nat-m, nit-ac, nux-v, par, puls, ran-b, rhus-t, sabad, scil, sep, sil, sulph.

- Panaritium: antho, ap, ars, flu-ac, hep, lach, merc, nat-s, rhus-t, sil.

- Pricking: colch.

- Ribbed; ridged, furrowed: ars, sabad.

- Sensitive: calc, con, hep, mag-s, merc, nat-m, nux-v, puls, sep, sulph.

- Soft: thuj.

- Splinters under, as of: calc-p, coc-c, colch, fl-ac, hep, nat-m, nit-ac, petr, plat, ran-b, sil, sulph.

- Splitting cracked: ant-c, ars, fl-ac, nat-m, ruta, sabad, sil.

- Spotted: alum, ars, nit-ac, sep, sil, spig, sulph, thuj.

- Suppuration: see *ulcerative pain*

- Thick: see *deformed* above

- Throbbing under: sulph

- Tingling in: colch.

- Ulcerated, onychia: alum, am-m, ant-c, ars, aur, bar-c, bell, borx, bov, calc, calc-f, caust, chin, cist, con, graph, hep, lach, lyc, merc, mur-ac, nat-m, nat-s, nit-ac, petr, ph-ac, plat, puls, ran-b, rhus-t, ruta, sabad, sec, sep, sil, sulph, sul-ac, sul-i, thuj.

- Ulcerative pain: am-m, bell, calc-p, caust, chin, graph, hep, kali-c, mag-s, merc, mosch, mur-ac, nat-m, nux-v, puls, ran-b, rhus-t, ruta, sep, sil, sul-ac, thuj.

- Yellow: ambr, ant-c, ars, aur, bell, bry, calc, canth, carb-v, caust, cham, chel, chin, con, ferr, hep, ign, lyc, merc, nit-ac, nux-v, op, plb, puls, sep, sil, spig, sulph.

■

Chapter-35

Diseases of the Sweat Glands

BROMHIDROSIS

Definition

Foul smelling perspiration is termed as bromhidrosis.

Etiology & Pathology

Certain drugs, chemicals (e.g. arsenic), food (especially garlic, valerian, asafetida, onions) and a few disease conditions (gout, diabetes, scurvy, typhoid, etc.) tend to give cause an odorous perspiration, especially due to the bacterial decomposition of apocrine sweat producing fatty acids with distinctive offensive odors. In a few cases, intranasal foreign body and chronic mycotic infection in the sinuses are other known causes.

Persons who have a strong smelling sweat tend to have a more potent and richer bacterial colonization, which again varies from person to person, depending on his or her race, work and social habits.

Clinical Features

The fetid perspiration is usually confined to the feet and axillae, though less commonly found to occur also on the genitals. It is often found that true bromhidrosis is usually not recognized by the patient himself, but is commented on by others. It is also found that the patients who usually come complaining of offensive axillary sweat actually have no offensive odor, but it is usually a sign of delusion, paranoia, phobia, or a lesion of the central nervous system.

Treatment

Treatment includes:

- Frequent cleaning or washing of the axillary regions, clothing and socks. Frequent changes of clothes and footwear and wearing of open chappals will also be of help.

- Excluding exposure to the causative agents; e.g. the particular drug, chemical, etc. and omitting strong-smelling food items (like garlic or onions) from the diet.

Differential Diagnosis

- 'Fish odor syndrome' is a metabolic disorder, where due to the excretion of trimethylamine, there is an odor of rotten fish coming from the eccrine sweat, urine, saliva and other secretions. The diagnosis is confirmed by testing for the metabolite in the urine. A diet low in choline and carnitine (sea fish, eggs, liver, peas, soya beans) is beneficial.

CHROMHIDROSIS

A very rare condition where the apocrine sweat is colored, which is especially strong or uncommon like blue, brown, green, black or red.

Etiology

- Ingested or injected drugs and elements (like iodides, copper, phosphorus, iron) tend to give rise to this condition.

- Also, elimination of products of metabolism (like indicans) tends to give rise to the colored sweat.

Clinical Features

At least 10% of the normal persons have a colored sweat, usually yellowish or greenish, but in this condition, localized areas of skin become markedly discolored, especially areas involving the face, axillae, groins, genitalia, abdomen, chest, etc. The colors may vary from dark yellowish to greenish and can also be brown, blue, violet or black in colour. The colored apocrine sweat is caused by the pigment lipofuscin, and it usually occurs in response to adrenergic stimuli.

'Eccrine chromhidrosis' is a condition where the normal clear eccrine glands tends to get pigmented due to chemicals, dyes, pigments or metals on the skin surface. For example, bluish green sweat of copper workers. At times there is secretion of bile through the eccrine sweat in patients with liver failure and marked hyperbilirubinemia.

Differential Diagnosis

'Pseudo-chromhidrosis' is a condition where the sweat is initially colorless, but it becomes colored after coming on the surface of the skin, either due to the action of the bacteria or due to the presence of dyes and chemicals from clothing, cosmetics, shoes, etc.

HAEMATOHIDROSIS

This is a rare condition where the sweat tends to be bloody, especially due to bleeding disorders, and is not related to sweat-gland activity.

HYPERHIDROSIS

Definition

Here is a condition where there is an excessive production of sweat, which can be either localized to one or several areas or can be of a generalized type. It can occur due to physiological or pathological reasons. It can be transient or permanent. Besides being an annoying and uncomfortable complaint, hyperhidrosis may interfere with social and occupational activities, which makes it a distressing ailment.

Etiology & Pathology

It can occur either due to changes in the sweat glands; due to pharmacological agents acting on the gland; due to an abnormal stimulation of the sympathetic pathway between the hypothalamus and the nerve ending; or due to overactivity of one of the three different 'centers' responsible for thermoregulatory, mental and gustatory sweating

Treatment

There is no particular treatment of this condition except for aiming to treat the underlying systemic disease; and to maintain a certain degree of general hygiene. One may also benefit by cutting down on hot, spicy food, tea, coffee, alcohol and tobacco. One needs to reduce the degree of emotional stress. Wearing the right kind of clothes is also important (esp. light-colored cotton ones), which helps facilitate the evaporation of the sweat and allow better cooling.

Prognosis

The prognosis of this condition is not very good, though there are isolated cases known of spontaneous recovery.

Complications

The excessive sweating can give rise to maceration of the skin, fungal infection, miliaria, intertrigo, secondary dermatitis, contact eczema and keratoderma.

Types

The following are the most frequent types seen:

GENERALIZED THERMOREGULATORY HYPERHIDROSIS

The amount of thermoregulatory sweating that each one of us has varies depending on a number of factors. Night sweats are a common clinical feature in this condition.

Etiology

- Generalized hyperhidrosis can occur due to physiological reasons – Exertion or vigorous exercises; emotional embarrassment; or in a hot humid environment.

- It occurs commonly in cases of febrile illnesses (esp. malaria) and shock.

- It can also occur in the following conditions as a result of hormonal disturbances – e.g. obesity, hyperthyroidism, hyperpituitarism, diabetes mellitus, during pregnancy and menopause.

- It may also occur in neurological conditions, Parkinson's disease, pheochromocytoma, hypoglycemia, alcohol intoxication, gout, salicylism, malignancies and infective processes (malaria, tuberculosis, brucellosis, lymphoma subacute bacterial endocarditis, etc.).

- Concussion and a few drugs (fluoxetine, pilocarpine) are also known to cause generalized hyperhidrosis.

PALMOPLANTAR (EMOTIONAL) HYPERHIDROSIS

In this condition, there is a localized hyperhidrosis, especially occurring on the palms, soles and axillae; and to a lesser extent on the face and groins. It usually begins around puberty, though it can also be seen in children; and one can often find a strong family history for the same. The parts can become cold, show a dusky hue (especially the palms) and can be offensive (especially the armpits). It can be a constant feature in the patient, occurring without any clear emotional trigger factor; or it can occur intermittently in phases, especially when in a warm room, or when anxious, stressed up or fearful.

Etiology

- It is an autosomal dominantly inherited feature in quite a few cases.
- It can also be an associated feature with Raynaud's phenomenon, reflex sympathetic dystrophy or after cold injury.

Complications

- Bromhidrosis (on the feet due to bacterial decomposition)
- Contact dermatitis.
- Intertrigo.
- Keratoderma of the palms and soles.
- Pompholyx.
- Ringworm infection, especially of the feet.

ASYMMETRICAL HYPERHIDROSIS

Etiology

- Hyperhidrosis can occur due to neurological lesions involving any part of the sympathetic pathway from the brain to the nerve ending. It usually occurs in association with other neurological symptoms or signs.
- It can also occur as a reflex action to visceral disturbances; or in an area adjacent to an area of anhidrosis; or around ulcers, nevi or tumors.
- Compensatory hyperhidrosis occurs in normal sweat glands when those elsewhere are not functioning because of neurological or skin disease, or after sympathectomy.

GUSTATORY HYPERHIDROSIS

In this condition there is physiological excessive perspiration in a few individuals on the upper lip, forehead, around the mouth and the nose, especially during or after the consumption of alcohol, tea, coffee, soups, tomato sauce, chocolate, and especially after hot or spicy food. Along with the increased sweating there can also be an associated vasodilatation of the area.

Etiology

- Besides the above stated physiological reasons, it may also occur in pathological conditions of the autonomic nervous system; due to a lesion in the central nervous system; or due to damage to and hyperactivity of the sympathetic nerves around the head and neck following an injury, abscess formation or after an operation (esp. on the parotid gland).

- It may also be caused due to sensory neuropathy (as after an attack of herpes zoster or with diabetes mellitus).

ANHIDROSIS

Definition & Clinical Features

Anhidrosis is the absence of sweat from the surface of the skin in the presence of an appropriate stimulus. The complaint thus causes the patient to feel a dryness of skin and the body's heat regulation system is so impaired that hyperpyrexia or heat stroke occurs on exposure to heat. A dysfunction at any step in the normal physiologic process of sweating can lead to decreased or absent sweating, which may be localized or generalized.

Etiology

Anhidrosis may be due to an abnormality of the sweat gland itself, or at any level in the nervous pathway.

A few of the common causes are:

- Organic lesions in the brain and spinal cord (due to sympathectomy, diabetes mellitus, syringomyelia, Horner's syndrome, leprosy, scleroderma, alcoholism, congenital sensory neuropathy, multiple myeloma, etc.).

- Hyperthermia.

- Ganglion-blocking and anticholinergic drugs.

- Aplasia or congenital ectodermal dysplasia.
- Ichthyosis.
- Congenital xeroderma.
- Scleroderma.
- Lymphoma.
- Miliaria profunda caused by sweat retention.
- Skin conditions like eczema, atopic dermatitis, lichen planus, or psoriasis (due to sweat-duct blockage).
- Sjögren's syndrome.

Complication

Patients coming with the complaint of decreased or absence of sweating, usually also complaint of an associated pruritis, fine papules and severe itching whenever they are exposed to heat in any form. Thus they may often be misdiagnosed as suffering from rash or urticaria. External cooling in such cases helps to resolve the symptoms temporarily.

MILIARIA

Miliaria is a condition where there is a retention of the sweat inside the eccrine sweat ducts due to occlusion of the pores, and this tends to give rise to an eruption that is common in the tropical countries and especially so in a hot, humid weather. Due to obstruction of the normal secretion of sweat from the sweat glands, there is a gradual back-up pressure developing that causes rupture of the sweat gland or the sweat duct at different levels. This results in an escape of the sweat into the adjacent tissue, which produces miliaria.

There are different **types** of miliaria, depending on the level and site of injury to the sweat gland or duct.

MILIARIA CRYSTALLINA (SUDAMINA)

Etiology

They are often seen in febrile illnesses of bedridden patients with profuse perspiration. It is also seen in cases of infants and children where, due to improper or overzealous clothing, there is less dissipation of heat and moisture.

Clinical Features

In this type, due to a superficial obstruction, the vesicles are small, clear and superficial without an inflammatory reaction. This condition is usually self-limited and short-lived, where the vesicles tend to rupture by the slightest trauma. Thus usually no treatment is necessary.

Clear, thin-walled vesicles, 1-2 mm in diameter, without an inflammatory areola, and symptomless, develop in crops, mainly on the trunk. In persistent febrile illnesses recurrent crops may occur. The vesicles soon rupture, and are followed by superficial branny desquamation.

MILIARIA RUBRA (PRICKLY HEAT OR HEAT RASH)

Etiology & Incidence

This condition tends to occur most frequently in hot and humid weather conditions, especially in the tropical countries. Some individuals are more prone to develop the affection than others; but besides this individual proneness, this condition tends to occur in infants and in individuals, who tend to sweat profusely, who are on the overweight side, who have sensitive skins and a low immunity. Local epidermal injury, friction or maceration also predisposes to this condition. It is commonly seen in those working in hot, stuffy rooms with improper ventilation and improper clothing.

Pathology

It is postulated that an increase in the bacterial flora of the skin could be responsible for the production of a slimy substance, which tends to block the pores of the sweat duct. This results in oozing of the sweat into the epidermal structure with the resultant formation of papulovesicles around the duct. Then there are parakeratotic plugs found on the skin due to keratinization of the intraepidermal part of the sweat duct, which tend to aggravate the obstruction.

Clinical Features

Here there is formation of separate and distinct, red, extremely itchy, erythematous papulovesicles, which tend to have a prickling, tingling and burning sensation in them. These discrete lesions then merge together becoming confluent on a bed of erythema. The intense itching and scratching may result in excoriations, pyoderma and eczema formation.

The most frequently affected sites are – the trunk, neck, cubital and popliteal fossae, inframammary areas (especially under pendulous breasts), abdomen (especially at the waistline) and the inguinal regions. The palms and soles are never affected.

One can note that this condition begins with hyperhidrosis of the part, which is later on followed by anhidrosis due to retention of sweat.

The typical lesions develop on the body, especially in areas of friction with clothing, and in flexures. They may also commonly be seen after occlusive therapy with polythene. The lesions are uniformly minute erythematous papules, which may be present in very large numbers. Characteristically, they lead to intense discomfort in the form of an unbearable pricking sensation. In infants lesions commonly appear on the neck, groins and axillae, but also occur elsewhere.

Diagnosis

- The characteristic seasonal appearance of the lesions in hot humid weather.

- The typical papulovesicular lesions with their characteristic distribution and itching, burning, prickling, etc. tends to confirm the diagnosis.

MILIARIA PROFUNDA

Etiology & Incidence

Miliaria profunda tends to occur after a severe attack or repeated bouts of miliaria rubra. They occur most frequently in the hot, humid weather of the tropical countries.

Pathology

It is usually a more severe condition, where there is an occlusion of the sweat duct in the upper dermis or the dermo-epidermal junction, followed by its rupture. Sweat retention occurs in the dermis with the production of flesh coloured dermal papules localized around a sweat pore.

Clinical Features

There are discrete, multiple, non-itchy, deep-seated, whitish or skin-colored papules occurring especially on the trunk and the extremities. Since they are almost skin-colored, they are best viewed from an oblique angle. Here all the sweat glands tend to be nonfunctional, except for the ones on the face, hands and the feet, where there may be a compensatory hyperhidrosis.

This nearly always follows repeated attacks of miliaria rubra, and is uncommon except in the tropics. The lesions are easily missed. The affected skin is covered with pale, firm papules 1-3 mm across, especially on the body, but sometimes also on the limbs. There is no itching or discomfort from the lesions.

Complications of Miliaria

- *Postmiliarial Hypohidrosis*: This condition invariably follows a bout of miliaria, where due to a hot environment and an occlusion of the sweat ducts and pores, there is a marked reduction in the quality and quantity of work performed. This is associated with marked irritability, anorexia, drowsiness, vertigo, and headache. In severe cases, the person may appear to be wandering as if in a sort of a daze.

• *Tropical Anhidrotic Asthenia*: This is a severe form of miliaria profunda, where there is a long-lasting occlusion of the sweat pores, resulting in fever, anhidrosis of the trunk with hyperhidrosis of the face, profound weakness and heat retention.

Treatment

The most effective treatment for miliaria is to place the patient in a cool environment. One needs to especially make a note of the following:

• Wear light-colored, loose, cotton clothing. Avoid anything synthetic or nylon.

• Have proper ventilation or air conditioning at the place of work or physical exertion.

• Have a balanced, nutritious diet with lots of fluids and fresh fruits.

• Avoid alcohol, tea, coffee, eggs, meat and hot, spicy food.

• Have frequent cold water baths, followed by thorough drying of the skin, especially at skin folds.

PERIPORITIS

Definition

Pyogenic inflammation of the sweat pore may result in the formation of abscesses of the sweat glands, which is termed as periporitis.

Synonym

It is also referred to as 'Miliaria pustulosa' in the initial stages (before abscess formation).

Clinical Features

It is usually always preceded by some skin ailment (like contact dermatitis, lichen planus, intertrigo, etc.) that has caused injury, destruction or blockage of the sweat duct. The pustules that tend to form are superficial, distinct and independent of the hair follicle; and may at times occur even several weeks after the disease has subsided.

The contents of the pustules are usually sterile, but secondary infection with staphylococcus aureus may result in true abscess of the sweat glands.

These tend to occur most frequently in areas like the skin folds, anterior surfaces of the extremities, scrotum and on the back (especially in cases of bed-ridden patients).

Differential Diagnosis

These are often confused as folliculitis or furuncles and can be distinguished from them clinically by a lack of any tendency to 'point', 'coldness' on touch and an absence of tenderness.

HIDRADENITIS

It is a condition characterized by a histological finding of an inflammatory infiltrate around the eccrine glands. It can be further divided into two types – neutrophilic eccrine hidradenitis and idiopathic plantar hidradenitis (recurrent palmoplantar hidradenitis).

NEUTROPHILIC ECCRINE HIDRADENITIS

It is usually seen in some leukemic patients within about 10 days of receiving chemotherapy. There is the formation of red, oedematous papules and plaques on the trunk, limbs, around the eyes and sometimes on the palms. Fever and neutropenia are associated complaints. Histologically one can find a dense neutrophilic infiltrate around and in the eccrine glands, and at times there can be an associated necrosis of the sweat glands.

RECURRENT PALMOPLANTAR HIDRADENITIS

It is usually seen in children and young adults, who complain of recurrent, red, painful nodules on the plantar surface of the foot (and rarely on the palms), making walking difficult. It is especially seen in cases where the child or the individual tends to walk too much.

HIDRADENITIS SUPPURATIVA

Definition

Suppurative hidradenitis is a chronic, painful and relapsing pyogenic infection of the apocrine gland follicles, where there is formation of chronic, often indolent, discharging abscesses due to subcutaneous extension (especially in the axillae and perineum), with induration, scarring, destruction of skin appendages and sinus formation.

Incidence & Etiology

This condition is usually seen in females, especially after puberty (since the apocrine glands are fully matured by then). Also low oestrogen levels in the patients tend to predispose them to the suppuration.

The predisposing factors that tend to lead to this condition are:

- Hyperhidrosis.
- Obesity .
- Recurrent personal or family history of acne, especially acne conglobata.
- Intertrigo.
- Synthetic or tight clothes, which prevent proper circulation of fresh air.
- Shaving, waxing or use of hair-removing creams.

The causative organisms usually responsible are Staphylococcus aureus, anaerobic Streptococci and Streptococcus milleri.

Pathology

Initially there are keratin plugs seen in the 'apocrine gland follicles', along with inflammatory changes within and around the apocrine glands. This results in a comedonal occlusion of the 'apocrine gland follicle' unit, which tends to obstruct the outflow of the apocrine gland in addition to that of the sebaceous gland, which initiates the formation of the hidradenitis. There is a secondary bacterial infection that occurs, which tends to cause suppuration, which then extends into the adjacent and subcutaneous tissues, and causes a resultant destructive scarring and fibrosis followed by fistula and sinus formation.

The cause of the initiating events remains unknown, but hormonal mechanisms are suspected.

Clinical Features

As this condition occurs in areas where apocrine glands are present, the axillae (esp. in females), groins and perineal regions (esp. in males), buttocks and upper thighs are most frequently affected. Other affected areas can be mammae (esp. around the areolae), neck, post-auricular areas and the back.

Intense itching and burning precedes the formation of the small, tender and painful, red, firm, subcutaneous nodules. Though these are firm initially, they later become fluctuant and very painful. Comedones surround the affected areas. The formation of pustules and the resulting suppuration can occur weeks or months after of the initial nodule formation. There is formation of indurated plaques or thick linear bands in the affected areas due to the subcutaneous extension. The inflammatory nodules often rupture externally leading to formation of abscesses or sinuses with discharge of fluid containing a thick, viscous, mucoid, suppurative, serous exudate with or without blood.

The severity and course of the symptoms vary from patient to patient and there can be partial remissions followed by frequent acute relapses. As the old lesions heal, recurrent new lesions keep forming, so that the course of the disease is often protracted. It may eventually lead to the formation of honeycombed, fistulous tracts with chronic infection. A probe inserted into a suppurating nodule will reveal a burrowing sinus tract, which may extend for many centimeters, running horizontally just underneath the skin surface.

Complications

* Ulcers or abscesses in the neighbouring structures.

* At times acute cellulitis with fever and toxicity may also follow.

* Anaemia, chronic malaise, depression, hypoproteinemia, amyloidosis, renal failure, interstitial keratitis and spondyloarthropathy are the consequence of chronic inflammations.

* Urethral, vesical and rectal fistulas.

* In a few long-standing cases, esp. in perineal affections, squamous cell carcinoma is known to occur.

Diagnosis

* The typical clinical presentation.

* Pus taken from the draining sinuses can be sent for culture, which will help reveal the Staphylococcus aureus or other gram-negative organism responsible.

Differential Diagnosis

* Common furuncles are typically unilateral and not associated with comedones, unlike hidradenitis.

* Ulcers in the axillary and inguinal lesions need to be differentiated from scrofuloderma, actinomycosis, granuloma inguinale or lymphogranuloma venereum.

* In cases of anogenital sinuses one needs to rule out Crohn's disease, sigmoidal diverticulitis, etc.

* Bartholin abscess also needs to be ruled out.

Treatment

- Maintaining local hygiene of the part with regular cleaning and drying is necessary.
- Keep hair in the affected parts short and dry.
- Obese patients need to loose some weight.

FOX-FORDYCE'S DISEASE

Etiology & Incidence

This condition tends to occur usually in females, especially after puberty to 35-40 years of age, but it can occur in males and children too.

Though there is no definite cause known to cause it, a few theories are proposed where obstruction of the apocrine glands and a few hormonal or endocrinal disorders can be held contributory.

Pathology

Histologically, a small vesicle is seen in the apocrine duct followed by an inflammatory lesion, which ruptures and the keratotic cells and lymphocytic infiltrate causes blockage of the apocrine duct and hair follicles. There is an associated spongiosis of the infundibulum at the site of entrance of the apocrine duct into the hair follicle.

Clinical Features

This is a chronic condition where there are multiple, discrete, pruritic, firm, papular eruptions in the axillae and pubic areas. Other areas affected are areolae, umbilicus, labia majora and perineum.

The main presenting complaint can be intense itching, esp. in the axillae, and to a lesser extent in the anogenital region and around the breasts. The characteristic feature of the itching is that it tends to get worse from emotional upset and not so much by heat. In a few cases there is no itching.

The itching is then followed by the skin-coloured, dome-shaped, papular eruptions in the typical sites.

There is no apocrine sweating occurring in the affected areas due to the apocrine duct blockage, and the density of hair in these areas is also low.

The disease runs a very prolonged course, and may persist until the menopause. There is a definite improvement in the symptoms during pregnancy.

GRANULOSIS RUBRA NASI

Definition

Granulosis rubra nasi is a rare familial condition seen in children, where the cartilaginous part of the nose, cheeks and chin are affected.

Etiology

Most cases are genetically determined, but the mode of inheritance is uncertain.

Pathology

Histologically, blood vessels are dilated and there is an inflammatory infiltrate about the sweat ducts.

Clinical Features

This condition usually begins anytime from the sixth month to ten years of age. The initial symptom is increased sweating over the nose, chin and cheeks. This is then followed by diffused erythema on the tip of the nose, cheeks, upper lip and the chin, which appear red or violet. Small dark red macules or papules or vesicles then form at the sweat-duct orifices.

This condition usually tends to subside spontaneously by puberty. Many cases are seen where there is a poor peripheral circulation and hyperhidrosis of the palms and soles.

ECCRINE NEVI AND TUMORS

SYRINGOMA

In this condition there are discrete, small, globular, yellowish or brownish papules, clustered especially on the eyelids and upper cheeks. It is a chronic, slowly developing condition, especially in females with Down syndrome. They can also be seen in the following areas – the axilla, abdomen, forehead, penis, and vulva.

Clear Cell Syringoma, a metabolic variant of this condition, is especially seen in diabetics.

Eruptive Syringoma is a condition where there are numerous shiny, rose-colored papules on the neck, chest, axillae, upper arms, and on umbilical region of the abdomen. It is a familial trait seen in Down syndrome and is known to occur in diabetic women.

HIDROCYSTOMA

These are discrete, chronic, non-inflammatory, symmetrically distributed, 1-3 mm, translucent, skin coloured, cystic lesions, occurring due to retention of sweat in the dermis. It usually occurs in hot weather, or in those people working around stoves or coming in contact with steam; so is especially seen in housewives, washerwomen and cooks.

POROMA

It is a benign, slowly growing, soft, reddish tumor occurring especially on the soles of the feet (rarely on the palms), which bleeds easily from the slightest of injury. This lesion characteristically grows and protrudes from a cup-shaped shallow depression in the skin.

Eccrine poromatosis is a variant of the above condition in which there are multiple lesions on both the palms and the soles associated with hidrotic ectodermal dysplasia.

POROCARCINOMA

Malignant changes may occur in chronic, long-standing cases of eccrine poromas, and is usually seen in small children by the age of 8-10 years. There is a blackish or bluish nodule, plaque formation or ulceration occurring in addition to the other clinical signs and symptoms of a poroma. These lesions are especially seen on the legs, feet, face and upper arms. In this condition the palms and soles are only rarely involved inspite of these areas having the highest concentration of eccrine glands. Mortality rate is high in cases of metastasis.

CHONDROID SYRINGOMA

In this condition there is a firm intradermal or subcutaneous nodule formation occurring especially on the face, which are usually asymptomatic and measuring 5 to 30 mm in diameter.

Homoeopathic Approach to Disorders of the Sweat Glands

Amongst all the disorders of the sweat glands, the following are the most common ones seen – Bromhidrosis, Hyperhidrosis, and Miliaria. Even though the lesion is at the level of sweat glands, it is purely the constitutional approach, which will really help the patient in the long run. Some points experienced in my practice are as follows

In hyperhidrosis, drugs like Calcarea, Calcarea Silicata, Silicea, Natrum Silicata, Baryta Carb, Baryta Silicata, have been extremely useful to me. The extent of improvement in hyperhidrosis will never be 100%, but atleast till 70% you can give relief to the patient. Perspiration on the palms is much more easier to control with homoeopathy than that on the soles. Long-term treatment of 5-10 years is sometimes required to treat the above disorder. Hence a lot of reassurance should be given to the patient.

As far as miliaria is concerned, unless it is very acute, I try to treat this with many home remedies. I do not feel it is worth treating it with homoeopathy unless very severe.

The following are a few home remedies that I tend to use in my practice:

- First of all I ask them to consume a lot of water throughout the day.
- The person should be put on a diet consisting of fresh juicy fruits, whole grain cereals and raw vegetables. He or she should avoid tea, coffee, white bread and starchy and sugary foods.
- I ask them to drink a lot of diluted limejuice, coconut water, buttermilk or lassi and water flavored with Khus grass roots. These decrease the overall heat in the body and thus prevent the prickly heat, and are also very useful for hyperhidrosis.

Consumption of almonds and grapes (especially dry grapes) are also very useful for these patients.

- Increased intake of Vitamin C by taking more of citrus fruits, black currents, green peppers, parsley, broccoli etc. is of help too.
- Fruit juice should be taken in plenty by these patients.
- Applying aloe vera pulp or sandalwood paste on the skin helps in cases of miliaria.

Improving the general state mental, physical and hygienic conditions. Also cutting down hot, spicy food, tea, alcohol and tobacco. Living in cool, fresh air, in loose thin clothing that allows evaporation of sweat, should be encouraged.

- Constant emotional stresses, strain and excitement must be avoided and physical exertion avoided.
- The cause or causes must be removed, for instant localized hyperhidrosis of feet, deformities like flat foot should be corrected. If there is obesity, the weight should be reduced.
- In cases of hyperhidrosis, one should wear sandals or chappals or open type shoes. Socks should be changed twice a day. Avoid nylon or woolen socks. Wearing of sleeveless shirt and blouse should be encouraged in cases of axillary hyperhidrosis.

Some Important Homoeopathic Remedies

Baryta carbonica: Fetid foot sweat toes and soles get sore, checked foot sweat, followed by lameness, tonsillar angina, etc. sweat increased in presence of strangers; offensive sweat of one (mostly left) side; sweat returned by eating, sweat returning every other evening; soles feel bruised at night, keep one awake; callosities on soles, which are painful on walking; cramps in soles of feet, < while walking or dancing.

Bryonia alba: Sweat in short spells and only on single parts; profuse and easily excited sweat, even when slowly walking in the cold open air; profuse night and morning sweat; sour or oily sweat, night and day; sour sweat at night, preceded by thirst; oppressive drawing in head when the sweat is about to terminate and succeeded by muddled condition of the head; vaporous exhalation of the skin from evening till morning.

Calcarea carbonica: Sweat during the slightest exercise, even in cold open air (Sep – sweat after the exercise, when sitting quietly); during first sleep; morning sweat; most profuse on head and chest; clammy night sweats, only on legs; foot sweat makes feet sore; feet cold and damp.

China officinalis: Copious, profuse oily sweat, easily excited during sleep or motion; exhausting night sweats, greasy sweat on the side on which he lies; increased thirst during sweat; partial cold sweat on face or all over body, with thirst; sweats easily especially at night in sleep; hectic fever, with profuse debilitating night sweats.

Hepar sulphur: Cold, clammy, frequently sour or offensive smelling sweat; perspires day and night, without relief, or first cannot sweat at all and then sweats profusely; night or morning sweat with thirst.

Hydrastis canadensis: Offensive sweat on genitals; excessive sweat of axilla and about genitals; clothing feels uncomfortable about groins.

Jaborandi: Copious sweating and salivation; profuse secretion from most of the glandular structures of the body, perspiration starts on forehead and face and then spreads all over body, most profuse on trunk, profound prostration after sweating; unilateral left sided sweat; profuse night sweats (Pilocarp).

Mercurius solubilis: Profuse sweat at night, towards morning with thirst and palpitations; from exertions, even when eating; evening in bed before falling asleep. Sour, offensive or cold clammy, oily (China) and causing burning of skin; with all pains, but giving no relief < by the weakness.

Phosphorus: Sweat mostly on head, hands and feet, or only on forepart of body, with increased urine, profuse clammy night sweats < during sleep (Samb- when awake, no sweat while sleeping), without relief.

Sambucus nigra: Dry, burning heat during sleep, giving way immediately on waking to profuse sweat, first on face and then extending over whole body, continuing more or less during waking hours; on going to sleep again the dry heat returns with cold hands and feet, but still he shuns uncovering; profuse, weakening sweat, day and night, lasts during the apyrexia.

Sepia officinalis: Free and sudden perspiration from a nervous shock or from exertion, the sweat, coming out after the exertion is over or the shock passed and when one is sitting quietly (Calc-sweat during exertion). Night sweat on chest, back and thighs, from above downwards to the calves, smelling sour offensive or like elder blossom; profuse morning sweat after awakening; offensive foot sweat, causing cold heels and soreness of toes; every third night sour, offensive sweat, like elder blossoms; crippled nails.

Silicea terra: Nocturnal head sweat keeps the child awake, profuse sweat of head, the body being dry or nearly so; copious offensive foot sweat, with rawness between toes and itching of soles, driving to despair; periodical sweat; debilitating, sour and offensive night sweats, mostly after midnight.

Stannum metallicum: Sweat comes on after he falls asleep, and as soon as he moves he is chilly on back and shoulders; often sequelae of weakening diseases, sweat smells, mouldy, musty, most profuse on neck, especially night and morning; hectic fever, anxious heat, as if sweat would break out.

Thuja occidentalis: Sweat, either of those parts, alone which are, covered (Bell, Chin, Spig) or of those alone which are uncovered, while covered parts are dry and hot; sweat. Most copious on upper part of body, except head; sweat on perineum; fetid sweat on toes, with redness and swelling of tips; on soles of feet; nails crippled, brittle or soft; sweat during sleep, but stops as soon as he awakens; oily, fetid sweat; sweetish odor exhaling from skin, accompanying abdominal or pelvic disorders, suppressed foot sweat.

REPERTORY

- **Sweat, in general:** acet-ac, agar, agn, alum, ambr, am-c, am-m, anac, ang, ant-c, ant-t, apis, arg-met, arn, ars, asar, aur, bar-c, bell, benz-ac, borx, bov, brom, bry, calad, calc, calc-p, camph, canth, caps, carb-an, carb-ac, carb-v, caust, cham, chin, cic, cina, clem, cop, colch, coloc, con, croc, cupr, cycl, dig, dros, dulc, euphr, ferr, fl-ac, gels, glon, graph, guaic, hell, hep, hyos, ign, iod, ip, jab, kali-c, kali-n, kreos, lach, lact-ac, laur, led, lith-c, lyc, màg-c, mag-m, mang, merc, mez, mosch, mur-ac, nat-c, nat-m, nit-ac, nux-m, nux-v, op, par, petr, phos, ph-ac, plat, plb, psor, puls, ran-b, ran-s, rheum, rhod, rhus-t, ruta, sabad, sabin, samb, sars, sec-c, sel, seneg, sep, sil, spig, spong, stann, staph, stram, sulph, sul-ac, tarax, thuj, valer, verat, viol-o, viol-t, zinc.

- **Absent (Inability to sweat):** Skin, dry, perspire, inability to: acet-ac, acon, alum, am-c, ambr, anac, apis, apoc, arg-met, arg-n, arn, ars, ars-i, bell, berb-a, bism, bry, calc, calc-sil, cham, chin, colch, con, crot-t, cupr, dulc, eup-pur, graph, hyos, iod, ip, kali-ar, kali-c, kali-i, kali-s, kali-sil, lach, laur, led, lyc, mag-c, maland, merc, merc-c, nat-c, nat-m, nit-ac, nux-m, nux-v, olnd, op, petr, ph-ac, phos, plat, plb, psor, puls, rhus-t, sabad, samb, sang, sars, sec, seneg, sep, sil, spong, squil, staph, sulph, thuj, thyr, verb, viol-o.

- **Exercising when:** arg-met, calc, nat-m, plb.
  - Perspiration.
  - Alternating sides: agar.
  - Right side: aur-m-n, bell, bry, fl-ac, jab, merc, nux-v, phos, puls, ran-b, sabin.
  - Left side: ambr, anac, bar-c, chin, fl-ac, jab, kali-c, phos, puls, rhus-t, spig, stann, sulph.
  - Ascending: arn, bell.
  - Anger, from: acon, bry, chin, cupr, ferr-p, lyc, petr, sep, staph.
  - Anxiety, during: acon, alum, alum-p, am-c, ambr, ant-c, arn, ars, ars-s-f, bar-c, bell, benz-ac, berb, bry, calc, calc-p, calc-sil, cann-s, carb-v, carbn-s, caust, cham, chin, chinin-ar, cic, cimx, clem, cocc, ferr, ferr-ar, fl-ac, graph, kali-bi, kali-n, kreos, marc, mang, merc, merc-c, mez, mur-ac, nat-ar, nat-c, nat-m, nat-p, nit-ac, nux-v, ph-ac, phos, plb, puls, rhus-t, samb, sel, sep, sil, spong, stann, staph, stram, sul-ac, sulph, tab, tarent, thuj, verat.
    - Evening: ambr, sulph.
    - Night: ars, carb-an, carb-v, nat-m.
    - Dinnera, after: calc.
  - Bloody: anag, arn, ars, calc, cann-i, cann-s, cham, chin, clem, cocc, crot-h, cur, hell, lach, lyc, nux-m, nux-v, petr.
    - Night: cur.
  - Coition, after: agar, calc, chin, graph, nat-c, sel, sep.
  - Colliquative: acet-ac, ant-t, ars, ars-h, camph, carb-v, chin, crat, eupi, ferr, iod, jab, lach, lyc, mill, nit-ac, psor, sec.
  - Conversation, from: ambr.
  - Critical: acon, bapt, bell, bry, canth, chlor, pneu, pyrog, rhus-t.

- Debilitating: acon, ambr, ant-t, arn, ars, bar-c, bry, calad, calc, camph, canth, carb-m, caust, chin, cocc, croc, dig, ferr, graph, hyos, iod, kali-n, lyc, merc, nat-m, nux-v, ph-ac, phos, psor, rhod, samb, sep, sil, stann, sulph, tarax, verat.
  - Delivery after: samb.
- Descending: sep.
- Drinking, after: aloe, ars, castm, chin, cham, cocc, con, kali-p, merc, puls, rhus-t, sel, sulph, sumb.
  - Amel: caust, chinin-s, op, phos, sil.
  - Warm drinks: bry, kali-c, mag-c, merc, phos, sil, sul-ac, sumb.
  - Wine: acon, apis, con, lach, op, sul-ac, thuj.
- Eating, while: ant-t, arg-met, ars, ars-s-f, bamb-a, bar-c, bar-s, benz-ac, borx, bry, calc, calc-sil, carb-an, carb-v, carbn-s, cocc, con, eupi, graph, guare, ign, kali-ar, kali-c, kali-p, kali-sil, merc, nat-c, nat-m, nit-ac, nux-v, ol-an, phos, puls, sars, sep, sil, sul-ac, valer, viol-t.
  - Amel: anac ign, lach, mez, phos, zinc.
  - Anxiety & cold perspiration: merc.
  - Eating, after: arg-met, ars, bry, calc, calc-sil, carb-an, carb-v, carbn-s, caust, chan, con, crot-c, crot-h, ferr, ferr-ar, graph, kali-c, kali-sil, laur, lyc, nat-n, nit-ac, nux-v, petr, ph-ac, phos, psor, sel, sep, sil, sul-ac, sulph, thuj, viol-t.
  - Amel: alum, anac, chin, cur, ferr, lach, nat-c, phos, rhus-t, sep, verat.
  - Breakfast: carb-v, grat.
  - Dinner: carb-an, dig, mag-n, phos, ptel, sep, thuj.
  - Warm food: bry, carb-an, carb-v, chan, ferr, kali-c, lach, mag-c, ph-ac, phos, puls, sep, sul-ac, thuj.
- Emotions, after: phys, rhus-t, sep.
- Excitement, after: ars-s-f, bamb-a, bar-c, graph, lach, phos.

- Face, of the whole body, except the: rhus-t, sec.
- Feet, except: chin, phos.
- Flatus, when passing: kali-bi.
- Fright, from: anac, bamb-a, bell, gels, lyc, op.
- Head, general perspiration except: bell, merc, mur-ac, nux-v, rhus-t, samb, sec, sep, thuj.
- Hot, lower limbs except: op.
- Lower limbs, except: lyc.
- Mental exertion: act-sp, aur, bell, borx, calc, calc-sil, graph, hep, hyos, kali-c, lach, lyc, nat-m, nux-v, phos, psor, sep, sil, staph, sulph, tub.
- Amel: ferr, nat-c.
- Music, from: sabin, tarent.
- News, from, unpleasant: calc-p.
- Occupation, during: berb.
- Odor
- Aromatic: all-c, benz-ac, guare, petr, rhod, sep.
- Bitter: dig, verat
- Blood: lyc
- Bread, white: ign
- Burnt: bell, bry, mag-c, sulph, thuj.
- Cadaverous, like: ars, art-v, lach, psor, pyrog, thuj.
- Camphor: camph.
- Cheesy: con, hep, plb, sulph.
- Coffee, like fresh: bamb-a.
- Drugs, like corresponding: asaf, ben, camph, carbn-h, chen-a, chinin-ar, iod, ol-an, phos, sulph, tab, ter, valer.
- Eggs, spoiled: plb, staph, sulph.
- Elder-blossoms: sep.

- Fetid: aesc, all-c, aloe, am-c, am-m, ambr, anac, arn, ars, aur-m, bapt, bar-c, bell, bov, canth, carb-ac, carb-an, carb-v, cimic, coloc, con, crot-h, cycl, daph, dios, dulc, eucal, euphr, ferr, fl-ac, graph, guaj, hep, kali-c, kali-p, lac-c, lach, led, lyc, mag-c, mag-m, med, merc, merc-c, nit-ac, nux-v, petr, phos, plb, psor, puls, pyrog, rhod, rhus-t, rob, sel, sep, sil, spig, staph, stram, sulph, tell, thuj, tub, vario, verat, zinc.
- Garlic: art-v, kalag, lach, sulph, thuj.
- Herring, pickled: vario.
- Honey: thuj.
- Leek: thuj.
- Lilac: sep.
- Mice: tub.
- Musk: apis, bism, mosch, puls, sulph, sumb.
- Musty: arn, cimx, merc, merc-c, nux-v, psor, puls, rhus-t, stann, syph, thuj, thyr.
- Offensive: acon, all-s, aloe, am-c, ambr, apis, arn, ars, ars-s-f, art-v, asar, aur-m, bamb-a, bapt, bar-c, bar-m, bar-s, bell, bov, bry, calc-sil, camph, canth, carb-ac, carb-an, carb-v, carbn-s, caust, cham, cimic, cimx, cocc, coloc, con, cycl, daph, dulc, euphr, ferr, ferr-ar, fl-ac, fink-b, graph, guaj, haliae-lc, hep, hyos, ign, iod, ip, kali-act, kali-ar, kali-c, kali-p, kali-sil, lach, led, lyc, mag-c, mand, med, merc, merl, mosch, murx, nat-m, nit-ac, nux-v, oci-sa, oena, petr, phos, plb, podo, psor, puls, pyrog, rheum, rhod, rhus-t, rob, sacch-l, sel, sep, sil, sol-t-ae, spig, stann, staph, stram, sulph, syph, tarax, tax, tell, vario, verat, wies, zinc.
- One side: bar-c.
- Morning: carb-v, dulc, merc-c, mist-v.
- Afternoon: fl-ac.
- Night: ars, carb-an, carb-v, con, cycl, dulc, euphr, ferr, graph, guaj, lyc, merc, mag-c, nit-ac, nux-v, puls, rhus-t, sep, spig, staph, tell, thuj.

-    Midnight: mag-c, merl.
-    Sleep during: cycl.
-    Cough after: hep, merl.
-    Exertion on: nit-ac.
-    Menses during: stram.
-    Motion, on: rupi, mag-c.
- Onions: art-v, bov, calc, kali-p, lach, lyc, osm, phos, sin-n, tell.
- Penetrating: bapt.
- Pungent: cop, gast, ip, sep, sulph, thuj.
- Putrid: bapt, carb-v, con, kali-p, led, mag-c, med, nux-v, psor, pulx, pyrog, rhus-t, sil, spig, staph, stram, verat.
- Rancid, at night: thuj.
- Rank: art-v, bov, cop, ferr, goss, lac-c, lach, lyc, sep, tell.
  -    Menses, during: stram, tell.
- Rhubarb: rheum.
- Sickly: chin, chinin-s, thuj.
- Smoky: bell.
- Sour: acon, alco, all-s, arn, ars, ars-s-f, asar, bapt, bell, bry, bufo, calc, calc-s, calc-sil, carb-v, carbn-s, caust, cham, chel, chin, cimx, cina, clem, colch, cupr, ferr-ar, ferr, ferr-m, fl-ac, gast, graph, hep, hyos, ign, iod, ip, iris, kali-c, kalm, lac-ac, lach, led, lyc, mag-c, merc, nat-m, nat-p, nit-ac, nux-v, pilo, psor, puls, rheum, rhus-t, ruta, samb, sep, sil, spig, staph, sul-ac, sul-i, sulph, sumb, tarent, tep, thuj, verat, zinc.
  -    Morning: bry, carb-v, iod, lyc, nat-m, rhus-t, sep, sul-ac, sulph.
  -    Forenoon: sulph.
  -    Afternoon: fl-ac.
  -    Night: arn, ars, asar, bry, carbn-s, caust, cop, graph, hep, iod, kali-c, lyc, mag-c, merc, nat-m, nit-ac, phyt, plect, sep, sil, sulph, thuj, zinc.
  -    Sleep, during: bry.

- Spicy: rhod.
- Sulphur: phos, sulph.
- Sulphuric acid: plb, staph, sulph.
- Sweetish: apis, ars, bamb-a, calad, merc, puls, sep, thuj, uran-n.
- Sweetish sour: bry, puls.
- Urine: benz-ac, berb, bov, canth, card-m, caust, coloc, ery-a, graph, lyc, nat-m, nit-ac, plb, rhus-t, sec, thyr, urt-u.
  - Horses: nit-ac, nux-v.
- Vinegar: iris.
- Vinous: sec.

- Oily: agar, arg-met, arn, ars, aur, bry, bufo, calc, chin, fl-ac, lyc, mag-c, med, merc, nat-m, nux-v, ol-j, petr, plb, psor, rhus-t, rob, sel, stram, sumb, thuj, thyr.
  - Daytime: bry.
  - Morning: bry, chin.
  - Night: agar, bry, croc, mag-c, merc.

- Profuse: abrot, acet-ac, acon, aesc, aeth, agar, alum, am-c, am-m, ambr, aml-ns, androc, ant-c, ant-t, anthraco, apis, arg-n, ars, ars-i, asar, asc-c, aur, aur-i, aur-m, aur-m-n, aur-s, bamb-a, bapt, bar-c, bell, ben, benz-ac, bol-la, bry, bufo, cact, calc, calc-ar, calc-i, calc-s, calc-sil, camph, canth, caps, carb-ac, carb-an, carb-v, carbn-s, carc, casc, castm, caust, cedr, cham, chel, chin, chinin-ar, chinin-s, chlor, cist, clem, coc-c, cocc, colch, coloc, con, cop, corn, crat, crot-c, cupr, dig, dulc, elaps, elat, esin, eup-per, eup-pur, ferr, ferr-ar, ferr-i, ferr-p, fl-ac, gels, granit-m, graph, guaj, hep, hyos, iod, ip, jab, kali-ar, kali-bi, kali-c, kali-n, kali-p, kali-s, lac-ac, lac-c, lach, lact, lith-c, lob, lob-e, lyc, mag-c, mang, merc, merc-c, mez, nat-ar, nat-c, nat-m, nat-p, nit-ac, nux-v, op, par, petr, ph-ac, phase-vg, phos, pisc, podo, psor, puls, pyrog, rhus-t, sabad, sal-ac, samb, sang, sars, sec, sel, sep, sil, spong, stann, staph, stram, sal-ac, sulph, tab, tarax, thuj, tub, valer, verat, verat-v, zinc, zinc-p.

- Daytime, during sleep: caust.
- Morning: acon, am-c, am-m, ars, bry, carb-v, caust, chin, chinin-s, dulc, ferr, fur-ar, mag-c, merc, nat-c, nat-m, nat-p, nit-ac, op, ph-ac, phos, puls, rhus-t, sep, sil.
  - Bed in: am-m, ferr.
  - Hot dry: cham, chin, op, phos.
  - Lasting all day: ferr.
  - Sleep during: chinin-s, puls.
  - Waking after: ferr, sep, sulph.
- Afternoon: fl-ac.
  - Heat, with: staph.
- Evening: bar-c, chel, con, fl-ac, samb, sars, sulph.
  - 19-1h, dry heat returns on going to sleep: samb.
  - Fever with high: con.
  - Lasting all night: bol-la.
  - Periodical every alternate evening: bar-c.
- Menses.
  - Before: hyos, thuj.
  - During: graph, hyos, murx, verat.
  - Beginning of, at the: bamb-a.
- Music, from: tarent.
- Periodical, night, alternate: bar-c, kali-n, nit-ac.
- Siesta during: caust, sel.
- Sitting quietly, while: kali-bi.
- Sleep, during: camph, carb-an, chin, chinin-s, con, dulc, merc, nat-c, op, phos, podo, thuj.
- Uncovered parts, except the head on: thuj.
- Waking, on: am-m, canth, chin, dros, ferr, lac-d, samb, sep, sulph.

- Walking, while: bry, canth, chinin-s, kali-c, merc, psor, sel, sep, sulph.
  - Air, in the open: caust, chin, lyc, ph-ac, rhod, sel, zinc.
  - Weather, warm: lyc.
  - Winter, during: carc.
- Rage, during: acon, ant-t, ars, bell, hyos, lyc, merc, nat-c, nat-m, nit-ac, nux-v, op, ph-ac, phos, puls, stram, verat.
- Sadness, from: calc-p.
- Salty deposits, after perspiration: sel.
- Sensation as if about to perspire, but no moisture appears: alum, am-c, bapt, borx, bov, calc, camph, cimx, croc, ferr, glon, ign, iod, nicc, phos, pop-c, puls, raph, sars, senec, stann, sul-ac, sulph, thuj, x-ray.
- Sexual excitement, with: lil-t.
- Single parts: acon, ambr, ars, ars-s-f, bar-c, bar-s, bell, bry, calc, calc-p, calc-sil, cann-s, caps, caust, cham, chin, con, hell, hep, ign, ip, led, lyc, merc, mez, nux-v, par, petr, plect, psor, puls, pyrog, rhus-t, sel, sep, sil, spig, spong, stann, sulph, thuj, tub, verat, zinc.
  - Side, lain on: acon, bell, bry, chin, nit-ac, nux-v, puls, sanic.
  - Side, not lain on: benz, thuj.
  - Front part of body: agar, ambr, anac, arg-met, arn, asar, bell, bov, calc, canth, cina, cocc, dros, euphr, graph, ip, kali-n, laur, merc, merc-c, nat-m, nux-v, phos, plb, rheum, rhus-t, ruta, sabad, sec, sel, sep, staph.
  - Lower part of body: am-c, am-m, apis, ars, asaf, aur, bry, calc, cinnb, cocc, coloc, con, croc, cycl, dros, euph, ferr, hyos, iod, kali-n, mang, merc, nit-ac, nux-v, phos, ran-a, sanic, sep, sil, thuj, zinc.
    - Touching each other, parts: nicc-s.
  - Upper part of body: acon, agar, anac, ant-t, arg-met, arn, asar, aza, bar-c, bell, berb, bov, calc, camph, canth, caps, carb-v, caust, cham, chin, cina, coc-c, dig, dulc, eup-per,

euphr, fl-ac, graph, guaj, ign, ip, kali-c, laur, mag-c, mag-m, mag-s, merc-c, mosch, mur-ac, nat-c, nit-ac, nux-v, op, par, petr, ph-ac, phos, plb, puls, ran-s, rheum, rhus-t, ruta, sabad, samb, sars, sec, sel, sep, sil, spig, stann, sul-ac, thuj, tub, valer, verat.

- Sleep, before: berb.
- Smoking: nat-m, thuj.
- Spots in: merc, ptel, tell.
- Staining, the linen: arn, ars, bar-c, bar-m, bell, benz-ac, calc, carb-an, carl, cham, chin, clem, dulc, graph, lac-c, lach, lyc, mag-c, med, merc, nux-m, nux-v, rheum, sel.
    - Bloody: anag, arn, ars, calc, cann-i, cham, chin, clem, cocc, crot-h, cur, dulc, hell, lach, lyc, merc, nux-m, nux-v, phos, sel.
      - Night agg: cur.
    - Blue: indg, iod, kali-i.
    - Brown: iod, nit-ac, sep, wies.
    - Brownish yellow: ars, bell, carb-an, graph, lac-c, lach, mag-c, sel, thuj.
    - Dark: bell.
    - Difficult to wash out: lac-d, mag-c, merc.
    - Green: agar, cupr.
    - Red: arn, calc, carb-v, cham, chin, clem, crot-h, dulc, ferr, gast, lach, lyc, nux-m, nux-v, thuj.
    - Yellow: ars, bell, ben-n, bry, cadn-s, carb-an, carl, chin, chinin-ar, crot-c, elat, ferr, ferr-ar, graph, guat, hep, ip, lac-c, lac-d, lach, mag-c, merc, rheum, sel, thuj, tub, verat.
    - White: sel.
- Sticky: sbies-c, agar, ant-t, anthraci, anthraco, ars, bamb-a, both, brom, cann-i, canth, caust, chlor, crot-h, ferr, fl-ac, hep, iod, kali-bi, kali-br, lach-n, op, phal, phos, plb, tab, tax.

- Evening: anthraco, fl-ac.
- Stiffening the linen: merc, nat-m, sel.
- Strangers, in the presence of: ambr, bar-c, lyc, sep, stram, thuj.
- Sudden: aml-ns, apis, ars, bell, carbn-s, clem, crot-h, hyos, ip, merc-cy, valer.
  - Afternoon: clem.
  - Disappearing suddenly, and: bell.
  - Walking in the open air with chilliness while: led.
- Symptoms.
  - Aggravated during perspiration: acon, ant-t, arn, ars, calc, calc-i, caust, cham, chin, chinin-ar, cimx, cinnb, cist, croc, eup-per, euphr, ferr, ferr-ar, form, ign, ip, kali-ar, lyc, med, merc, mur-ar, nat-ar, nat-c, nux-v, op, phos, psor, puls, rhod, rhus-t, sep, spong, stram, sulph, verat, wye.
  - After perspiration: acon, ant-t, calc, cham, chin, con, ip, merc, ph-ac, phos, puls, sep, sil, staph, sulph.
  - Amel, during perspiration: acon, aesc, aeth, apis, ars, bapt, bell, bov, bry, calad, camph, canth, chan, chinin-s, cimx, clem, cupr, elat, eup-per, gels, graph, hep, lach, lyc, nat-m, psor, rhus-t, samb, sec, stront-c, thuj, verat.
    - Headache except the: nat-m.
    - Which is aggravated: ars, chinin-s, eup-per.
- Talking: ambr, gink-b, graph, iod, sil, sulph.
  - Public, in: bamb-a.
- Taste, salty: nat-m, sel.
- Thighs, except: lyc.
- Uncovered parts, on: bell, puls, thuj.
- Vexation, after: acon, bry, cham, lyc, petr, sep, staph, verat.

- Warm: acon, ant-c, asar, ben, camph, carb-v, cham, cocc, dig, dros, ign, kali-c, kreos, lach, led, nat-m, nux-v, op, phos, puls, sep, sil, staph, stram, thuj, verat.
  - Convulsions with: sil.
  - Epilepsy after: sil.
  - Evening: anac, puls.
  - Hot exertion from: limest-b.
  - Morning alternate: ant-c.
  - Night: staph, thuj.
  - Periodical: carb-v.
  - Room: carb-v, cist.
  - Sitting, in: asar.
  - Somnolence, with: op.
  - Stool; becomes cold & sticky after: merc.
  - Unbearable: plan.
  - Uneasiness, causing: calc, cham, nux-v, puls, sep, sulph.
  - Waking amel: thuj.
- Wash off, difficult to: merc, mag-c, lac-d, sep.
- Washing amel.: thuj.
- Wind, aggravates, cold: cur.
- Writing, while: borx, hep, kali-c, psor, sep, sulph, tub.

Location

- **Head, scalp:** aesc, agar, anph, anac, ant-t, apis, ars-i, bamb-a, bar-c, bar-i, bar-m, bar-s, bell, benz-ac, borx, bov, bufo, calc, calc-i, calc-p, calc-s, calc-sil, camph, carb-v, carbn-s, caust, cham, chin, cimx, clem, cycl, dig, eup-pur, gamb, glon, graph, grat, guaj, hep, iod, ip, kali-c, kali-m, kali-p, kali-sil, kali-s, laur, led, lyc, mag-c, mag-m, merc, mez, mosch, mur-ac, nat-m, nit-ac, nux-v, ol-m, olnd, op, petr, ph-ac, phel, phos, plb, psor, puls, pyrog, rheum, sabad, sep, sil, spig, staph, stram, stry, sul-i, sulph, tab, tarent, thuj, valer, verat-v, zinc, zinc-p.

- Daytime: ol-an, stram.
  - And night: sulph.
- Morning: bamb-c, calc, cann-s, dulc, hep, mez, nat-m, nux-v, sep.
- Rising on: nat-m.
- Forenoon: mag-c.
- Afternoon: bamb-a.
- Evening: anac, bar-c, calc, mag-m, mur-ac, sep, sil.
  - Lying down, after: petr.
- Night: bov, bry, calc, carb-an, chin, coloc, hep, hydrog, kali-c, merc, nat-m, nit-ac, rhus-t, sanic, sep, sil.
  - Midnight: ph-ac, rhus-t.
- Bed in: bry.
- Breakfast, after: par.
- Chill after: sulph.
- Clammy: cham, merc, nux-v.
- Cold: acon, ant-t, benz-ac, bry, bufo, calc, camph, carb-v, cina, cocc, con, dig, hep, lob, merc, merc-c, nux-v, op, petr, phos, podo, tub, verat.
  - Air in: calc.
  - Room in: calc.
- Coughing, on: ant-t, calc, ip, merc, sil, tarent.
- Eating, while: calc, nux-v, petr.
- Epilepsy, before: caust.
- Except the head: bell, merc, mur-ac, nux-v, rhus-t, samb, sec, sep, thuj.
- Excitement, with: bamb-a.
- Fetid: calc, merc, puls, staph.
  - One side: nux-v, puls.
- Headache, with: bamb-a, calc, mez, phys, sil, sulph.

- Heat, during: sep.
- Honey, smelling like: thuj.
- Hot: calc, cham, cimic, con, op, podo.
- Menses, during: cham, merc, phos, verat.
- Mental exertion: kali-c, kali-p, ph-ac, ran-b.
- Musk like odor: apis, sulph.
- Musty: nat-m.
- Oily: bry, hura, merc.
- Only the head: acon, am-m, calc, cham, kali-m, phos, puls, rheum, sabad, sanic, sep, sil, spig, stann.
- Painful part: sil.
- Reading while: nat-s.
- Sensation as if: gink-b.
- Sleep.
    - During: bamb-a, bry, calc, calc-p, cham, cic, lyc, merc, podo, sanic, sep, sil.
    - Falling asleep, on: graph, sep, sil, tarax.
- Soup after: phos, rheum.
- Sour: bry, cham, hep, merc, rheum, sep, sil.
- Stool during: ptel.
- Uncovered parts: thuj.
- Waking on: ph-ac.
- Walking after: calc, carb-v, merc.
    - Air in open: borx, calc, chin, graph, guaj, phos, thuj.
- Washing after: graph.
- Forehead: acet-ac, acon, aeth, agar, aml-ns, anag, ant-t, ars, ars-i, asaf, bapt, bell, brom, bry, cact, calc, calc-i, calc-sil, camph, cann-i, carb-v, chin, cic, cupr, guaj, hep, ip, kali-bi, kali-c, laur, led, merc-c, nat-ar, nat-c, nit-ac, op, phos, ran-s, sars, stann, sulph, tab, valer, verat, vesp, zinc.

- Morning: ambr, ang, dios, kali-c, nux-v, phys, stann, staph.

- Noon: ferr-i, nat-m, valer.

- Evening: anac, carb-v, chin, ol-an, puls, ran-b, sars, senec.

- Night: bry, calc, cann-s, chin, crot-t, sacch.

- Anxiety, as from: nux-v, verat.

- Burning: nat-c.

- Chill, during: acon, bry, calc, chin, cina, dig, led, nat-s.

- Clammy: acet-ac, acon, carb-an, cina, colch, hep, op.

- Cold: acet-ac, acon, ars, bell, bry, cact, calc, canth, caps, carb-v, chin, cina, cocc, colch, croc, cupr, dig, dros, gels, glon, hell, hep, ip, kali-bi, kali-p, lach, laur, merc, op, phyt, plb, sec, staph, sulph, tab, verat, zinc.

  - Icy cold: lachn.

- Cough during: ant-t, ars-s-f, ip, verat.

- Diarrhoea, during: sulph.

- Easy: rheum.

- Eating, while: carb-v, nit-ac, nux-v, sul-ac, sulph.

- Fever, during: ant-t, cann-i, dig, ip, mag-s, sars, staph, verat.

- Greasy: coloc, hydr, psor.

- Headache, during: cist, glon, kali-c, ph-ac, phyt, sulph.

- Hot: cham, chin.

- Menses, during: phos, verat.

- Motion, during: valer.

- Offensive: led, sil.

- Sleep, during: cham.

- Sour: led.

- Sticky: cann-i, cham, cocc.

- Stool after: crot-t, ip, merc, nat-c, verat.
- Storm, during approach of a: nat-c.
- Vomiting: ant-c, mag-c, phos.
- Walking in open air while: guaj, led, merc, nux-v.
- Warm: acon, act-sp, anac, camph, cham, glon, phys, psil, puls.
- Occiput: anac, ars, bamb-a, calc, chin, ferr, mag-c, mosch, nit-ac, nux-v, ph-ac, sanic, sep, sil, spig, stann, sulph.
  - Sleep during: sanic.
  - Walking while: sulph.
- Sides.
  - One side: ambr, bar-c, nit-ac, nux-v, puls, sulph.
  - Painless side: aur-m-n.
- Temples: ars-s-f, crot-c.
  - Cough agg.: ars-s-f.
- Vertex: ruta.
- **Eyebrows and eyelids:** calc-p.
- **Ears:** calc, olnd, puls, zinc.
  - Behind the ears: cimic.
- **Nose:** bell, cimx, cina, cinnb, laur, nat-m, rheum, ruta, teucr, tub.
  - Morning: cimx.
  - Cold, around nose: chin, rheum.
- **Face:** acet-ac, acon, aesc, aeth, agar, alum, alum-p, am-c, am-m, ambr, amyg, ant-t, apis, arg-met, arg-n, arn, ars, ars-h, aur, aur-ar, aur-s, bamb-a, bapt, bell, benz-ac, borx, bry, calc, calc-p, calc-s, calc-sil, camph, caps, carb-ac, carb-an, carb-v, carbn-s, cham, chin, chinin-ar, chion, cic, cina, cocc, colch, coloc, con, crot-h, cupr, cupr-s, dig, dros, dulc, elaps, ferr, ferr-ar, ferr-p, fl-ac, glon, guaj, hell, hep, hydr-ac, hyos, ign, ip, jab, kali-ar, kali-bi, kali-c, kali-i, kali-m, kali-p, kali-s, kali-sil, kreos, lach,

lachn, laur, lyc, lyss, mag-c, med, merc, mez, morph, mosch, mur-ac, nat-c, nat-m, nat-s, nux-v, ol-an, op, ox-ac, par, petr, phos, psor, puls, rheum, rhus-t, sabad, samb, sars, sec, sep, sil, spig, spong, stann, staph, stram, stry, sul-ac, sulph, tab, tarent, tell, thuj, til, valer, verat, verat-v, vip.

- Right: alum, puls.
- One side: alum, ambr, bar-c, nux-v, puls, sulph.
- Morning: ars, bamb-a, chin, nit-ac, puls, ruta, sulph, verat.
- Forenoon: phos.
- Noon: cic.
- Afternoon: bamb-a, con, ign, samb.
  - 16 hours: bamb-a
- Evening: hura, psor, puls, sars, spong.
  - House, in: mez.
- Night: dros, hep, sulph.
  - Midnight: plat, rhus-t.
  - 2 hour: ars.
- Anxiety, with: nat-c.
- Bee sting, from: sep.
- Cold: acon, aeth, agar, ant-c, ant-t, aur, ars, ars-s-f, aur, aur-ar, aur-s, bell, benz-ac, bry, cact, cadm-s, calc, çalc-p, calc-s, camph, caps, carb-ac, carb-an, carb-v, carbn-s, chin, chinin-ar, cina, coc-c, cocc, crot-h, cupr, dig, dros, euph-l, ferr, glon, hell, hep, hura, ip, kali-bi, lach, lachn, lob, lyc, merc, merc-c, morph, mur-ac, nat-m, nux-v, op, ox-ac, phos, plat, puls, pyrog, rheum, rhus-t, ruta, sabad, samb, sec, sep, spig, spong, staph, stram, sul-ac, sulph, tab, verat, verat-v, zinc-m.
  - Diarrhoea: apoc.
  - Forehead: acet-ac.
  - Mouth around: chin, rheum.
- Convulsions, during: cocc.

- Coughing, when: tarent.
- Dinner, during: carb-an.
  - After: sulph.
- Drinking, after: cham.
- Eating: ign, ham, sulph.
  - After: alum, cham, nat-s, psor, viol-t.
  - Warm food: mag-c, sep.
- Eructations during: cadm-s.
- Exertion, after: sil.
  - Slightest exertion, from: bamb-a, sulph.
- Except the face: rhus-t, sec.
- Eyes, under: con.
- Flatus, when passing: kali-bi.
- Heat, during: alum, ars, bell, cham, chel, dros, dulc, lach, psor, puls, sep, spong, valer.
- Lips.
  - Lower: rheum.
  - Upper: acon, coff, kali-bi, kali-c, med, nux-v, rheum, sin-n, thuj.
- Motion during: psor, valer.
- Offensive: puls.
- Only face: calc, con, ign, phos.
- Palpitation: ars.
- Scalp, and: puls, valer, verat.
- Side.
  - Lain on: acon, act-sp, chin .
  - Not lain on: sil, thuj.
- Sitting, while: calc.
- Sleep.
  - Before: calc.

- During: med, prun, sep, tab .
- Going to sleep, on: sil.
- Spots on, eating, during: ign.
- Standing: eupi.
- Stool, after: com.
- Supper, during: calc.
- Waking, on: bamb-a, puls.
- Walking: borx, valer, verat.
  - Air open: guaj.
- Warm food & drink: Sep, sul-ac.

- **Stomach,** pit of, at: bell, borx, hyos, kali-n, nux-v, ol-an, sec.
- **Abdomen:** ambr, anac, arg-met, arg-met, arg-n, caust, cic, cocc, dros, merc, phos, plb, rhus-t, sel, staph, sulph, thuj.
  - Forenoon: arg-met.
  - Night: anac, cic, dros, staph, sulph and chest, on abdomen: arg-met, cocc, phos, sel.
  - Coition after: agar.
  - Cold: dros.
  - Exercise during: ambr.
  - Heat during: arg-met.
  - Walking after: caust.
  - Hypochondria: caust, conv, ign, iris, verat.
  - Hypogastrium, while sitting: sel.
  - Inguinal region: ambr, canth, iris, sel, sep, thuj.
  - Umbilicus, spreading from: rhus-t.
- **Anus and perineum:** agar, alum, bell, brass-n-o, carb-an, chin-b, con, hep, kali-c, psor, rhus-t, thuj.
  - Morning: thuj.
  - Night: kali-c.

- Stool before & during: sep.
- Acrid: arum-t.
- **Male genitalia:** acet-ac, agn, alum, alum-p, am-c, ars, ars-i, ars-s-f, asc-t, aur, aur-ar, aur-i, aur-s, bar-c, bell, calad, calc, canth, carb-an, carb-v, carbn-s, carl, con, cor-r, fl-ac, gels, hep, hydr, ign, iod, lachn, lyc, mag-m, merc-i-f, merc, mez, petr, ph-ac, puls, sel, sep, sil, staph, sulph, thuj.
  - Morning: aur.
  - Evening: carbn-s.
  - Night: bell.
  - Burnt smells as if: thuj.
  - Cold: carb-v.
  - Exertion after: sep.
  - Offensive: aloe, ars-met, calc-sil, fago, fl-ac, hydr, iod, nat-m, psor, sars, sep, sulph.
    - Pungent smell as if: dios, fl-ac .
    - Sweetish smell as if: thuj.
  - Penis: lachn, nat-m, nit-ac, thuj.
  - Scrotum: acon, agn, alum-sil, am-c, aur, aur-s, bar-c, bar-s, bell, calad, calc, calc-p, calc-sil, carb-an, carb-v, carbn-s, caust, con, cupr-act, daph, dios, gels, ham, hep, hydr, ign, iod, lachn, lyc, mag-m, merc, mez, nat-s, petr, psor, rhod, sel, sep, sil, staph, sul-i, sulph, thuj, ust.
    - One side: thuj.
    - Morning: thuj, ust.
    - Evening: nat-s, sil.
    - Night: ham, mag-m.
    - Strong odor: dios.
    - Sweetish odor: thuj.
    - Thighs between: cinnb.

- **Female genitalia:** carb-v, gink-b, lyc, merc, petr, sel, thuj.
  - Offensive: Sulph.
- **Chest:** agar, anac, ant-t, arg-met, arn, asar, bamb-a, bell, ben, bov, calc, calc-p, calc-sil, canth, cedr, chel, cocc, crot-c, dros, euphr, glon, graph, hep, ip, kali-n, lyc, merc, merc-c, nit-ac, op, petr, ph-ac, phos, plb, rhus-t, sabad, sec, sel, seneg, sep, sil, spig, stry, tab, thuj, verat.
  - Daytime: petr.
  - Morning: bamb-a, bov, cocc, graph, kali-n.
  - Forenoon: arg-n.
  - Afternoon, 17-21 hours: chel.
  - Evening, walking, while: chin, sabad.
  - Night: agar, anac, arg-met, arg-n, bamb-a, bar-c, bell, calc, kali-c, nit-ac, sep, sil, stann, sulph.
    - Midnight: nat-m, ph-ac.
      - After: lyc.
      - 4 hours: sep.
      - 5-6 hours: bov.
    - Sleep: euphr.
    - Waking, on: canth.
  - Abdomen & chest, only on: arg-met, cocc, phos, sel.
  - Axilla: all-c, aloe, asaf, asar, bov, bry, cadm-s, calc, caps, carb-ac, carb-an, carb-v, carbn-s, carc, cedr, chel, cur, dulc, gink-b, gymno, hep, hydr. hyos, kali, kali-p, kali-s, lac-c, lach, lappa, lour, lil-t, merc-c, nat-m, nit-ac, ox-ac, petr, phos, psil, rhod, sabad, sanic, sel, sep, sil, squil, sul-ac, sulph, tab, tell, thuj, tub, verat, viol-f, zinc.
    - Daytime: dulc.
    - Evening: sabad.
    - Night: sulph.
    - Acrid: sanic.

- Brown: lac-c, thuj.
- Cold: lappa.
- Coldness during: tab.
- Cold air in: bov.
- Copious: sanic, sel.
- Eat holes in the linen: iod, psor, sep, sil.
- Frosty deposit in the hair, with: sel, thuj.
- Garlic, like: bov, kali-p, lach, osm, sulph, tell.
- Heat during: zinc.
- Offensive: apis, bov, carb-ac, con, dulc, gink-b, hep, hydr, lac-c, lach, lyc, merc-c, nit-ac, nux-m, osm, petr, phos, rhod, sel, sep, sil, sulph, tell, thuj, tub.
    - Menses
        - During: stram, tell.
        - Between: sep.
- Onions: bov.
- Red: arn, carb-v, dulc, lach, nux-m, nux-v, thuj.
- Sour smelling: asar.
- Yellow: lac-c.
- Chilliness during: sep.
- Coition after: agar.
- Cold: agar, camph, canth, hep, cocc, lyc, merc, petr, seneg, sep, stann.
- Mammae: arg-met, arn, bov, calc, hep, kali-n, lyc, plb, rhus-t, sel, sep.
    - Between, fetid: nux-m.
    - Morning: bov, cocc, graph, kali-n.
    - Night: agar, bar-c, calc, kali-c, lyc, sil, stann, sulph.
- Menses during: bell, kreos.
- Offensive: arn, carc, euphr, graph, hep, lyc, phos, sel, sep.
- Oily: arg-met.

- Profuse: carc.
- Red: arn.
- Sternum: graph .
    - Morning: graph.
- Walking rapidly: nit-ac.
- **Back:** acon, anac, ars, ars-s-f, bufo, calc, calc-s, calc-sil, camph, casc, caust, chin, chinin-s, coff, dig, dulc, ferr, guaj, hep, hyos, ip, kali-bi, lac-c, lach, laur, led, lyc, morph, mur-ac, nat-c, nat-p, nit-ac, nux-v, par, petr, ph-ac, phos, puls, rhus-t, sabin, sep, sil, stann, stram, sulph.
    - Daytime while at rest: petr.
    - Morning: chim.
    - Evening: mur-ac.
    - Night: anac, ars, calc, coc-c, coff, guaj, lyc, sep, sil.
        - Midnight after: hep.
        - 3 hours: rhus-t.
        - 4 hours waking at: petr.
    - Cervical region: anac, ars, calc, calc-sil, cann-s, chel, chin, elaps, ferr, fl-ac, mag-c, med, mosch, nit-ac, nux-v, ph-ac, phel, sep, sil, spig, stann, sulph.
        - Daytime: ph-ac.
        - Morning: nux-v, stann, sulph.
        - Evening: fl-ac.
        - Night: calc, sulph.
        - Menses, before: nit-ac.
        - Motion, least: chin.
        - Sleep
            - Amel: samb.
            - In: calc, lach, ph-ac, phos, sanic.
            - Walking: camph.
        - Chill during: cann-s.

-    Cold: acon, chin, colch, cub, ph-ac, sep.
-    Cough, during and after: cub.
-    Eating, after: card-m, par.
-    Emissions, after: sil.
-   Lumbar: asaf, brass-n-o, clem, hyos, sil .
  -    Night: sil.
  -    Cold: plan.
  -    Menses, before: nit-ac.
-   Menses.
  -    Before: nit-ac.
  -    During: kreos.
-   Motion, on: chin.
-   Sacrum: plan.
  -    Cold: plan.
-   Sleep, during: tab.
-   Stool, during effort at: kali-bi.
-   Waking, on: hep.
-   Walking, on: caust, lac-ac, lach, nat-c, petr, phos, rhus-t, sep.
  -    Rapidly: nit-ac.
- **Extremities:** aur, aur-m, carb-v, con, cupr, glon, lac-ac, ol-j, op, plb, stram.
  -    Left arm & left leg: lac-d.
  -    Morning: carb-v, con.
  -    Night: calc, carl, con, kali-n.
  -    Clammy: ars, cact, chinin-s, lil-t, merc-c, nux-m, op, phos, plb, tab.
    -    Menses should appear, when: lil-t.
  -    Cold: ars, asaf, aur, aur-m, bell, cact, calc-sel, canth, dros, lach, lachn, merc-c, morph, ox-ac, phos, sec, spong, stram, tab, verat, verat-v.

- Menses during: ars, phos, sec, verat.
- Stool during: gamb.
- Paralyzed limb: ars, caust, cocc, merc, rhus-t, stann.
- Joints: Am-c, ars, bell, bry, calc, dros, led, lyc, mang, nux-v, ph-ac, rhus-t, sars, stann, sulph.
  - Elbow, flexure of: sep.
  - Morning: am-c, lyc.
  - Cold: rhus-t.
  - Only: am-c, ars, bell, bry, calc, dros, led, lyc, mang, nux-v, ph-ac, rhus-t, stann, sulph.
  - Painful: am-c, lyc.
  - Bends of: carc, sep, zinc.
    - Morning: lyc.
    - Night: sars.
- Lower limbs: ars, asaf, borx, calc, coc-c, coloc, con, croc, hep, hyos, kali-n, mang, merc, nux-v, phos, rhod, sec, sep, ter verat, zinc, zinc-p.
  - Morning: lyc.
    - Bed in: rhod.
      - Waking after: con, sep.
    - Evening.
      - In bed: ter.
    - Night: am-c, ars, calc, coloc, con, kali-n, mang, merc, rumx, ter, zinc.
    - Except the lower limbs: lyc.
    - Fetid: phos.

Foot: scon, am-c, am-m, ang, apis, arn, ars, ars-i, bar-c, bar-i, bar-n, bell, benz-ac, brom, bry, calc, calc-i, calc-s, camph, cann-s, canth, carb-an, carb-v, carbn-s, carc, caust, cham, chel, coc-c, cocc, coff, coloc, croc, cupr, cycl, dros, euph, fago, fl-ac, graph, hell, hep, hura, hyper, ind, iod, ip, jab, kali-ar, kali-bi, kali-m, kali-p, kali-s, kalm, kreos, lac-ac, lach, lact, led, lyc, mag-m, mang, med, merc, mez, mur-ac, naja, nat-ar, nat-c, nat-m, nat-p, nit-ac, ox-ac, petr, ph-ac, phos, phyt, pic-ac, plb, podo, psor, puls, rhus-t, sabad, sabin, sanic, sec, sel, sep, sil, squil, staph, sul-i, sulph, tarent, thuj, verat, zinc, zinc-p.

- Left: cham, nit-ac.
- Right: plect, sulph.
- Daytime: pic-ac.
  - Morning: am-m, bry, coc-c, euphr, lyc, merc, sulph.
- Bed in: bry, lach, merc, phos, puls, sabin.
- Rising after: am-m.
- Forenoon: fago.
- Afternoon: graph, lac-ac, plect.
- Evening: calc, coc-c, cocc, graph, mur-ac, pic-ac, podo.
- Bed in: calc, clem, mur-ac.
- Night: coloc, mang, merc, nit-ac, staph, sulph, thuj.
- Midnight, before 2-3 hours: hura.
- After 2 hours: ars.
- Waking on: mang.
- Back of: iod.
- Burning, with: calc, lyc, mur-ac, petr, sep, sulph, thuj.
- Carrion, like: sil.
- Chill, during: cann-s.
- Clammy: acon, calc, cann-i, pic-ac, sep, sulph.
- Cold: acon, ars, ars-i, ars-s-f, bar-c, bell, benz-ac, calc, calc-p, calc-s, calc-sil, canth, carb-v, carbn-s, caust, cimic, cocc, cupr, dig, dros, fago, graph, hep, hura, ind, ip, kali-c, kali-m, kali-p, kali-s, laur, lil-t, lyc, mang-m, med, merc, mez, mur-ac, nit-ac, ox-ac, phos, pic-ac, plb, psor, puls, sanic, sec, sep, sil, squil, staph, stram, sulph, thuj, verat.

- Room: calc.
- Constant: sil, thuj.
- Diarrhea, during: sulph.
- Except the feet: chin, phos.
- Excoriating: bar-c, calc, carb-v, coff, fl-ac, graph, hell, iod, lyc, nit-ac, ran-b, sanic, sec, sep, sil, squil, zinc.
- Destroys shoes: sil.
- Heat during: ars.
- Heel: ol-an, phos, thuj.
- Injuries of spine in: nit-ac.
- Leather, like sole: cob.
- Menses, before & during: calc.
- During, from severity of pain: verat.
- After: calc, lil-t, sep, sil.
- Offensive: am-c, am-m, anan, arg-n, ars, ars-i, ars-s-f, arund, bamb-a, bar-c, bar-s, bufo, but-ac, calc, calc-s, carb-ac, carbn-s, carc, chlol, cob, coloc, cycl, fl-ac, graph, kali-c, kali-sil, kalm, lyc, nat-m, nit-ac, petr, phos, plb, psor, puls, rhus-t, sanic, sec, sep, sil, staph, sulph, tell, thuj, zinc, zinc-p.
- Profuse: ars, arund, but-ac, carb-an, carb-v, carbn-s, carc, cench, cham, coloc, fl-ac, graph, ind, ip, kali-c, kreos, lac-ac, lach, lyc, merc, naja, nit-ac, petr, phyt, psor, puls, sabad, sal-ac, sanic, sep, sec, sil, staph, sulph, thuj, zinc.
- Rotten eggs: staph.
- Sitting while: bell.
- Sole: acon, am-m, arn, calc, chel, fago, fl-ac, hell, kali-c, maland, merc, nat-m, nit-ac, nux-m, petr, plb, puls, sabad, sil, sulph.
- Cold: acon, sulph.
- Itching: sil, sulph.
- Making sole raw: bar-c, calc, nit-ac, sil.

- Offensive: petr, plb, sil.
- Sour: calc, calc-sil, cob, nat-m, nit-ac, sil.
- Evening: sil.
- Sticky: calc, kali-c, lyc, sanic.
- Stool after: sulph.
- Suppressed: am-c, apis, ars, bad, bar-c, bar-m, bar-s, cham, coch, colch, cupr, form, graph, haen, kali-c, lyc, merc, nat-c, nat-n, nit-ac, ol-an, ph-ac, phos, plb, puls, rhus-t, sal-ac, sel, sep, sil, sulph, thuj, zinc, zinc-p, swelling of feet, with graph, iod, kali-c, kreos, lyc, petr, ph-ac, plb, sabad.
- Urine, like: canth, coloc.
- Waking on: mang.
- Walking while: carb-v, graph, nat-c.
- Warm: led.
- Winter, during, agg.: arg-n, med.
- Knee: am-c, ars, bry, calc, clem, dros, led, lyc, plb, sep, spong, sulph.
- Night: ars, carb-an.
- Circumscribed: clem.
- Cold: ars.
- Fever, after: plb.
- Swelling with: lyc.
- Popliteus: bry, bufo, carb-an, con, dros, ign, sep.
- Leg: agar, am-c, ars, bry, calc, calc-p, caps, coc-c, coloc, euph, hyos, kali-bi, mang, merc, mez, nux-v, petr, podo, psor, puls, rhod, rumx, sep, stram, sulph, thuj, til.
- Right: coc-c.
- Morning: ars, euph, sulph.
- Waking on: coloc.
- 5 hours: sulph.

- Evening, in bed: agar, ter.
- Night: agar, am-c, calc, coloc, kali-bi, mang, merc, rumx, sulph, thuj.
- Clammy: rumx.
- Cold: caps, euph, merc, phos, psor, thuj .
- Except the legs: lyc.
- Fetid: phos.
- Inner surface: agar.
- Sticky: calc.
- Menses during: calc, lil-t.
- Menstrual colic during: ant-t.
- Nates: thuj.
- Paralyzed limbs: stram.
- Thigh: acon, ambr, ars, borx, caps, carb-an, coloc, crot-t, dros, eup-pur, euph, hep, hyos, kali-bi, merc, nux-v, ran-g, rhus-t, sep, sulph, thuj.
- Morning: ruph, rhus-t, thuj.
- Night: carb-an, coloc, merc, sep.
- Midnight after: ars, nux-v.
- Cold: crot-t, merc, sep.
- Except the thigh: lyc.
- Sleep, at beginning of: ars.
- Spots in: caps.
- Walking in open air: caps.
- Sensation of: caps.
- Between: aur, cinn-b, hep, nux-v.
- Morning: carb-an, nux-v.
- Night: aur, carb-an.
- Corrosive: cinnb.

- Offensive: cinnb.
- Walking while: ambr, cinnb.
- Inner surface of: sulph, thuj.
- Near genitals: thuj.
- Male genitals: crot-t.
- Offensive: crot-t.
- Toes: acon, arn, clem, kali-c, lach, phyt, puls, sep, sil, squil, tell, thuj, zinc.
- Between: acon, anac, arn, bar-c, carb-v, clem, cob, cupr, cycl, ferr, fl-ac, kali-c, kali-sil, lyc, nit-ac, puls, sep, sil, squil, tarax, thuj, zinc.
- Evening: cem.
- Offensive: bar-c, cob, cycl, fl-ac, kali-c, lyc, nit-ac, puls, sep, sil, thuj, zinc.
- Rawness causing: bar-c, carb-v, fl-ac, graph, nit-ac, panic, sep, sil, zinc .
- Morning in bed: lach.
- Under toes: phyt, tarax.
- Walking while: graph.
- Upper limbs: agar, asaf, asar, bry, caps, guave, hyos, ip, jab, merc, petr, ph-ac, stann, stront, zinc.
- Night: ol-j.
- Coition after: agar.
- Cold & clammy: cinc.
- Fingers: agn, ant-c, bar-c, carb-v, ign, rhod, sulph.
- Between: sulph.
- Tips: carb-m, carb-v, phos, sep, sulph.
- Forearm: petr.
- **Hand:** acon, agn, ambr, aml-ns, anac, ant-t, ars, ars-i, bamb-a, bar-c, bar-i, bar-s, bell, brom, calc, calc-i, calc-s, camph, canth,

caps, carb-v, carbn-o, carbn-s, caust, chan, chel, cina, cit-v, cocc, coff, coloc, con, cupr, dig, dirc, dulc, fago, ferr, fl-ac, glon, graph, guave, hell, hep, hura, ign, iod, ip, kali-bi, kreos, lac-ac, laur, led, lith-c, lyc, marb-w, merc, merc-c, naja, nat-ar, nat-c, nat-m, nat-p, nit-ac, nux-v, oena, ol-m, op, osc-ac, petr, ph-ac, phel, phos, phys, pic-ac, puls, pyrus, rhod, rhus-t, sanic, sars, sep, sil, spig, stict, sul-i, sulph, syph, tab, thuj, tub, verat, zinc, zinc-p.

- Daytime: nit-ac, ol-an, pic-ac.

- Morning: lyc, phos, puls, sulph.

- Bed in: phos.

- Rising after: puls.

- Forenoon: fago.

- Noon until evening, daily: lac-ac.

- Afternoon: bar-c.

- Evening: glon, ign, sulph.

- Lying down before: sulph.

- Night: coloc.

- Air, open: agn.

- Alternately in one or the other: cocc.

- Anxiety with, accompanied by trembling hand: granit-m.

- Back of hand: lil-t, lith-c.

- Cold: lil-t, chion, zinc-s.

- Exercising while: thuj.

- Between the fingers: sulph.

- Chill during: eup-per, ip, puls.

- Clammy: anac, ars, carb-ac, ind, lyc, merc, nux-v, phos, pic-ac, plan, pyrog, spig, sulph, zinc.

- Cold: acon, ambr, ant-c, ant-t, ars, ars-i, ars-s-f, atro, bell, brom, calc, calc-s, calc-sil, canth, caps, carb-ac, cham, cimic, cina, cocc, ferr, hep, iod, ip, kali-bi, kali-cy, lach,

kali-sil, lyc, lil-t, merc-c, morph, nit-ac, nux-v, osc-ac, petr,
ph-ac, phos, phyt, pic-ac, plb, psor, rheum, rhus-t, sanic,
sars, sec, sep, spig, sulph, tab, thuj, tub, verat, verat-v, zinc,
zinc-p.

- Warm room in: ambr.
- Coldness, during internal: tab.
- Cold nose, with: nux-v.
- Copious: bamb-a, ip, kali-sil, naja, nat-c, nit-ac, sil.
- Coughing, on: ant-t.
- Dysmenorrhea: tarent.
- Excitement, from: bamb-a.
- Exhausting: nat-c.
- Heat, with: nit-ac.
- Injuries of the spine: nit-ac.
- Itching, with: sulph.
- Migraine, during: calc.
- Offensive: calc-s, coloc, hep, nit-ac.
- Only on: agn, verat.
- Ophthalmia: brom, card-s, calc, con, dulc, fl-ac, gymno,
  ind, iod, led, petr, sulph.

- **Palm:** acon, agar, all-c, all-s, am-m, aml-ns, anac, ant-t, bar-c,
  bar-i, bar-s, brom, bry, cadm-s, calc, calc-i, calc-p, camph, cann-
  i, caps, carb-v, caust, cench, chan chel, coff, con, dig, dulc,
  fago, ferr, fl-ac, glon granit-m, gymno, hell, hep, hyos, ign,
  ind, iod, jatr-c, kali-c, kali-s, kali-sil, kreos, laur, led, lib-t, lob,
  lyc, manc, merc, naja, nat-m, nit-ac, nux-v, petr, phos, psor,
  rheum, rhus-t, sep, sil, spig, sulph, tab, tarent, tub.

- Daytime: dulc.
- Morning: am-m.
- Afternoon: bar-c.
- Evening: tab.

- Night: psor.
- Midnight after: merc.
- Clammy: anac, coff, spig.
- Cold: acon, calc-sil, cham, coff, con, hydrog, nux-v, rheum, spig, sul-i, tub, zinc-i.
- Coldness, during: gran.
- Back; during coldness on: all-c.
- Back of hand, with coldness of: hell.
- Cough during: naja.
- Exertion on: calc, psor.
- Pressed together when: rheum.
- Room in: caust.
- Soup, after: phos.
- Walking in open air: nux-v, rhus-t.
- Prolapsus uteri: lil-t.
- Rising on: am-m, fago.
- Sitting, while: calc.
- Sleep on going to: ars.
- Stool, after: sulph.
- Sulphur, odor of: coloc.
- Walking in open air: agn.
- Writing while: coff.
- Inner side of upper limbs: arn.
- Shoulder: chin.
- Coition after: agar.
- Under, dinner amel: phos.
- Wrist: petr, syph.

Chapter-36

Some of the Homeopathic Medicines for Diseases of Skin

ACETICUM ACIDUM

Look of the skin

Pale, waxen appearance of the skin.

On examination

Dry, hot skin or bathed in profuse sweat.

Ailments from

Grief.

Emotional excitement.

Sphere of action

Legs, joints.

Pathology

Condylomata, excrescences, herpetic, gangrene, ulcers, warts, scurvy.

Modalities

General

Agg.: Night, lying on the back.

Amel.: After eating, lying on abdomen.

Particular

Agg.: Cold.

Discharge

Moist.

Eruptions

- Desquamating.
- Condylomata: Flat.
- Ulcers: Bleeding.
- Warts: Flat.

Itching

Burning after scratching.

Sensation

Burning.

Concomitants

Mentals

Irritable.

Worried about business affairs.

Generals

Family history of tuberculosis.

Wasting and debility.

Pale, lean persons with lax, flabby muscles.

ALUMINA

Look of the skin
Chapped and dry tettery appearance of the skin.

On examination
Chapped skin.

Ailments from
Anger with anxiety.

Anger with silent grief.

Anticipation.

Bad news.

Celibacy.

Disappointment.

Hurry.

Mortification.

Scorned being.

Surprises.

Sphere of action
Fingers, extremities.

Pathology
Acne; blisters; cracks; cicatrices; eczema; herpes; impetigo; psoriasis; scabies; lupus; vitiligo; urticaria; ulcers; warts; gangrene.

Modalities
General
Agg.: Periodically, afternoon, from potatoes, morning on awaking, warm room.

Amel.: Open air, from cold washing, evening and alternate days, damp weather

Particular

Eruptions   - < Warmth of bed, < Winter.

Itching   - < Warmth, < Warmth of bed, < Scratching,
                    > Scratching, > Evening in bed.

Discharge

Moist, yellow discharge; scratching.

Eruptions

Bleeding, coppery, crusty, burn, phagedenic, painful, scaly; bran like, worse after scratching, suppurated, vesicular and confluent.

- Acne: Sore as if excoriated, stinging.
- Cicatrices: Itching.
- Cracks: Deep, bloody, washing after, in winter.
- Herpes: Burn, chapping, corrosive, crusty, dry, itching, moist, spreading, stinging, suppurated.
- Scabies: Suppurated.
- Urticaria: Nodular, scratching after.
- Ulcers: Fungous, indolent, spongy, indurated, painful, itching, unhealthy.

Itching

Biting, burning, must scratch until it bleeds, scratching; changes place on scratching, itching unchanged by scratching, smarting, spots, tickling, aggravated on becoming warm.

Sensation

Burning, gnawing pains – worse after scratching, as if tense, constricted.

Concomitants

Mentals

Answers - reflects long before answering.

Anxiety as if he has not done his duty.

Anxiety with hurry.

Anxiety as if time is set.

Cannot look at blood.

Confused as to personal identity.

Fear of loss of reason.

Time passes slowly.

Moody.

Resignation.

Slowness of mind.

Suicidal tendency.

Time passes to slowly.

Generals

Chilly.

Dryness.

Slow functions.

Numbness of soles.

Tendency to catch cold.

Tendency to paretic muscular states.

Potatoes aggravates.

APIS MELLIFICA

Look of the skin

Dermographia, dryness, desquamation, inelasticity, waxy appearance of the skin. Dry and hot skin alternates with gushes of sweat.

On examination

Old, dirty appearing; red, black or bluish discoloration.

Ailments from

Bee sting.

Suppressed sexuality.

Sexual excess.

Anger.

Grief.

Bad news.

Sphere of action

Scalp, lids, ears.

Pathology

Boils, chicken pox, carbuncles, cellulitis, eczema, erysipelas, herpes, lichen planus, measles, erythema nodosum, scarlatina, urticaria.

Modalities

General

Agg.: Warmth of any kind - warm room, heat of fire, warm bath, all intolerable, touch, pressure.

Particular

Itching	-	< Cold air, < Scratching, < Warmth of bed, < Evening, < Burning, < Heat, > Warmth, > Scratching.
Eczema	-	< Heat, > Exposure to air.
Eruptions	-	< Before, during and after menses, < Cold air, < Heat.
Rash	-	< Change of weather, < Coming into warm room from open air, < Over heated when
Urticaria	-	< Night, < Change of weather, < During and after chill, < Shellfish, < Warm, < After exercise.

Discharge

Discharges are offensive.

Eruptions

Suppressed eruptions; rough eruptions on perspiring parts; red stinging eruptions; shiny red eruptions; allergic eruptions.

- Bites: Swelling after bites, sensitive and sore.
- Urticaria: Worse in the night; seen in patients suffering from asthma; worse after chill, during fever, during perspiration, from warmth and exercise; nodular.
- Erysipelas: Edematous, sensitive to touch. Phlegmatous. Traumatic and chronic, recurring periodically. Pinkish, rosy or purplish hue - especially face - travels from right to left.
- Ulcers: Sarcomatous and painful.

Itching

Itching on perspiring parts. Aversion to heat. Burning, stinging, smarting and soreness.

Sensation

Prickling sensation.

Concomitants

Mentals

Busy, industrious people, better when occupied.

Fruitlessly busy.

Jealousy.

Awkward, clumsy and fidgety.

Says is well when sick.

Generals

Right sidedness.

Effects of suppression of any kind.

Oedematous swellings.

Thirstlessness.

ARNICA MONTANA

Look of the skin

Black and blue.

On examination

Dry, excoriated.

Ailments from

Abused, after being sexually.

Bad news.

Excitement, emotional.

Grief.

Mental shock.

Money, from losing (causes psoriasis).

Sphere of action

Extremities, back, shoulders.

Pathology

Abscess, acne, boils, cracks, decubitus ulcers, carbuncles, eczema, herpes zoster, measles, erysipelas, intertrigo, purpura hemorrhagica, psoriasis, pustules, tubercles, urticaria, and ulcers. It is a great prophylactic for pus formation.

Modalities
General

Agg.: Least touch, motion, rest, wine, damp cold.

Particular

Erysipelas   - < After scratching.

Itching   - < Scratching or > Scratching.

Discharge

Fetid pus, bloody discharge.

Eruptions

Eruptions in blotches, biting, burning, on injured parts, itching, worse after scratching, with symmetrical swelling, with tearing pain, tense, ecchymosis, asymmetrical eruptions. Typical Koebner's phenomenon.

- Abscess: Chronic, incipient, pus, bloody, recurrent, fetid.
- Boils: Painful, blood boils, small crops. Recurrent tendency to boils.
- Acne: Very painful, small, splinter like pain, stinging, tensive.
- Urticaria: Nodular.
- Erysipelas: Scratching after, with swelling.
- Ulcers: Bluish, bleeding, crawling with, dirty, itching, inflamed, pulsating, varicose ulcers, swollen, tense, tingling.

Itching

Biting, burning, crawling, itching on scratching changes place, must scratch until it is raw, itching unchanged by scratching, in spots, stinging.

Sensation

Sore, lame, bruised feeling.

Concomitants

Mentals

Agoraphobia from mental strain or shock.

Aversion to being approached by persons.

Censorious.

Company aversion to.

Delusion he is well .

Fear of death when alone.

Fear of doctors.

Fears touch or approach of anyone.

Frightened easily.

Indifference, inability to work.

Morose.

Sensitive to noise and pain.

Talking loudly in sleep.

Generals

Desires: Vinegar, sour food, whiskey.

Aversion Tobacco, meat, milk, soup.

Excess of energy in children.

ARSENICUM ALBUM

Look of the skin

Dry, dirty, shrivelled, seared.

On examination

The lesions are scaly, hard, rough, thickened and inelastic.

Ailments from

Suppression - from mercury or sulphur ointment.

Sphere of action

Scalp, face, extremities, nails.

Pathology

Acne, anesthesia, cicatrices, comedones, carbuncles, eczema, herpes, gangrene, lichen planus, measles, intertrigo, leprosy, psoriasis, pemphigus, ulcers, urticaria.

Modalities

General

    Agg.: Cold food, fruit, fat, night, especially midnight to 3
        a.m.

    Amel.: Warmth.

Particular

Itching	- > Warmth even with scalding water, > Bleeding, > Scratching, < Undressing, < Scratching, < Night.
Eruptions	- < Fish, < Night, < Warmth.
Urticaria	- < Night, < Cold air, < Fish, > Warmth, > Exertion.
Psoriasis	- < Night, < Heat, < Menses.
Eczema	- < Night, < Open air, < Undressing. > Heat, > Warm bathing.
Acne	- < Cold air, < Warm weather.
Herpes	- < Cold or open air. > Warm applications, > Heat, > Night.

Discharge

    Corrosive discharge.

Eruptions

    Acuminate eruptions. Suppressed eruptions. Eruptions are blackish, bleeding and desquamating. White or black crusty eruptions. Eruptions are ulcerated and suppurating. Eruptions alternate with internal respiratory symptoms. Eruptions appear from exposure to cold air and on becoming cold. Eruptions are worse after scratching. Burning after scratching. Swelling after scratching. Vesicular eruptions including black and bloody vesicles.

- **Acne and vesicles:** Burning violently.
- **Ulcers:** Chronic with burning, with cutting pain and bloody, brown, white, yellow, grey or green discharge. Discharges are

corrosive, offensive, tenacious and watery; putrid, ichorous, copious. Itching around ulcers. Jagged margins with lardacious base.

- **Psoriasis:** Bland eruptions without itching. Thick and whitish. Hard skin and cracked. Burning with marked itching.
- **Warts:** Burning, suppressed. Warts surrounded by ulcers.

Itching

It alternates with burning. Must scratch till it bleeds or until it is raw. Itching without eruptions and formication.

Sensation

Sensation as of worms under the skin.

Concomitants

Mentals

Insecurity, dependence.

Fearfulness: Death, poverty, disease, being alone, robbers, cancer.

Fastidious: Orderly and conscientious. Censorious.

Miserly, possessive.

Restless.

Anguish.

Generals

Restlessness.

Acridity, burning sensation and acrid discharges.

Periodicity.

Desires: Fat, sour things, old drinks in frequent sips, sweets.

Aversion: Sweets, fat, farinaceous foods.

ARSENICUM BROMATUM

Sphere of action

Face, mouth.

Pathology

Acne, herpes, warts, excrescences, dandruff.

Modalities

General

Agg.: Spring in.

Particular

Acne   - < Spring in.

Discharge

Moist.

Eruptions

- Moist, fetid eruptions affecting the corners of the mouth.
- Acne: In young people; acne rosacea with violent papules. Acne on nose

Concomitants

Generals

White tongue.

Cancerous affections.

Enlarged spleen.

Diabetes mellitus.

Distorted nails.

Diabetes with acne.

Diabetes with emaciation.

Hodgkin's disease.

Swollen and indurated glands.

ARSENICUM IODATUM

Look of the skin
Dry skin, with scales.

On examination
Dry and scaly appearance of the skin. There is marked exfoliation of skin in large scales.

Ailments from
Mental exertion.

Sphere of action
Beard, face, extremities.

Pathology
Acne; abscess; bubo; eczema; herpetic; impetigo; lichen; measles; excrescences; erysipelas; psoriasis; urticaria; ulcers; purpura hemorrhagica.

Modalities
General
Agg.: Bathing, cold.
Amel.: Eating after.

Particular
Itching   - < Night, < Undressing when.
Eczema   - < Washing.

Discharge
The discharge is fetid, watery, dry, moist and corrosive.

Eruptions
Boils: Crusty, coppery, desquamating, scaly, serpiginous, whitish, suppurated.

- Acne: Hard, shotty, indurated base with pustules at apex
- Eczema: Watery, oozing, itching
- Ulcers: Bleed, cancerous, indolent, indurated, painful, sensitive, suppurating.

Itching

It is worse in the night, when undressing with burning and stinging sensation.

Concomitants

Mentals

Answering, aversion to answer.

Bulimia.

Cheerful.

Confusion of mind.

Fastidious.

Indifference to loved ones.

Indifference to the surrounding.

Startling sleep during.

Timid children.

Generals

Desires - alcoholic drinks, stimulants, milk.

Aversion - fish.

Chorea.

Dropsy.

Hot patient yet aggravated by draft of cold air.

BELLADONNA

Look of the skin

Scarlet red.

On examination

The skin is dry, hot, glossy, swollen and sensitive.

Ailments from

Alcoholism.

Ambition deceived.

Anger.

Fright, fear.

Grief.

Indignation.

Love disappointed.

Mental exertion.

Mortification.

Reproaches.

Scorned being.

Silent grief.

Sphere of action

Face, scalp, behind ears, extremities, chest and back.

Pathology

Abscess, acne, comedones, dermatitis, erysipelas, psoriasis, scarlatina and urticaria.

Modalities

General

Agg.: Heat of sun, draft of air, afternoon, lying down, motion, pressure, touch, company, suppressed perspiration, 3 p.m., washing hair.

Amel.: light covering, bending backward, semi-erect, rest in bed, standing.

Particular

Itching   - < scratching.

Acne   - < before menses.

Boils & abscesses - < touch, < jarring, < spring.

Discharge

The discharges are hot and scanty.

Eruptions

Eruptions are fiery red; blotches; shiny. Red streaks are seen after scratching. Dry burning eruptions with desquamation. Moist eruptions, worse on scratching. Suppressed eruptions. Swelling of affected parts. Vesicles are inflamed and painful. Vesicles appear after scratching.

- Psoriasis: With inflamed, hot and swollen skin. Fever and enlarged lymph nodes with generalized aching.

- Acne: Very itchy, hard and indurated. Oozing and moist after scratching.

- Abscess: Boils deep in the skin. The swelling is from deep under the skin. Bright red and remarkably hot to touch. Terribly painful and usually throbbing boils.

- Urticaria: Violent, sudden outbreaks of red, hot, painful urticaria with metrorrhagia.

Itching

Itching with stinging.

Sensation

Throbbing pains with sensation of heat.

Concomitants

Mentals

Energetic and plethoric with an intense temperament.

F- 53

Aggressive.

Desire to bite, kick, strike, and pull hair (especially in children).

Strikes head against the wall with anger.

Fear of animals, dogs.

Fearlessness, audacity.

Quarrelsome.

Generals

Sudden, violent onset.

Right sided.

Sensitive to light, jar, noise.

Thirstless.

BERBERIS VULGARIS

Look of the skin

Bluish; white; brown; yellow (jaundice); wrinkled.

On examination

Circumscribed pigmentation or brown patches are seen.

Ailments from

Abused, after being, sexually.

Quarrelling.

Sphere of action

Extremities and around the anus.

Pathology

Eczema, warts.

Modalities

General

Agg.: Motion, jarring, standing, rising from sitting position, fatigue, urinating, twilight, darkness.

Particular

Itching	- < wandering, < night, < scratching, > cold air, > cold, > water application.
Eruptions	- > cold bathing.

Eruptions

Eruptions leave circumscribed pigmentation or brown patches. Eruptions appear in patches and blotches. The pustules are painful and red. Herpetic eruptions.

Itching

Itching with burning.

Wandering itching.

Sensation

Bubbling sensation; biting; burning.

Concomitants

Mentals

Indifference.

Listless, apathy.

Sees forms in the dark.

Mentally exhausted.

Indifference and weariness of life.

Generals

Radiating pains.

Numbness.

Left sided.

Affinity for kidneys.

Skin diseases in elderly, gouty people.

Skin diseases in women whose domestic affairs tired and fret.

Warts - small.

BOVISTA LYCOPERDON

Look of the skin

Goose flesh; puffy skin; red; yellow.

On examination

There are cracks on skin. Blunt instruments leave deep impression on skin.

Ailments from

Abuse of cosmetics.

Emotional excitement.

Skin diseases in children who have a strong family history of skin diseases.

Sphere of action

Extremities.

Pathology

Acne, corns, eczema, hemorrhage, rheumatism, urticaria and warts.

Modalities

General

Agg.: menses, full moon, hot weather, wine, coffee, getting warm, cold food.

Amel.: Bending double, hot food, eating.

Particular

Urticaria   —   < morning on waking, < warmth and exercise, < with diarrhoea, < after excitement, < during menses, < night after bathing, < bathing.

Itching   —   < on getting warm, < undressing, < scratching, < night.

< warmth of bed.

> scratching.

Discharge

The discharge is thick, tenacious, yellow, pustular (oozing), ichorus with formation of scabs and crusts.

Eruptions

Herpetic eruptions, cracks and burning eruptions. Eruptions are seen after scratching; eruptions bleed after scratching. The eruptions are either dry or moist, worse after scratching. Oozing scabs. Burning vesicles. There is puffiness of affected parts. Unhealthy skin, every scratch festers. Eczema of the hands and hollow of the knees.

- Acne - covering the entire body.
- Urticaria - covering the whole body with diarrhoea or metrorrhagia. Delirium with urticaria.
- Eczema - moist with formation of thick crusts or scabs.
- Ulcers - burning, painful, crusty, and deep.
- Warts - inflamed, painful, suppurative.

Itching

Scratching leads to bleeding. He must scratch until it bleeds or until it is raw. Itching is accompanied with burning.

Sensation

Shooting pain experienced in the entire body. There is sensation of enlargement of parts of the body.

Concomitants

Mentals

Awkward in speech and action, stammers and drops things.

Confusion.

Loquacity.

Open hearted.

Quarrelsome.

Weak memory - slowness of understanding and comprehension.

Mental symptoms from sexual excess.

Generals

Tendency to puffiness.

Desires - wine, milk, cold water and cold drinks.

Aversion - cooked food, milk, warm food.

CALADIUM SEGUINUM

Look of the skin

Red spots, dry red strip down the centre of the tongue, widening upto the lip.

On examination

Formication.

Ailments from

Sexual excess.

Tobacco.

Sphere of action

Genitals.

Pathology

Acne, eczema, herpetic, pustules, urticaria.

Modalities

General

Agg.: Motion, coition after, sudden noise, lying, lying on left side.

Amel.: After sleeping in time, short sleep, cold air, open air.

Particular

Itching   - < evening, < evening, bed in, < scratching.
                     > cold, cold air.

Eruptions   - > discharges.

Eruptions

Burning, dry, itching, scaly, suppressed, vesicular, skin disease of people who chew tobacco or smoke cigarettes.

- Herpetic - burning, itching.
- Urticaria- alternating with asthma.

Itching

Crawling, stinging sensation. Itching after insect bite, unchanged by scratching, aggravated on becoming warm in bed.

Sensation

Sensation of cobweb.

Concomitants

Mentals

Anxiety about his health.

Courageous.

Delusion rocking.

Fear of cutting himself while shaving.

Fear of infections.

Fear of being injured.

Helplessness.

Generals

Faintness aggravated after lying.

Desires - tobacco.

Aggravation - discomfort after pickled fish.

Loss of fluids.

CALCAREA CARBONICA

Look of the skin

Withered, wens, wrinkled and shrivelled; freckles.

On examination

Dry, cracks.

Ailments from

Anticipation.

Anxiety.

Bad news.

Business failure.

Cares and worries.

Death of loved ones - child, parent, friends.

Egotism.

Money from losing.

Sexual excess.

Failure.

Excitement emotional.

Accident, from sight of an.

Sphere of action

Occiput, scalp, flexures, face.

Pathology

Abscess, cracks, decubitus, ecchymoses, eczema, herpetic, impetigo, intertrigo, gangrene, leprosy, molluscum contagiosum, acne, lupus, nevi, keloid, moles, ringworm, psoriasis, scabies, scarlatina, ulcers, warts, urticaria.

Modalities

General

Agg.: exertion (mental or physical), ascending, cold in every form, water, washing, moist air, wet weather, during full moon, standing.

Amel.: Dry climate and weather, lying on painful side.

Particular

Eruptions	- < winter, < washing.
	> cold air.
Eczema	- < winter, < repeated washing.
	> scratching.
Cracks	- < winter, < washing.
Urticaria	- < damp weather, < milk.
	> cool or open air.
Itching	- < morning in bed, < evening in bed, < scratching,
	< bathing warm or hot.
	> scratching.

Discharge

Bloody, offensive discharge like rotten eggs; scanty, sour smelling, corrosive, copious, ichorus discharge.

Eruptions

Crusts and scabs with bland pus; in patches, vesicular, dry, desquamating, crusty, bleeding, burning, clustered, dry, biting.

- Herpetic - burning, chapping, circinate, corrosive, crusty, dry, itching, suppressed.
- Acne - crust with itching, moist, scratching, sore, green.
- Eczema - elevated, folds of skin, grape shaped.
- Impetigo - inflamed, itching.
- Leprosy - mealy, milk form.
- Molluscum contagiosum - painful, papular patches.
- Pemphigus - phagedenic.
- Psoriasis - diffusa, inveterata, pustules, scarlet.
- Scabies - bleeding, dry, moist, suppressed by mercury and sulphur by; scaly.
- Tubercles.
- Urticaria.
- Erysipelas.
- Condylomata.
- Ulcers - bleeding, areola red, bluish, burning, cancerous, crusty, deep and dirty.
- Warts - fleshy, had, hollow, horny, indented, inflamed, old, painful, pulsating, red, round, small, smelling like old cheese, suppurating, soft.

Itching

Biting, burning, crawling, jerking, on perspiring parts, stinging, smarting, must scratch until it becomes raw, changes place on scratching.

Sensation

Electric sparks as if, anesthesia, bubbling, burning, chapping, coldness.

Concomitants

Mentals

Depressed, melancholic or doubting.

Many fears and anxieties - dogs, dark, death, disease, poverty, insanity, animals, spiders.

Obstinate.

Slowness.

Responsibility.

Sensitive to hearing about cruelties.

Fear of her condition being observed.

Hopelessness of ever getting well.

Generals

Chilly.

Sour perspiration.

Flabbiness.

Desires - eggs, indigestible things, chalk, ice cream, starchy food, oysters, sweets, salt and sour.

Aversion - meat, milk, slimy food, fat and coffee.

CALCAREA SULPHURICA

Look of the skin

Dryness, cracks, unhealthy.

On examination

Dry, unhealthy.

Ailments from

Envy, jealousy.

Sphere of action

Hands, arms, scalp, feet, knees, face.

Pathology

Acne, cracks, eczema, intertrigo, impetigo, herpetic, ulcers, urticaria, warts, psoriasis.

Modalities

General

    Agg.: From change of weather.

    Amel.: Open air

Particular

Cracks	- < winter, < after washing.
Intertrigo	- < warmth of bed.
	> scratching.
Eczema	- < winter, < night, < emotional stress, < repeated washing.
	> scratching.
Itching	- < warmth of bed.
	> scratching.

Discharge

Moist, yellow, offensive, albuminous discharge.

Eruptions

Burning, crusting, desquamating, yellow crust, dryness and cracks.

- Herpetic - itching.
- Psoriasis - pustules, rash, scaly, suppurating.
- Urticaria - vesicular, excoriation, formication.
- Intertrigo - itching.
- Ulcers - bleeding, burning, cancerous, crusty, deep, fistulous, foul, indolent, indurated, painful, pulsating.
- Eczema - dry, sharply demarcated, yellow crusty eruptions with infection and inflammation.

Itching

Itching with burning.

Sensation
Burning.

Concomitants

Mentals
Fear of birds and dark.

Jealousy.

Forsaken feeling.

Lamenting because he is not appreciated.

Generals
Tendency to suppuration.

Abscess.

Fistulae.

Tendency to croup in children.

Desires - green fruits.

CARBO ANIMALIS

Look of the skin
Goose flesh and nevi are seen.

On examination
Cracks.

Ailments from
Sexual excess.

Sphere of action
Hands, face, extremities, neck, axilla, groin, mammae.

Pathology
Abscess; acne rosacea; blisters; cicatrices; carbuncles;

excrescences; herpetic; erysipelas; urticaria; ulcers; scabies; warts; varicose veins.

Modalities

General

Agg.: After shaving, loss of animal fluids.

Particular

Cicatrices   - < weather change.

Erysipelas   - < after scratching.

Itching   - < scratching, < evening in bed.

                       > scratching.

Discharge

Yellow, offensive after scratching.

Eruptions

Coppery, crusty, scratching after, scaly bran like, suppurated, tense, flat, hard, itching.

- Acne - itching.
- Abscess - incipient.
- Herpetic - burning, crusty, itching, moist.
- Tubercles - burning, itching, red.
- Urticaria - nodular, scratching after.
- Erysipelas - children, newborns.
- Excrescences - fungus, medullary swelling, inflamed, puffy bunches.
- Ulcers - bleed, bluish, cancerous, crusty, scratching after, burning.
- Warts - itching.

Itching

Evening - bed in, biting, burning, unchanged by scratching, stinging, on becoming warm in bed.

Sensation

Burning, coldness.

Concomitants

Mentals

Anxiety at night.

Aversion to company.

Avoids conversation.

Desire to be alone.

Fear of crowd, people.

Fear in dark.

Taciturn.

Prostration of mind.

Weepy.

Melancholic.

Generals

Ailments from weaning milk.

Chilly.

Induration of glands.

Cancerous affections.

Impaired hearing.

Offensive perspiration.

Marked weakness.

Aversion to fat.

Fat aggravates.

Fish aggravates.

Desires - eggs, pickles.

Uncovering aversion to and aggravates.

CARCINOSIN

Look of the skin
Brown.

On examination
Brown liver spots are seen.

Ailments from
Abuse.

Anger.

Anticipation.

Domination.

Fear, fright.

Grief.

Mental shock.

Reproaches.

Rudeness of others.

Sphere of action.

Face, extremities.

Pathology
Eczema, keloid, moles, nevi, warts.

Modalities
General
Agg.: sea side.

Amel.: sea side.

Particular
Eczema -   > sea side.

Eruptions - > air.

Discharge

Bloody and offensive discharge.

Eruptions

Brown, bloody and suppressed eruptions.

- Eczema - suppressed.
- Warts - cylindrical, fleshy, small and soft.

Itching

Itching without eruptions.

Concomitants

Mentals

Conscientious, fastidious, perfectionist, duty-bound.

Industrious.

Sympathetic.

Sensitive to sensual impressions.

Obstinate children.

Affectionate.

Anticipatory anxiety.

Liking for animals.

Loves thunderstorms and dancing.

Desire for travel.

Generals

Family history of cancer, tuberculosis and diabetes.

Blue sclera.

Café-au-lait complexion.

Fear of dark.

Desires-fat, eggs, chocolates, spicy, butter, fruit, salt, sweets, ice-cream, vinegar.

Aversion- fat, eggs, sweets, fruits, milk.

F- 54

CICUTA VIROSA

On examination

Numbness, swelling, thick, bruised, hard, coldness.

Ailments from

Anticipation.

Bad news.

Accidents.

Injury, head injury.

Mental symptoms from.

Mental shock.

Quarrelling.

Sphere of action

Scalp, face, hands.

Pathology

Acne, eczema, ecthyma, herpetic, lupus, impetigo, psoriasis, urticaria, ulcers.

Modalities

General

Agg.: from touch, draughts, concussion, tobacco smoke, milk.

Particular

Itching - > scratching.

Discharge

Yellow, offensive, ichorous, and copious discharge.

Eruptions

Burning, confluent, crusty, smarting, suppressed, suppurating, with swelling.

- Herpetic - burning, crusty, itching, mealy, moist, suppurating.
- Psoriasis - diffusa.
- Acne - confluent, lenticular.
- Eczema - itching without.
- Impetigo - itching, mealy, painful.
- Pustules - confluent, red, scaly.
- Urticaria - nodular, scratching after.
- Ulcers - crusty, elevated with indurated margins, painful, phagedenic, painless, sensitive, suppurating, swollen.

Itching

Burning; eruptions without itching may be seen.

Sensation

Anaesthesia, coldness, burning.

Concomitants

Mentals

Childish, simple behaviour.

Suspicious.

Fear of men.

Hatred, contempt.

Violent.

Sympathetic.

Aversion to company.

Horrible things and sad stories affect her profoundly.

Generals

Tendency to convulsions, jerking and twitching.

Desires - chalk, charcoal and indigestible things, raw potato, cabbage and alcohol.

Aggravation - milk.

Chilly.

CLEMATIS ERECTA

Look of the skin

Withered appearance.

On examination

Unhealthy, thick, dry, wrinkled.

Ailments from

Grief.

Homesickness.

Sphere of action

Occiput and lower limbs.

Pathology

Acne, abscess, eczema, impetigo, erysipelas, psoriasis, scabies, small pox, rupia, rhus poisoning, ulcers.

Modalities

General

Agg.: night, warmth of bed.

Amel.: open air, perspiring.

Particular

Eruptions   - < after washing in cold water, < full moon.

Itching   - < night, < warm on becoming, < bed warmth
                  > bathing, > cold water, > scratching, > heat
                  of stove.

Impetigo   - < night, < warmth, < warmth of bed, <
                  washing in cold water.

Discharge

Corrosive, green, ichorus, offensive, scanty, watery, yellow discharge.

Eruptions

Blisters, burning, crusty, moist, desquamating, painful, phagedenic, vesicles - itching or painful, watery or yellow; dry burning.

- Eczema – herpetic, circinate, spreading, dry, itching, crusty, moist, scaly and corrosive.
- Acne - sore, as if elevated.
- Psoriasis - diffusa, inveterata.
- Pustules – yellow, itch like rash.
- Scabies - dry, fatty, moist, scaly, bran like, serpigenous.
- Small pox - suppressed, suppurating, vesicular.
- Condylomata.
- Ulcers - burning, cancerous, crusty, deep, elevated with indurated margins, itching, painful, phagedenic, sensitive, spongy, suppurating, tense, unhealthy.

Itching

Burning, itching without eruptions, itching unchanged by scratching, stinging.

Sensation

Burning, prickling.

Concomitants

Mentals

Sensitive to all external impressions.

Homesickness.

Aversion to company yet dreads being alone.

Fear of solitude, being alone.

Fear of misfortune.

Quiet disposition.

Generals

Affinity for glands, especially testes.

Right sided.

Effects of suppressed gonorrhea.

COPAIVA OFFICINALIS

Look of the skin

It appears as if bitten by an insect.

On examination

It is hard like parchment. Dry and hot.

Sphere of action

Abdomen, mucus membranes, face, hands and genitals.

Pathology

Acne, eczema, measles, roseola, scabies, urticaria, erysipelas.

Modalities

General

Agg.: cold.

Particular

Urticaria   - < night.

Itching   - < touch.

Eruptions

The eruptions are confluent, elevated, itching, lenticular, mottled. Pemphigus; pustules; rash – scarlet red; vesicular; bullous; liver spots; large red blotches all over the body, with constipation and some fever; tormenting eruptions only between fingers, and on both forearms as far as bend of elbow;

- **Acne:** Small, red, slightly itching pimples on the upper part of the forehead, on hairy scalp, above the ears and on the occiput; acne of long duration, with much disfigurement of face.

- **Eczema:** Consisting of small vesicles, itching and pricking with severe inflammation in parts. Denuded epithelium.

- **Pemphigus vulgaris:** Here the mucous membrane is first affected then the skin. There is presence of excessive foetid discharge. Presence of pemphigus in people having past history of gonorrhoea.

- **Urticaria:** Night; in children; chronic urticaria with constipation; urticaria during fever, after gastric upset. Nodular, rosy, large giant urticaria. Urticaria after eating shell fish.

Itching

Stinging sensation, violent; itching and pricking in skin; annoying itching with severe inflammation in parts denuded of epithelium.

Sensation

As if bitten by an insect.

Concomitants

Mentals

Anxiety, health about – own health.

Business aversion to.

Company aversion to.

Contradiction aggravates.

Dwells on past disagreeable occurrences.

Fancies lascivious.

Hysteria.

Fear death of.

Mental exertion aggravates.

Generals

Desires – onions raw.

Aggravation - shellfish.

Paralysis - after disappearance of nettle rash.

CORNUS CIRCINATA

Look of the skin

Yellow, earthy appearance.

On examination

Chronic yellow discolouration of the skin.

Sphere of action

Face, mouth.

Pathology

Eczema, urticaria, ulcers.

Modalities

General

Agg.: forenoon, scratching, rubbing.

Particular

Itching -   < night.

Eruptions

Burning, dry, vesicular eruptions.

• Eczema - vesicular.

Itching

Paroxysmal.

Concomitants

Mentals

Confusion of mind, worse morning after rising.

Indifference, apathy to agreeable things.

Petulant.

Sadness with sleepiness.

Generals

Desires - sour food, pastries.

Aversion - bread.

Side - right.

Skin complaints associated with chronic hepatitis.

CROTON TIGLIUM

Look of the skin

Skin adherent to the bone.

On examination

Rough, coldness.

Ailments from

Summer.

Rhus poisoning.

Sphere of action

Genitals, face, hands.

Pathology

Acne, eczema, ecthyma, herpetic, impetigo, scabies, urticaria.

Modalities

General

Agg.: Summer, touch, night and morning, washing.

Amel.: open air.

Particular

    Herpetic   - < scratching.

                       > gentle rubbing.

    Itching   - < night, < scratching.

                       > gentle rubbing, > warmth.

Discharge

Moist, sticking.

Eruptions

Eruptions alternate with internal affections, pain in the limbs and with respiratory symptoms. Blotches, burning, crusty, desquamating, discharging, vesicular, pustular, inflamed.

- Acne - pustules, inflamed, itching, red, scurfy, ulcerated.
- Impetigo - itching.
- Scabies - symmetrical.
- Urticaria - nodular, rosy, vesicular.

Itching

Intense, burning, stinging, alternates with burning.

Sensation

As if hidebound.

Concomitants

Mentals

Anxiety and fear usually associated with diarrhea.
Selfish.
Egotism.

Generals

Diarrhea that is worse from least food or drink.

DULCAMARA

Look of the skin
Freckled.

On examination
Hard callosities, cold, dry, thick, inelastic, parchment like.

Ailments from
Being chilled while hot.
Damp weather.
Suppressed discharges, sweat, eruptions.
Mercury poisoning.

Sphere of action
Face, lips, hands and fingers.

Pathology
Acne, eczema, chicken pox, impetigo, measles, psoriasis, scabies, herpetic, urticaria, scarlatina, ulcers, warts, lichen planus, purpura.

Modalities
General
Agg.: Night, from cold, cold damp weather, rainy weather.

Amel.: Moving about, external warmth.

Particular

Urticaria	- < cold air, < damp weather, < autumn.
	< menses, < from scratching.
	< from sour stomach.
	> warmth, > cold washing.
Herpetic	- < cold air, < damp air, < before menses.
Warts	- < cold washing.
Psoriasis	- < itching.

Acne	- < scratching after.
Eczema	- < cold weather.
Eruptions	- < cold weather, < washing, < winter.
Itching	- < night, < after eating, < warmth of bed, < cold air.

OR

> warmth, > undressing.

| Measles | - < before and during menses . |

Discharge

Scanty, yellow, pus, white.

Eruptions

Bleeding, blisters, blotches, boils break out, burning, painful, pemphigus, petechiae, crusty, desquamating.

- Herpetic - bleeding, all over the body, burning, circinate, clusters, dry, itching, mealy, moist, spreading and suppurating.
- Eczema - elevated.
- Impetigo - itching.
- Lichen planus - mealy.
- Measles - petechiae, painful.
- Acne - itching, painful.
- Psoriasis - diffusa, pustules, itching, red coloured, ulcerated, scruffy.
- Scabies - bleeding, dry, moist, suppressed, scaly.
- Scarlatina - suppressed, scaly.
- Urticaria - nodular.
- Purpura - thick.
- Condylomata.
- Ulcers - bleeding, cancerous, indolent, indurated, painful, painless, phagedenic, swollen, suppurating.

- Warts - flat, fleshy, hard, horny, large, pedunculated, small, smooth.

Itching

Burning, wandering, stinging, violent, worse during sleep, unchanged by scratching, itching of old people.

Sensation

Biting - fleas of, burning and coldness.

Concomitants

Mentals

Bossy, quarrelsome.

Anxiety about others.

Over-concerned about her family.

Scolding without being angry.

Generals

Aversion - coffee.

Paralysis single parts.

EUGENIA JAMBOS

Look of the skin

Cicatrices.

On examination

Inflamed area around the lesions especially the acne.

Ailments from

Tobacco toxicity.

Sexual excesses.

Sphere of action

Face, nails, toes.

Pathology

Simple rosacea or indurated acne, fissures, felons, panaritium, cicatrices, stab wounds.

Modalities

General

Agg.: Exposure to sun, closing eyes, evening, night, right side, after coition.

Amel.: After urination, smoking, coffee.

Particular

Acne   - < during menses.

Eruptions

* Acne - pustular with indurated papules. Surrounding skin is inflamed and painful. Sore as if excoriated.
* Fissures - especially between the toes.
* Wounds - emergency stab wounds, bleeding profusely. Old wounds and scars reopen and are painful.
* Ulcers - cracks between and above the toes.
* Panaritium - skin recedes from the thumbnail and contains pus. Desquamation and suppuration of the skin round the nail of the thumb.

Sensation

Old wounds become painful again. Internal pinching pains here and there. Crawling, titillating pains.

Concomitants

Mentals

Talkative but indolent.

Generals

Nightly cramps in soles of feet.
Extreme desire for tobacco.

EUPHORBIUM OFFICINARUM

Look of the skin
Yellow.

On examination
Sore skin.

Sphere of action
Cheeks, face, coccyx.

Pathology
Decubitus ulcers; excrescences; erysipelas; herpes zoster; pustules; condylomata; gangrene; ulcers; warts; carcinoma; carbuncles.

Modalities
General
Agg.: Bending, beer, ascending, turning in bed, changing position.

Particular
Ulcers   - < with scratching.

Eruptions
Biting, bleeding, boils, burning, desquamating, flat, scratching after, vesicular.

- Erysipelas – with swelling vesicular.
- Ulcers - black, gangrenous, indolent, painful, suppurating.

Itching
Biting, burning; unchanged by scratching; in spots, stinging, tickling.

Sensation
As if a thin cord is lay under the skin.

Concomitants

Mentals

Acute mania.

Art ability for.

Anxiety about future.

Delusion, someone is walking before and after.

Delusion – every thing appears larger than he is.

Generals

Beer aggravates.

Cancerous affections.

Children – complaints in.

Warm drinks aggravates.

FALCON PEREGRINUS DISCIPLINATUS

Look of the skin

Wrinkled and shrivelled Look of the skin.

On examination

Cracks and dryness.

Ailments from

Abused, after being sexually.

Anger suppressed.

Domination, long time from.

Mortification.

Scorned being.

Sexual excitement.

Shame.

Sphere of action

Face, mouth, extremities.

Pathology

Acne, eczema, psoriasis.

Modalities

General

Agg.: Cold.

Amel.: Air - open air, in mountains, wet weather.

Particular

Eczema   - < water, < hot weather.

Eruptions

* Bleeding, gritty.
* Acne - bleeding, inflamed, itching, painful.
* Eczema - eczema on hands, like blisters, quite big, like bubbles under the skin, quite painful, not red, odd patches, but quite a lot of blisters.

Concomitants

Mentals

Art ability for.

Absent minded.

Abstraction of mind.

Activity desires.

Cursing – from contradiction.

Delusion he has neglected his duty.

Delusion he is under superhuman control.

Delusion he is trapped.

Generals

Desires - tobacco, beer, chocolate and sugar.

Aversion - coffee, tomatoes, cucumber.

Obesity.

FERRUM ARSENICOSUM

Look of the skin

It is pale, greasy, dropsical and yellow.

On examination

Dry, cold.

Ailments from

Hemorrhages.

Loss of fluids.

Abuse of quinine.

Sphere of action

Face.

Pathology

Eczema, impetigo, psoriasis, ulcers.

Modalities

General

Agg.: Lying, dry weather, open air, walking, morning, night.

Eruptions

Eczema, impetigo, psoriasis, lepra, liver spots.

- Ulcers – burning.
- Warts – withered.
- Nails – blue discoloration of the fingernails.

Sensation

There is a sore or burning sensation. Coldness of the skin.

Concomitants

Mentals

Confusion of mind.

Hysteria.

Discontented.

Conscientious about trifles.

Late – always too late.

Mood – changeable.

Generals

Anaemia.

Desires - bread.

Aversion - bread.

Constipation.

History of abuse of quinine for treatment of rheumatoid arthritis and malaria.

Liver is enlarged.

Emaciation.

Varicose veins.

FLUORICUM ACIDUM

Look of the skin

Unhealthy appearance.

On examination

Skin is hard like callosities.

Ailments from

Anticipation.

Celibacy.

Debauchery.

Mental exertion.

Sphere of action

Bones, glands, joints.

Pathology

Abscess, acne, cicatrices, decubitus ulcers, psoriasis, excrescences, keloid, nevi, ulcers, warts, eczema, herpes.

Modalities

General

Agg.: Warmth, morning, warm drinks.

Amel.: Cold , while walking, open air, cold bath.

Particular

Ulcers   - < warmth.
                > cold application.

Eruptions   - < warmth.

Itching   - < evening, < march month of.
                < spring in, > scratching.

Discharge

Fetid.

Eruptions

Blotches, crusty, desquamating, dry, hard, itching, scaly eruptions.

- Abscess - chronic, acrid pustular discharge.
- Cicatrices - break open, elevated, hard, itching, scaly.

- Tubercles - mucus, suppurating, syphilitic, ulcerating.
- Ulcers - cancerous, painful, cold, fistulous, indolent, indurated – shining margins, surrounded by pimples, varicose ulcers.
- Warts - dry, flat, hard, painful.

Itching

Itching of old people; in spots and perspiring parts.

Sensation

Burning.

Concomitants

Mentals

Anxiety for others.

Aversion to friends, parents, wife, family members.

Indifference towards loved ones.

Inability to realize responsibility.

Buoyancy.

Dancing in children.

Delusion of impending danger.

Delusion everything is meaningless.

Delusion repulsive, fantastic.

Elated and gay.

Fear of open spaces.

Fear of strangers.

Fear of suffering.

Generals

Craving - cold water, stimulants, pickles.

Aversion - coffee.

Aggravation - melons.

Amelioration - coffee.

FULIGO LIGNI

On examination

Distension of vessels on hands and feet.

Sphere of action

Glandular system, mucus membrane, epidermis, mouth, tongue, genitalia - scrotum.

Pathology

Eczema, tetters, epithelioma, cancer, chronic ulcerations of malignant types, growths.

Eruptions

* Ulcers - cancerous, bleeding, obstinate, indolent, non-healing and malignant.

Itching

Itching of genitalia.

Concomitants

Mentals

Sadness.

Thoughts of suicide.

Generals

Cancerous affections.

GRAPHITES

Look of the skin

Freckles, flabby, wrinkled, shrivelled, unhealthy look of the skin.

On examination

Hard like callosities, desquamating, dry, rough, chapping, cracks.

Ailments from

Anticipation.

Grief.

Sorrow.

Mental stress in office work.

Discord between friends, chief, subordinates.

Sphere of action

Hands, fingertips, bend of elbows and knees, behind ears, lips, scalp, and genitalia.

Pathology

Acne, eczema, cracks, psoriasis, leprosy, cicatrices, scabies, warts, ulcers, impetigo.

Modalities

General

Agg.: Warmth, at night, during and after menstruation.

Amel.: dark, from wrapping up.

Particular

Psoriasis	- < night, < heat, < menses.
Eczema	- < night, < heat, < becoming heated in bed.
Acne	- < before menses.
Eruptions	- < winter, < before and during menses. > bathing.
Itching	- < night, < warmth of bed, < during and before menses, < scratching.
Impetigo	- < evening, < night, < before storm.

Discharge

Honey like, glutinous, brown, pale red, corrosive discharge.

Eruptions

Alternating with internal affections, in patches, blisters, blotches, desquamating, phagedenic.

- Boils - burning, crusty, dry, foetid, honey, moist, allergic to hay.
- Impetigo - itching.
- Leprosy - mealy.
- Eczema - elevated, fetid, fleabites like folds of skin, granular, gritty, herpetic.
- Acne - burning, itching, moist, painful.
- Psoriasis - diffusa, red pustules.
- Scabies - dry, moist, suppressed, blood filled with burning, vesicular.
- Warts - horny, itching, smell like old cheese, stinging.

Itching

Burning and prickling with itching; must scratch until it is raw, without eruption, wandering itch.

Sensation

Sting of insects, cutting, gnawing, sore, tearing.

Concomitants

Mentals

Indecisive, timid, lacking confidence.
Fastidious.
Conscientious about trifles.
Fidgety.
Changeable mood.
Weeps from music.
Dullness and anxiety on waking.

Generals

    Chilly, sensitive to drafts.

    Prone to flushes of heat.

    Obesity.

    Tendency to fissures.

    Aversion - fish, sweet, meat, salt.

    Desires - chicken, beer.

HEPAR SULPHUR

Look of the skin

    Wrinkled, shrivelled, unhealthy.

On examination

    Coldness.

Ailments from

    Anger, suppressed.

    Discords between parents or friends.

    Mental shock.

Sphere of action

    Hands, fingers, face, scalp, mouth, lips, folds of skin, feet.

Pathology

    Acne, abscess, cellulitis, cicatrices, cracks, carbuncles, impetigo, herpetic, intertrigo, lupus, scabies, scarlatina, tubercles, urticaria, condylomata, ulcers, warts, wens.

Modalities

General

    Agg.: Draught, uncovering, dry air, winter.

    Amel.: damp, warmth.

Particular

Eruptions	- < winter, < scratching.
Urticaria	- < after scratching.
	> warmth, > exercise.
Erysipelas	- < after scratching.
Ulcers	- < after scratching.
Itching	- < morning on rising, < wool, < undressing, < cold air.
	> scratching, > warmth.

Discharge

Fetid, thin, acrid discharge.

Eruptions

Cracks and painful sensitive. Inflammation, suppuration, can be dry, moist, pimples, pustules, scabs, vesicles or patches, fetid, especially in folds, dry, itching, scaly, scratching after.

- Herpetic- burn, chapping, circinate, corrosive, crusty, suppurating, zoster-zona.

- Cicatrices- painful.

- Carbuncles - burn.

- Acne- itching, scratching after.

- Scabies - dry, suppurating.

- Urticaria- chill before, chill after, fever - prodrome, nodular, scratching after.

- Erysipelas- swelling with, vesicular.

- Ulcers- bleed, burn, cancerous, crawling with, crusty, foul, inflamed, pimples surrounded with, sensitive, scratching after, unhealthy, jagged margins with.

- Warts - bleed, burn, inflamed, painful, sensitive to touch, small, smell like old cheese, sting, suppurated.

Itching

Must scratch until raw, burning, chill during, jaundice during, crawling, stinging.

Sensation

Sticking, splinter pains, burning.

Concomitants

Mentals

Hypersensitive and vulnerable to everything.

Irritable, impatient, hurried.

Impolite, unpleasant nature.

Threatening.

Violent anger.

Impulse to stab or kill.

Wants to set things on fire.

Dreams of fire.

Generals

Sensitive to pain.

Offensiveness.

Splinter like pains.

Desires - vinegar, sour, spices, pungent tastes, and fats.

Aversion - cheese, fats.

HIPPOZAENINUM

Look of the skin

Swelling.

On examination

Articular, non-fluctuating swellings – nodules.

Sphere of action

Arms, face.

Pathology

Abscess, actinomycosis, carbuncles, eczema, decubitus, ulcers.

Discharge

Unhealthy corrosive discharges.

Eruptions

Boils, papular, pustules; erythema, erysipelatous or phlegmonous processes, abscesses, pustules, and ulcers are spread so extensively over surface of body that hardly any part remains free. Good drug for carbuncles; malignant, phagedenic skin diseases. Actinomycosis.

- Abscess – deep or — of brain, liver, lungs. Surrounding subfascial abscesses the numerous layers are pale, discoloured and readily torn; large abscesses upon different regions of the body, with inflamed lymphatic vessels and glands.

- Pustules – of size of pea often arise in large numbers, bursting by discharging a thick, mucous, sanguineous pus, often emitting an offensive odour.

- Ulcers- bluish, cancerous, deep, indolent, malignant, unhealthy. Ulcers have no disposition to heal, livid appearance. New abscesses are constantly forming in vicinity of the ulcers, especially about joints. Ulcers often penetrate so deep as to lay bare the tendons and bone. Ulcers deep, lard-like fundus, elevated, pectinated edges, slow healing, leaving a star-shaped white scar.

- Erysipelas - malignant particularly if attended by large formations of pus, and destruction of parts.

- Tubercles – on the alae nasi size; of a millet seed to a pea, firm texture, gray, yellowish or reddish, in lungs.

- Tumours - fluctuating tumours in muscular tissue.

Concomitants

Mentals

Restlessness - move about constantly.

Generals

Aversion - sweets.

Aggravation – alcoholic drinks.

Septicemia.

Swelling of glands.

HYDROCOTYL ASIATICA

Look of the skin

Thickened skin.

On examination

Exfoliation of skin.

Sphere of action

Extremities, palms, soles, chest.

Pathology

Acne, eczema, impetigo, leprosy, lupus, elephantiasis, psoriasis gyrata and diffusa, pemphigus.

Modalities

General

Agg.: Sitting, standing.

Discharge

Offensive.

Eruptions

Papular, bullous, scaly, dry, circular spots with scaly edges.

- Herpetic.
- Acne.
- Tubercles.
- Urticaria.
- Erysipelas.
- Condylomata.
- Ulcers – phagedenic.
- Warts.

Itching

Intolerable itching especially of soles.

Concomitants

Mentals

Cheerful.

Communicative.

Loquacious.

Confiding.

Ennui, tedium.

Fear, people of.

Hopeful.

Vivacious.

Optimistic.

Generals

Aversion - tobacco, liquid food.

Recurrent tendency to cellulites.

Enlarged and tender lymph nodes.

ICHTHYOLUM

Look of the skin
Red.

Sphere of action
Face, chin, genitals.

Pathology
Acne rosacea, erysipelas, eczema, psoriasis, pruritis.

Eruptions
Crops of boils, eczema, chronic, scaly, itching, pruritis during pregnancy.

Itching
During pregnancy.

Concomitants

Mentals
Irritable.

Depressed.

Alcoholism.

Forgetful.

Lack of concentration.

Generals
Bad effects of alcoholism.

Chronic rheumatism.

Skin diseases particularly related to chronic renal failure.

Aggravation – tobacco.

IGNATIA AMARA

Look of the skin
Dry.

On examination
Sensitive, burning, coldness.

Ailments from
Anger.

Bad news.

Death of loved ones.

Disappointed love.

Disappointment

Homesickness.

Honour wounded.

Indignation.

Jealousy.

Mental shock.

Mortification.

Position loss of.

Reproaches.

Silent grief.

Sphere of action
Eyes, mouth, vagina.

Pathology
Abscess, intertrigo, decubitus, measles, tubercles, ulcers, urticaria, eczema.

Modalities

General

Agg.: Morning, open air, after meals, coffee, smoking, liquids, external warmth, sweets.

Amel.: while eating, traveling, change of position.

Particular

Itching   - < during fever, < when overheated.

                   < on warm becoming.

                   > scratching, > with pain.

Urticaria   - < during fever, < during chill.

Discharge

The discharge is scanty, painful, pulsating, inflamed and suppurating.

Eruptions

Dryness, cracking; blotches or vesicles; boils, burning, itching, smarting, stinging.

- Urticaria - nodular.
- Decubitus - dry.
- Ulcers - burning.

Itching

Stinging, burning, and sticking. Itching changes place on scratching. Crawling on painful parts and tickling.

Sensation

Swollen; sensation as if a mouse were under the skin; as of an ant crawling on the skin.

Concomitants

Mentals

Alternating and contradictory states.

Conscientious.

Consolation aggravates.

Easily offended.

Defensive.

Fear of birds.

Idealistic.

Romantic.

Indignation, sensitive to injustice.

Involuntary sighing.

Sadness cannot weep.

Sensitive.

Silent grief.

Somatization of anxiety and grief.

Suppressed anger, anger with silent grief.

Sympathetic.

Generals

Sensation of lump in various organs of the body.

Paradoxical symptoms.

Desires sour, bread, butter, cheese, sour, fruit.

Aversion - meat, tobacco.

Hyperaesthesia of all senses.

Faintness on excitement.

JUGLANS CINEREA

Look of the skin

Red.

Sphere of action

Lower extremities, sacrum, and hands.

Pathology

Eczema, herpes, impetigo, lichen, pustules, ringworm, scarlatina, urticaria, erysipelas, erythema.

Modalities

General

Agg.: Walking, warmth.

Amel.: On getting heated, scratching, on rising in the morning.

Particular

Itching   - < when overheated, < being heated with over exertion.

> with scratching.

Discharge

Moist.

Eruptions

Itching, in patches, pemphigus, suppurating.

- Urticaria - nodular.

Itching

Burning, over heated when, spots, wandering.

Concomitants

Mentals

Company aversion to.

Memory, weakness of memory.

Restlessness at night.

Sadness.

Generals

Emaciation.

Flushes of heat alternating with chills.

Skin disease associated with liver disorders.

JUGLANS REGIA

Ailments from

Puberty, complaints in.

Sphere of action

Axilla, scalp, face, ears.

Pathology

Acne, abscess, comedones, carbuncles, icthyma, eczema, pustules, herpes, impetigo, ringworm, purpura.

Modalities

General

Agg.: With motion.

Amel.: Stool after.

Particular

Itching   - < night, < washing, < undressing.

Discharge

Fetid.

Eruptions

Eruptions are like flea bites, itching, vesicular.

- Herpetic - itching.
- Pustules - burning, covered with green spots.
- Purpura - idiopathica.
- Ulcers - chancre like.

Itching

Itching violently especially at night; redness after itching.

Sensation

Sore feeling.

Concomitants

Mentals

Concentration difficult.

Confusion ameliorated by eating.

Laziness.

Delusion flying.

Delusion floating.

Delusion head is floating.

Generals

Growth in length too fast.

Stools ameliorate[2].

Desires - cold water.

Aversion - wine, tobacco.

Aggravation - fat .

Farrington says – Juglans regia is one of the best remedies in tinea cruris and capitis, where itching is intense at night, so the patient has difficulty in sleeping. Perspiration always influences the itching.

KALIUM SULPHURICUM

Look of the skin

Dry, cracked.

On examination

Inflammation, cold, dry.

Ailments from

Sexual excess.

Sphere of action

Axilla, neck, hands.

Pathology

Abscess, acne, cracks, eczema, erysipelas, herpetic, intertrigo, measles, psoriasis, scabies, urticaria, ulcers, warts.

Modalities

General

Agg.: Evening, heated room.

Amel.: Cool, open air.

Particular

Eruptions	- > bathing.
Itching	- < warmth, < warmth of bed.
	> scratching.

Discharge

Moist, yellow.

Eruptions

Scaly desquamating, burning, yellow scales, crusty, dry, blisters, suppurating.

- Eczema - suppurating.
- Herpetic - itching.
- Urticaria - nodular.
- Ulcers - bleed, bluish edge, burn, crusty, indolent, pulsating, suppurating.
- Warts – painful.

Itching

Burning, crawling, stinging sensation; burning after scratching.

Sensation

Burning.

Concomittants

Mentals

Proper, rigid, inflexible attitude.

Hurried and irritable.

Fear of death, falling, people.

Consolation aggravates.

Anxiety ameliorated in open air.

Full of cares for others.

Delusion she is disgraced.

Frightens easily.

Restlessness during menses.

Generals

Tendency to suppuration.

Desires - sweets, sour.

Aversion - bread, eggs, fats, fish, meat and warm things.

Aggravation - fish.

LACHESIS MUTUS

Look of the skin

Flabby; freckled.

On examination

Swelling; dry skin.

Ailments from

Alcoholism.

Anger.

Bad news.

Death of loved ones.

Debauchery.

Egotism.

Fortune, from reversal of.

Fright, menses during.

Grief.

Jealousy.

Love disappointed.

Marital torture.

Mental exertion.

Mortification.

Discords between chief and subordinate, friends or parents.

Excitement emotional.

Sphere of action

Left side of the body, genitals, face, extremities, left side of face.

Pathology

Acne, abscess, cellulitis, cicatrices, cracks, blisters, carbuncles, ecchymoses, eczema, erysipelas, excrescence, gangrene, herpetic, leprosy, lupus, measles, naevi, small pox, scarlatina, purpura hemorrhagica, tubercles, ulcers, urticaria, warts.

Modalities

al

Agg.: After sleep, left side, spring, warm bath, pressure or constriction, hot drinks, appearance of discharge.

Amel.: Warm application.

Particular

Acne   - < before menses, < at menopause.

Abscess   - < spring, < before menses.

Erysipelas   - < after scratching.

Cellulitis	- < heat, < pressure, < touch, < tight clothing.
Herpes	- < heat, < night.
'Genital herpes	- < before menses.
Eczema	- < in spring.
Ulcers	- > warmth.
Itching	- < night, < in spring, < scratching, < on becoming heated.

Discharge

The discharges are bloody or yellow and worse after scratching.

Eruptions

Eruptions are usually seen on hairy parts. Blotches, cracks, vesicles, pustules, black suppuration, fetid, swelling, scaly, smarting, burning, desquamating, worse after scratching.

- Herpetic - itching, chapping, corrosive, burning, moist, red, suppressed.

- Eczema - alternating with asthma.

- Cicatrices - bleeding, blue, break open, painful.

- Measles - accompanied by dark brown discoloration of the root of the tongue.

- Acne – seen in drunkards. Painful.

- Carbuncles – with small purple vesicles around the lesion.

- Small pox - black.

- Scarlatina - accompanied by salivation, saliva is viscid. Gangrenous.

- Tubercles - hard, itching, painful, red, soft.

- Urticaria - nodular, worse after scratching.

- Erysipelas - spreading from left to right; accompanied by trembling of tongue; gangrenous, with vesicular swelling.

- Gangrene - cold.

- Ulcers - black, bleeding, burning, cancerous, with crawling sensation. Old ulcers reopen. Unhealthy ulcers. Mercurial ulcers. Mucosal margins; painful, phagedenic ulcers surrounded by pimples worse after scratching.
- Warts - flat, hard, painful, small.

Itching

Biting; burning; crawling. Eruptions without itching seen in drunkards. Scratching violent - must scratch until it is raw. Itching in spots, violent and stinging.

Sensation

Biting – as if ants were biting; burning.

Concomitants

Mentals

Loquacious.

Extrovert.

Passionate.

Exuberant.

Suspicious, envious, jealous.

Mentally active, good memory, theorizing.

Religious, superstitious beliefs.

Fanaticism.

Fear of snakes.

Generals

Hot, worse on becoming heated and in warm rooms.

Left sided.

Purplish discoloration.

Desires - indigestible things, meat, alcoholic drinks, beer, fruits, coffee, farinaceous foods, flour, cold food.

Aversion - bread, cooked food, milk.

LYCOPODIUM CLAVATUM

Look of the skin

It appears withered, waxy, wrinkled, shrivelled. Freckles.

On examination

Chapping, cold, dry skin.

Ailments from

Abuse.

Anger suppressed with indignation.

Silent grief.

Anticipation.

Cares and worries.

Death of loved ones.

Disappointment.

Domination.

Egotism.

Excitement, emotional.

Failure.

Rudeness of others.

Scorned being.

Grief.

Mortification.

Sphere of action

Scalp, hands, nipples, nose, lips, behind ears.

Pathology

Acne, abscess, blisters, condylomata, ecthyma, eczema, herpetic, impetigo, erysipelas, intertrigo, lupus, naevi, psoriasis, scarlatina, scabies, tubercles, urticaria, ulcers, warts.

Modalities

General

Agg.: Right side, 4-8 p.m., heat, warm room, hot air, bed.

Amel.: Motion, after midnight, from warm food and drink, on getting cold, from being uncovered.

Particular

Erysipelas	- < after scratching.
Urticaria	- < after scratching, < warmth, < exercise.
Itching	- < warmth, < evening, < perspiring.
Eruptions	- < after scratching, < warm weather.
Cracks	- < washing after.
Psoriasis	- < summer.
	> winter, > open air.
Ulcers	- < warm applications, < scratching.
	> cold application.

Discharge

Moist pustular discharge after scratching. Discharge is white, yellow, destroying hair and foetid.

Eruptions

Eruptions with concomitant urinary, gastric or hepatic troubles. Crusty eruptions on perspiring hairy parts. Eruptions dry, bleeding, crusty, burning, coppery, painful, papular, vesicular, swelling, inflamed, itching, mealy.

- Herpetic - bleeding, burning, chapping, corrosive, crusty, dry, indolent, itching, mealy, moist, patches, scaly, suppurated, stinging, yellow.
- Acne - itching, smarting.
- Tubercles - itching, painful, wart shaped.
- Urticaria - nodular.
- Erysipelas - right to left, receding with swelling.

- Condylomata - dry, itching, pediculated.
- Ulcers - black, bleed, burning, cancerous, deep, dirty, fistulous, flat, foul, gangrenous, indolent, inflamed, indurated margins, unhealthy, varicose.
- Warts - bleeding, indented, inflamed, isolated, jagged, moist, painful, pedunculated, pulsating, stinging.

Itching

Biting, burning, crawling; on perspiring parts; scratching – must scratch until it is raw; smarting; in spots; violent, stinging and tearing.

Sensation

Anesthesia; biting, burning, prickling sensation.

Concomitants

Mentals

Haughty, arrogant, dictatorial persons. These types of behaviour are seen as here they feel safe and there is compensation for underlying emotions.

Lack of confidence, cowardice.

Intellectual types.

Intolerant of contradiction.

Fear of responsibility and anything new.

Tendency to anticipatory anxiety.

Helplessness.

Anxiety about health.

Generals

Desires - sweets, olives, warm food and drink.

Aversion - beans, peas, oysters.

Aggravation - onions, oysters, cabbage, fasting.

MALANDRINUM

Look of the skin

Scaly, greasy.

On examination

Dry.

Ailments from

Ill effects of vaccination.

Sphere of action

Lower half of body, hands, feet, face, upper lip.

Pathology

Keloid, impetigo, measles, rupia, small pox, herpes zoster.

Modalities

Particular

Itching   - < cold weather, < washing.

Discharge

Moist discharges. Greasy, oily fatty skin and discharges.

Eruptions

Dry, scaly, itching, greasy. Recurrent tendency to abscesses, as one heals another appears.

Itching

Burning, terrible, scalded sensation.

Sensation

Stinging.

Concomitants

Mentals

Dullness.

Generals

Cancerous affections.

Delayed healing.

History of repeated vaccinations.

MERCURIUS SOLUBILIS

Look of the skin

Withered, wrinkled, shrivelled.

On examination

Cracks, dry, rough.

Ailments from

Disappointment.

Ambition, deceived.

Anger, indignation with.

Egotism.

Fright.

Mental shock.

Mortification.

Sexual excess.

Surprises, pleasant.

Sphere of action

Folds of skin, face.

Pathology

Acne, cicatrices, cracks, chicken pox, eczema, erythema, herpetic, impetigo, measles, gangrene, scabies, psoriasis, scarlatina, small pox, tubercles, urticaria, purpura, condylomata, intertrigo, ulcers, warts.

Modalities

General

Agg.: Night, perspiration, heat or cold, right side.

Particular

Eruptions	- < exertion, < winter, < on hairy parts.
Impetigo	- < warmth of bed.
Acne	- < scratching after.
Ulcers	- < warmth.
Itching	- < warmth, < wool, < scratching, < perspiration, < undressing, < evening, < night. > scratching.

Discharge

Fetid, offensive, bloody, moist, corrosive, destroying hair.

Eruptions

Moist, bleeding, thick crusts, vesicular or pustular eruptions. Deep, bloody cracks. Ulceration and suppuration. Eruptions on hairy parts, on folds of skin. Desquamating and dirty.

- Acne- burn, crust with, itching, smarting, ulcerated.
- Scabies - bleeding, dry, fatty, moist.
- Scarlatina- accompanied by salivation.
- Tubercles- burn.
- Urticaria- nodular, scratching after.
- Gangrene - cold.
- Ulcers- bleed, burn, cancerous, deep, crusty, dirty, fistulous, foul, fungus, itching, salt, rheum like, sarcomatous, pimples surrounding with, unhealthy.
- Warts - suppurating.

Itching

Old people; scratch - raw -must scratch until it is, smarting, spots, violent, voluptuous, wandering, warm becoming on, itch without eruptions. Itching can be intense and distressing.

Sensation

Sticking, night, stings of insects.

Concomitants

Mentals

Instability and over-sensitivity.

Closed, unconfident people.

Delusion that everyone is an enemy.

Easily offended.

Stammering.

Violent impulses.

Internal hurried feeling with slowness of execution.

Anarchist, disobedience, defiance.

Generals

Sensitive to weather changes and draughts.

Offensiveness.

Glandular affections, salivation.

Trembling and restlessness.

Desires - bread, butter, lemons.

Aversion - sweets, coffee, salt, fats.

NATRIUM MURIATICUM

Look of the skin

The skin appears waxy, wrinkled and shrivelled.

On examination

The skin is rough and greasy.

Ailments from

Abuse.

Anger, indignation with.

Anticipation.

Bad news.

Business failure.

Cares, worries.

Death of loved ones- parents or friends of.

Depressing - emotional.

Disappointment.

Excitement.

Fear, fright.

Grief.

Wounded honour.

Love disappointed.

Marital shock.

Mortification.

Reproaches.

Rudeness of others.

Scorned being.

Sexual excess.

Shame.

Silent grief.

Suppression.

Sphere of action

Hair margins, between fingers, groin, where thighs rub, scalp, joints, ankles, hands, bends of knees and elbows, chin and nose, genitals, eyelids, flexures.

Pathology

Acne, blisters, cicatrices, cracks, chicken pox, eczema, erysipelas, excrescences, intertrigo, herpetic, measles, impetigo, lupus, leprosy, measles, psoriasis, small pox, scabies, tubercles, urticaria, ulcers, warts.

Modalities

General

Agg.: Warm room, lying down, about 10 a.m., at seashore, mental exertion, consolation, heat, talking.

Amel.: Open air, cold bathing, going without regular meals, lying on right side, tight clothing.

Particular

Eczema	- < heat, < menses, < exertion, < sea bathing, < excess salt.
	< after grief or suppressed emotions.
	> cold.
Psoriasis	- < sea bathing, < after scratching, < emotional stress, < overheating.
	< from exercise.
Urticaria	- < before menses, < seaside, < rubbing.
Simple herpes	- < emotional stress, < acute illness or fever, < exposure to sun.
Genital herpes	- < coition.
Itching	- < perspiration, < undressing, < on becoming warm, < wool.
	< exertion, < touch.
Eruptions	- < seaside, < excessive salt, < sun, < exertion, < before menses.

Discharge

The discharge is corrosive, destroying the hair. It is glutinous, thin, white or yellow pus like. Scratching aggravates the condition.

Eruptions

On hairy and perspiring parts; granular; gritty; dry; vesicular; crusty; clustered; desquamating; pemphigus; phagedenic. The eruptions are worse from exposure to sun. Scaling of the lesions is seen after scratching. Eruptions appear from being overheated.

- Herpetic - burning, chapping, circinate, crusty, dry, during fevers, itching, moist, patches, scaly, suppressed, zoster-zona
- Cicatrices - break open, painful, and red.
- Eczema - worse seaside, raw, red and inflamed.
- Measles - accompanied by salivation
- Acne - itching, worse after scratching
- Scabies - suppressed
- Urticaria - aggravated during chill, after exercise, from scratching, warmth and exercises; violent, nodular.
- Ulcers - bleed, burn, with crawling sensation, deep, fistulous, inflamed, itching, painful, pulsating, swollen, sensitive, suppurating, surrounded with vesicles.
- Warts - painful, sensitive to touch.

Itching

Biting, burning, crawling, jerking, seen in spots and perspiring parts, worse after exertion when touched on becoming warm.

Sensation

Sensation as from electric sparks; sting of insects; prickling; sticking.

Concomitants

Mentals

Desire to be alone yet fear of rejection.

Self-reliant.

Dwells on past disagreeable occurrences.

Resentful.

Avoids causing and being hurt.

Defensive.

Sympathetic.

Guilt.

Consolation aggravates.

Closed, reserved, serious.

Generals

Desires - salt, bitter, bread, fish, oysters, chocolates, coffee.

Aversion - salt, fat, coffee, fish, bread, chicken, slimy.

NITRICUM ACIDUM

Look of the skin

Dark freckles.

On examination

Unhealthy, dry, chapping appearance.

Ailments from

Anxiety.

Discords between chief and subordinate, parents and friends.

Excitement - emotional.

Fright.

Grief from mental shock.

Reproaches.

Sphere of action

Face, lips, hands, fingers, genitals, scrotum, anus.

Pathology

Abscess, acne, carbuncles, condylomata, cicatrices, decubitus, ecthyma, eczema, erysipelas, herpetic, impetigo, intertrigo, keloid, leprosy, lupus, moles, nevi, psoriasis, rupia, scabies, scarlatina, small pox, tubercles, urticaria, ulcers, warts.

Modalities

General

Agg.: touch, evening and night, cold climate, hot weather, from slight causes.

Amel.: gentle motion.

Particular

Urticaria	- < after scratching, < cold air and open air, < warmth and exercise.
	< after washing.
Psoriasis	- < night, < winter, < change of weather.
Erysipelas	- < after scratching.
Genital herpes	- < after coition.
Warts	- < washing, < rubbing.
Itching	- < cold air, < undressing.
	> scratching, > warmth.
Eruptions	- < cold air.

Discharge

Foul, acrid, corrosive, pus discharge, discharging after scratching.

Eruptions

Eruptions especially on hairy parts, crusts, in patches, bleeding, worse after scratching, vesicles, scaly spots, swelling, smarting, sensitive to touch.

- Cracks - deep, bloody.
- Carbuncles - stinging.
- Acne - gnawing, itching, hard, inflamed, painful scratching after, ulcerated.

- Scabies - suppressed.
- Scarlatina - accompanied by cracked tongue, dryness of tongue.
- Tubercles - burn, itch, mucus, red, suppurating.
- Urticaria - nodular.
- Condylomata - bleeding, broad, burn, dry, moist, offensive, pediculated, suppressed.
- Ulcers - bleeding - touched when, burning, cancerous, deep, dirty, fistulous, flat, foul, jagged margins with, zigzag, lardaceous, unhealthy, scratching after.
- Warts - bleeding, washing from, horny, indented, inflamed, jagged, large, moist, old, painful, pedunculated, soft, and suppressed, stinging.

Itching

Burning, must scratch until it bleeds, itch changes place on scratching, spots, stinging, crawling.

Sensation

Prickling, burning.

Concomitants

Mentals

Anxiety about health.

Fear of death.

Resentful, hatred, bitter, revengeful.

Dwells on past disagreeable occurrences.

Tormenting thoughts.

Anger with cursing.

Discontented.

Quarrelsome.

Sensitive to all external impressions.

Selfish.

Generals

Coldness.

Splinter like pains.

Strong urine.

Affinity for angles and muco-cutaneous junctions.

Desires - fat, salt, lime, fish.

Aversion - cheese, meat.

PETROLEUM

Look of the skin

Freckled.

On examination

Rough, hard, thickened skin, dryness, cracks, coldness.

Ailments from

Anger.

Chemical and dyes.

Coal tar products.

Contradiction.

Fright.

Grief.

Mortification.

Vexation.

Sphere of action

Hands, fingers, palms, heels, scrotum, genitals, skin folds, occiput.

Pathology

Abscess, cracks, cicatrices, eczema, erysipelas, herpes, impetigo, moles, nevi, psoriasis, scabies, ulcers, warts, acne, leprosy, urticaria.

Modalities

General

> **Agg.:** Dampness, before and during thunderstorm, riding in cars, passive motion, in winter, eating, mental state.
>
> **Amel.:** Warm air, lying with head high, dry weather.

Particular

Eczema	- < winter.
Psoriasis	- < winter, < cold weather, < dry weather.
Herpes	- < cold weather, < winter.
Eruptions	- < winter, < scratching.
	> bathing, > warmth.
Itching	- < night, < open air, < morning in bed.
	> warmth, > bathing

Discharge

Offensive, corrosive, bloody, moist discharge.

Eruptions

Biting, bleeding, blister, blotches, excoriating, offensive, suppurating, swelling.

- Herpetic - burning, chapping, corrosive, crusty, dry, itching, suppurating.
- Psoriasis - inveterata, burning, itching, red rash.
- Scabies - dry, moist, scaly, bran like, ichthyosis, smarting, stinging.
- Urticaria - nodular, rosy, vesicular, black.
- Condylomata.
- Ulcers - areola indurated, red, burning around margins, cancerous, cold and deep, fungous, indolent, indurated.
- Warts - burning, painful.

Itching

Burning, smarting. Itching of orifices, must scratch until raw, biting, during chill, without eruptions.

Sensation

Burning, biting, pressing, stitching and tearing.

Concomitants

Mentals

Irritable, fiery temperament.

Quarrelsome.

Confusion - loses way in well known streets.

Weakness of memory.

Irresolution.

Forgetful.

Discouraged.

Timid and bashful.

Anxiety in a crowd.

Easily offended.

Anger at trifles.

Aversion to company.

Generals

Emaciation.

Tendency to suppuration.

Weak extremities.

Lack of vital heat.

Offensive perspiration.

Nausea riding in a car.

Diarrhea only in the daytime.

Ravenous appetite with diarrhea.

Desires - dainties, beer and sweets.

Aversion - fat and meat.

PHOSPHORUS

Look of the skin

There is withered, waxy and wrinkled appearance of the skin.

On examination

Rough swollen, unhealthy, dry and hard, parchment like.

Ailments from

Anger.

Silent grief with anticipation.

Cares, worries.

Celibacy.

Excitement, emotional.

Fear, fright menses during.

Grief.

Jealousy.

Love, disappointed.

Mental exertion.

Moral excitement.

Mortification.

Music.

Scorned, being.

Sexual excess.

Sphere of action

Palms, soles, elbows, knees, legs and eyebrows.

Pathology

Abscess, acne, blisters, cicatrices, cracks, eczema, ecchymoses, gangrene, erysipelas, herpetic, impetigo, intertrigo, keloid, leprosy, psoriasis, measles, scarlatina, small pox, tubercles, purpura, rubella, ulcers, urticaria, warts and nevi.

Modalities

General

Agg.: Touch, warm food or drink, change of weather, from getting wet in hot weather, evening.

Amel.: cold, > open air, > washing with cold water.

Particular

Eruptions - < after scratching, < washing.

Urticaria - < after bathing.

Ulcers - < during menses.

Itching - < night, < during menses, < scratching, < undressing, < wool,

< warm - bed on becoming, < during sleep > scratching.

Acne - < scratching after.

Discharge

White-yellow, offensive, scanty discharge.

Eruptions

Biting, burning, confluent, coppery, crusty, moist, desquamating, dry, scaly, smarting, stinging, suppressed, with swelling, tense, painful, papular, patches, phagedenic.

- Blisters - burn, blotches.
- Cracks – decubitus, dirty.
- Cicatrices - bleeding, break open, painful, coldness, contraction.
- Eczema - elevated, flat, granular, gritty.
- Herpetic - burning, circinate, corrosive, crusty, dry, itching, mealy, moist, patches, scaly.
- Impetigo - itching.
- Acne - painful.
- Psoriasis - pustules, rash.
- Urticaria - nodular, vesicular.

- Gangrene - moist.
- Purpura - itching, associated with formication.
- Ulcers - indurated, bleeding edges, burning, cancerous, deep, fistulous, fungus, painful, itching, pulsating, surrounded by pimples, sensitive, unhealthy, wart shaped.
- Warts - burning, itching, painful, surrounded by ulcers in a circle.

Itching

Burning, biting, crawling, paralysed parts in. Stinging and tickling; must scratch until it is raw or bleeds.

Sensation

Anesthesias, biting, burning; sensation as if bone were adherent to the skin; as if skin were loose and hanging.

Concomitants

Mentals

Open, expressive, extrovert.

Loves company.

Affectionate, tactile.

Consolation ameliorates.

Fear of dark, ghost, being alone, disease, cancer, and thunder

Sympathetic, anxiety for others.

Selfish even though sympathetic.

Becomes indifferent to loved ones.

Feelings 'out of sight, out of mind'.

Generals

Sensitive to weather and temperature changes.

Desires - spicy, salt, cold things, fish, ice cream, wine, chocolate.

Aversion - warm food and drink, tomatoes, fish, milk, sweets, vegetables and fruits.

PIX LIQUIDA

Look of the skin

Dry and cracked appearance of the skin along with bleeding.

On examination

Baldness; scaly eruptions on back of hands.

Ailments from

Bad effects of local applications in skin disease.

Bad effects of tobacco.

Sphere of action

Back of hands.

Pathology

Alopecia, acne, eczema, psoriasis.

Modalities

Particular

Itching   - < scratching, < night.

Discharge

Foul smelling dark coloured discharges.

Eruptions

Eruptions associated with intolerable itching and bleeding after scratching. Bleeding ceases when itching. Dry and cracked skin and scaling of the lesions. Eczema, alopecia, psoriasis and acne.

• Eczema- acute eczema. The eruption is scaly, and is attended with intolerable itching. It usually affects the back of the hands. The lesions bleed after scratching. Associated with sleeplessness.

Itching

There is intolerable itching. Scratching till it bleeds.

Sensation

Burning,

Concomitants

Generals

Dark-coloured urine.

Sleeplessness.

Bronchial irritation after influenza.

Chronic bronchitis.

Pain referred to the third left costal cartilage, as it joins the rib.

Expectoration of a purulent matter of offensive odour.

Foul taste and a constant vomiting of blackish fluid with pain in stomach.

POLYGONUM PERSICARIA

Ailments from

Menopause.

Sphere of action

Skin, mucus membrane, lower extremities.

Modalities

General

Agg.: Cold weather, cold drinks.

Particular

Amel.: Perspiration.

Eruptions

- Ulcers- old indolent and flat.

Concomitants

Mentals

Irritability with sadness.

Dread of death.

Generals

Epilepsy.

Coldness of tip of nose.

Disturbed sleep.

Trembling from exercise.

Desires – cold drinks.

PSORINUM

Look of the skin

Dirty, wrinkled, shrivelled Look of the skin.

On examination

Unhealthy, dry, rough and thick.

Ailments from

Anticipation.

Excitement emotional.

Grief.

Love disappointed.

Mental exertion.

Sexual excess and excitement.

Sphere of action

Folds of skin, hands, nose, forehead, behind ears.

Pathology

Acne, cracks, eczema, erysipelas, condylomata, herpetic, keloid, leprosy, ringworm, psoriasis, scabies, ulcers, urticaria, warts.

Modalities

General

Agg.: coffee, change of weather, in hot sunshine, from cold.

Amel.: heat, warm clothing, summer, eating after.

Particular

Eczema	- < night, < cold, < undressing, < heat of bed, < winter, < bathing, < from wool. > warmth.
Psoriasis	- < from washing dishes, < washing in cold water, < winter, < after vaccination, < cold air, < heat of bed, < night, < wool.
Acne	- < menses, < coffee, < fats.
Eruptions	- < winter, < washing, < spring.
Itching	- < undressing, < warm becoming on, < warmth of bed, < wool.

Discharge

Pus, thick, thin, white and yellow, offensive discharge.

Eruptions

Bleeding, burning, coppery, crusty, desquamating, dirty, dry, scaly, serpigenous, suppurating, spring in suppressed, vesicular, papular, pemphigus, phagedenic, fetid.

- Herpetic - burning, dry, indolent, moist, scaly.
- Acne - itching, pocks.
- Pustules - indolent.

- Scabies - dry, suppressed by mercury and sulphur.
- Urticaria - after violent exercise, warmth aggravates.
- Erysipelas - traumatic.
- Keloid - lousiness.
- Condylomata - itching and moist.
- Ulcers - deep, itching.
- Warts - itching, moist.
- Eczema - suppurating and offensive.

Itching

Biting, despair from itching, eruptions without, scratching, must scratch until it bleeds and raw.

Sensation

Prickling.

Concomitants

Mentals

Forsaken feeling.

Hopeless despair.

Pessimistic.

Fear of poverty.

Manifest with - no ambition, will power, energy, love, success, faith, etc.

Anxiety, forebodings.

Dull, difficulty in thinking.

Generals

Chilly.

History of suppression.

Foul discharges.

Lack of reaction and recurrence of complaints.

After effects of acute disease.

Feels well before an attack.

Constant hunger.

Aversion - tomatoes, pork.

RHUS TOXICODENDRON

Look of the skin

Unhealthy, wrinkled, shrivelled Look of the skin.

On examination

Hard, thickening, chapping.

Ailments from

Getting wet while perspiring.

Straining.

Over lifting.

Sphere of action

Arms, hands, genitals, legs, thighs, face and neck

Pathology

Blisters, carbuncles, cellulites, chicken pox, cracks, eczema, acne, erysipelas, gangrene, lupus, impetigo, measles, herpetic, psoriasis, pustules, purpura, roseola, rupia, scabies, small pox, scarlatina, tubercles, urticaria, ulcers, warts, wens, fissures, intertrigo, excrescences.

Modalities

General

Agg.: During sleep, cold, wet, rainy weather, after rain, night, during rest, drenching, lying on back or right side.

Amel.: Warm, dry weather, motion , walking, change of position, rubbing, warm applications.

Particular

Eczema   - < morning in bed, < cold, damp weather, < getting wet < becoming heated in bed.

> running scalding hot water over the eruptions.

Psoriasis   - < heat of bed, < washing, < scratching.

> scalding hot water.

Urticaria   - < getting wet, < cold air, < autumn, < rubbing, < fever.

> during the sweats, > scalding hot water.

Erysipelas   - < after scratching.

Herpetic   - < night .

> warmth or hot bathing, > constantly moving.

Ulcers   - < night, < after scratching.

Itching   - < morning in bed, < scratching, < cold air, < perspiration and on perspiring parts, < wool, < hairy parts.

> scratching, > warmth, > hot bathing.

Eruptions   - < cold air, < winter, < spring, < change of weather, < perspiring parts, < after scratching.

Fissures   - < after washing.

Discharge

Moist, corrosive, greenish, ichorus discharge destroying hair and worse after scratching.

Eruptions

Eruptions alternates with dysentery, tightness of chest and asthma. Biting blisters, blotches, boils, clustered, crusty, desquamating, dry, excoriating, foetid, grape-shaped, hairy parts on, petechial, phagedenic, pemphigus, scaly, vesicular.

- Herpetic - alternates with chest complaints and dysenteric stools. Burning, chapping, corrosive, dry, itching, moist, scaly, suppurating, tearing.
- Zoster - zona.
- Acne - bleeding, burning, hard, after scratching feel sore as if excoriated.
- Psoriasis - diffusa, inveterata.
- Pustules - black, cracked, inflamed, malignant.
- Erysipelas - gangrenous, swelling with, vesicular.
- Ulcers - biting, black, bleeding, cancerous, bruised, burning, cold feeling, crawling, crusty, cutting with, deep, fistulous, foul, gangrenous, indolent, inflamed, itching, phagedenic, surrounded with pimples, sensitive
- Warts - bleed, burn, indented, inflamed, jagged, large, moist, old, painful, pedunculated, small, stinging.

Itching

Biting, burning, on perspiring parts, crawling, jerking, scratching until it is raw, itching unchanged by scratching, smarting, tickling, stinging.

Sensation

Anesthesia, biting, burning and bruised.

Concomitants

Mentals

Restless especially at night.

Narrow minded people.

Dwells on past especially at night.

Superstitious.

Fearful of ghosts, death, people being hurt.

Forsaken feeling.

'Causeless' weeping.

Wants to go home.

Anxiety about business.

Generals

Desires- milk, oysters, sweets.

SALICYCLICUM ACIDUM

Sphere of action

Extremities.

Pathology

Herpes zoster, urticaria, purpura, gangrene.

Modalities

General

Agg.: night, touch.

Amel.: open air.

Particular

Itching   - > scratching.

Eruptions   - > scratching.

Eruptions

Vesicular, itching.

- Purpura - idiopathic.
- Ulcers - indolent, inflamed.

Itching

Better by scratching.

Concomitants

Mentals

Absentminded.

Desire to be quiet.

Mildness.

Silent grief.

Restless.

Generals

Caries of bone.

Diabetes mellitus accompanied by Kimmelstein Wilson syndrome.

Wound - gangrene of.

Side - left.

SANICULA AQUA

Look of the skin

Dirty, greasy, brownish, wrinkled.

On examination

Cracks.

Skin about the neck wrinkled, hangs in folds.

Ailments from

Cares, worries.

Sphere of action

Head, hands, fingers.

Pathology

Abscess, eczema, herpetic circinate, tinea cruris.

Modalities

General

Agg.: Moving arms backwards, touch, riding in a car, motion, jar stepping, warm room.

Particular

Cracks -   < in winter.

Itching -   < scratching, < night.

Discharge

Pus is thick and acrid.

Eruptions

Boils slowly maturing.

- Abscess - acrid, thick pus.
- Urticaria - exercise, exertion, from – violent.

Concomitants

Mentals

Absentminded.

Anger in children at trifles.

Constantly changing occupation.

Cursing.

Company aversion to.

Darkness aversion to.

Delusion hated by others.

Delusion forsaken.

Generals

Intolerance of clothing.

Rickets.

Desire for open air.

Allergic constitution.

Desires – sweets, meat, eggs, milk, ham, bacon, fat ham, salt.

SARSAPARILLA OFFICINALIS

Look of the skin

Unhealthy, flabby, withered, wrinkled and shrivelled Look of the skin.

On examination

Cold, chapping, dry.

Ailments from

Vaccination.

Losing money.

Sphere of action

Palms, hands, feet, genitals.

Pathology

Acne, eczema, cracks, erysipelas, herpetic, impetigo, psoriasis, roseola, scabies, ulcers, urticaria, warts.

Modalities

General

Agg.: Thinking of his complaints, dampness at night, in spring, before menses, at close of urination.

Amel.: darkness.

Particular

Eruptions	- < washing, < spring, < summer, < before and during menses.
	< warmth of bed, < after vaccination.
Acne	- < after scratching, < when warm.
Cracks	- < after washing.
Itching	- < from warmth, < night, < morning, < scratching or > scratching.

Discharge

Moist discharge after scratching.

Eruptions

Boils, burning, dry, patches, pemphigus, scaly, worse after scratching, smarting, suppurated, swelling with, vesicular.

- Herpetic - burning, chapping, crusty, dry, itching, patches, suppurating
- Cracks - burning, deep, bloody, new skin cracks and burns
- Scabies - suppurating
- Erysipelas – with swelling
- Gangrene - old people in
- Ulcers - black, burn, cancerous, crusty, deep, gangrenous, herpetic, indolent, inflamed, itching, phagedenic, pulsating, suppurating, varicose ulcers
- Warts - dry, inflamed, small.

Itching

Burning, scratching, changed or unchanged by scratching, smarting, stinging.

Sensation

Burning.

Concomitants

Mentals

Changeable moods.

Forsaken feeling.

Offended easily.

Cheerful.

Dullness, mental exhaustion.

Sadness with despair.

Anger about former vexations.

Impatience from itching.

Delusion he is friendless.

Dwells on past disagreeable occurrences and recalls old grievances.

Generals

Marasmus.

Gouty tendency.

Suppressed gonorrhea.

Desires - cold drinks, cold food, juicy and refreshing things.

Aggravation - warm food, spicy.

SELENIUM COLLOIDALE

Look of the skin

Unhealthy.

On examination

Dry, scaly.

Ailments from

Anger.

Debauchery.

Mental exertion.

Sexual excess.

Sphere of action

Palms, folds of skin, ankles, genitals, between fingers and finger joints.

Pathology

Acne, comedones, herpes zoster, scabies, urticaria, ulcers, seborrhoea oleosa.

Modalities

General

Agg.: After sleep, in hot weather, draught of air, coition.

Particular

Itching   - < evening, > scratching.

Discharge

Moist discharge after scratching.

Eruptions

Biting, blotches, desquamating, dry, flat, itching, painful, smarting, suppurate, vesicular, worse after scratching.

* Acne - scratching after, sore as if excoriated.
* Scabies - fatty, suppurated by mercury and sulphur.
* Urticaria - nodular, worse after scratching.
* Tubercles - humid.
* Ulcers - indolent, burn deep, fistulous, flat, indurated, itching, painful, sensitive, superficial, suppurated, unhealthy.

Itching

Evening, biting, burning, crawling, of folds, in spots, stinging, tickling

Concomitants

Mentals

Extreme sadness with melancholy.

Mental labour fatigues.

Lascivious thoughts.

Generals

Great debility after exhausting diseases.

Sexual atony with impotency.

SILICEA TERRA

Look of the skin

Withered, waxy, wens.

On examination

Unhealthy, dry, cold, swelling, thick and flabbiness.

Ailments from

Anger.

Anticipation.

Contradiction.

Egotism.

Excitement emotional.

Fear, fright.

Friendship deceived.

Mental exertion.

Mental shock.

Mortification.

Sphere of action

Folds of skin, hairy parts, flexures, scalp, between fingers, occiput, and cervical region.

Pathology

Acne, abscess, cracks, cicatrices, eczema, carbuncles, chicken pox, herpetic, keloid, lupus, moles, nevi, impetigo, psoriasis, ulcers, warts, blisters.

Modalities

General

Agg.: New moon, morning, from washing, during menses, uncovering, lying down, damp, cold.

Amel.: Warmth, summer, wet or humid weather.

Particular

Itching   - < undressing, < daytime, < evening.

Ulcers   - > warmth.

Impetigo   - < cold.

                 > warm wraps.

Discharge

White-yellow pus like discharge.

Eruptions

Biting, blackish, burning, crusty, desquamating, dry, fetid, flat.

- Herpetic - burning, chapping, corrosive, crusty, dry, itching, mealy, moist patches, scaly.

- Ulcers - indurated, black, bleeding, bluish, burning, cancerous, crusty, cold, deep, fistulous, flat, gangrenous, painful.

- Warts - fleshy, hard, inflamed, large, painful, pedunculated, pulsating, soft, stinging, suppurating.

- Cicatrices - shining, break open, depressed, nodules, painful.

Itching

Stinging, tearing, spots, tickling after scratching, voluptuous, wandering.

Sensation

Stings of insects, burning.

Concomitants

Mentals

Abstracted.

Anticipation.

Yielding.

Nervous and excitable.

Obstinate, headstrong children.

Fixed ideas, thinks only of pins, fears them, searches and counts
   them.

Sensitive to all impressions.

Brain fag.

Generals

Ill effects of vaccination.

Tendency to suppurative processes.

Chilly, lack of vital heat.

Prostration of mind and body.

Intolerance of alcoholic stimulants.

Aversion - meat, warm food.

SULPHUR

Look of the skin

Dirty look, freckles.

On examination

Chapping, cicatrices, cracks, rough, dry and scaly.

Ailments from

Embarrassment.

Vaccination.

Exposure to dyes and chemicals.

Egotism.

Eruptions suppressed.

During full moon, decreasing moon.

Sphere of action

Extremities, scalp, genitals, back, chest and neck.

Pathology

Abscess, eczema, herpes zoster, impetigo, gangrene, psoriasis, purpura hemorrhagica, keloids, nevi, scabies, ringworm, urticaria, warts, ulcers, carbuncles, molluscum contagiosum, chicken pox, leprosy, measles, pemphigus, blisters, acne.

Modalities

General

Agg.: 11 a.m., alcoholic stimulants, periodically, standing, washing, bathing, at rest, warmth in bed, in morning.

Amel.: Dry, warm weather, lying on right side, from drawing up affected limbs.

Particular

Eczema	- < night, < on becoming heated, < bathing. > cold application.
Psoriasis	- < night, < bathing, washing, < heat of bed
Urticaria	- < night, < heat of bed, < exercise. > cold air, > cold application.
Herpes	- < heat, < night.
Impetigo	- < bathing, < heat, < night.
Eruptions	- < water, < after scratching.
Itching	- < warmth, < warmth of bed, < washing, < scratching, < walking in open air, < wool. > scratching.

Discharge

Blackish, bloody, copious, green, offensive cheese like, sour, putrid, thin, watery, whitish-yellow, corrosive, glutinous discharge; pus- yellow fetid; with maggots.

Eruptions

Alternating with respiratory complaints, vesicular, blood filled vesicles, burning, confluent, humid, itching, suppurated, ulcerated, yellow, feels to break out, crusty, green yellow suppurated.

- Herpetic - burning, chapping, circinate, corrosive, scaly, suppurated, chapped and moist.
- Boils - blood boils, another boil appears as soon as-first one heals. Periodical, slowly maturing and small boils.
- Acne - burning, inflamed, itching, moist, painful.
- Ulcers - black, black based with margins, bleeding edges, burning when touched, cancerous, crusty, deep, indolent, indurated, inflamed, itching around ulcers.
- Warts - burning, in young girls, hard, horny, inflamed, itching, painful, small.

Itching

Bleeding after scratching; itching of drunkards; itching in old persons without eruptions; on perspiring parts; itching alternates with burning.

Sensation

Anesthesia, biting, burning.

Concomitants

Mentals

Theorizing, intellectual.

Selfish, egotism.

Critical.

Lazy, tendency to take shortcuts.

Very forgetful.

Generals

Hungry at 11 a.m.

Stoop shouldered.

Offensiveness.

Uncovers feet.

Desires- chocolates, spices, fat, alcohol, sweets, apples, ice cream.

Aversion- eggs, fish, sweets, vegetables.

F- 59

SULPHUR IODATUM

Look of the skin
Freckles.

Ailments from
Anticipation.

Excess of alcohol.

Sphere of action
Ears, nose, urethra, face, lips, neck, arms, scalp.

Pathology
Acne, abscess, eczema, herpes, lichen planus, psoriasis, excrescences, urticaria, ulcers, sycosis barbae.

Modalities
General
Agg.: Touch, cold, lying, moon - full moon, motion.

Amel.: standing, air open, winter.

Discharge
Moist.

Eruptions
Desquamating, scaly, suppurating, papular.

- Ulcers - bleeding, cancerous, indolent, indurated, sensitive, spongy, suppurating.

Itching
Barber's itch; burning.

Concomitants
Mentals
Cowardice.

Hurry in movements, occupation and at trifles.

Indifference, apathy.

Suspicious.

Restless.

Generals

Desires – alcoholic drinks, pickles, lemon and lemonade.

Sides - right.

THIOSINAMINUM

Look of the skin

Thick.

On examination

Adhesions from old wounds.

Sphere of action

Scar tissue, glands, cornea, ear.

Pathology

Restrictive adhesions, strictures, scar tissues, tumours, enlarged glands, cicatrices, lupus, urticaria, keloid, dupytren's contracture.

Itching

Itching, together with mental irritability.

Sensation

Stinging sensation like pin pricks.

Concomitants

Generals

Weakness.

Tinnitus.

THUJA OCCIDENTALIS

Look of the skin

Filthy appearance of the skin, freckles, brown spots.

On examination

Gooseflesh thickened skin, hard callosities, dryness, indurations and nodules.

Ailments from

Vaccination.

Suppressed and cured sexually transmitted disease.

Sphere of action

Genitals, thigh, face, forehead, upper-lip, abdomen, chest.

Pathology

Acne, chicken pox, condylomata, carbuncles, eczema, erysipelas, herpetic, lupus, moles, nevi, psoriasis, rupia, tubercles, scabies, sarcoma, smallpox, ulcers, warts, abscess, urticaria.

Modalities

General

Agg.: Night, from heat of bed, 3 a.m. And 3 p.m., from cold damp air, after breakfast, fat, coffee, vaccination.

Amel.: left side, while drawing up a limb.

Particular

Psoriasis	- < cold bathing.
Herpetic	- < evening.
Eruptions	- < after scratching.
Itching	- < evening, < at night, > scratching
Erysipelas	- < after scratching.
Urticaria	- < after scratching.

Discharge

Moist, corrosive, yellow discharge worse after scratching.

Eruptions

Biting, burning, boils, painful, patches, itching, pemphigus, mealy, scaly, suppressed, swelling, on covered and perspiring parts, crusty, dry vesicles, coppery, desquamating.

- Herpetic - burning, circinate, crusty, dry, itching, mealy, moist, scaly, suppurating, stinging, whitish, zoster-zona.
- Acne - bleed, close together, moist
- Psoriasis - diffusa
- Eczema - flat
- Urticaria - nodular
- Condylomata - bleeding, broad, burning, dry, fan shaped, horny, itching, moist, offensive, pediculated, rapidly growing
- Moles - itching and stinging
- Ulcers - biting, bleed, black base, burning, cancerous, crawling, deep, dirty, fungous, inflamed, isolated, itching, jagged, large, moist, old, painful, pedunculated, red, sensitive to touch, small, smell like old cheese, soft, stinging, suppurating.

Itching

Biting, burning, crawling, painful, stinging, without eruption, on perspiring parts.

Sensation

Biting and burning.

Concomitants

Mentals

Reserved, secretive person.

Confused.

Fixed ideas, fanaticism.

Questioning, doubtful, sceptical.

Perfectionism, fastidious.

Sensitive to music.

Hurried.

Generals

Left sided.

Worse at 3 a.m. and 3 p.m.

Tendency to warts, growths and excrescences.

Oily skin.

Sweet perspiration.

Sweat on uncovered parts.

Desires - salt, tobacco, onions.

Aversion - onions, meat, tobacco, potatoes.

Aggravation - onions, potatoes, tea, fat.

USTILAGO MAYDIS

Look of the skin

Copper coloured spots.

On examination

Dry, loss of hair and nails.

Ailments from

Abused after, being sexually.

Sphere of action

Extremities, genitals.

Pathology

Eczema, naevi, psoriasis, urticaria.

Modalities

General

    Agg.: Touch.

    Amel.: Menses.

Particular.

    Itching   - < night.

    Eruptions   - < touch.

Discharge

    Moist.

Eruptions

    Tendency to small boils, coppery spots.

    Psoriasis - internally and externally.

Itching

    Night.

Sensation

    As if boiling water is running along the body.

Concomitants

Mentals

    Amativeness.

    Aversion to company.

    Company aversion to.

    Delusion is caught in wires.

    Discontented with everything.

    Fancies lascivious.

    Irritable when questioned.

    Irritable when spoken to.

    Menses after, mental symptoms.

Generals

Desires - hearty, heavy food, apples, sour food.

Amelioration - apples.

Side - left.

Anaemia.

Weakness.

Weakness emissions after.

Weakness after sexual excess.

Weakness from talking.

Skin disease associated with menstrual irregularities.

VINCA MINOR

Look of the skin

Redness.

On examination

Redness and soreness of skin on slight rubbing.

Ailments from

Anger.

Mental exertion.

Sphere of action

Face, head, legs, hands, genitals.

Pathology

Eczema, ulcers.

Modalities

General

Agg.: Coffee, < during menses.

Discharge

Offensive discharge.

Eruptions

Fetid, granular, itching, crusty.

Itching

Burning, corrosive.

Concomitants

Mentals

Suppressed anger.

Mental exertion aggravates.

Fear death of with sadness.

Fear of misfortune.

Anger with red face and red tip of tongue.

Generals

Weakness.

Trembling externally from mental exertion.

VIOLA TRICOLOR

Look of the skin

Chapped.

On examination

Dry, excoriated, cracked skin with thick scabs.

Ailments from

Suppressed eruptions.

Sphere of action

Face, head.

Pathology

Abscess, acne, boils, eczema, herpes, impetigo, pustules, ringworm, urticaria, ulcers. One of the few specific remedies for atopic eczema and impetigo in childhood.

Modalities

General

Agg.: Winter, sitting, night.

Amel.: Open air.

Particular

Itching   - > scratching,

Eruptions   - < night.

Discharge

Yellow pus and tenacious, gummy discharge that mattes the hair together worse after scratching.

Eruptions

Biting, burning, crusty, worse after scratching. Dry, itching, phagedenic patches. Suppressed, suppurating eruptions.

- Herpetic - burning, chapping, corrosive, crusty, dry, itching, moist, stinging, suppurating.
- Pustules - green, fetid, painful, yellow
- Eczema - children in
- Boils - large and small.
- Urticaria - nodular.
- Ulcers - crusty, itching, suppurating, unhealthy.

Itching

Biting, burning, crawling, stinging.

Sensation

Intolerable itching and burning worse in the night.

Concomitants

Mentals

Anxiety after eating.

Anxiety about future.

Cowardice.

Discontented with everything.

Discontented with himself.

Mental emotional symptoms after eating.

Fear after eating.

Hypochondriacal in the daytime and cheerful in the evening.

Impatient.

Sadness ameliorated in the evening.

Vivacious.

Generals

Children, complaints in.

Dropsy, internal dropsy.

Rhus tox. resembles Viola tricolor in many of its skin symptoms.

XEROPHYLLUM ASPHODOIDES

Look of the skin

The skin is rough and cracked.

On examination

Feels like leather.

Sphere of action

Knees, genitalia, female genitalia – labia.

Pathology

Eczema, poison oak, erythema, dermatitis, herpes, erysipelas, erythema nodosum.

Modalities

General

Agg.: Afternoon, evening.

Amel.: Morning, moving the affected part.

Particular

< application of cold water.

Eruptions

Blisters, little lumps. Dry eruptions. Vesication with intense itching. Dermatitis surrounded by inflammation.

- Erythema – with vesication and intense itching.
- Abscess – blisters like lumps.
- Dermatitis – especially around knees, with swelling of inguinal glands behind the knees.
- Inflammation – it resembles poison oak.

Itching

Intense itching with stinging and burning. Sensitive skin.

Concomitants

Mentals

Poor concentration.

Forgets names, makes spelling mistakes – writes last letters of words first.

Generals

Glands behind knees swollen.

Chapter-37

Cases

The following cases demonstrate various approaches. The cases have been edited due to shortage of space; only symptoms on which the specific drug was prescribed is discussed, and in some cases only a few local remedies are discussed trying to show their failure and success where ever possible. This may seem to the reader quite contrary to what I had already written but I have to confess that many times in out patient department where there is time constraint and due to patients poor educational back ground history taking and symptoms analysis becomes very poor. I have given my conclusion at the end of the case. Not all the cases given below has been treated by me, some cases are by classical authours like Burnette (cases with excessive vaccination), Boger, Kent, Nash Lippe, etc.

CORNS

CASE 1

Mrs. S.P. aged 42 years, consulted me for multiple, painful corns on the soles of both the feet, present since the last four years. She was in great agony due to the pain. In the past when the corn used to be painful she used to consult a pedicurist who in turn would scrape the skin and remove the corn. Since the corns occurred recurrently, she decided to start with some homeopathic treatment.

On examination, I found the corns were very tender, even to the slightest touch. They were hard and were rough to feel.

Her other symptoms were:

- Menorrhagia with dysmenorrhea - sometimes she fainted due to pain.
- Constipation with frequent ineffectual urging.
- She was a chilly patient.
- Headache by strong odors.
- She was depressed due to her condition.

I selected *Hepar sulph. 1M* as the remedy for her, since the corns were very sensitive to touch. After a week she reported that she had only partial relief. I repertorized the case taking all the above symptoms and selected *Ignatia.* A few infrequent doses were given in the 200th potency followed by placebo, which not only removed the pain but also gave her relief in her menstrual symptoms and headache.

Time and again I have verified that whenever *Hepar sulph.* fails or acts partially in cases of painful tender corns, drugs like *Ign., Sulph., Ran-s.,* usually cures the condition

CASE 2

A young man came to consult me for painful corns on both the palms. He was going to a gymnasium and used to lift heavy weights. Due to the constant friction of his palms with the iron rods, he developed corns on them. There was a burning sensation in the corns. He had no other characteristic symptoms. I had prescribed to him *Radium bromatum 200C* for a prolonged period. Gradually his corns started disappearing.

The characteristic indication for its use was a *burning sensation in the corn.*

CASE 3

A lady consulted me for painful corn on her soles. On examination I found that around the corns there were small blisters with ulceration. Also, the corns were very tender to touch. The patient received from me *Ranunculus scleratus 30C* on the characteristic indication *'Painful corns with ulceration and formation of blisters'*.

I have personally verified this on many occasions that *Ran-s.* dissolves the corn if there is presence of blisters or ulcers around them.

CRACKS

CASE 1

A lady, of over 60 years, came to me with the complaints of cracks on her hands, which were painful and discharging serum and blood. There were pustules on her hands along with this. The patient had this complaint since the last four years, along with some boils on the body. On the above indications *Petroleum 30C* was given. After ten days, the cracks and pustules on her hands had greatly improved. After a further ten days, there was more improvement.

At the next visit she said that there was no further improvement and her hands had become hot and were burning. Based on these symptoms I gave her a few doses of *Sulphur 200C* infrequently with placebo. With the above course of medicines, the condition of her hands came back to normal within two months time.

CASE 2

A lady came to me with palms that were deeply cracked all over. She had this complaint since the last three years, approximately after the time of giving birth to her child. There was intense itching and burning pain in the palms and soles. This was troublesome to her especially in her sleep and compelled her to put her hands and feet out of the blanket. Based on these symptoms I gave her *Sulphur 200C*.

By the next fortnight, there was much relief in the sensation of heat in her hands and feet as also in the itching. I gave a few doses of placebo and promised to see her again next Sunday. By her next visit, about a month later, the skin on her hands had almost regained its natural tone and colour. About a week later there was an appearance of an eczematous patch between index finger and thumb on the left hand. There was itching worse at night, warm room, warm application, but great relief in itching and eczema if exposed to open air. I gave her a single dose of *Psorinum 200C* and her eczema cleared off within a week's time. *Sulphur* followed by *Psorinum* have been confirmed by me number of times especially if eczema is better by exposure to open air.

CHILBLAINS

CASE 1

A lady, in her mid-20's, came to me with her complaint of chilblains, occurring since many years. With no other characteristic indications in her case, I prescribed to her *Petroleum 30C*, which kept her free of this complaint in the successive winter months.

Petroleum as a drug is very useful in cases of itching chilblains and cracked, chapped hands with burning pain and an intolerable itch, especially in the winter months.

CASE 2

A lady came to me with the complaints of chilblains since the last 5-6 years, worse from the slightest of cold weather. She had a strong desire for fats and salts. Based on these symptoms I selected *Nitricum acidum* for her, which gave her a lot of relief.

CASE 3

A lady came to be with chilblains on her hands and feet, which were swollen bright red with complaints of burning and itching. There were marked cracks, which bleed easily. She was extremely chilly and was known for her quick temper and hypersensitivity. I prescribed to her *Nux vomica 200C*, which cured the case within a few infrequently given doses.

HERPES

CASE 1

Here is a case where the patient came to me saying that she had developed a 'bad rash' on her sacrum, which went down the back between the nates, all the way to her labia. This was no rash, but was a case of a pustular form of herpes. It caused her a lot of itching and the pain was so severe as to cause her to faint at times. She could not lie on her back. With further history, it was found that she had been vaccinated three to four times in the past. I gave her *Variolinum 200C* based on these symptoms and called her after a week.

By her next visit she was much more comfortable and the eruptions had reduced in number and severity. She said that within three days time after the first dose, she could lie on her back without any pain. She was extremely grateful and surprised at the same time. On examination I found that there were still a few dry pustules present on the skin, but these were just scabby without any inflammation or pain. I did not repeat the dose, but just waited and watched. She felt much better within a month's time, with no new formation of scabs or pustules.

Dr. Burnett, a great homeopath, has written very often about the benefits of using the remedy *Variolinum* (a medicine made from small-pox pus that is sterilized and potentized) in cases of herpes. He has said that it tends to wipe out the eruptions and its resultant neuralgic pain.

CASE 2

Here is a case of an elderly lady with a chronic and severe form of herpes, with lesions that were inflamed, extremely tender and ulcerated, present on both her breasts. She was much better within a few doses of the remedy *Ranunculus bulbosus*, in the 30th potency.

CASE 3

A patient of herpes genitalis case to me, with lesions on and around the labia, occurring chronically every 2-3 months since many years. She was a dark skinned, slim woman who had two miscarriages, both in the third month of pregnancy. She also complained of an intermittently occurring whitish-yellow vaginal discharge, which caused a lot of itching in the area. The herpetic lesions characteristically got worse before and after her menses. She had her menarche at the age of 19 years, and her menstrual cycle occurred irregularly every 2-3 months. She was pretty anxious about her not being able to conceive and also worried that her herpetic lesions would get worse in case she did manage to get pregnant. She was known to get easily irritated and was very often depressed and would avoid conversation or communication of any kind. She had a strong desire for pickles, lemons and sauerkraut. Based on the above symptoms I gave her *Sepia 200C*, two doses.

She came back after a fortnight saying that she had a regular menstrual cycle a week after the first dose. Also the herpetic lesions had erupted during that time, but were not as severe as they used to be. I gave her placebo and asked her to come back after 2 months.

After 2 months, her herpetic lesions were much better, and also the purulent vaginal discharge had stopped occurring. She had a regular menstrual cycle during both the months.

Sepia is known to be a very deep-acting remedy. Farrington has mentioned that when the vaso-motor nerves are inactive the skin is more liable to the effects of irritation and particularly to herpetic eruptions, which *Sepia* cures. *Sepia* is a well-known remedy for herpetic lesions on the abdomen, genitals or around the lips.

The mental-emotional picture of Sepia is often one of indifference to those loved best; irritability and sadness with anxiety toward evening. It is particularly adapted to delicate females with rather fine skin, sensitive to all impressions, usually with dark hair; the face is apt to be sallow, and the eyes surrounded by dark rings.

CASE 4

This is one more case of chronic and recurrent herpes labialis in a young girl. The herpetic eruptions, occurring every 2-3 months, were associated with fever and chills. She had a lot of grief due to her boyfriend and his family, who mistreated her. She had a marked desire for salty and spicy food.

I gave her *Natrium mur. 200C*, two doses a month for two months. Her lesions became much better after the second dose and she has not had another attack of herpes after that for almost a year.

Natrium mur. is a well-known remedy in cases of herpetic eruptions arising from any kind of stress or psychic disturbance. The lesions are especially marked around the lips and the genitals (like in cases of *Sepia*). Farrington has stated that herpes labialis accompanied by chills (that are worse around 10 a.m.) and fever, are especially characteristic of *Natrium mur.* Herpes in cases of *Natrium mur.* occurs in both males and females, whereas *Sepia* tends to affect especially the females.

CASE 5

Here is a case of a 43-year-old man with a history of recurrent herpetic lesions on the glans penis, almost every 2-3 months. There were no characteristic mental symptoms that he was revealing due to his secretive nature, but he had a marked tendency towards easy but foul perspiration, and was sensitive to both cold and heat. I prescribed to him *Mercurius vivus 1M*, one dose a week.

Follow-up

The patient came back after a month and was put on Sac Lac.

He reported a decrease in the size and number of lesions. By the third month after the last dose, he had two small eruptions on the glans, which went away after one more dose of the medicine, and there has been no recurrence after that.

The remedy *Mercurius vivus* is a useful remedy for herpes in cases of males especially. Mentally the patient may complain of a weakened memory and at times a feeling as if 'is losing his reason'. *Mercury is an addition in my repertory as one of the secretive remedy.* In General there is a tendency to free perspiration and sensitivity to both cold and heat.

CASE 6

This is a case of herpes genitalis, who came to me with an eruption on his penis, present since about 10 years, and which would get worse in the summer months. He complained of a burning pain in the urethra when urinating. There was a history of sexual exposure. An associated complaint that he had was that of insomnia, since he was pretty much worried and stressed about his health.

There was a strong family history of hypertension, especially in the paternal side.

Personal History

He had a very poor appetite, though he could not tolerate hunger very well. He would feel very weak and giddy on an empty stomach.

He was fond of chicken, fruit, ice cream, milk and sweets. He would always lie on the right side when sleeping. As regards his sexual sphere, he practiced masturbation almost everyday.

Life Situation

The patient was born and brought up in Bihar. He finished his MBA and came to Bombay for a job.

He tends to be short tempered, getting angry easily if contradicted, or in situations where people are rude to him. When angry he tends to scream and throws things, or at times just remains in solitude. If it is his own fault he apologizes, or else he waits for the opposite person to talk.

He is very fearful of being alone in the dark.

He is obstinate and dominating.

He is very sentimental, crying easily when watching emotional scenes on television or movies. He weeps easily when he misses his family.

He likes to be consoled.

He had a history of disappointment in love. He was very disturbed mentally during this time, due to which he visited a prostitute.

Rubrics taken in his case were:

- Fear, phobia, alone of being, in darkness.
- Anger, contradiction from.
- Anxiety, conscience of.
- Rage, fury, striking.
- Ailments from love, disappointed.
- Male, masturbation disposition to.
- Sleep, position, right side on.
- Desires, chicken.
- Desires, ice cream.
- Desires, fruit.

Treatment

On this basis *Phosphorus* 1M was prescribed and repeated every 15 days.

Follow-up

In two months his skin complaints were 60% better. *Phosphorus* was later raised up to C.M during the course of treatment for permananent cure.

WARTS

CASE 1

A young Gujarati boy, aged 20 years old, came to me with multiple warts on the palms, fingers and feet, present since the last five years. He was a student studying in Commerce College and he used to cut/cauterize his warts whenever it became painful or whenever he found the site to be looking ugly.

The following were the characteristic symptoms seen in his case:

- The warts were flat, hard and tender to touch.
- Profuse perspiration from the slightest exertion.
- Tendency to catch cold very easily.
- He was very talkative and a happy-go-lucky type of person. He was not very much interested in studies as he wanted to learn and practice carpentry; but because his father didn't like the idea, he was forcibly advised to join a commerce college. He also had difficulty in concentration and comprehension. He had an inability to perform any intellectual task.
- Appetite was voracious.
- He was weak physically, and his stomach would get disordered easily, especially after consuming any milk products.

Line of Treatment given

For a week he was given placebo, during which time the case was repertorized. Then he was given the remedy *Natrum carb 1M,* 3 doses for 21 days. Within a fortnight all the warts had disappeared. So he was advised not to repeat the last dose. Until very recently he was under my observation and had not developed any new warts.

CASE 2

A 43-year-old man consulted me in March 1987 with two chief complaints

- Left sided renal calculus since April 1985.
- Multiple warts around the mouth, nose, thumb and extremities.

Other characteristic features seen in his case were:

- Craving for lime.
- Difficulty in digesting milk.
- Nausea after eating. Occasional bouts of bitter or sour vomiting.
- Burning micturition with urine of a strong odour.
- Psychologically, he had a fear of death due to his illness. He was easily frightened. Got vexed at trifles. Occasionally developed fits of rage with despair.
- He had a strong family history of asthma, DM and IHD and a past history of cataract and typhoid.
- His IVP taken on June and November 1985 showed large opaque calculus in the left upper ureter.

Treatment

He was prescribed *Nitricum acidum 30,* four pills twice a day for a week, followed by *Nitricum acidum 200,* once in three days for 15 more days.

Follow-up

For 2 months the patient did not report to us. It was only in June 1987, when he had an attack of bilious headache that he came back to us, and we inquired about his warts and to our surprise not a single wart was present. There was also no recurrence of the renal colic.

CASE 3

A 9 years old kid was brought to me in May 1988 for a wart on the middle phalanx of the left index finger. He had noticed this only 4 months back. Being a student of the 4th standard, he was very conscious of this wart and would pick on it continuously.

The following characteristic symptoms were taken into consideration:

- Extreme restlessness.
- Stubborn – always retaliates to authority.

- Short tempered, becomes angrier when contradicted.
- Disorderly and very haphazard in his work.
- Desire for cold milk, ice cream, chocolates, and potatoes.
- Aversion to meat and spicy food.
- Profuse perspiration.
- Dreams of ghosts – fearful.
- Nocturnal enuresis.

Treatment

After detailed study of this case, *Tuberculinum bovinum 10M*, one dose every alternate day, was prescribed for a period of seven days.

Follow-up

On his second visit there was slight improvement – the wart had decreased in size. So he was put on *Tuberculinum bov.* 10M one dose every fourth day for one month. Since they were to migrate to Australia his mother was most adamant to get rid of the wart as fast as possible. To speed up the healing a specific prescription was given and the drug was *Lac-c. 200*, 4 pills once a week for 2 weeks. This was chosen since *Lac-c.* was the only remedy with 3 marks in Kent's repertory under 'warts on the fingers'.

CASE 4

This is a case of venereal warts. This female patient was treated for gonorrhoea 18 months back with sulphonamides, with apparently a very quick and successful result. There had been no discharge at all since then, but recently, she noticed crops of warts on the vulva that were increasingly spreading. She had a strong aggravation from tea and coffee as this lead to stomach upset, she loved to put extra garlic on some selected dishes. She was always covering her body to warm himself. On examination these were typical condylomata acuminata.

Treatment

She was given the drug *Thuja 30C*, four pills three times a day, for a week.

Follow-up

She came back after a fortnight with no change in her lesions. Then one dose of *Thuja CM* was given and within three months all her warts had disappeared and there has been no recurrence of it as yet.

THUJA (ARBOR VITAE)

The main action of this drug is on the skin and genito-urinary organs producing conditions, which correspond to Hahnemann's sycosis, where the chief manifestation is the formation of wart-like excrescences on the mucous membranes and the cutaneous surfaces.

It has been extolled for its effects in suppressed gonorrhoea and vaccination, and is the drug of choice in vaccinosis when constitutional effects following vaccination are extreme. There is no doubt that here it acts specifically and quickly. One had always felt that a simple experiment to prove the efficacy of potencies would be to administer potencies of *Thuja* for some weeks before vaccination and observe how many cases would show complete resistance to vaccination with cowpox.

A .patient (like *Nat-sulph.*) has a hydrogenoid constitution, i.e., is susceptible to damp humid atmosphere. Its pains (like *Rhus tox.*) are worse in damp weather and get better in dry weather.

The mental symptoms of *Thuja* are strange, rare and peculiar, e.g. the patient feels that there is a strange person at his side; or that there is something alive in the abdomen, etc.

The skin is greasy like *Nat-mur.* and *Psorinum*. Chronic catarrhal states of the eyes, nose, and ears are covered by Thuja in the eyes – styes and tarsal tumours; ears – polypi and chronic discharge; nose – ulceration and conditions resembling ozaena. The teeth decay next to the gums as in pyorrhea.

Thuja is recommended for tea drinkers' dyspepsia and has an aggravation from eating onions. The stool recedes like Silicea and there are, of course, the anal warts.

In the male, *Thuja* is quoted for enlargement of the prostate and for chronic epididymitis and indeed both may be a result of gonorrheal infection. In the female, *Thuja* covers many manifestations of chronic pelvic infection (not necessarily gonorrheal) and again, the warts of vulva and vagina already mentioned. Papillomata of the larynx are of course again covered in the Thuja constitution.

In the limbs the peculiar symptom of 'legs feel like glass or wood' should be remembered and was the guide to the use of *Thuja* in Dr. Fergie Wood's famous 'brittle man'.

Thuja sweats only on the uncovered parts, unlike *China* and *Pulsatilla,* which sweat only on covered parts.

The skin manifestations have already been described but all sorts of blotches, brown spots, even naevi are noted in the picture besides the warty growth so typical of the drug.

Thuja (like *Leuticum*) is worse at night, (like *Sulphur*) from the heat of the bed and (like *Kalium carb.*) at 3 a.m. and 3 p.m.

CASE 4

This is a case of plantar warts in a 46-year-old woman. She had warts on the left foot since about twenty years before she presented to me. She would keep cauterizing the warts off and on but they started to get worse since the last six months.

They were extremely painful and tender, making it very difficult for her to walk too. There was a sensation of pin-prick and a stabbing pain, which would get worse on lying down and when keeping the legs raised up and extended; the pain would be better on letting the leg hang down. A concomitant symptom with these plantar warts was recurrent and chronic sinusitis.

Treatment

Conium 200C, two doses, was prescribed on the basis of the peculiar Modalities, and the result was a beautiful cure within two weeks. I was confident of the prescription though Conium was not listed under warts or corns in any repertory.

CASE 5

This is a case of warts on the tongue and left tonsil, in a five-year-old girl, since the past three months. The warts were soft, non-bleeding and not painful or tender. They were growing and were more marked on the left side of the tongue.

Other characteristic features seen in her case were:

- She had a tendency to catch colds easily right since her birth.
- She was a hot patient throwing off covers even in winter months and was averse to any tight clothing around the neck.

Treatment

I had given to her *Lachesis 1M*, but there was no change in her warts.

Follow-up

Then she came back to me during one of the episodes of her cold, wherein she had a thick yellow, stringy nasal discharge, and blocked nose that was better in open or cold air.

Treatment

I gave her *Kali sulph. 6C*, four doses.

Follow-up

It was noticed that within 4-5 days a slight reduction had taken place in the size of the warts. Of course the coryza was cured with *Kali sulph.* 6C within this period.

Treatment

She was kept on *Kalium sulph.* 6C, four times a week and gradually the warts were cured in about two months time.

CASE 6

During one of my foreign visits, I had a 35-year-old patient, with a fair complexion, blue eyes and a mild disposition, who was into farming and fruit growing as a family business.

Family history

He had a very strong family history of alcoholic consumption, with two sisters and an uncle dying of its bad effects. Also, one of his own children, aged two years, died last summer due to marasmus. His parents were both living and well now, though both were subjected to recurrent attacks of erysipelas about once a year.

Chief complaint

As long as he remembers has had a wart on the left cheek, near the angle of the mouth, about the size of a small pea. It never gave him any trouble until last September, when, for some unknown reason, it began to grow rapidly. At the end of two months it had grown about one inch in length, and as thick as the little finger, and had already begun to ulcerate and discharge thin, acrid and badly smelling pus; occasionally it would bleed so profusely, as to be somewhat alarming. It was during one of these attacks that he called the attention of a physician to it, who diagnosed it as a cancerous wart, and advised immediate excision. Not satisfied with his decision he consulted two others, who gave him similar advice, when he was advised to consult me about it. On examination of it carefully I came to the conclusion that it was cancer; the ulceration had already reached the cheek, which was very much swollen, infiltrated and angry; with a tendency of the tissues to contract around the growth.

Treatment

From the character of the discharge, which was thin, watery and excoriating, with the intense burning, constant thirst, and the nightly restlessness and aggravation after midnight, I prescribed *Arsenicum album CM*, two doses for a week.

Follow-up

At the end of one week he returned, with most of his complaints having had improved. The discharge had nearly ceased, the inflammation lessened, the growth had now begun to contact at the base, the excessive thirst had reduced, and the nightly restlessness was also much better. At the end of the second week it had dried up so much that it looked as if it was burnt. The contracted lesion, which had gone still further at the base, so that with a slight touch the lesion broke off from the cheek, followed by a slight hemorrhage. There was no medicine given and at the end of the third week I considered the case as cured, but the only regret was that the diagnosis was not cofirmed by a biopsy!!

CASE 7

There was an adolescent girl who came to me with huge warts on her fingers of both the hands, since almost over a year. There were five warts on right index finger and one on the right middle finger. On the left hand there was a small wart on the index finger. She often complained of pain in legs and headache on returning from school for which she was given frequent painkillers. She would get constipated easily, especially when travelling. There was a history of worms since her childhood and eczema on left foot 6 months back. Based on the above symptoms and a few other characteristic traits, I gave to her *Calcarea phos. 10M* one dose in two weeks, for 2 months.

Within a month two warts on her right index finger had fallen off and the remaining ones had considerably reduced in size. By the next month, all the warts had fallen off and most of her complaints were better. The frequency of her headaches had also reduced.

CASE 8

This is a case where the person had multiple warts on the chin and neck since about two years. The warts were soft, pedunculated and fleshy, but had become very tender and would bleed easily when shaving. Cauterization was tried a number of times, but the recurrence rate kept increasing. After further history it was revealed that he had been re-vaccinated two years back, after which the warts had increased in number and size.

I gave him *Thuja* 200C, one dose every month. Within about two months all his warts disappeared completely.

CASE 9

This is a case of a 40-year-old man having almost about 30-35 warts on the face and neck, which were black in color, variable in size and soft in consistency. He also had a few other small warts all over his body. All these came up within a short span of 4-6 months. Being a high executive, he tried to get himself treated over here and even in the United States but to no avail. The warts came back with vigor. He even tried homeopathy from a number of doctors, but with no positive result.

Past history

He had a past history of scabies, boils, blisters, fungus infection toes, occasional vaccinations and inoculations.

Family History

Father died early, cause not known; mother normal.

He was a hot patient, and would sweat easily and profusely, having a foul odor. He was a short and obese man, of 5 feet and weighing about 82 kgs.

No other symptoms were available but he gave a strong history of using a lot of Cortisone preparations, both orally and locally, for his skin condition.

Treatment

I gave him *Cortisone* 200C, one dose a week, for three weeks.

Follow-up

After three weeks he came back with not much change in his physical condition.

Constitutionally, he looked like a *Calcarea carb.* patient, but he had already been given an innumerable number of medicines before he came to me. So I thought of trying a new remedy called *Calcarea calcinata 30C* in repeated doses.

Follow-up

Within about 15 days, 50% of the warts disappeared and some became smaller in size.

The same remedy was repeated in the 200C potency, but given infrequently, about once in 2 weeks.

The patient came back after two months, saying that all the warts over his body had completely disappeared. All those who were working with him were really surprised with this magic cure. I have tried this remedy in some other cases also with a good deal of success.

CASE 10

This is another case of multiple warts in a 12-year-old child, who came to me with his mother. He had about 20-25 warts on his hands, sides of the fingers and legs, since the past six months or so. Most of the warts were fairly large, hard and jagged and two or three were soft.

Being Anglo-Indian and believer in the Modern Science, the mother consulted the Government Doctor. He naturally being ignorant of any other better treatment applied Silver Nitrate over all the warts. The result was that the poor fellow's skin was burnt, but the warts remained as they were. I asked the mother to wash them nicely with soap and warm water and apply nothing externally, and just watch the wonderful effects of homeopathic treatment.

I could not elicit many characteristic symptoms even after taking a careful case history, but I could find that the boy while in a boarding school at Deolali was inoculated every year against smallpox, also sometimes against Typhoid, Cholera and lastly he had taken B.C.G. inoculation. I had seen several such cases in my practice suffering from the ill effects of vaccination, and I presumed that these warts were due to the same.

Treatment

I gave the patient a single dose of *Thuja 1M*.

Follow-up

There was no improvement in his condition for about one fortnight. One evening he came alone and told me that while playing and whenever he injured his legs the warts began to bleed and asked me to stop the bleeding. This gave me a clue and I put him on *Causticum 30C*, twice a day.

Within eight days he told me that he found the warts had disappeared like magic effect of the minimum dose and told the Government Doctor about the result. But alas, the doctor refused to believe that so many warts could disappear so soon with just oral medicine, and no external applications. This is the modern trend of thought.

CASE 11

One day in a children's clinic, a child came with large and flat warts on the tongue, inside the cheeks and a few scattered at other places. The child had been given *Thuja 30C* in the past without any effect. Then whooping cough and other treatment had intervened; but always the warts persisted. They had been previously operated on in an adjacent hospital – cauterized and cut away but had recurred.

Dr. Nash got out his pocket case and put a few tiniest globules of *Thuja CM* on the child's tongue. A month later, all the warts had disappeared except a very small excrescence, which a dose of *Thuja 10M* (the highest potency then procurable) finally caused to disappear.

CASE 12

Though warts are not dangerous as a rule, they can be unsightly and troublesome to the patient, especially if they are situated in areas like around the eyes, inside the mouth or anus, etc.

Dr. Burnett gives a case of a middle-aged man, who complained of long-standing indigestion, epigastric pain and distress. He also complained of a very uncomfortable sensation in his anal region, which was found to have a number of small warts arranged almost in a ring around the orifice. The patient had an old history of exposure to gonorrhea and had also taken several vaccinations. This then led to the prescription of *Thuja 30*, in infrequent doses, which quite cured the dyspepsia and also the anal warts; for when again examined, the warts had quite disappeared.

ECZEMA

CASE 1

This is a case of a 25-year-old patient who suffering from eczema and asthma, where the episodes of both tend to alternate with each other. He had eczema right since the age of 7 years, which was suppressed by applying the various ointments and lotions. He was then fine for a few years, but then had an episode of fever with severe cough, for which he was hospitalized and diagnosed as having pneumonia, which was subsequently treated with antibiotics. Then once at about midnight, he woke up suddenly from his sleep with cough and breathlessness. He was then diagnosed as having asthma, for which allopathic medicines were given with no relief. Then one fine day he suddenly found himself to be cured of his asthma, but then his eczematous eruptions started to come back. He went to a local doctor who gave some ointments, after which his asthma came back. The patient by now was fed up with this alternating affair and in despair he came to me for help.

After taking his case in detail, the following characteristic symptoms were found:

- His asthma used to get worse in the night, especially around midnight, with the attacks lasting till morning. There was a spasmodic pain in the chest with rattling of mucus. During the attack he couldn't sleep and had to be sitting near an open window. Open air used to relieve him of his distress.

- His eczema was extremely itchy, relieved only by scratching, which would be followed by burning. The eruptions and itching would get worse from heat.

- He was a hot patient with a strong desire for open air. He would wear thin clothes even in the very cold winter days. He would not take covers during sleep.

- He was a light sleeper, waking up from the slightest of noise.

- He would consume a lot of water, and his appetite in comparison was much smaller.

- He had a strong craving for sweets.

- His family history revealed a history of eczema in the mother, asthma in his sister, and gout in the father.

Treatment

His case was repertorized and then he was put on *Sulphur 30C* for two months.

The patient gradually improved in his complaints, but had a bad health again after two months, and then he was put on *Sulphur 200C*.

For three months he was on the same medicines, and was gradually improving with reduction in the frequency and intensity of the attacks of both the eczema and the asthma.

Again after three months, the patient's condition came to a standstill and so *Sulphur 1M* was chosen and given for two months. There were no more attacks of eczema or asthma for two months and the patient stopped coming for his follow-up.

Within two months after stopping the medicines, his attack of asthma came on again, though it was not as severe, and *Sulphur 1M* was repeated and this treatment was continued for four more months. Then the patient was asked to report back in case he had any complaints again.

So for over 6 months he went without medicines, and was fine. Then he came back one day with a little bit of itching in the various parts of the body, but there were no eczematous lesions seen. He also complained of a slight breathlessness in the middle of the night since the last seven days.

We re-studied his symptoms and found that – He still wanted open air when breathless, but this was only in the summers. When he came back to me, it was July and it was a rainy season, during which time, he was not comfortable in open air and if it would get very windy he had to close the windows. Last time when he came, sweating was of no characteristic importance; but at this time he perspired profusely from his scalp, especially at night.

Based on the above symptoms Calcarea Carb was selected for him, which was found to be present in the following symptoms:

- Longing for fresh air, which inspires, benefits, strengthens.
- Aversion to cold air; sensitive to cold, damp air.
- Head sweats profusely while sleeping.

Also, *Calcarea carb.* complements the remedy *Sulphur* very well, so *Calcarea carb.* 1M was given and the patient was asked to come back after 15 days. The patient did not feel much change and so the potency was increased and *Calcarea carb.* 10M was selected and given for 15 days.

The patient came back after that with a smiling face. He felt much better in all his symptoms and had no itching of the skin, or any breathlessness at night.

The remedy was repeated once a month for three months, and the patient remained in good health.

CASE 2

This is a case of a 9-year-old child who is suffering from eczema behind both the knees since she was a year old. She was already given all kinds of treatment but to no avail. Infact the eczema from behind the knees was suppressed and then came on onto the child's abdomen. The child was brought to me and the mother said that the eczematous lesions would get better every time the child was taken near the seashore. I gave the child a dose of *Medorrhinum 200*, and asked them to report back to me within a month's time.

The parents came back to me with the child after a month and they reported that they found a considerable reduction in the size and number of the eczematous lesions. I put the child on placebo and within the next 2-3 months the whole skin got cleared of eczema. The child was monitored for almost a year, but there was no reported recurrence in her.

CASE 3

This is a case of weeping eczema since 10 years, with lesions especially between the fingers, and a few lesions all over the body. The patient complained of intense itching. The patient was given four doses of *Parotidinum 200C* by *Dr.Nash*, to be taken once in 4 days. After three weeks the patient was cured of all the lesions.

CASE 4

This is a case of eczema at the wrists, bends of the elbows and armpits, behind the ears and on the scalp, accompanied by abscesses affecting the bones. Nothing would relieve the eruptions, which would recur again and again. The patient complained of intense itching, that would even prevent sleep, with constant desire to scratch.

The patient was given one dose of *Psorinum 10M*.

The patient initially complained of an increase in the size of the patches, and then within 2 weeks time, the patches reduced in size and number and gradually within a month the skin became completely clear.

CASE 5

This is a case of eczema in a lady having it since the last 25 years, for which innumerable treatments and light therapy was tried, with no relief. The lesions were especially at the bends of the elbows and knees, thighs, hands (knuckles) and feet also between the webs of the toes. The skin over the lesions would become hyper-pigmented, dry and hard with fissures and at times would ooze out a watery but sticky fluid. The lesions would be worse during the winter season and warm or hot applications would relieve the itching. Thus the patient would always take a warm water bath. Temperamentally the patient would be very depressed and of a worrying type. She was anxious about her prolonged illness and had no peace of mind due to intense itching. Along with this she also complained of a dull memory since the past few months.

Her past history revealed an operation she had of her hernia, cataract and fracture of the right wrist. She had herpes opthalmicus three years back.

The patient received a dose of *Sepia 200C* and was asked to report after two weeks. She came back after that time, saying that the skin lesions had improved and that the hyperpigmentation had started to reduce over the lesions. The patient was then put on placebo and asked to report after a month. Then, when the patient came in next, after a month, she said that the lesions were very much better in intensity and number, with a marked reduction in the distressful itching. She was put on placebo again for 3 months.

After 4 months the patient came back saying that the itch is better on the flexures, but have become slightly worse on the knuckles and the feet, with a slight oozing. A single dose of *Sepia 200* was given.

Then she came back after a month with absolutely a clear skin with no lesions on it. The roughness and hyper-pigmentation had also cleared up and she was looking much more happy than she had when she first came in.

CASE 6

An infant was brought to me with a generalized eczema all over the body, present since she was 10 days old. All sorts of ointments and external applications had been tried onto her, which would suppress the lesions at one place and bring it on at another. This infact was very fat, chubby, had a sweaty scalp, no teeth, was constipated, and would catch cold all the time. She would not crawl.

The medicine that I prescribed was *Calcarea carb.*, starting from 1M potency and went up all the way to 50M, at infrequent intervals and helped cure the case in less than four months. Besides the eczematous lesions, the child started having a normal growth of her teeth and she stopped getting the recurrent cold affections she was prone to having.

CASE 7

This was a case of a 19-year-old patient suffering from eczema since the past 5 years, with intense itching, getting worse at night, especially when going to bed. After taking the case history, when I examined the patient, I noticed that the muco-cutaneous junctions of the body were red. There was also an offensive odor from his body.

I prescribed to him two doses of *Sulphur 200C* by *Dr.Kent*, each dose to be taken at an interval of a fortnight, and asked him to come over after a month and show me. The patient came back to me after a month, completely cured of his eczema.

CASE 8

This is a case of atopic eczema in a 6-year-old child, present since the last two years. The eczema was generalized and had spread to all over the body, but was especially marked around the mouth. The eruptions were pustular in type with a reddish erythema around them. A few eruptions were ulcerated and were discharging a thin watery fluid. The itching was so violent that the child would go on scratching even if the surface bled profusely. Itching was worse at night, by exposure to heat and during the rainy season.

I started the child on *Bacillinum 200C*, based on the strong family history of pleurisy with effusion. This had no effect on the skin but the dry cough that the child chronically suffered from disappeared.

The next prescription I gave was *Arum triphyllum 30C*, based on the intolerably violent itching that made the child scratch till the part became raw and bled.

CASE 9
Eczema and Goitre Cured
(Dr. Truman Coates)

A graduate of 'Old School' in 1888, although willing, yet anxious, to accept the good wherever found and knowing our limitations, a few years ago I strayed into neighboring pastures led by a case of very stubborn eczema in a woman of middle life. The trouble at times, especially after becoming heated from undue work in sunshine, covered her face, hands, exposed parts of her arms, the skin being very red and exasperatingly itchy and thick.

After repeated failures in my efforts and of those to whom I applied for assistance, I sought for help in the domain of Hahnemann, when I was recommended to give *Skookum chuck* 3x, four tablets a day and to my surprise and our thankfulness the case was cured in two weeks, the lady never had an itchy skin again and the skin cleared up entirely. If we have anything in our school that will do this, it was my misfortune to never find it.

A year ago a lady of fifty-seven years came to me for relief from a pain in her right brow, toward the temple, attacking her at frequent periods nearly all her life. Three years previously I corrected her eyestrain with lenses, which dissipated at least half of her suffering. I gave *Magnesia phos.*, somewhat irregularly for a few weeks, with but partial relief from pain, but to our surprise and real joy a goiter on right side, in size very noticeable even through an ordinary collar was gone; not a vestige was left. I at once began research for such and found in Dr. Vondergoltz's

Biochemical Manual; *Magnesia phos.* is the second remedy he recommends for goiter. To this day the goiter is not to be seen.

I might continue relating further results, further results, especially in nasal catarrh and adenoids in cases of children from eight to seventeen years, but the foregoing is likely enough for my maiden effort in new company.

A woman, twenty-seven years of age, for four weeks suffered from a dry, papulous, violently itching eczema of neck, upper part of chest and wrist, during six weeks prior to the outbreak of the eczema, the patient became sleepless, lying awake for hours. Upon one dose of *Coffea* 200, which covered both disorders the eczema disappeared within a week, the sleeplessness the next night. The patient was told that the remedy was administered for the eczema; the disturbance of sleep was purposely not mentioned.

In this method remedies, which cover several disorders, are given to the patient and the patient is told that they are given for one of them. The influence on the other disturbances can thus critically be observed and any suggestive influence is avoided.

CASE 10

Infantile Dermatitis

Master N. aged 1 year 8 months, in June 1965 developed eczema relieved by local application of Hydrocortisone. In September 1965 eczema relapsed again on the left cheek and was treated similarly. In November 1965 spread to both the cheeks, abdomen, back, legs and arms with violent itching day and night. Face was swollen, moisture on scratching, and the patient did not want to cover. The child craved for indigestible substances like pencil, chalk, earth. Stools were hard, at times streaked with blood. Fissure in Ano.

Family History

Sister – Psoriasis; Mother – Alopecia Areata, Mother's sister – Asthma; Father – Urticaria and Grandfather – Diabetes. There was a strong history of allergy in the family.

The following drugs were given *Graphites* 30, *Acidum nitricum* 200, *Kalium sulph.*, *Lachesis, Sepia, Rhus-tox, Ratanhia, Pulsatilla*, but ultimately it was *Arum triphyllum* 200 by Dr.Nash to which he responded and the eczema started clearing up.

CASE 11

A 72-year-old man came in complaining of an obstinate eczema that he had since the past 40 years, which extended all the way from his feet to the genitals, the trunk, and lastly to the eyelids and scalp. He had tried applying many ointments to suppress these eruptions. After 20 years when finally after the use of all the superficially acting ointments and lotions, his eczema subsided, but he then started suffering from frequent influenza, followed by bronchitis, which gradually turned into an asthmatic episode. He also complains of a loud, paroxysmal cough that tends to be either loose or dry. The patient is frequently disturbed in his sleep by his cough and after 5 in the morning he cannot sleep at all. On examination, lots of loud rhonchi are heard in the chest.

Gradually, he also started suffering from rheumatism, especially of the shoulders, hands and lower limbs. The winter season was the worst period for him, when he had atleast one to two attacks of lumbago and sciatica, without mentioning attacks of bronchitis and asthma. There were numerous nodosities around the articulations of both hands and fingers. The toes nails were very much thickened. His tendon reflexes were not very marked.

Now since the past 2 years he has a pityriasic erythema on the scalp, dry eczema of the eyelids and conjunctivitis. The skin all over the body is extremely dry and covered with little white scales, especially abundant on the limbs.

His solar plexus and the liver region are tender to touch. There is a mild hepatomegaly with gastric ptosis. The patient has no appetite and was usually always constipated.

After a detailed case taking I arrived at the remedy *Sulphur* for him, which I gave to him in the *30C* potency, one dose every week for a month. The patient came back after that saying that he could sleep better since his cough had disappeared and his breathing was better. He could climb stairs with less difficulty and his appetite had returned. He could also evacuate almost 2-3 times a day, with the stools being of normal consistency. The only major complaint he had was that his rheumatic pains had got worse. I still put him on placebo and asked him to return after another month.

He came back after a month with a more active mind. The itching and erythema of the scalp had disappeared. The scales on the eyes were reducing in intensity. The rheumatic pains though were a bit stronger in the hands and the feet. Also the way he would perspire earlier with worsening of his eczema was the characteristic feature.

"An extraordinary thing, doctor, my previous perspirations and my eczema of 20 years ago, on the genitals, hands and feet have returned. I don't want to recommence this remedy of yours." I warn my patient and tell him to abstain from any external medicinal application and I speak to him of the law of cure explaining to him that his symptoms are following exactly the desired direction.

From the above downward (the head is better, the lower parts of the body worse).

From within outward (the cough, asthma, breathing, digestive functions are very much improved, whilst the extremities show serious aggravation).

And in the reverse order of the coming of the symptoms (reappearance of the previous eczema and perspiration) Of course, I gave Placebo.

On April 2, I see my patient again. He declares that his state has rapidly improved, until a recent journey during which he indulged in an indiscretion of diet, which brought a strong aggravation of all skin symptoms. The rheumatism is better but has not completely disappeared. I order a dose of *Sulphur* 200 and Placebo. (The duration of *Sulphur* 30 was 10 weeks).

On July 6, the patient returns to thank me. He is cured and wishes to make me endorse his opinion.

URTICARIA

CASE 1

Urticaria Appearing Annually

Mrs. S. about forty years old, wife of a prominent clergy man in the city, consulted me for annually appearing paroxysms of urticaria, or whatever you may be pleased to call it. On the thirteenth day of May every year for seven years she had been seized with a burning and itching of the skin that would nearly drive her to distraction. I saw her in bed with one of these attacks with her entire surface and here eyes closed with oedema of the lids. The hives were so confluent and not a spot of healthy integument could be seen. The whole paroxysm lasted twenty-four hours. She seemed to be in terrible distress and exclaimed every moment. "I shall die this time, surely." She semed suffocating and was throwing off the covers. It seemed from her movements and speech that her skin felt as if on fire. There was no perceptible thirst and time was precious, and I am satisfied that I made waste by my haste in giving her dose of *Apis 200* which has no effect. But the paroxysm passed off and another year rolled by, when she called on me, as I requested her to do, a month before the expected paroxysm. I then learned more of her symptoms. I learned that when the eruption was out distinctly in nearly all the attacks she had found that heat calmed her terrible distress and ameliorated the itching and burning. While she craved cold and had even thrown the covers off she was made worse by it, but when she had retained presence of mind and covered herself warmly with clothing she soon became quiet and the paroxysm terminated with less suffering. This being the case *Apis* could not be her similimum, and I could now understand clearly why I had failed to interrupt the paroxysm and bring about a feeling of contentment so usual in such cases. I have quieted such patient very frequently in an hour, and plainly as a result of a homeopathic remedy, but this case furnished me with no evidence of curative action of my selected remedy. With the symptoms as given and the new modality I gave her one dose of *Rhus rad.200* bided my time ten days before the expected paroxysm. Within a few hours after taking the remedy she declared that her 'spell' was coming on; but it was only the shadow, the paroxysm never appeared again. She missed it two years and she is in better health than ever. She remarked to me one day, "Doctor, your powders have made a new woman of me." She had been treated allopathically, physiologically, electrically, pathologically, and with all very badly. This may not have been urticaria. Some of the wise heads of the old school told her it was from eating strawberries, and she refrained from these luxurious fellows and still did not miss the paroxysm. One told her one thing and another disputed his. What was it? I don't know, neither do I care. Perhaps some pathologist could inform me as to the scientificity of my prescription, I simply know that when comparing the pathogenesis found in the Symptomen Codex I found a picture of the disease to be cured, and that is enough for me. The highest potency at hand was administered and never repeated. The slight aggravation usual to such work followed, and then I was contented to await results. I am contented with such results, and so will any man who knows how to apply the law – the simillimum, the smallest dose, the dynamized drug. In this way shall we become the most useful to our patrons.

CASE 2

A girl, aged 20, having urticaria, Pressure urticaria, since many years. Has taken many medicines, allopathic, ayurvedic. They did not help much. After stopping of the medicines urticaria comes up again. The symptoms were such that, she could have urticaria whenever she wanted; i.e., by scratching with a pointed thing like a nail or a pencil, eruption would come up, if a staright line is drawn eruption would come up in a straight line; if a circle is drawn, eruption would come up in a circle form. If the wristwatch is tight on the wrist, eruption round the wrist would come up, elevated and itching around the wrist. That would remain for a few minutes to an hour or two. Even without pressure, urticaria would come up, mostly in the evening or night, and would come in different parts of the body each time. She was about to be married and that made me joke with her. "When you go to your husband's home, we will write on your hand "To Kamlesh, with Love". That comment of mine brought tears in her eyes, and she started weeping. I was embarrassed, I said sorry, but she would not stop weeping. The parents who accompanied her told me that she had, of late, become very sensitive and cries often, without any reason; especially when anyone jokes about her or with her. Past history of measles, strong attack, but no after effects. The age at that time was 17. After measles, the first menses came up. Hot patient, always better in cold weather. Wants to wear thin clothes; Thirst – less, takes only two glasses of fruit juices, water intake, almost nil; even in summer. Appetite good, but can't have steaming hot food, even would take tea when it gets cold. Would prefer cold dishes than hot dishes. Menses – very irregular; sometimes early, sometimes late. Flow also, sometimes profuse, sometimes scanty.

Referring to Allen's Key Notes on Pulsatilla

1. The first serious impairment of health is referred to puberty age.
2. Menses – Derangement at puberty. Irregular, intermittent flow. Delayed first menses.
3. Symptoms ever changing; no two attacks alike

Treatment was started with *Puls.1M* every week, three doses for 11/2 months; and S.L. in between days t.d.s. Then Puls. 10M. and S.L. in identical way for another one month. No more urticaria. Completely all right.

CASE 3

A Little Known Remedy 'Bombyx'

I met with a case of urticaria, which I am sending to you for publication in your esteemed Journal. Nearly two months back (on August 21) my grandson, about one and half years of age, suffered from urticaria, caused by a particular type of mosquito bite (type not known) with the following symptoms "Intense irritation of the whole body, hard, large red spots on the whole body, very thick, hardly leaving any space, starting from the buttocks, the whole body swollen, burning heat of the skin. Temp. 103 deg. F, accompanied by severe yawning, no thirst, appetite diminished. He slept only in the lap of the mother; frequent urination." I administered him *Rhus tox. 6*, every two hours, but no relief. On 22nd I referred the case to another homeopath of my locality, who also tried 4 to 5 remedies (names not known), but no improvement. Since there was no improvement, the other members of the family thought to change to allopathy, but I boldly resisted the move and consulted Therapeutic index in Pocket Manual of Homeopathic Materia Medica. Meanwhile, I noticed one more symptom, viz. very acute constipation. From Therapeutic Index I selected *Bombyx* (after studying it in the Dictionary of Practical Materia Medica, I decided on it). I got *Bombyx* 30 from the market after a great search and with only two powders at 5 hours interval the boy became normal.

CASE 4

This is a case of a 50 years old lady who came with the complaint of urticaria on 16-3-98

She was suffering from it since two years when it started on her legs. There appear pinkish purplish patches with heat of parts with itching followed by burning. The complaints are worse at night, from perfumes, tight clothes and tight shoes; and better by scratching, from cold water and ice.

She has taken cetzine, polaramine, colestone and incidal for her urticaria.

Associated Complaints

The skin of her finger tips ahs become dry and rough.

Also suffering from hypertension since two years for which she is taking tenormin and calciguard.

Past History

Dysentery, hysterectomy, appendicectomy, depression, skin

reaction after stopping oral contraceptive pills that she was taking for 3 years – she developed pustules all over with brown pus of fishy odor. She took cortisone and later homeopathy for the same.

Family History

Father – hypertension, eczema, renal failure, expired at 67 years.

Mother – optic atrophy.

Personal History

Appetite: Good.

She tends to over eat when she is nervous.

Thirst: 4-5 glasses ofcold water.

Desires: Eggs^2, sour, fried foods^2, salads, raw onions.

Stool: Loose stools from spicy foods and pickles.

Perspiration: Profuse on chest – under mammae and palms when she is nervous.

Menstrual history: Past history of heavy bleeding with dark clots, 25 days cycle lasting for 8-10 days. Occasional leucorrhea which was profuse and whitish.

In 1998 the bleeding was profuse for 42 days and medicines did not help. Hysterectomy was done.

After hysterectomy – hot flushes, palpitations and an increase in nervousness.

Thermal: Hot.

Sleep: Position – left side, curled up position, cannot sleep on the back.

Sound sleep.

Wakes up with a start on seeing a dream.

Dreams: Falling from a high place. Death of people.

Mind and life situation: Born and brought up in Bombay. She had a very happy childhood.

Father was an automobile engineer and mother was a housewife. The patient was an average student with more interest in languages. She did her BA and secretarial course. She fell in love with a boy whom she knew since her school days and got married in 1971.

The patient is basically sympathetic and affectionate by nature. She usually tends to feel quite insecure especially when alone. Initially she was a very carefree and jovial person, but now she has become pessimistic and timid. She cannot mix with people easily. She likes cooking and household work. She avoids taking responsibility as far as possible since she has a poor self-confidence and cannot take her own decisions. She is always afraid whether her husband will agree with her decision. She has a fear of losing her family members especially her mother. She says " What will happen to me after my mother death or after my daughters marriage?" she dislikes crowds and closed rooms especially when alone. She gets scared of pain and suffering. She weeps on seeing others in pain but avoids weeping in front of others because she feels that people will make fun of her. She feels that other women look down upon her since she is only a housewife and has no career. So sometimes she prefers to be alone.

Her husbands nature is exactly the opposite of her. He is very short tempered, dominating and doesn't like any interference in his work. He will blow up even if the patient reminds him twice about anything. When angry he shouts and becomes abusive. At times the patient argues with him but doesn't succeed and cries. Sometimes she would think about leaving the house but then she would think about her daughters future. She is also very insecure since she is not earning. Her husband is a self made man. He had a bitter childhood due to his step father. His parents didn't approuve of the marriage, so they stayed at the patients house with her parents. The major problem started when he had an extramarital affair 6 years ago and then that other woman ditched him. So he has become extremely irritable and doesn't trust women, not even his wife. He will ask his wife to give an account of the money she spends. He accuses the patient of things which don't concern her. He would insult her in public and friend circles. He would threaten her about a divorce. He loves his daughter a lot but is very strict with her. The patient can't express her feelings in front of him. He has no faith in the patient and does not show any affection towards her. Patient likes to be consoled and needs sympathy. The death of her father in 1985 also left a great impact on her. She suffered from amenorrhea for 3 months after her father's death.

Her basic feeling is that she has lost the faith and affection of her husband on whom she was completely dependant. This makes her feel insecure, pessimistic and have a low self-esteem about herself.

She has turned towards religion and prays a lot everyday. If she fails to pray even a single day she feels guilty.

Rubrics

- Affectionate.
- Delusion, deserted, forsaken is.
- Delusion, deserted, forsaken is, care for her no one would.
- Elusion, despised is.
- Delusion, affection of friends has lost.
- Delusion, confidence in him, his friends have lost all.
- Religious.
- Fear of misfortune.

Discussion

In this case the basic feeling of the patient has been converted ito rubrics. These rubrics were given highest marks. The other symptoms lie more in the periphery and so should not be given so much importance. If one would repertorize this case by using all the rubrics, remedies like *Nat-m., Puls., Ign., Bar-c.* and even *Lac-c.* would come into the picture. But her basic feeling is not covered by any of these remedies.

25-3-98 *Hura* 1M was prescribed.

The patient improved progressively until 22-4-98 when the urticaria got aggravated again with all the itching and redness. So one more dose was prescribed.

29-4-98 Patient is feeling much better and the intensity of the symptoms has reduced a lot.

ERYTHEMATOUS RASHES

CASE 1

(Steven Johnson Syndrome)

It was an evening of first August 1986; I was busy seeing patients at my clinic. A young gentleman entered my chamber with a request to see his ailing mother who was in a critical condition lying in a hospital with no hopes of recover. At first, I refused to go since I had a painful experience about the Hospital Staff who never co-operate with a homeopath; moreover the people contact a homeopath only in such dying moments. But on his insistently requesting me, I ultimately agreed.

Next day, while accompanying him to hospital, he told me that his mother was a diabetic and had developed some skin problem, which appeared in the form of eruptions over her chest. Those eruptions were very painful. The family doctor diagnosed it was Herpes zoster and had treated her but without improvement. Other specialists were consulted too, but nothing helped. A leading skin specialist was called in, but his medicine had severe reaction over her whole body. At this stage she was hospitalized. Days passed without even relief, rather she became worse. All sorts of medicines (some of them imported) were tried but in vain.

When I reached the hospital, the Staff nurse and a Houseman accompanied me. They thought me to be a dermatologist, since every other day some new doctor was visiting her. She was lying quietly as if in Coma, looking like a burn's case. Her whole body was painted with gentian violet. There were lots of blisters, small and large, some of them broken with peeling of skin and serous discharge.

Her eyes were half open and filled with exudates from the necrosed margins of her eyes, which looked as if bitten by a rat. Her face was swollen with signs of inflammatory changes inside her mouth and nasal tract as well; her lips were necrosed and swollen. On the whole, it was looking as if she had been thrown into a boiler. It was a horrible sight to look at.

She was in toxic condition an advanced stage of shock. The drip was on, she was breathing with difficulty since there was some pleural effusion as well. The urine output was scanty since there were inflammatory changes in the kidneys and bladder also. She was last seen by a very famous dermatologist who had diagnosed this group of symptoms – as Stevens Johnson Syndrome.

Stevens-Johnson Syndrome is a condition where mucosa and skin are involved. It gives rise to various groups of symptoms. Mucosal involvement may be oral, ocural or genital. The bullae, which form, lead to extensive ulceration and pseudo-membrane formation, hemorrhagic crusts, purulent or catarrhal conjunctivitis. Whereas skin involvements give rise to variable size of large and small bullae which contain clear or hemorrhagic fluid with severe constituticnal symptoms. Allopathic treatment is with antibiotics and steroids of adrenocorticotropic hormones (ACTH). The prognosis is grave, spontaneous recovery rare and severe cases are always fatal.

For homeopathy it was a simple case. Though she was in a stage of shock she responded well to every question. She told that she felt as if she is lying on burning sand. She was thirsty but could not drink. Every attempt was very painful. She could not eat nor see because of constant oozing of stuff in to her eyes. She could hardly eat or pass stools. She could hardly pass a few drops of urine, which caused severe cutting and burning pains.

She was disgusted with everything, i.e. to eat, to drink, to see and to urinate. Guided by those symptoms, a few doses of *Cantharis*

30 t.d.s. was given for 3 days – with great relief in 24 hours. The same day her mental condition improved. The next day she could drink and urinate. Third day she could eat and pass stool. The recovery was very rapid. On fourth day she wanted to go home. A patient who a couple of days ago were in dying condition was asking to go home. The hospital authority did not believe that this remarkable improvement was the result of homeopathic medicine.

By the time she went home within a week the bullae had dried completely and she was discharged from the hospital against medical advice.

After going home the burning pains while passing urine recurred again and she was given a few more doses of Cantharis. Skin was not falling off in the same way as when one removes his socks or hand gloves. Natural healthy skin was forming. She could see, eat, drink, pass stool and urinate without any difficulty. All this happened in a week's time and she resumed her routine work. She was later treated for diabetes according to her constitution.

FURUNCULOSIS

CASE 1

A woman of 30 years suffered from boils in the ears, alternating from one ear to the other. Chemotherapy helped to clear up the boils but did not stop recurrence. She had no freedom from boils for more than a week or two at a time. The following symptoms were present dislikes consolation, could not weep, even when she lost her mother who died from cancer of the uterus. Nausea and vomiting at the beginning of her periods. Dragging down at M.P. Headache before a thunderstorm. Tired in the morning, better in the evening. Profuse offensive axilliary perspiration. *Natrium mur.* and *Gelsemium* have sadness but cannot weep. *Sepia*, however, which contains *Natrium mur.*, seemed to be much more indicated. The patient was given *Sepia* 30, 200, 1m, 10m, which was followed by three weeks freedom, after which another relapse. *Carcinosinum*

30, 200, 1m was given. It was followed by a severe aggravation lasting about a week and then has been followed by complete freedom for three years.

CASE 2

A lady of 39 years of age; a very successful person in life, working as a P.A. to the top most boss of a reputed company; well respected and feared. She had an injury on her toe and developed a sore, which would bleed easily with the slightest injury. When she had been to London, she had it removed by surgery. She was told that the name of the disease is *Pyogenic Granuloma*; it's benign in nature, so she should not worry.

After sometime she developed a red mass on upper lip, which would also bleed on slightest injury. She was told that this was recurrence of her old complaint, only difference being that now it has come up on the face, and advised excision.

This difference was nothing to the advising doctor, but it made a hell of a lot of difference to the patient. Advice of best doctors in India and abroad was taken. All were unanimous in their opinion "Get it operated. You need not fear, though, because it is a harmless condition; but may keep, on recurring even after operation". But its appearance on lip made a lot of difference to the patient.

So she wanted to try homeopathy at this stage, but she had no time to come and see me. She sent her brother only with the news that she has "Pyogenic Granuloma", and I should give some medicine for her. I asked her brother to ring her up from my clinic and I talked to her. The symptoms which I got were as follows; over and above the ones narrated above.

The patient has had vaccination, all sorts of vaccinations many times, as she has to travel a lot.

Fond of warm drinks. Desire for milk but it disagrees, gives flatulence in abdomen and diarrhoea; so she adds coffee in it. Desire for sweets, very fond of chocolates.

Chilly person. Has to sit in an air-conditioned office but is uncomfortable in it. She covers herself properly when in the office. When at home she does not want breeze or fan.

I asked the brother about her mental attributes. He could not say anything that could be of help; but he said, "She is very fastidious; fastidious in office work, fastidious in what she wears; and fastidious at home, finding fault with little things."

The meaning of fastidious in the dictionary is – Squeamish, scrupulous, critical.

Treatment was started with *Sulphur* 30 tds. for three months. No change. *Sulphur* 200 tds. for another three months. 50% improvement. Repeat. Altogether *Sulphur* was given for 8 months. When the tumour was gone, the patient was asked to continue for two more months. No recurrence.

CASE 3

Mrs.B. age 30 years had large suppurating pustules on the hands, particularly near the ends of the fingers. Has had eight or ten within a few weeks, and several more forming at present. Itching of body, particularly while in bed. *Psorinum* 30 in repeated doses of which some half dozen were given during a few days, preventing the development of those just beginning, and healing those which were suppurating within ten days.

CASE 4

B. age 3 months; pustules and boils on head, particularly on the scalp; scalp had a dirty look and emitted an offensive odour; fine red eruption on the body, forming small white scales. Pustules on the hands. *Psorinum* 30. Odour removed in 24 hours. Eruption began to improve in a few days. Heard from the child several weeks late; quite well and skin in much better condition; pustules and boils had disappeared; rash still on neck and one arm; later reports show continued improvement.

CASE 5

Abscess

January 3rd, a woman 55 years age, came to hospital because of an abscess in left axilla; just starting to discharge. She was given *Tarentula cubensis* CM, three doses and a compress of *Hypericum*. Two days later it was well. No pain; no discomfort; no induration; a slight redness round, and a scrap of dressing adhering to the actual spot where it had discharged. People seemed rather surprised.

Seen again January 19th. Slight recurrence three days ago and very slight discharge. Dry now, but a tiny area of induration and two reddish spots that might be a threat of more, so *Tarentula cub.* was repeated.

CASE 6

Boil

One of our doctor reports, "About a week ago saw a girl with large boil on cheek, with hard center and bluish discoloration. Gave *Tarentula cubensis*, and heard a few das later that it had disappeared with discharging."

CASE 7

Abscess on face

A middle-aged gentleman had an abscess on the side of the face just in front of the ear. Suppuration was advanced and the fluctuation was marked. *Silicea* had done some good, as it has controlled the pain. A surgeon aspirated the cavity several times, but it continued to refill. After three weeks there was no abatement. The integument took on a new feature, becoming bluish, mottled, with great burning and sharp cutting pains. The hardness was extending and opening gave out a bloody thin excoriating fluid of foul smell. He was chilly and nauseated and had symptoms of pyaemia. After one dose of *Tarentula cubensis* 12x, an immediate change for the better took place, no more pus formed, and he was well in ten days. The discoloured localization became a bright red and then faded to the natural colour. The nausea and General pyaemic symptoms were greatly relieved within twelve hours. No more medicine.

CASE 8

Carbuncle on the Back of the Neck

A lady aged about thirty, suffered greatly from a carbuncle on the back of the neck. She had applied many domestic medicines and obtained no relief. The tumefaction seemed destined to suppurate. It was mottled bluish and the pain was intense, knife cutting and burning. She felt terribly sick even to vomiting and at night she was delirious. Her eyes were staring, and she had fever; the tongue was foul and breath fetid. There was great tension in the scalp and muscles of the face. She begged for morphine to stop that burning and cutting.

Tarentula cubensis 12x, one dose produced improvement quite immediately, and the angry looking tumefaction failed to complete its work; it did not suppurate. The discoloration was gone in two days and the hardness soon disappeared. She regained her normal state very rapidly and she said to me a short time ago, that she never had her old headaches since that swelling left her, showing how deeply the medicine affected her whole system. If the part is mottled bluish, growing dark, with those symptoms, *Tarentula cubensis* must be the most appropriate remedy.

You see, therefore, that *Tarenula cubensis* is not a specific for an abscess, bubo or carbuncle, but only when it is bluish, mottled with great burning and sharp cutting pains. When you have these you cannot go wrong.

IMPETIGO

CASE 1

Impetigo – Sepia 30

June 25th 1872. A little girl, 3.1/2, fleshy leucophlegmatic, for three years has had impetigo, consisting of a thick, putrid smelling, pustular eruption covering the scalp like a skull-cap, surrounding the eyes, on the face, and appearing on the genitals. A papular eruption is scattered all over the body, with pustules here and there. Much itching. After scratching the scalp it bleeds. The hair is agglutinated. Excretion probably albuminous. Urine putrid when first voided. The impurities of the blood seek an outlet through the skin and kidneys. Bowels regular. *Sepia* 30, July 1st – Better every way. July 15th – General improvement; urine normal; scalp smells less putrid; face and genitals healed. August 19th – Profuse scalp-sweat and impetigo. *Calcarea carb*. 85m. Impetigo soon afterwards disappeared and the child was well.

In this case, the putrid urine and offensive impetigo indicated the putrescent state of the blood. On constitutional grounds *Calcarea carb.*, was first prescribed without apparent benefit, the case growing worse, as it did previously without medicine. Afterwards the putridity of the urine suggested *Sepia*, which nearly cured the patient. Finally the occurrence of profuse head-sweat indicated the appropriate time for administering *Calcarea carb;* which completed the cure.

Eruptive disease, are called skin diseases on account of their location. But they originate in certain diseases of the blood of which they are symptomatic and they are occasioned by the elimination from the blood of various impurities through the skin.

ACNE

The superiority of homeopathic treatment over the local applications and alternative drugs of the allopaths may be shown by a few illustrative cases.

CASE 1

Mary, employed in the hospital, came to the clinic affected with acne. The eruption came out since she had worked in the laundry, never troubled in this way before. Menses had been missed twice, her feet were cold and damp all the time; she complained of them without being asked about it. *Calcarea carbonica* worked about magically, in three weeks her face was perfectly smooth and well (Dr. Burnette).

CASE 2

A.S.30 years old, acne for several years. Owing to chronic rheumatic pains, had drunk a great deal of whisky, which, he says always relieved his pains, but made his face a good deal worse. The pains were worse during quiet and relieved by motion. He is weak and complains that he can do little work because his strength gives out. All liquor stopped and *Rhus 30* given. He was well in about ten weeks (Dr. Burnette).

CASE 3

J.B.16 years old, acne simplex on both sides of the face. Glands on the sides of the neck somewhat enlarged; skin generally yellowish; an unusual condition was that the skin of the face was very sensitive to touch. Acne is not usually a painful or sensitive disease. The sensitiveness, enlarged glands and pustules led to the prescription of *Hepar suph*. Report in three weeks showed much improvement, fell back during fourth week probably from the discontinuance of the remedy. It was then represcribed, with improvement (Dr.Burnett).

CASE 4

K.E. 22 years old, acne simplex. Yellowish and unhealthy skin; every little injury suppurates; always worse during and after menses; glands of neck enlarged. *Hepar sulph.* was given for about six weeks, with disappearance of eruption and better health generally.

The symptoms in these two cases in different sexes were about the same and called for the same remedy.

Neither of these cases is fully reported, but *Hepar*, has sensitiveness to touch, glandular swellings, suppuration, unhealthy skin and yellow complexion (Dr. Nash).

CASE 5

G.C.22 years old, acne for several years; has taken Sulphur salts and other home remedies for it; takes cold easily, takes wine often; has suffered from suppuration of the glands of the neck, *Baryta carb.* – cured (Dr.Nash).

CASE 6

Man aged 25 years. Had syphilis; has taken much Iodide of Potash. Some weeks ago an eruption came upon his face. He considered it a return of his old trouble, which so affected him that he had serious thoughts of throwing himself in the lake. On the mental condition he was given *Aurum*, which removed the eruption in about two months.

Other remedies have cured cases to their credit – namely *Nux vomica, Graphites, Lycopodium, Ledum* and *Pulsatilla.* Many more are placed in the repertories under acne (Dr. Kent).

CASE 7

This is a case of Miss S.R.A., a 26 years old unmarried lady, who came with a complaint of acne on 26-2-98.

Chief Complaint

Location	Sensation	Modalities
Skin – face Since 5-7 years Since 3-4 years	Increased facial hair growth. Pimples with scars.	< Before menses. < When tense. < Chocolates. < Butter, cheese. < Oily fried food. < Ice cream.
Since 5 months	Itching without eruptions of the whole body, more on hands.	< Night. > Hot water.
Scalp	Dandruff. Hairfall.	

Associated Complaints

Generalities: Vertigo from hunger.

Head: Headache < Eyestrain from computer.

Past History

Not significant.

Family History

Maternal grandfather – cancer throat.

Younger sister – piles.

Personal History

Appetite: Normal. Hungry more in the evening.

Thirst: 5-6 glasses/ day. Prefers cold.

Craving: Spicy[3], ice cream[2], fish, prawns, pickles, fruit.

Aversion: Milk.

Stool: Normal.

Urine: Normal.

Perspiration: Profuse on armpits and back.

Thermal state: Ambithermal.

Sun < Rash on face.

Menstrual history

FMP- 12 years. Has a 28 days cycle lasting for 5-6 days. The bleeding is regular, moderate, bright red and clotted.

Before menses: Pain in abdomen.

During menses: Pain in breasts.

After menses: Leucorrhea, clotted, stains sometimes difficult to wash.

Mental History and Life Space

Patient was born in Mangalore and brought up in Mulund. In school she was an average student. She scored lass in std. X and took up commerce. After her Third Year Bachelor of commerce, she took up a secretarial job and has been working there was the past 4 years.

As a child she was very scared of her parents, especially her mother who was very strict. But her parents and sisters were very loving and caring.

By nature the patient is quite reserved; can't make friends easily; feeling uncomfortable to speak to unknown people; does not like to open up. She will open up only if the opposite person is friendly and she can trust him. The patient was in love with a married man with whom she had split up a year back. She refused to give information on this front; only said that her trust had been broken. Now she doesn't want to trust anybody. Felt that people have taken advantage of her.

Feels nervous when speaking to men. Has fear of the opposite sex. She also has a fear of lizards.

She has a poor confidence level. She is also quite conscious of the way she dresses or the way she talks and behaves. She always wants to do something different from others.

She weeps easily, especially when reprimanded. Prefers to cry alone but feels better if consoled.

She is very sensitive to rudeness. Will keep quiet but will keep thinking about it for months or even years but later will see to it that she gets back and insults that person.

Gets irritated very soon, especially when somebody makes fun of her. But will keep quiet. Since the disappointment in love, she gets angry on petty matters. When angry she gets trembling of the whole body. She loves listening to music.

Sleep

Sleeps on sides. More on the left than on the right.

When mentally disturbed, does not get sleep till 2-3 am and wakes up by 6 am.

Dreams

Occasionally of friends.

Rubrics

- Generalities, food and drink, spices, condiments, piquant, highly seasoned food.
- Generalities, food and drink, ice cream desires.
- Generalities, food and drink, fruit desires.
- Mind, music ameliorates.
- Mind, reserved.
- Mind, timidity, public, about appearing in.
- Mind, weeping, tearful mood, reproaches from.
- Mind, Ailments from, disappointment, deception.
- Mind, brooding.

Remedy

Natrium mur. 1M II x 2 for 15 days.

Follow up

28-3-98

Acne >

Itching >

Dandruff and hairfall SQ

Rx Nat-m. 1M, II x 2 / 15 days.

11-4-98

Pimples increased ? < sun

Body itching restarted

Dandruff – scalp itching

Rx Sac Lac x 6 days.

18-4-98

Pimples <
Itching >

Dandruff and hairfall SQ

Rx Nat-m. 1M II x 2 / 15 days.

25-4-98

Perspiration on body offensive

Rx Nat-m. 1M II doses / 6 days.

9-5-98

Itching of body >>

Pimples on face + since 7 days

Size decreased

Intensity decreased

Dandruff and hairfall SQ

Perspiration offensive SQ; Stains yellow

Rx Nat-m. 1M II x 2 / 15 d

6-6-98

Pimples recurred on face since 15 days
Hairfall and dandruff SQ

Perspiration offensive stains yellow.

Rx Nat-m. 10M I dose / 10d

4-7-98

Pimples on forehead and cheek recurred

Hairfall SQ

Dandruff decreased

Perspiration does not stain but offensive

Rx Nat-m. 10M I dose / 15 d

19-7-98

Pimples come on and off

Hairfall and dandruff SQ

Perspiration >>

Rx Nat-m. 10M I dose/15 d.

1-8-99

Pimples new ones come up

Dandruff >

Hairfall SQ

Rx Nat-m. 10M II doses/10 d.

29-8-98

Pimples – new ones appeared

Dandruff

Rx Nat-m. 10M II doses / 15 d.

19-9-98

Acne >

Dandruff >

Hairfall SQ

Rx Nat-m. 10M II doses / 15 days.

CASE 8

This is a case of a 31-year-old lady who came with the complaint of acne and headaches on 7-5-98.

She was getting acne from the age of 17-18 years. The acne was cystic in nature and very painful. They are pustular with yellowish pus and blood. It leaves scars.

Her eruptions leave scars.

She also suffers from throbbing headaches since the past 1-11/2 years. Headaches start from the frontal region and spreads all over. The headaches are worse in the sun, from bad news, from excitement, after a head bath especially if she sits under the fan.

Associated Complaints

Worms in stools since 6-8 months.

Itching in anal region worse after stool for hours.

Burning in the anal region worse from sitting, better by standing, walking, and cold-water application.

Past History

Jaundice.

Epilepsy (class 3 to class 9).

Family History

Father- IHD.

Paternal grandfather – MI.

Personal History

Appetite: Good, she has a habit of nibbling.

Thirst: 5-6 glasses of cold water, she feels thirsty on waking up in the morning.

Desires: Fish3, sour3 (pickles and raw mangoes).

Aversion: Milk.

Aggravation: Shellfish – loose stool.

Farinaceous food: Flatulence > eructation.

> Passing flatus.

Stool: Travelers constipation, has to strain whether soft or hard stool.

Perspiration: Upper lip, axilla.

Sexual sphere: Sensitivity of vaginal area to coition, which is very painful.

Sleep: Sound, in any position.

Disturbed by light, wants total darkness.

Dreams: Accidents, frightful, someone dying.

Menstrual History

FMP- 12 years; LMP - 26-5-98

Her periods are irregular, and bright red.

She has a 30 - 60 days cycle which lasts for 4 days.

Before menses - irritability, leucorrhea (white occasionally water)

Severe pain in abdomen before and on the first day of menses.

Ambithermal.

Mind and Life Space

Born and brought up in Bombay. Since the age of 11-12 years she stayed in a boarding school in Bandra because the area in which they lived was not very good. She used to feel very home sick but gradually she adjusted.

Father was working as an officer in the mill. He was short-tempered but very affectionate. Patient was very close to her father. He would give his whole salary to his stepmother. So the patient's mother had to work in the Gulf to support the family, occasionally there were fight between the parents. Patient got along very well with her brothers and her parents. Her family is the most important for her than anything else.

She was an average student, but weak at maths. She finished her graduation and got the job of a steno secretary.

She got married in Dec. '96. 4 months after marriage, her husband lost his job due to fights between the partners. He refused to do anything illegal and so one of the partners started spoiling his name. Some girls would call up at home and tell the patient that her husband had an affair with them. She was under a lot of stress. She didn't tell her parents since she didn't want them to get tense. Later her husband got a good job with a good pay but her insecurities and fears still persist.

She would feel depressed after her marriage as she was away from her family.

When the telephone rings she has a fear of bad news. She can't see accidents. She also has a fear of dogs, cockroaches, lizards, and high places. If her husband doesn't return on time, she starts getting anxious and gets negative thoughts with a fear that something bad will happen. She is very sensitive to criticism and once she feels hurt she breaks the relation totally. She gets irritated if someone taunts her. She feels like striking in anger and shouts and says nasty things. She doesn't feel like talking to that person again and wants to be left along. She dislikes consolation. She tends to weep easily on seeing someone suffering or someone in pain.

She feels nervous in new places or when she has to deal with strangers.

She wants everything to be in order otherwise she feels anxious and loses her temper. She wants everything to be done fast.

She trusts people easily and has been cheated even by her friends. She always remembers the person who has offended her. She feels that she should get even with that person. Her greatest grief in life is that her mother was not present when she and her family needed her the most.

Likes listening to music, watching TV, reading. Hates stitching, cooking.

Music has a very soothing effect on her.

Rubrics

- Desires, fish.
- Desires, sour.
- Aversion milk.
- Aggravation, shellfish.
- Rectum, itching, stool, after.
- Head, pain, sun, from exposure to.
- Fear misfortune of.
- Fear, high places, of.
- Fear, dogs, of.
- Homesickness.
- Fastidious.
- Music ameliorates.
- Anger, taciturnity with.
- Anger violent.

Remedy and Follow-up

Nat-m. 1M I dose on 2-6-98.

Nat-m. 1M was repeated twice in a month.

9-7-98.

Acne >>

Headache, which she used to get almost everyday, has now reduced to once a week. The headache is less in intensity and frequency.

Menses irregular.

Worms – SQ.

TINEA

CASE 1

Tinea capitis

Lady aged 55, had an eruption involving the greater part of the scalp and ears, extending over the forehead. The scabs are large and thick, and of a yellowish–greenish colour; the hair is matted,from which pus exudes; the forehead is fiery red; the parts involved itch, and are very painful. The patient is irritable, and although there is no general disturbance of the health, yet she says she does not feel well. When quite young she had an attack of tinea capitis, which was treated 'scientifically'. On the break of this suppressed tinea she was under old school treatment, but this time it would be suppressed, and all the applications had only the effect of making her more ill. She received one dose of *Mezereum 1M.* On reporting at the expiration of one week I found a decided change in the character of the eruption; the redness on the forehead disappeared to a great extent. She said she felt better as to her general health than she had for a long time previously. She had for the week three discharges daily of bright red blood from the rectum; these discharges were profuse, no pain or no especially weakness was noticed. She received but this one dose of the remedy, she steadily improved, and the eruption gradually disappeared as she states she feels as well as she did when she was a young girl.

The thickness and colour of the scabs called my attention to *Mezereum. Lycopodium* has moist scabs; *Rhus* eruptions destroy the hair, eating it off in the progress of the eruption, there is a crusty eruption under *Staphysagria*, but we have a peculiar symptom of *Staphysagria* wanting; when scratching the itching changes its place, but the part becomes more humid. (Dr.Burnett)

VITILIGO

CASE 1

This is the case of a 14-year-old girl (student) who came with the complaint of hypo-pigmented spots on the knees and left upper eyelid since 5-6 years. She gets itching on these spots occasionally.

Associated Complaints

Constipation – has to strain a lot due to dry hard stool.

Past history

    Worms.

    Diarrhoea.

Family History

    Sister: Hypo-pigmented spots.

    Father: Gall stones, gastric ulcer.

    Mother: Asthma.

    Paternal grandfather: Diabetes, myocardial infarct.

    Paternal grandmother: Hypertension.

    Maternal grandfather: Asthma, myocardial infarct.

    Maternal grandmother: Diabetes.

Personal History

    Appetite: Good, feels very hungry in the evening.

    Thirst: 7-8 glasses / day. Prefers cold water; after meals.

    Desires: Cold drinks[3], chocolate[2].

    Aversion: Chicken.

    Perspiration: Face-upper lip, axilla; offensive.

    Thermal: Hot patient.

    Sleep: Position – back.

    Dribbling of saliva occasionally.

    Talking in sleep occasionally.

    Dreams- examinations, friends.

Menstrual History

    FMP: 12 years.

    She has a regular 28 days cycle lasting for 3-4 days with moderate bleeding.

MIND AND LIFE SITUATION

    [Observation – patient talks like an elderly person. She gives vague answers in the presence of her parents]

Since childhood she is in the habit of talking to her parents with aggressive speech. She has the habit of putting the handkerchief in her mouth.

She says that she is very short tempered and prefers to be left alone when she is depressed or angry. If anyone offends her she remembers it for a long time. She thinks about taking revenge but she controls herself.

She feels very bad when her parents are quarrelling and starts weeping.

She feels anxious about her family and about her health. She has a lot of anticipatory anxiety before exams and before results. She usually tries to achieve perfection in her work. She repents if something goes wrong. If she decides to do something she will achieve it. Once when she didn't do well in her studies she poked herself with a pin.

Her mother doesn't understand her viewpoint. Her mother blames her for spending too much money. Patient loves to wear good clothes and perfumes. Her hobbies are painting and dancing – loves fast music and dances to it when alone.

She likes to have a change in life, doesn't like routines. She doesn't like closed rooms and gets irritated in crowded places.

Rubrics
- Desires, cold drinks, water.
- Desires, chocolate.
- Aversion, chicken.
- Sleep, position, back on.
- Sensitive, oversensitive, music to.
- Dancing.
- Consolation aggravates.
- Anger, irascibility, trifles at.

Remedy and follow-up
26-3-96
    Rx Nat-m. 200 II x 8 / 60 days.

15-5-96

Rx ct all / 30days.

12-6-96

Very slight pigmentation on right upper eyelid.
Increase on both knees.
New patches on right thumb and left nostril.
Slight itching occasionally.
Constipation SQ.

Rx Nat-m. 1M I dose every15 days / 75 days.

7-9-96

Spots on eyelid >.
New spots on fingers.

Rx ct all / 90 days.

12-1-97

Left lower eyelid hypo-pigmented spot increased.
New hypo-pigmented spots on fingers SQ.
No itching.
No constipation.

Rx Nat-m. 1M II x 8 / 60 days.

18-3-97

New hypo-pigmented spots on right
pinna and sight sole.
Old spots SQ.

Rx Nat-m. 10M I x 4 / 60 days.

1-5-97

Rx ct all / 30d.

19-6-97

Rx Nat-m 10M II x 8 / 60 days.

10-8-97

New lesion behind ears.
Right elbow >
Right finger >

Eyelids SQ
Knees SQ
Ankles SQ
Constipation SQ
        Rx ct all / 60 d.

11-10-97 to 28-10-98
        Rx ct all.

12-12-98
        Rx Nat-m. 10 M. III x 8 / 60 days.

21-1-99
        Rx ct all / 60 d.

20-3-99
No new spots
Ankles and eyelids SQ
Elbow and knee >
        Rx Nat-m. 10M. IV x 8 / 60 days.

26-5-99
Improvement in lesions over both knees and left upper eye
lid.
No new spots.
No constipation
        Rx Nat-m. 10 M II x 4 / 30 days.

6-6-99 to 9-8-99
Pigmentation of eyelids SQ
Knees >
No new spots.
No constipation
Pimples off and on
        Rx ct all.

■

Word Index